Speech–Language Pathology Assistants

A RESOURCE MANUAL

Third Edition

Speech–Language Pathology Assistants

A RESOURCE MANUAL

THIRD EDITION

Jennifer A. Ostergren, PhD, CCC-SLP
Margaret Vento-Wilson, PhD, CCC-SLP

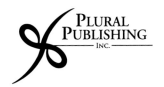

PLURAL
PUBLISHING
INC.

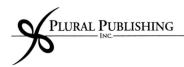

9177 Aero Drive, Suite B
San Diego, CA 92123

e-mail: information@pluralpublishing.com
Website: https://www.pluralpublishing.com

Typeset in 10.5/13 Palatino by Flanagan's Publishing Services, Inc.
Printed in the United States of America by Integrated Books International

Library of Congress Cataloging-in-Publication Data

Names: Ostergren, Jennifer A., author. | Vento-Wilson, Margaret, author.
Title: Speech-language pathology assistants : a resource manual / Jennifer
    A. Ostergren, Margaret Vento-Wilson.
Description: Third edition. | San Diego, CA : Plural Publishing, Inc.,
    [2024] | Includes bibliographical references and index.
Identifiers: LCCN 2022046675 (print) | LCCN 2022046676 (ebook) | ISBN
    9781635504156 (paperback) | ISBN 1635504155 (paperback) | ISBN
    9781635504163 (ebook)
Subjects: MESH: Speech-Language Pathology--methods | Allied Health
    Personnel | Language Disorders--therapy
Classification: LCC RC424.7 (print) | LCC RC424.7 (ebook) | NLM WL 21 |
    DDC 616.85/5--dc23/eng/20221202
LC record available at https://lccn.loc.gov/2022046675
LC ebook record available at https://lccn.loc.gov/2022046676

Contents

Part III. Treatment for Specific Populations and Disorders

Preface

Speech-language pathology assistants (SLPAs) are "support personnel who, following academic and/or on-the-job training, perform tasks prescribed, directed, and supervised by American Speech-Language-Hearing Association (ASHA) certified speech-language pathologists (SLPs)" (ASHA, n.d., para. 2). The use of SLPAs and support personnel is not new. As early as the 1970s, support personnel in the field of speech-language pathology were being used and regulated by different states in the United States (ASHA, n.d.). ASHA has had guidelines for the use of support personnel since 1969. Expansion in the use of SLPAs continues to increase as professionals in the field look for ways to contain costs and expand clinical services (ASHA, n.d.). ASHA maintains and periodically updates formal policy and guidelines on the training, use, and supervision of SLPAs. In 2020, ASHA also created a formal certification for SLPAs (C-SLPA) (Council for Clinical Certification in Audiology and Speech-Language Pathology of the American Speech-Language-Hearing Association, 2020).

CONTENT

This book is written specifically for SLPAs, addressing their unique needs. It is intended to be a practical resource on a wide range of topics that SLPAs may find of value. It does not cover normal processes of communication or communicative disorders in depth. Rather, it is intended as a "what now" or real-world perspective offering technical and clinical procedure suggestions for SLPAs, including SLPA professional issues and ethics, and instruction in workplace behaviors, such as implementing treatment and collecting and summarizing data. Specialized topics applicable to SLPAs, such as augmentative and alternative communication, cultural and linguistic diversity, play and literacy in therapy, speech sound remediation, and autism spectrum disorder are also included to extend SLPAs' foundational knowledge to real-world applications. This book is written for individuals with a variety of SLPA experience and training. It is our hope that SLPAs with all levels of experience and background will find tools and resources of value to them in this book. If you are an SLPA who has been in the field for many years, this book may offer you a fresh perspective on your role and ideas for continuing to refine your skills. If you are an SLPA just starting your career, this book offers you important information to take with you on your journey. If you are an SLPA in training, the book provides you with information relevant for your training, particularly to your clinical practicum and future employment as an SLPA.

ORGANIZATION

The first six chapters cover broad topics, including an overview of the roles and responsibilities of SLPAs and their supervisors. The initial chapters also cover professional conduct, ethics, cultural and linguistic diversity, and topics important to the health and safety of SLPAs and the individuals they serve. Within these sections, ASHA documents are a cornerstone when referencing policies, procedures, rules, and regulations applicable to SLPA practice. At present, there is considerable variability between states' regulations applicable to SLPAs. As such, ASHA, as the sole national organization for the profession in the United States, serves as an important and primary resource on the topic. That is not to say that SLPAs should ignore state regulations. Rather, as will be discussed, SLPAs must be cognizant of both ASHA and individual state regulations. References and suggestions for accessing state-specific information are provided. Furthermore, given the dynamic nature of policies and procedures, readers should view the information in this book as an overview of regulations and policies in place at the time of publication. The reader is referred to ASHA's website, at https://www.asha .org, for the most recent information.

The next six chapters of the book are organized as "skill development" chapters. These chapters cover a specific set of skills needed by SLPAs across a wide variety of settings. They include the important topics of data collection, note writing, therapy implementation techniques for individual and group sessions, and a newly added chapter on the use of behavioral principles. Throughout each skill development chapter, helpful tips and applicable references and resources are provided, with the major emphasis on providing information that will be of value in actual clinical work as an SLPA.

The remaining seven chapters include treatment foundations and suggestions for specific populations, including newly added chapters on early intervention, language interventions for children, and foundational knowledge for working with adults with acquired neurologic disorders. This is not an exhaustive list of all the populations and disorders SLPAs may encounter in their clinical work. Rather, these chapters serve as additional considerations for common populations and disorders SLPAs might encounter.

COMPANION WEBSITE

This book has a companion website with important forms SLPAs can use in their clinical work. These forms can be freely modified and copied. Explanations about the content on the companion website are embedded within the chapters of the book. The following symbol denotes where the content of the companion website is referenced.

REFERENCES

American Speech-Language-Hearing Association (ASHA). (n.d.). *Frequently asked questions: Speech-language pathology assistants (SLPAs)*. https://www.asha.org/associates/SLPA-FAQs/

Council for Clinical Certification in Audiology and Speech-Language Pathology of the American Speech-Language-Hearing Association. (2020). *2020 Standards for ASHA Speech-Language Pathology Assistants Certification*. https://www .asha.org/certification/2020-slpa-certification-standards/

Acknowledgments

First and foremost, we would like to thank the many speech-language pathologist assistants (SLPAs) who work in concert with speech-language pathologists (SLPs) out in the field supporting individuals with communicative needs. We would also like to acknowledge the essential role of both the educators who share their knowledge and passion with their students and the supervising SLPs who provide clinical guidance and mentoring to the next generation of SLPAs. The American Speech-Language-Hearing Association and field of speech-language pathology are clearly strengthened by the unique contributions of all these professionals.

In this edition, we have tried to capture what is most important for clinicians working in the field, whether it be with children or adults, in a private practice, a hospital, a home, or an educational setting. This was accomplished in no small way by the generous contributions of the chapter authors, who gave unselfishly of their time and expertise. These contributors include those outside our field, those who work in and alongside the field, and those firmly entrenched in the field. The contributors also represent practitioners and academics to ensure a balance of the theoretical and the practical. The collective experience and knowledge of the authors provide SLPAs with a firm foundation in the mix of the *science and art* that is the practice of speech-language pathology.

We would also like to thank Plural Publishing and the publishing team for their commitment to excellence, their attention to detail, and for setting a high bar for their authors and readers.

Contributors

Sara M. Aguilar, MA, CCC-SLP
Chapter 16
Sara M. Aguilar is a school-based speech-language pathologist in Southern California. Her professional areas of interest include augmentative and alternative communication, early literacy intervention, and supervision and training of support personnel. She has published and presented on the training, supervision, and use of SLPAs in California. Sara is a recipient of the Contemporary Issues in Communication Sciences and Disorders Editor's Award at the 2012 American Speech-Language-Hearing Association conference.

Carley B. Crandall, MA, CFY-SLP
Chapter 19
Carley B. Crandall currently works as a Clinical Fellow in home health and private practice. She graduated from California State University, Long Beach with honors, obtaining her BA in Communicative Disorders and her MA in Speech-Language Pathology. Carley's clinical experience involves adults and children across the spectrum of school-based, private, inpatient, outpatient, community-reintegration, and home-care settings. She has a research background in traumatic brain injury, neurogenic communication disorders, and evidence-based practices in augmentative and alternative communication.

Stephanie P. Davis, MA, CCC-SLP, BCBA
Chapter 11
Stephanie P. Davis is a dually certified speech-language pathologist and behav-ior analyst, whose career began in the public school system. Currently employed in a pediatric hospital, she specializes in patients with challenging behaviors, prioritizing caregiver coaching, AAC, data collecting, and collaborating with members of multidisciplinary teams. She holds an MA in Communicative Disorders from California State University, Long Beach and an MA in Special Education from Ball State University.

Sarah Guzzino-Herrick, MA, CCC-SLP
Chapter 12
Sarah Guzzino-Herrick is a speech-language pathologist in Southern California. She received her BA and MA degrees in speech-language pathology at California State University, Long Beach. Sarah worked as an SLPA while in graduate school and was offered the opportunity to participate in the first edition of *Speech-Language Pathology Assistants: A Resource Manual*. She coauthored *Group Therapy* during her last semester of graduate school.

Pei-Fang Hung, PhD, CCC-SLP
Chapter 6
Pei-Fang Hung is an Associate Professor and Department Chair in the Department of Speech-Language Pathology at California State University, Long Beach. Her research interests are aphasia management, neurogenic cognitive-communication disorders, and language impairments related to early dementia. She is a trilingual speech-language pathologist who holds certificates and licenses in both the United States and Taiwan and has extensive clinical experience working with

people with neurogenic speech and language disorders.

Carolyn Conway Madding, PhD, CCC-SLP
Chapter 5

Carolyn Conway Madding, Professor Emerita, formerly Chair of the Department of Speech-Language Pathology at California State University Long Beach, is a Fellow of ASHA and an ASHA Minority Champion and received the Diversity Award from the California Speech-Language-Hearing Association. She is bilingual, founded the Linguistically Different Clinical Practicum and initiated courses in diversity at CSULB, and has presented and published nationally and internationally on bilingualism and linguistic and cultural diversity within the profession of speech-language pathology.

Stephanie L. Peterson, MA, CCC-SLP
Chapter 7

Stephanie L. Peterson has experience as a speech-language pathologist within the school and clinical settings and part-time lecturer in the Department of Speech and Language Pathology at CSULB. Her specialties include AAC, data collection, teletherapy, and collaboration. She has taught a variety of courses at CSULB, including SLPA, Child Language Disorders, and Speech Sound Disorders. Currently, she is working as a program specialist supporting multidisciplinary special education teams and overseeing a grant to support secondary special education students.

Jodi Robledo, PhD, BCBA
Chapter 17

Jodi Robledo is a Professor in Special Education at California State University San Marcos (CSUSM) and serves as the Program Coordinator of the Education Specialist Credentials and Master of Arts in Special Education Programs, the Program Director for the Applied Behavior Analysis Certificate of Advanced Study, and the Associate Director of the School of Education at CSUSM. Dr. Robledo has referred journal publications, several book chapters, and numerous national conference presentations.

Lei Sun, PhD, CCC-SLP
Chapter 13

Lei Sun is a full professor in the Department of Speech-Language Pathology at California State University Long Beach. She completed her BA and MA in Taiwan before changing the career path to become a speech-language pathologist. Dr. Sun speaks Mandarin Chinese as her primary language and is an English-language learner. Dr. Sun is passionate about developmental language disorder, language-based learning disability, speech sound disorders, and multicultural/multilingual issues.

PART I

Defining Roles: Speech–Language Pathology Assistants (SLPAs)

CHAPTER 1

Defining Roles: SLPAs

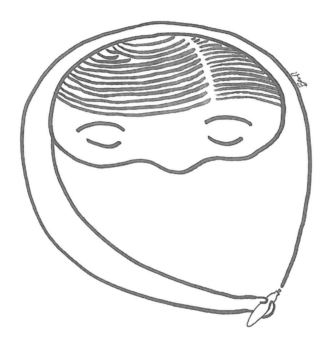

*Confidence, like art, never comes from having all the answers;
it comes from being open to all the questions.*

—Earl Gray Stevens

The American Speech-Language-Hearing Association (ASHA) defines SLPAs as "speech-language pathology assistants are support personnel who, following academic coursework, fieldwork, and on-the-job training, perform tasks prescribed, directed, and supervised by ASHA-certified speech-language pathologists" (ASHA, n.d.-a, Defining Speech-Language Pathology Assistants, para 1.).

SLPAs are not independent practitioners but rather work specifically under the direction and guidance of a qualified speech-language pathologist (SLP) to increase the availability, frequency, and efficiency of services provided by the SLP. SLPAs provide services in a wide variety of settings. These settings include but are not limited to the following (ASHA, 2022, Practice Settings, para. 1):[1]

- Public, private, and charter elementary and secondary schools
- Early intervention settings (e.g., homes, preschools, daycare settings)
- Hospitals (inpatient and outpatient)
- Residential health care settings (e.g., long-term care and skilled nursing facilities)
- Nonresidential health care settings (e.g., adult daycare, home health services, and clinics)
- Private practice settings
- University/college clinics
- Research facilities
- Corporate and industrial settings
- Student's, patient's, or client's residences

SLPAs differ from other support personnel, such as speech and language aides, instructional aides, paraprofessionals, and communication aides, both in the level of training and in the amount of supervision and oversight they receive. According to ASHA (n.d.-a.), "Aides, for example, have a different, usually narrower, training base and more limited responsibilities than speech-language pathology assistants" (Defining Speech-Language Pathology Assistants, para. 2).

The use of SLPAs is not new in the field of speech-language pathology. ASHA has had documents addressing support personnel since as early as the 1960s. The role of the SLPA in the field of speech-language pathology continues to evolve, however, given changes in health and educational service delivery models, increases in the number of individuals diagnosed with communication disorders, expansion in the scope of services

provided by SLPs, and the rising costs of providing these services.

ASHA (2022) outlines that "some tasks, procedures, or activities used to treat individuals with communication and related disorders can be successfully performed by individuals other than SLPs if the persons conducting the activity are properly trained and supervised by ASHA-certified and/or state-credentialed SLPs" (Executive Summary, para. 3). This chapter outlines recommendations for the training and use of SLPAs. Recommendations for the supervision of SLPAs are summarized in Chapter 2.

Internationally, there is variability in professional classification, services provided, and the use of assistants in the field of speech-language pathology. For individuals interested in obtaining information about SLPAs outside of the United States, ASHA maintains a summary of international SLP professional organizations (this information is also available at https://www.asha.org/members/international/intl_assoc/). These organizations are a good starting point for discovering if SLPAs exist at similar levels in other parts of the world. The International Association of Logopedics and Phoniatrics is also a source of information on this topic (http://www.ialp.info/).

In the United States, regulations for the training, use, and supervision of support personnel vary from state to state. The governing bodies that regulate or oversee the use of SLPAs also vary from state to state. In some locations, a state's department of education (or similar educational body) establishes and oversees specific requirements for SLPA training, use, and supervision in school settings. In some locations, state licensing boards regulate SLPA training, use, and supervision in nonschool settings. And in some cases, educational setting-specific requirements overlap with those of noneducation requirements, but in others they differ.

As an SLPA, if you are working in a setting that requires formal licensure, certification, or registration for support personnel, it is imperative that you adhere to any applicable laws, regulations, and procedures. Not doing so could compromise the care of the individuals you serve and place you and your supervisor in legal jeopardy for actions outside your state's standards. SLPAs should familiarize themselves with the most recent regulations in their locations. Realize as well that state standards may change annually or without notice. Hence, it is your responsibility as an SLPA to be familiar with, and stay abreast of, the most recent regulations in your location.

ASHA's State Advocacy Team maintains a page on ASHA's website that summarizes each state's requirements, including requirements for support personnel (ASHA, n.d.-b.). This is a valuable resource for SLPAs. SLPAs should also go directly to the website of their state's regulating body for information regarding SLPA regulations, laws, and procedures. An Internet search using terms, such as the name of your state plus speech-language pathology assistant, support personnel, registration, certification, or licensure, will likely yield the contact information you need.

ASHA is the national professional organization in the United States in the field of speech-language pathology. ASHA's primary policy document outlining recommend training, use, and supervision of SLPAs is the *Speech-Language Pathology Assistant Scope of Practice* (ASHA, 2022). This document is available

in Appendix 1–A. This and other important documents pertaining to SLPAs can be retrieved from ASHA's website (http://www.asha.org/). This includes ASHA's "Frequently Asked Questions" section on its website with current and helpful information about SLPAs and ASHA "practice portals" for professionals to access ASHA resources and policies on specific topics. The practice portal on the subject of SLPAs (http://www.asha.org/ Practice-Portal/Professional-Issues/Speech-Language-Pathology-Assistants/) is highly valuable for current information on topics related to support personnel.

Lastly, keep in mind that the information discussed in this book applies to documents published by ASHA at the time this book was written. As an SLPA, you should make ASHA's website a favorite on your homepage for ready access. Similar to state regulations, ASHA policies and documents change over time. As such, it is critical that you keep abreast of recent information from ASHA applicable to SLPAs. Following a description of ASHA's recommended use and training of SLPA, the final section of this chapter describes a recently created ASHA certification for SLPA (C-SLPA).

SLPA MINIMUM QUALIFICATIONS

As noted earlier, required training and education will vary by state, but ASHA's SLPA scope of practice recommends that SLPAs complete an "approved course of academic study, complete a supervised clinical experience, successfully pass the ASHA Assistants Certification Exam, meet credentialing requirements for the state in which they practice, and receive orientation as well as on-the-job training of SLPA responsibilities specific to the setting" (ASHA, 2022, Minimal Qualifications of an SLPA, para. 1). There are three educational pathways for doing so (ASHA, 2022, Minimal Qualifications of an SLPA, para. 2):[1]

1. Completion of an SLPA program from a regionally accredited institution (e.g., an associate's degree, a technical training program, a certificate program), or
2. Receipt of a bachelor's degree in communication sciences and disorders from a regionally accredited institution AND completion of ASHA education modules, or
3. Receipt of a bachelor's degree in a field other than communication sciences and disorders AND completion of ASHA education modules AND successful completion of coursework from a regionally or nationally accredited institution in all of the following areas:
    - Introductory or overview course in communication disorders
    - Phonetics
    - Speech sound disorders
    - Language development
    - Anatomy and physiology of speech and hearing mechanisms

Following completion of one of the above pathways, ASHA's scope of practice stipulates each of the following (ASHA, 2022, Minimal Qualifications of an SLPA, para. 3):[1]

1. Completion of a supervised clinical experience that consists of a minimum of one hundred (100) hours

under the direct supervision of an ASHA-certified SLP. The supervising SLP must meet all ASHA certification and supervising requirements and state credentialing requirements.
2. Achieve a passing score on the ASHA Assistants Certification Exam.
3. Meet all state credentialing requirements.

SLPA DUTIES AND RESPONSIBILITIES

ASHA expectations for SLPAs working in the field of speech-language pathology include performing only those tasks that are prescribed by an SLP and adhering to all applicable guidelines and regulations, including state licensure and related rules regarding SLPAs in specific settings. Specifically, ASHA states that SLPAs are expected to do the following (ASHA, 2022, Expectations of an SLPA, para. 1):[1]

- Adhere to all applicable state laws and rules regulating the practice of speech-language pathology.
- Adhere to the responsibilities for SLPAs specified in this scope of practice document and in state requirements.
- Avoid performing tasks or activities that are the exclusive responsibility of the SLP.
- Perform only those tasks approved by the supervising SLP.
- Work only in settings for which the SLPA has been trained and in which state regulations allow for SLPA employment.
- Deliver services only with an ASHA-certified and state-

licensed SLP providing direct and indirect supervision on a regular and systematic basis. Frequency and type of supervision should be based on the SLPA's competencies and the caseload need, both of which are determined by the supervising SLP.

- Conduct oneself ethically within the Assistants Code of Conduct (ASHA, 2020) and state ethical codes.
- Self-advocate for needed supervision and training and for adherence to this SLPA scope of practice and other requirements.
- Provide culturally responsive services while communicating and collaborating with students, patients, clients, the supervising SLP, colleagues, families, caregivers, and other stakeholders.
- Actively pursue continuing education and professional development activities.
- Obtain information regarding availability and need for liability insurance.

ASHA's (2022) document makes a specific point of highlighting those activities SLPAs should not engage in, as they are specifically outside an SLPA's scope of service (Box 1–1). If you find yourself in a situation during your training or at any point during the course of your employment as an SLPA where you engage in (or are asked to perform) any of these activities, this is a clear warning sign that you should seek immediate assistance in addressing the issue. Chapter 3 discusses ethical dilemmas such as this and recommendations for resolving ethical conflict.

Now that you know what an SLPA must not do, ASHA's 2022 scope of practice document also outlines activities that are within the scope of responsibilities of an SLPA, including duties in the areas of service delivery, administrative support, and prevention and advocacy.

Service Delivery

In the area of service delivery, ASHA recommends that SLPAs identify themselves to clients, clients' families, and fellow service providers, both verbally and in writing, and wear a name badge (ASHA, 2022). Furthermore, as discussed in Chapter 3, SLPAs are expected to conduct themselves ethically, maintain client confidentiality, and adhere to all federal and state regulations in the provision of services in schools and medical settings. Provided SLPAs are under the direction of a qualified SLP and given adequate training and supervision, Box 1–2 outlines ASHA's recommendations for activities within the scope of an SLPA related to service delivery. SLPAs "may not perform tasks when a supervising SLP cannot be reached by personal contact, phone, pager, or other immediate or electronic means" (ASHA, 2022, Minimum Requirements in Frequency and Amount of Supervision, para. 9). Furthermore, the purpose of an SLPA is to support the SLP in the provision of services, not to increase the caseload numbers of the SLP. ASHA recommends that SLPAs have liability insurance as protection for malpractice during service provision. Your employer may provide this insurance for you, or you may be expected to independently acquire liability insurance. This should be done prior to providing services to clients.

Box 1–1. Activities Outside an SLPA's Scope of Practice
(ASHA, 2022, Responsibilities Outside the Scope of SLPAs, para. 1)[1]

The SLPA should *NOT* engage in any of the following activities:

- Representing themselves as the SLP
- Interpreting assessment tools for the purpose of diagnosing disability, determining eligibility or qualification for services
- Administering or interpreting feeding and/or swallowing screenings, checklists, and assessments
- Diagnosing communication and feeding/swallowing disorders
- Developing or determining the feeding and/or swallowing strategies or precautions for students, patients, and clients
- Disclosing clinical or confidential information (e.g., diagnosis, services provided, response to treatment) either orally or in writing to individuals who have not been approved by the SLP to receive information unless mandated by law
- Writing, developing, or modifying a student's, patient's, or client's plan of care in any way
- Making referrals for additional services
- Assisting students, patients, and clients without following the individualized plan of care prepared by the ASHA-certified SLP
- Assisting students, patients, and clients without access to supervision
- Selecting augmentative and alternative communication (AAC) systems or devices
- Treating medically fragile students, patients, and clients without 100% direct supervision
- Performing procedures that require specialized knowledge and training (e.g., vocal tract prosthesis shaping or fitting, vocal tract imaging)
- Providing input in care conferences, case conferences, or any interdisciplinary team meeting without the presence or prior approval of the supervising SLP or other designated SLP
- Providing interpretative information to the student, patient, client, family, or others regarding the student's, patient's, or client's status or service
- Signing or initialing any formal documents (e.g., plans of care, reimbursement forms, reports) without the supervising SLP's co-signature
- Discharging a student, patient, or client from services

Box 1–2. SLPA Scope of Responsibility: Service Delivery
(ASHA, 2022, Service Delivery, para. 1)[1]

- Self-identifying (e.g., verbally, in writing, signage, titles on name badges) as an SLPA to students, patients, clients, families, staff, and others
- Exhibiting compliance with federal, state, and local regulations, including the Health Insurance Portability and Accountability Act (HIPAA), the Family Educational Rights and Privacy Act (FERPA), reimbursement requirements, and state statutes and rules regarding SLPA education, training, and scope of practice
- Administering and scoring screenings for clinical interpretation by the SLP
- Assisting the SLP during assessment of students, patients, and clients (e.g., setting up the testing environment, gathering and prepping materials, taking notes as advised by the SLP)
- Administering and scoring assessment tools that (a) the SLPA meets the examiner requirements specified in the examiner's manual and (b) the supervising SLP uses to verify the SLPA's competence in administration, exclusive of clinical interpretation
- Administering and scoring progress monitoring tools exclusive of clinical interpretation if (a) the SLPA meets the examiner requirements specified in the examiner's manual and (b) the supervisor has verified the SLPA's competence in administration
- Implementing documented care plans or protocols (e.g., individualized education plan [IEP], individualized family service plan [IFSP], treatment plan) developed and directed by the supervising SLP
- Providing direct therapy services addressing treatment goals developed by the supervising SLP to meet the needs of the student, patient, client, and family
- Adjusting and documenting the amount and type of support or scaffolding provided to the student, patient, or client in treatment to facilitate progress
- Developing and implementing activities and materials for teaching and practice of skills to address the goals of the student, patient, client, and family per the plan of care developed by the supervising SLP
- Providing treatment through a variety of service delivery models (e.g., individual, group, classroom based, home

based, cotreatment with other disciplines) as directed by the supervising SLP

■ Providing services via telepractice to students, patients, and clients who are selected by the supervising SLP

■ Documenting student, patient, or client performance (e.g., collecting data and calculating percentages for the SLP to use; preparing charts, records, and graphs) and reporting this information to the supervising SLP in a timely manner

■ Providing caregiver coaching (e.g., model and teach communication strategies, provide feedback regarding caregiver-child interactions) for facilitation and carryover of skills

■ Sharing objective information (e.g., accuracy in speech and language skills addressed, participation in treatment, response to treatment) regarding student, patient, and client performance to students, patients, clients, caregivers, families, and other service providers without interpretation or recommendations as directed by the SLP

■ Programming AAC devices

■ Providing training and technical assistance to students, patients, clients, and families in the use of AAC devices

■ Developing low-tech AAC materials for students, patients, and clients

■ Demonstrating strategies included in the feeding and swallowing plan developed by the SLP and sharing information with students, patients, clients, families, staff, and caregivers

■ Assisting students, patients, and clients with feeding and swallowing skills developed and directed by the SLP when consuming food textures and liquid consistencies

In addition, SLPAs who use multiple languages (based on their training and experiences in working with multilingual students, patients, or clients and their families) may also:

■ Assist the SLP with interpretation and translation in the student's, patient's, or client's first language during screening and assessment activities exclusive of clinical interpretation of results.

■ Interpret for students, patients, clients, and families who communicate using a language other than English, when the provider has received specialized training with interpreting skills in the student's, patient's, or client's first language.

■ Provide services in another language for individuals who communicate using a language other than English or for those who are developing English-language skills. Such services are based on the provider's skills and knowledge of the language spoken by the student, patient, or client.

SLPAs who speak multiple languages can find serval valuable resources in advancing their skills and competency in this area within ASHA's Practice Portal devoted to Bilingual Service Delivery (located at https://www.asha.org/practice-portal/professional-issues/bilingual-service-delivery/). Chapter 5 also offers additional information and resources in this area.

Administrative Support

In addition to providing clinical services, SLPAs may provide administrative support to their supervisors, including the activities listed in Box 1–3.

Prevention and Advocacy

SLPAs may also assist their supervisors in activities related to the prevention of communicative disorders and advocacy for individuals with communicative disorders and their families. Box 1–4 highlights activities within the scope of responsibilities of an SLPA in this area.

CULTURALLY RESPONSIVE PRACTICES

ASHA highlights the critical importance of SLPAs meeting the needs of the individuals they serve in "a space of mutual understanding and respect" and in a culturally responsive manner (ASHA, 2022). Specifically, offering culturally responsive services is the "explicit use of culturally based care and health knowledge in sensitive, creative, and meaningful ways" (Leininger, 2002, p. 84, as cited in ASHA, 2022, Culturally Responsive Practices, para 2). This requires that SLPAs (ASHA, 2022, Culturally Responsive Practices, para 2):[1]

- Adjust communication style and expectations to meet the needs of clients, patients, and students from different cultural groups and to provide services in a culturally responsive manner.

Box 1–3. SLPA Scope of Responsibility: Administrative Support
(ASHA, 2022, Administrative Support, para. 1)[1]

- Assist with clerical duties and site operations (e.g., scheduling, recordkeeping, maintaining inventory of supplies and equipment).
- Perform safety checks and maintenance of equipment.
- Prepare materials for screening, assessment, and treatment services.

> **Box 1–4. SLPA Scope of Responsibility: Prevention and Advocacy**
> (ASHA, 2022, Prevention and Advocacy, para. 1)[1]
>
> ■ Present primary prevention information to individuals and groups known to be at risk for communication and swallowing disorders.
> ■ Promote early identification and early intervention activities.
> ■ Advocate for individuals and families through community awareness, health literacy, education, and training programs to promote and facilitate access to full participation in communication—including addressing the social determinants of health and health disparities.
> ■ Provide information to emergency response agencies for individuals who have communication, swallowing, and/or related disorders.
> ■ Advocate at the local, state, and national levels for improved public policies affecting access to services and research funding.
> ■ Support the supervising SLP in research projects, in-service training, marketing, and public relations programs.
> ■ Participate actively in professional organizations.

■ Provide information to families and staff regarding the influence of first language on the development of communication and related skills in a second language (under the direction of the supervising SLP).
■ Develop an understanding of the family dynamic from a cultural perspective to effectively engage in meetings surrounding intake, discussions of the therapy plan of care, and other communication scenarios surrounding practices for addressing communication concerns.
■ Engage in continuing education and training opportunities focusing on the assessment and intervention process when working with individuals from culturally and linguistically diverse backgrounds.

Becoming a culturally responsive practitioner takes time and requires proactive training and engagement for all SLPAs. Chapter 5 offers key information in the area. ASHA also offers several important resources on this topic, including a Practice Portal devoted to Cultural Competence (located at https://www.asha.org/practice-portal/professional-issues/cultural-competence/).

SLPA JOB DESCRIPTION: A DAY IN THE LIFE OF AN SLPA

After reading lists of duties and responsibilities, many SLPAs in training often still ask, "What will my job be like as an SLPA?" This is a valid question to ask but a difficult one to answer. The settings in which SLPAs work are highly variable, as are the populations of individuals for which SLPAs provide services. Equally variable is the nature of tasks SLPAs perform in these different settings. Appendix 1–B recounts several stories, collected from SLPAs throughout the United States, that tell of a "Day in the Life" of a specific SLPA. Lastly, Appendices 1–C and 1–D contain sample job descriptions for SLPAs in medical and educational settings, respectively. Each of these documents sheds a light on different roles of an SLPA. Ultimately, learning firsthand by meeting and speaking directly with SLPAs and SLPs themselves is one of the best ways to explore the field of speech-language pathology and the roles of SLPAs.

COMPETENCY ASSESSMENT

Webster's dictionary defines competent as "having requisite or adequate ability or qualities" or "having the capacity to function or develop in a particular way" (Merriam-Webster, 2003). Being a competent SLPA requires knowledge and the practical application of this knowledge in the execution of specific tasks (i.e., skill). In all settings, on-the-job-training is required to develop your knowledge and skills as an SLPA. To be competent in the performance of your duties in a specific work environment, you need additional knowledge and skills beyond what you learned in a training program to become an SLPA.

In the field of speech-language pathology, assessment based on competency is often used. As discussed in Chapter 2,

it is your supervisor's responsibility to outline what specific competencies are required for you to operate effectively as an SLPA in your unique setting (ASHA, 2022). Your supervisor is also responsible for creating a mechanism for assessing your competency in these areas and for developing ways to improve your knowledge and skills to required levels. As an SLPA, it is your responsibility to be aware of the knowledge and skills required of you and to strive for competency in all areas.

Appendix 1–E (and the companion website of this book) contains an example of a competency-based measurement, given the responsibilities within the scope of an SLPA (ASHA, 2022).

Note that it uses a continuum to rate competency in the responsibilities of an SLPA on a scale from does not meet (1) to far exceeds requirements (5). Table 1–1 contains a description of performance levels for this scale. It is important to remember, however, when descriptions of competency include the word *independent*, this does not mean SLPAs are performing any activity without the supervision of an SLP (e.g., operating as an independent clinician). Rather, this designation means that, under a supervising SLP's guidance, an SLPA has obtained a level of competency that allows her or him to operate with proficiency in the task described. Appendices 1–E to 1–I contain additional evaluation tools and forms recommended by ASHA for documenting the presence and degree of core proficiency levels for SLPAs.

These competency-based assessments illustrate an important point to consider throughout your career as an SLPA. Competency reflects your level of performance at any given point in time, for a specific set of circumstances (e.g., a specific task, client, and setting). You will likely not be

Table 1–1. Examples of Competency-Based Assessment Levels (ASHA, 2013)

Does not meet	Requires education and training at the introductory level
Needs improvement	Requires input from supervisor or other resource for routine cases.
Meets requirements	Demonstrates proficiency independently in most cases: independently seeks resources for additional support
Exceeds requirements	Independently demonstrates proficiency for routine to complex cases
Far exceeds requirements	Demonstrates proficiency at all levels of complexity; able to serve as a role model to other staff

equally competent across everything you do as an SLPA. That is completely normal. In fact, to expect that you will be perfect and exceed competencies in everything you do misses the potential of this type of assessment.

In each setting, additional, more specific competencies will be required, beyond the basic framework of SLPA responsibilities and job duties outlined by ASHA. For example, there are specific knowledge and skills needed to work with young children with autism spectrum disorder (ASD). These may be similar in some respects but different from the knowledge and skills needed to work with adults with aphasia. Similarly, if you are working in a school setting, there may be specific competencies needed that differ from those of a medical or private practice setting. As an SLPA, when you enter a training or employment setting, it is critical that you review all competency assessment tools applicable to you and ask your supervisor about the range of specific knowledge and skills required of you in that unique setting.

Beyond minimal competency, as an SLPA, you should always strive for higher levels of performance in all areas

of knowledge and skill applicable to your role. Your goal should be to continue to improve and enhance your knowledge and skills throughout your career. SLPAs who recognize there is always room for improvement and who seek ways to improve their performance are those who reach the highest levels of performance as an SLPA. ASHA also stipulates that SLPAs must "actively pursue continuing education and professional development activities" (ASHA, 2022, Expectations of an SLPA, para. 1). Furthermore, many state regulating bodies specifically outline the amount and nature of continuing education required for SLPAs to maintain licensure, certification, or registration in that state. You should be familiar with what is required in your state.

It is your responsibility to seek out appropriate continuing education opportunities. You can work with your supervising SLP to identify these opportunities, but ultimately you are responsible for initiating them. Chapter 4 offers suggestions for self-assessment and reflection to evaluate your own skills and abilities and then, importantly, identify avenues for improvement and formal continuing education.

ASHA CERTIFICATION

In 2020, ASHA created a certification for SLPAs (C-SLPA) (Council for Clinical Certification in Audiology and Speech-Language Pathology of the American Speech-Language-Hearing Association, 2020). This purpose of this certification is to (Introduction, para 2):

■ Help improve patient/client access to speech-language pathology services by creating a pipeline of qualified professionals who meet uniform standards of competency and are committed to delivering high-quality care.
■ Establish a uniform standard for the knowledge and skill level expected of assistants.
■ Ensure that all ASHA-certified assistants meet the same rigorous requirements.

The foundations of the requirements for becoming a C-SLPA are based on the above ASHA's scope of practice recommendations (ASHA, 2022), but becoming a C-SLPA is a "voluntary, entry-level credential recognizing SLPAs who have met established criteria and standards of practice to deliver high quality clinical service" (ASHA, n.d.-c., Purpose, para 1.). This designation indicates to employers, consumers, licensing boards, and third-party payers that a C-SLPA demonstrates clini-

cal skills and knowledge needed to practice as an SLPA (as per ASHA standards).

The process for receiving a C-SLPA includes completion of:

1. An eligible degree
2. Prerequisite courses
3. Online modules (or equivalent coursework) in the area of ethics, universal safety precautions, and patient confidentiality
4. Fieldwork/clinical hours requirements

Certification also requires that an applicant pass a national certification examination for SLPAs. Once certified, C-SLPA must adhere to the Assistants Code of Conduct (ASHA, 2020) and complete a certification maintenance assessment module every 3 years.

C-SLPA is a national, *voluntary* professional credential. It is separate from any state licensing/registration requirements. At this point, SLPAs may ask, how is a C-SLPA and state licensure/state registration as an SLPA different? This is a good question and one that warrants clarification. Table 1–2 offers some differentiating details.

Individuals interested in becoming a C-SLPA can find additional information on the process and requirements for application at https://www.asha.org/certification/about-assistants-certification/. This includes a *Speech-Language Pathology Certification Handbook* with all applicable details.

Table 1–2. Differences Between ASHA Certification and State Licensure/Registration

ASHA Certification (C–SLPA)	State Licensure/Registration
Voluntary/optional	Required in some states
SLPAs must meet ASHA eligibility requirements to obtain ASHA certification.	SLPAs must meet state eligibility requirements to obtain licensure/registration.
ASHA certification requirements are set by ASHA (not state licensing agencies).	Licensing requirements are set by state agencies (not ASHA).
ASHA maintains one national requirement for certification.	Licensing requirements vary from state to state.
Certification alone does not guarantee employment.	Licensure alone does not guarantee employment, but in some states, licensure is required to work as an SLPA.

REFERENCES

American Speech-Language-Hearing Association. (n.d.-a.). *Frequently asked questions: Speech-language pathology assistants (SLPAs).* https://www.asha.org/assistants-certification-program/slpa-faqs/

American Speech-Language-Hearing Association. (n.d.-b.). *ASHA state-by-state.* http://www.asha.org/advocacy/state/

American Speech-Language-Hearing Association. (n.d.-c.). *Speech-language pathology assistants certification handbook.* https://www.ashaassistants.org/

American Speech-Language-Hearing Association. (2020). *Assistants code of conduct* [Ethics]. www.asha.org/policy

American Speech-Language-Hearing Association. (2022). *Speech-language pathology assistant scope of practice.* http://www.asha.org/policy

Council for Clinical Certification in Audiology and Speech-Language Pathology of the American Speech-Language-Hearing Association. (2020). *2020 Standards for ASHA speech-language pathology assistants certification.* https://www.asha.org/certification/2020-slpa-certification-standards/

Merriam-Webster. (2003). *Merriam-Webster's collegiate dictionary* (11th ed.).

CHAPTER ENDNOTE

1. American Speech-Language-Hearing Association (2022). *Speech-language pathology assistant scope of practice.* Available from http://www.asha.org/policy. Copyright 2022 American Speech-Language-Hearing Association. All rights reserved. Reprinted with permission.

APPENDIX 1–A
ASHA Speech–Language Pathology Assistant Scope of Practice (ASHA, 2022)

ABOUT THIS DOCUMENT

This Scope of Practice for the Speech-Language Pathology Assistant (SLPA) was developed by the American Speech-Language-Hearing Association (ASHA) Ad Hoc Committee to Update the Scope of Practice for Speech-Language Pathology Assistants (hereafter, "the Ad Hoc Committee"). In January 2021, the ASHA Board of Directors approved a resolution for the development of the ad hoc committee to complete this task. Members of the committee were Jerrold Jackson, MA, CCC-SLP (chair, Texas), Tyler T. Christopulos, PhD, CCC-SLP (Utah), Erin Judd, C-SLPA (Minnesota), Ashley Northam, CCC-SLP (Oregon), Katie Orzechowski, MS, CCC-SLP (Illinois), Jennifer Schultz, MA, CCC-SLP (South Dakota), Nancy Thul, MS, CCC-SLP (Minnesota), Nicole Wilson-Friend, C-SLPA (California), and Lemmietta McNeilly, PhD, CCC-SLP (ex officio). Linda I. Rosa-Lugo, EdD, CCC-SLP, Vice President for Speech-Language Pathology Practice, served as the Board liaison. The composition of the Ad Hoc committee included ASHA-certified speech-language pathologists (SLPs) and SLPAs with specific knowledge and experience working with/as support personnel in clinical practice in schools, health care, and/or private practice settings.

This document is intended to provide guidance for SLPAs and their SLP supervisors regarding ethical considerations related to the SLPA practice parameters. It addresses how services performed by SLPAs should be utilized and what specific responsibilities are within and outside their roles of clinical practice. This information was developed by analyzing current practice standards, certification requirements, methods of academic and clinical training (from academic program directors, clinical educators, etc.), and feedback from stakeholders in communication sciences and disorders. Given that standards, state credentialing (e.g., licensure, etc.), and practice issues vary from state to state, this document's purpose is to provide information regarding ASHA's guidelines for the use of SLPAs for the treatment of communication disorders across practice settings.

DEDICATION

In loving memory of Steve Ritch, whose dedication, commitment, and perseverance contributed to ensuring integrity and quality in addressing the topic of SLPAs within the ASHA structure.

ACKNOWLEDGMENTS

We would like to acknowledge others who provided feedback and insights that aided in the development of this document. The Ad Hoc Committee would also like to acknowledge the expertise shared by Marianne Gellert-Jones, MA, CCC-SLP (Pennsylvania), Ianessa Humbert, PhD, CCC-SLP (Washington, D.C.), and Rosemary Montiel, C-SLPA (California).

EXECUTIVE SUMMARY

ASHA has identified critical shortages of speech-language pathologists (SLP) in all regions of the country, particularly in school settings. These shortages impede the ability of individuals with communication and related disorders to reach their full academic, social, and emotional potential. The use of speech- language pathologist assistants (SLPAs) is an essential element of aiding those professionals who provide services and individuals who rely on such services. It is the position of ASHA that the use of any support personnel be done with the explicit purpose of support for the SLP rather than used as an alternative.

This scope of practice presents minimum recommendations for the training, use, and supervision of speech-language pathology assistants. SLPAs perform tasks as prescribed, directed, and supervised by ASHA-certified and/or state-credentialed SLPs. Support personnel can be used to increase the availability, frequency, and efficiency of services.

Some tasks, procedures, or activities used to treat individuals with communication and related disorders can be successfully performed by individuals other than SLPs if the persons conducting the activity are properly trained and supervised by ASHA-certified and/or state-credentialed SLPs. The use of evidence as well as ethical and professional judgment should be at the heart of the selection, management, training, supervision, and use of SLPAs.

This scope of practice specifies the minimum qualifications and responsibilities for an SLPA and delineates the tasks that are the exclusive responsibilities of the SLP. In addition, the document provides guidance regarding ethical considerations when SLPAs provide clinical services and outlines the supervisory responsibilities of the supervising SLP.

INTRODUCTION

The *Scope of Practice for the SLPA* provides information regarding the training, use, and supervision of assistants in speech-language pathology—a designation that ASHA established to be applicable in a variety of work settings. Training for SLPAs should be based on the type of tasks specified in their scope of responsibility. Specific education and training may be necessary to prepare assistants for unique roles in various professional settings.

ASHA has addressed the topic of support personnel in speech-language pathology since the 1960s. In 1967, the ASHA Executive Board established the Committee on Supportive Personnel and, in 1969, the document ASHA Legislative Council (LC) approved the document *Guidelines on the Role, Training and Supervision of the Communicative Aide*. In the 1990s, several entities—including committees, a task force, and a consensus panel—were established and the LC approved a position statement, techni-

cal report, guidelines, and curriculum content for support personnel. In 2002, ASHA developed an approval process for SLPA programs, and in 2003 ASHA established a registration process for SLPAs. Both were discontinued by vote of the LC because of fiscal concerns. In 2004, the LC approved a position statement on the training, use, and supervision of support personnel in speech-language pathology. Since then, the number of SLPAs has increased primarily in schools and private practice settings. ASHA members in many states continue to request specific guidance from ASHA. In 2016, the ASHA Board of Directors (BOD) completed a feasibility study for the standardization of requirements for assistants; that study demonstrated strong support for certifying assistants, across all stakeholders. The ASHA BOD voted to approve the Assistants Certification program in 2017. In December 2020, the ASHA Assistants Certification Program launched; this program sets standards for the practices and operations for SLPAs as well as for audiology assistants.

This document does not supersede federal legislation and regulation requirements or any existing state credentialing laws, nor does it affect the interpretation or implementation of such laws. The document may serve, however, as a guide for the development of new laws or, at the appropriate time, for revising existing licensure laws.

STATEMENT OF PURPOSE

The purpose of this document is to define what is within and outside the scope of responsibilities for SLPAs who work under the supervision of properly credentialed SLPs. The following aspects are addressed:

- parameters for education and professional development for SLPAs
- SLPAs' responsibilities within and outside the scope of practice
- varied practice settings
- information for others (e.g., special educators, parents, consumers, health professionals, payers, regulators, members of the general public) regarding services that SLPAs perform
- information regarding the ethical and liability considerations for the supervising SLP and the SLPA
- supervisory requirements for the SLP and the SLPA.

MINIMUM REQUIREMENTS FOR AN SLPA

An SLPA must complete an approved course of academic study, complete a supervised clinical experience, successfully pass the ASHA Assistants Certification Exam, meet credentialing requirements for the state in which they practice, and receive orientation as well as on-the-job training of SLPA responsibilities specific to the setting.

The minimum educational, clinical, and examination requirements for all SLPAs are outlined in the subsections below:

Three Educational Options

1. Completion of an SLPA program from a regionally accredited institu-

tion (e.g., an associate degree, a technical training program, a certificate program).

or

2. Receipt of a bachelor's degree in communication sciences and disorders from a regionally accredited institution AND completion of ASHA education modules.

or

3. Receipt of a bachelor's degree in a field other than communication sciences and disorders AND completion of ASHA education modules AND successful completion of coursework from a regionally or nationally accredited institution in all of the following areas:

   - introductory or overview course in communication disorders
   - phonetics
   - speech sound disorders
   - language development
   - language disorders
   - anatomy and physiology of speech and hearing mechanisms

Additional Requirements

In addition to having satisfied one of the above three educational options, the SLPA must also meet all the following three requirements:

1. Completion of a supervised clinical experience that consists of a minimum of one hundred (100) hours under the direct supervision of an ASHA certified SLP. The supervising SLP must meet all ASHA certification and supervising requirements and state credentialing requirements.
2. Achieve a passing score on the ASHA Assistants Certification Exam.

3. Meet all <u>state credentialing require-ments</u>.

Expectations of an SLPA

The following list details of the roles and performance expectations of an ASHA-certified SLPA:

- Adhere to all applicable state laws and rules regulating the practice of speech-language pathology.
- Adhere to the responsibilities for SLPAs specified in this scope of practice document and in state requirements.
- Avoid performing tasks or activities that are the exclusive responsibility of the SLP.
- Perform only those tasks approved by the supervising SLP.
- Work only in settings for which the SLPA has been trained and in which state regulations allow for SLPA employment.
- Deliver services only with an ASHA-certified and state licensed SLP providing direct and indirect supervision on a regular and systematic basis. Frequency and type of supervision should be based on the SLPA's competencies, and the caseload need, both of which are determined by the supervising SLP.
- Conduct oneself ethically within the *ASHA Assistant's Code of Conduct* (ASHA, 2020b) and state ethical codes.
- Self-advocate for needed supervision and training and for adherence to this SLPA scope of practice and other requirements.

- Provide culturally responsive services while communicating and collaborating with students, patients, clients, the supervising SLP, colleagues, families, caregivers, and other stakeholders.
- Actively pursue continuing education and professional development activities.
- Obtain information regarding availability and need for liability insurance.

RESPONSIBILITIES WITHIN THE SCOPE OF PRACTICE FOR SLPAs

The supervising SLP retains full legal and ethical responsibility for students, patients, and clients served but may delegate specific tasks to the SLPA. The SLPA may execute components of services as specified by the SLP in the plan of care. Services performed by the SLPA are only those within the scope of practice and are tasks that the SLPA has the training and skill to perform as verified by the supervising SLP. The SLP must provide appropriate and adequate direct and indirect supervision to ensure quality care for all persons served. The amount of supervision may vary depending on the case's complexity and the SLPA's experience. Under no circumstances should the use of an SLPA's services (a) violate the *ASHA Code of Ethics* (2016a) or the *ASHA Assistants Code of Conduct* (2020b) or (b) negatively impact the quality of services. An SLPA's services are designed to enhance the quality of care provided by the SLP.

Decisions regarding the tasks that are appropriate to assign to the SLPA should be made by the supervising SLP in collaboration with the SLPA. The SLPA is responsible for communicating their knowledge, experience, and self-assessment of competence with specific skills to the supervising SLP. It is the SLP's responsibility to observe the SLPA performing specific tasks; to provide feedback regarding clinical performance; to recommend or provide education and training to develop skills to meet the needs of the students, patients, and clients served; and to validate the SLPA's competence. The SLPA's competence in practice areas can be determined by observations, collaboration between the supervising SLP and the SLPA, as well as other resources deemed significant by the supervisor/supervisee pair.

If the SLPA has demonstrated the necessary competencies and the supervising SLP provides the appropriate amount and type of supervision, the SLPA may engage in or assigned to perform the following tasks:

- service delivery
- culturally responsive practices
- responsibilities for all practitioners
- responsibilities for practitioners who use multiple languages
- administration and support
- prevention and advocacy.

Service Delivery

The SLPA should engage in the following activities when performing necessary tasks related to speech- language service provision:

- Self-identifying (e.g., verbally, in writing, signage, titles on name badges, etc.) as an SLPA

to students, patients, clients, families, staff, and others.
- Exhibiting compliance with federal, state, and local regulations including: The Health Insurance Portability and Accountability Act (HIPAA), the Family Educational Rights and Privacy Act (FERPA); reimbursement requirements; and state statutes and rules regarding SLPA education, training, and scope of practice.
- Administering and scoring screenings for clinical interpretation by the SLP.
- Assisting the SLP during assessment of students, patients, and clients (e.g., setting up the testing environment, gathering and prepping materials, taking notes as advised by the SLP, etc.).
- Administering and scoring assessment tools that (a) the SLPA meets the examiner requirements specified in the examiner's manual and (b) the supervising SLP uses to verify the SLPA's competence in administration, exclusive of clinical interpretation.
- Administering and scoring progress monitoring tools exclusive of clinical interpretation if (a) the SLPA meets the examiner requirements specified in the examiner's manual and (b) the supervisor has verified the SLPA's competence in administration.
- Implementing documented care plans or protocols (e.g., individualized education plan [IEP], individualized family service plan [IFSP], treatment

plan) developed and directed by the supervising SLP.

- Providing direct therapy services addressing treatment goals developed by the supervising SLP to meet the needs of the student, patient, client, and family.
- Adjusting and documenting the amount and type of support or scaffolding provided to the student, patient, or client in treatment to facilitate progress.
- Developing and implementing activities and materials for teaching and practice of skills to address the goals of the student, patient, client, and family per the plan of care developed by the supervising SLP.
- Providing treatment through a variety of service delivery models (e.g., individual, group, classroom-based, home-based, co-treatment with other disciplines) as directed by the supervising SLP.
- Providing services via telepractice to students, patients, and clients who are selected by the supervising SLP.
- Documenting student, patient, or client performance (e.g., collecting data and calculating percentages for the SLP to use; preparing charts, records, and graphs) and report this information to the supervising SLP in a timely manner.
- Providing caregiver coaching (e.g., model and teach communication strategies, provide feedback regarding caregiver-child interactions) for facilitation and carryover of skills.

- Sharing objective information (e.g., accuracy in speech and language skills addressed, participation in treatment, response to treatment) regarding student, patient, and client performance to students, patients, clients, caregivers, families and other service providers without interpretation or recommendations as directed by the SLP.
- Programming augmentative and alternative communication (AAC) devices.
- Providing training and technical assistance to students, patients, clients, and families in the use of AAC devices.
- Developing low-tech AAC materials for students, patients, and clients.
- Demonstrating strategies included in the feeding and swallowing plan developed by the SLP and share information with students, patients, clients, families, staff, and caregivers.
- Assisting students, patients, and clients with feeding and swallowing skills developed and directed by the SLP when consuming food textures and liquid consistencies.

CULTURALLY RESPONSIVE PRACTICE

Cultural responsiveness has been described as providing individuals "with a broader perspective from which to view our behaviors as they relate to our actions with individuals across a variety of cultures that are different from our own" (Hyter & Salas-Provance, 2019, p. 7).

Engaging in culturally responsive practices refers to the "explicit use of culturally based care and health knowledge in sensitive, creative, and meaningful ways" (Leininger, 2002, p. 84). It is important to remember that cultural and linguistic backgrounds exist on a continuum and not all individuals will exhibit characteristics of one group at any given time. Practitioners must meet the student, patient, client, and their families or caregivers in a space of mutual understanding and respect.

Not only is the supervising SLP responsible for engaging in these practices, but they should also train and provide support for the SLPA to develop these skills.

RESPONSIBILITIES FOR SLPs AND SLPAs

All practitioners have the following responsibilities related to cultural and linguistic supports:

- Adjust communication style and expectations to meet the needs of clients, patients, and students from different cultural groups and to provide services in a culturally responsive manner. For more information, see the ASHA Practice Portal on *Cultural Competence* [ASHA, n.d.-b].
- Provide information to families and staff regarding the influence of first language on the development of communication and related skills in a second language (under the direction of the supervising SLP).
- Develop an understanding of the family dynamic from a cultural

perspective to effectively engage in meetings surrounding intake, discussions of the therapy plan of care and other communication scenarios surrounding practices for addressing communication concerns
- Engage in continuing education and training opportunities focusing on the assessment and intervention process when working with individuals from culturally and linguistically diverse backgrounds.

Responsibilities for Practitioners Who Use Multiple Languages

Based on prior training and experiences in working with multilingual students, patients or clients and their families, the SLPA may engage in the following tasks:

- Assist the SLP with interpretation and translation in the student's, patient's, or client's first language during screening and assessment activities exclusive of clinical interpretation of results. For more information, see *Issues in Ethics: Cultural and Linguistic Competence* (ASHA, 2017) and the ASHA Practice Portal Page on *Bilingual Service Delivery* (ASHA, n.d.-a)
- Interpret for students, patients, clients, and families who communicate using a language other than English, when the provider has received specialized training with interpreting skills in the student's, patient's, or client's first language. For more information, see *Issues in Ethics:*

Cultural and Linguistic Competence (ASHA, 2017) and the ASHA Practice Portal Page on *Bilingual Service Delivery* (ASHA, n.d.-a)

■ Provide services in another language for individuals who communicate using a language other than English or for those who are developing English language skills. Such services are based on the provider's skills and knowledge of the language spoken by the student, patient, or client. For more information, see *Issues in Ethics: Cultural and Linguistic Competence* (ASHA, 2017) and the ASHA Practice Portal Page on *Bilingual Service Delivery* (ASHA, n.d.-a).

Administrative Support

Depending on the setting, adequate training, and guidance from the supervising SLP, the SLPA may:

■ assist with clerical duties and site operations (e.g., scheduling, recordkeeping, maintaining inventory of supplies and equipment);
■ perform safety checks and maintenance of equipment, and
■ prepare materials for screening, assessment, and treatment services.

Prevention and Advocacy

Depending on the setting, adequate training, and guidance from the supervising SLP, the SLPA may

■ present primary prevention information to individuals and groups known to be at risk for communication and swallowing disorders;
■ promote early identification and early intervention activities;
■ advocate for individuals and families through community awareness, health literacy, education, and training programs to promote and facilitate access to full participation in communication—including addressing the social determinants of health and health disparities;
■ provide information to emergency response agencies for individuals who have communication, swallowing, and/or related disorders;
■ advocate at the local, state, and national levels for improved public policies affecting access to services and research funding;
■ support the supervising SLP in research projects, in-service training, marketing, and public relations programs; and
■ participate actively in professional organizations.

RESPONSIBILITIES OUTSIDE THE SCOPE OF PRACTICE FOR SPEECH–LANGUAGE PATHOLOGY ASSISTANTS

There is potential for misuse of an SLPA's services, particularly when responsibilities are delegated by other staff members (e.g., administrators, nursing staff, physical therapists, occupational therapists, psychologists, etc.) without the approval of the supervising SLP. It is highly recommended that this *ASHA SLPA Scope of Practice* as well as the *ASHA Code of Ethics* (ASHA, 2016a) and the *ASHA Assistants Code of Conduct* (ASHA, 2020b) be reviewed with all personnel involved when employing an SLPA. It should be emphasized that an individual's communication and/or related disorders and/or other factors may preclude the use of services from anyone other than an ASHA-certified and/or licensed SLP. The SLPA should not perform any task without the approval of the supervising SLP. The student, patient, or client should be informed that they are receiving services from an SLPA under the supervision of an SLP.

The SLPA should NOT engage in any of the following activities:

- representing themselves as the SLP;
- interpreting assessment tools for the purpose of diagnosing disability, determining eligibility or qualification for services;
- administering or interpreting feeding and/or swallowing screenings, checklists, and assessments;
- diagnosing communication and feeding/swallowing disorders;
- developing or determining the feeding and/or swallowing strategies or precautions for students, patients, and clients;
- disclosing clinical or confidential information (e.g., diagnosis, services provided, response to treatment) either orally or in writing to individuals who have not been approved by the SLP to receive information unless mandated by law;
- writing, developing, or modifying a student's, patient's, or client's plan of care in any way;

- making referrals for additional services;
- assisting students, patients, and clients without following the individualized plan of care prepared by the ASHA certified SLP;
- assisting students, patients, and clients without access to supervision;
- selecting AAC systems or devices;
- treating medically fragile students, patients, and clients without 100% direct supervision;
- performing procedures that require specialized knowledge and training (e.g., vocal tract prosthesis shaping or fitting, vocal tract imaging);
- providing input in care conferences, case conferences, or any interdisciplinary team meeting without the presence or prior approval of the supervising SLP or other designated SLP;
- providing interpretative information to the student, patient, client, family, or others regarding the student's, patient's, or client's status or service;
- signing or initialing any formal documents (e.g., plans of care, reimbursement forms, reports) without the supervising SLP's co-signature;
- discharging a student, patient, or client from services.

PRACTICE SETTINGS

Under the specified guidance and supervision of an ASHA-certified and/or state-credentialed SLP, SLPAs may provide services in a wide variety of settings, which may include, but are not limited to, the following:

- public, private, and charter elementary and secondary schools
- early intervention settings (e.g., homes, preschools, daycare settings)
- hospitals (inpatient and outpatient)
- residential health care settings (e.g., long-term care and skilled nursing facilities)
- nonresidential health care settings (e.g., adult daycare, home health services, and clinics)
- private practice settings
- university/college clinics
- research facilities
- corporate and industrial settings
- student's, patient's, or client's residences

ETHICAL CONSIDERATIONS

ASHA strives to ensure that its members and certificate holders preserve the highest standards of integrity and ethical practice. ASHA maintains two separate documents that set forth the fundamentals of ethical conduct in the professions. The *ASHA Code of Ethics* (2016a) sets forth the fundamental principles and rules deemed essential for SLPs. This code applies to every individual who is

(a) an ASHA member, whether certified or not, (b) a nonmember holding the ASHA Certificate of Clinical Competence, (c) an applicant for membership or certification, or (d) a Clinical Fellow seeking to fulfill standards for certification.

The *ASHA Assistants Code of Conduct* (2020b) sets forth the principles and fundamentals of ethical practice for SLPAs. The Assistants Code of Conduct applies to all ASHA-certified audiology and speech-language pathology assistants, as well as applicants for assistant certification. It defines the SLPA's role in the provision of services under the SLP's supervision and provides a framework to support decision-making related to the SLPA's actions. The Assistants Code of Conduct holds assistants to the same level of ethical conduct as the supervising SLP with respect to responsibilities to people served professionally, the public, and other professionals; however, it does not address ethics in supervision and other duties that are outside the SLPA Scope of Practice.

It is imperative that the supervising SLP and the SLPA are knowledgeable about the provisions of both codes and that they behave in a manner consistent with the principles and rules outlined in the ASHA Code of Ethics and the ASHA Assistants Code of Conduct. Because the ethical responsibility for students, patients, and clients—or for subjects in research studies—cannot be delegated, the supervising SLP takes overall responsibility for the actions of any SLPA when that SLPA is performing their assigned duties. If the SLPA engages in activities that violate the Assistants Code of Conduct, then the supervising SLP may be found in violation of the Code of Ethics—if it is found that adequate oversight has not been provided.

The following principles and rules of the Code of Ethics specifically address issues that are pertinent when an SLP supervises SLPAs in the provision of services or when conducting research. Failure to comply with principles and rules related to supervisory activities in the Code of Ethics or failure to ensure that the SLPA complies with the Assistants Code of Conduct could result in a violation of the Code of Ethics by the supervisor.

Principle of Ethics I, Rule of Ethics A

Individuals shall provide all clinical services and scientific activities competently.

Guidance

The supervising SLP must ensure that all services, including those provided directly by the SLPA, meet practice standards, and are administered competently. The supervising SLP is responsible for providing training as needed or requested by the SLPA, identifying the services that the SLPA is competent to perform, monitoring the provision of those services to ensure quality of care, and intervening to correct the actions of the SLPA as needed.

Principle of Ethics I, Rule of Ethics D

Individuals shall not misrepresent the credentials of aides, assistants, technicians, support personnel, students, research interns, Clinical Fellows, or any others under their supervision, and they shall inform those they serve professionally of the name, role, and professional credentials of persons providing services.

Guidance

The supervising SLP must ensure that students, patients, clients, caregivers, and research subjects are informed of the title and qualifications of the SLPA. This is not a passive responsibility; that is, the super-

visor must make this information easily available and understandable to the students, patients, clients, caregivers, and research subjects and not rely on the individual to inquire about or ask directly for this information.

Principle of Ethics I, Rule of Ethics E

Individuals who hold the Certificate of Clinical Competence may delegate tasks related to the provision of clinical services to aides, assistants, technicians, support personnel, or any other persons only if those persons are adequately prepared and are appropriately supervised. The responsibility for the welfare of those being served remains with the certified individual.

Guidance

The supervising SLP is responsible for providing appropriate and adequate direct and indirect supervision to ensure that the services provided are appropriate and meet practice standards. The SLP must consider student, patient, or client needs and the SLPA's knowledge and skills to determine what constitutes appropriate supervision, which may be more than the minimum required in state regulations. The SLP must document supervisory activities and adjust the amount and type of supervision to ensure that the Code of Ethics and Assistants Code of Conduct are followed.

Principle of Ethics I, Rule of Ethics F

Individuals who hold the Certificate of Clinical Competence shall not delegate tasks that require the unique skills, knowledge, judgment, or credentials that are within the scope of their profession to aides, assistants, technicians, support personnel, or any nonprofessionals over whom they have supervisory responsibility.

Guidance

The supervising SLP is responsible for monitoring the professional activities performed by the SLPA and ensuring that they remain within the guidelines set forth in the ASHA SLPA Scope of Practice and applicable state and facility guidelines. In some cases, ASHA requirements may differ from state regulations. ASHA requirements do not supersede state licensure laws or affect the interpretation or implementation of such laws. The supervising SLP should ensure that the highest standards of ethical conduct are maintained.

Principle of Ethics II, Rule of Ethics A

Individuals who hold the Certificate of Clinical Competence shall engage in only those aspects of the professions that are within the scope of their professional practice and competence, considering their certification status, education, training, and experience.

Guidance

The supervising SLP is responsible for ensuring that they have the skills and competencies needed to provide appropriate supervision. This includes completion of required continuing education in supervision and may include seeking additional continuing education in supervision to remain current in this area.

Principle of Ethics II, Rule of Ethics E

Individuals in administrative or supervisory roles shall not require or permit their professional staff to provide services or conduct research activities that exceed the staff member's certification status, competence, education, training, and experience.

Guidance

The supervising SLP must ensure that the SLPA only performs those activities that are defined as appropriate for the level of training and experience and in accordance with applicable state regulations and facility guidelines. If the SLPA exceeds the practice role that has been defined for them, the SLP must intervene to correct the actions of the SLPA as needed.

Principle of Ethics III, Rule of Ethics D

Individuals shall not defraud through intent, ignorance, or negligence or engage in any scheme to defraud in connection with obtaining payment, reimbursement, or grants and contracts for services provided, research conducted, or products dispensed.

Guidance

States and third-party payers (e.g., insurance, Medicaid) vary in their policies regarding recognition of SLPAs as approved service providers, rate of reimbursement for assistant-level services, and other policies. The supervising SLP and SLPA are jointly responsible for knowing and understanding federal and state regulations and individual payer policies, billing for services at the appropriate level, and providing the amount and type of supervision required by the payer when billing for SLPA services.

Principle of Ethics IV, Rule of Ethics I

Individuals shall not knowingly allow anyone under their supervision to engage in any practice that violates the Code of Ethics.

Guidance

Because the SLPA provides services as an extension of those provided by the certified SLP, the SLP is responsible for ensuring the SLPA adheres to the Assistants Code of Conduct and monitoring the performance of the SLPA.

LIABILITY ISSUES

Individuals who engage in the delivery of services to persons with communication and swallowing disorders are potentially vulnerable to accusations of engaging in unprofessional practices. Therefore, ASHA recommends that SLPAs secure liability insurance as a protection for malpractice. SLPAs should consider the need for liability coverage. Some employers provide it for all employees. Other employers defer to the employee to independently acquire liability insurance. Some universities provide coverage for students involved in practicum and fieldwork. Obtaining or verifying liability insurance coverage is the SLPA's responsibility and needs to be done prior to providing services.

GUIDELINES FOR SLPA SUPERVISION OF SLPAs

For SLPAs to practice, a supervising SLP must be identified. The following indicates considerations for the supervising SLP:

- qualifications for the supervising SLP
- expectations of the supervising SLP
- considerations for the ratio of SLPs to SLPAs
- requirements for frequency and duration of supervision.

Minimum Qualifications for Supervising SLP

The minimum qualifications for an SLP to supervise the SLPA include the following:

- Hold the Certificate of Clinical Competence in Speech-Language Pathology (CCC-SLP) from ASHA and/or possess the necessary state-credentials
- Completion of a minimum of 9 months of experience after being awarded ASHA certification (i.e., completion of the 9-month Clinical Fellowship followed by 9 months of experience)
- Completion of a minimum of 2 hours of professional development in clinical instruction/supervision
- Adherence to state guidelines for supervision of the SLPA

■ It is recommended that the professional development course taken in clinical instruction or supervision include content related to the supervision of SLPAs

Expectations for the Supervising SLP

In addition to the minimum qualifications listed above, the following are additional roles and behavior that are expected of the supervising SLP:

■ Adhere to the principles and rules of the ASHA Code of Ethics (ASHA, 2016a)
■ Adhere to applicable licensure laws and rules regulating the practice of speech-language pathology
■ Conduct ongoing competency evaluations of the SLPAs
■ Provide and encourage ongoing education and training opportunities for the SLPA consistent with competency and skills required to meet the needs of the students, patients, and clients served
■ Develop, review, and modify treatment plans for students, patients, and clients that the SLPA implements under the supervision of the SLP
■ Make all case management decisions
■ Adhere to the supervisory responsibilities for SLPs
■ Retain legal and ethical responsibility for all students, patients, and clients served

■ Maintain an active interest in collaborating with SLPAs

Supervision of SLPAs

The relationship between the supervising SLP and the SLPA is paramount to the welfare of the student, patient, or client. Because the clinical supervision process is a close, interpersonal experience, the supervising SLP should participate in the selection of the SLPA when possible. It is the SLP's responsibility to design and implement a supervision system that protects the students', patients', and clients' care and that maintains the highest possible standards of quality. The amount and type of supervision must meet (a) minimum requirements as specified in this document and (b) state requirements. Supervision must be based on (a) the needs, competencies, skills, expectations, philosophies, and experience of the SLPA and the supervisor; (b) the needs of students, patients, and clients served; (c) the service setting; (d) the tasks assigned; and (e) other factors. More intense supervision, for example, would be required in such instances as the orientation of a new SLPA; initiation of a new program, equipment, or task; or a change in student, patient, or client status (e.g., medical complications). Functional assessment of the SLPA's skills with assigned tasks should be an ongoing, regular, and integral element of supervision. SLPs and SLPAs should treat each other with respect and should interact in a manner that will provide the best possible outcomes for student, patient, and client care. It is also critical that the SLP and SLPA understand that their language, culture, and experiences will be different within the dyad and across the triad (SLP, SLPA, and patient, client, and student). It is expected that the practitioners stay grounded in cultural responsiveness and culturally responsive practices when engaged in all aspects of interactions.

As the SLP's supervisory responsibility increases, overall responsibilities will change because the SLP is responsible for the students, patients, and clients as well as supervision of the SLPA. Therefore, adequate time for direct and indirect supervision of the SLPA(s) and caseload management must be allotted as a critical part of the SLP's workload. The purpose of the assistant level position is not to significantly increase the caseload size for SLPs. The specialized skills should be utilized to support the SLP with the care of individuals on the SLP's caseload. Under no circumstances should an assistant have their own caseload.

Diagnosis, treatment, and support of the students, patients, and clients served remains the legal and ethical responsibility of the supervisor. Therefore, the level of supervision required is considered the minimum level necessary for the supervisor to retain direct contact with the students, patients, and clients. The supervising SLP is responsible for designing and implementing a supervisory plan that protects consumer care, maintains the highest quality of practice, and documents the supervisory activities.

SLP-to-SLPA Ratio

The supervising SLP should determine the appropriate number of assistants whose practice can be supervised within their workload. Although more than one SLP may provide supervision of an SLPA, it is recommended that the SLP not supervise or be listed as a supervisor for more than three full-time equivalent (FTE) SLPAs in any setting. The number of SLPAs who can be appropriately supervised by a single SLP will depend on a variety of factors including caseload characteristics, SLPA experience, and SLP experience. The SLP is responsible for determining how many SLPAs can be supervised while maintaining the highest level of quality for services provided. When multiple SLPs supervise a single SLPA, it is critical that the supervisors coordinate and communicate with each other so that they collectively meet minimum supervisory requirements and ensure that they maintain the highest quality of services.

Requirements for the Frequency and Amount of Supervision

Supervision requirements may vary based on a variety of factors. The amount and type of supervision required must be consistent with (a) the SLPA's skills and experience; (b) the needs of the students, patients, and clients; (c) the service setting; (d) the tasks assigned; and (e) the laws and regulations that govern SLPAs. To ensure adequate and appropriate supervision, the supervising SLP should outline their expectations in collaboration with the SLPA. As the relationship continues to develop over time, the SLP/SLPA team can decide how and to what extent supervision is needed.

Before the SLPA begins to provide support independently, the supervising SLP must have first contact with all individuals on the caseload. "First contact" includes establishing rapport, gathering baseline data, and securing other necessary documentation to begin (or continue) the plan of care for the student, patient, or client. As the SLP/SLPA team dynamic continues to develop beyond the initial onboarding, minimum ongoing supervision must always include documentation of direct supervision provided by the SLP for each student, patient, or client at least every 30–60 days (depending on frequency of visits/sessions and setting).

The SLP can adjust the amount of supervision if they determine that the SLPA has met appropriate competencies and skill levels in treating students, patients, and clients who have a variety of communication disorders. Data on every student, patient, and client serviced by the SLPA should be reviewed by the supervisor in regular intervals and can be considered "indirect supervision." Supervisors should arrange designated days and times of day (morning or afternoon) in such a way that all students, patients, and clients receive direct contact with the supervising SLP.

The supervising SLP must accurately document and regularly record all supervisory activities, both direct and indirect. Further, 100% direct supervision (synchronous or "live" telesupervision is acceptable) of SLPAs for medically fragile students, patients, or clients is required.

The supervising SLP is responsible for designing and implementing a supervisory plan, which ensures that the SLP maintains the highest standard of quality care for students, patients, and clients. A written supervisory plan is a tangible way to document progress and outline the practices of the supervising SLP and the SLPA. Care of the student, patient, or client remains the supervisor's responsibility.

Direct supervision means in-view observation and guidance while the SLPA is performing a clinical activity. This can include the supervising SLP viewing and communicating with the SLPA via telecommunication technology as the SLPA provides clinical services, this scenario allows the SLP to provide ongoing immediate feedback. Direct supervision does not include reviewing an audio- or video-recorded session later.

Supervision feedback should provide information about the quality of the SLPA's performance of assigned tasks and should verify that clinical activity is limited to tasks specified in the list of an SLPA's ASHA-approved responsibilities. Information obtained during direct supervision may include, but is not limited to, data relative to (a) agreement (reliability) between the SLPA and the supervisor on correct or incorrect recording of target behavior, (b) accuracy implementing assigned treatment procedures, (c) accuracy recording data, and (d) ability to interact effectively with the student, patient, or client during presentation and implementation of assigned procedures or activities.

Indirect supervision does not require the SLP to be physically present or available via telecommunication while the SLPA is providing services. Indirect supervisory activities may include (a) reviewing demonstration videos; (b) reviewing student, client, or patient files; (c) reviewing and evaluating audio- or video-recorded sessions; and/or (d) conducting supervisory conferences either in person or via telephone and/or live, secure virtual meetings. The SLP will review each care plan as needed for timely implementation of modifications.

An SLPA may not perform tasks when a supervising SLP cannot be reached by personal contact, that is, phone, pager, or other immediate or electronic means. If, for any reason (i.e., maternity leave, illness, change of jobs) the supervisor is no longer available to provide the level of supervision stipulated, then the SLPA may not perform assigned tasks until an ASHA-certified and/or state-licensed SLP with experience and training in supervision has been designated as the new supervising SLP.

Any supervising SLP who will not be able to supervise an SLPA for more than 1 week will need to (a) inform the SLPA of the planned absence, (b) notify the employer or site administrator that other arrangements for the SLPA's supervision of services need to be made while the SLP is unavailable, and (c) inform the students, patients, or clients that their speech-language services will be rescheduled.

In some instances, multiple SLPs may supervise the SLPA. Those doing so must give special consideration to, and think carefully about, the impact that this supervisory arrangement may have on service providers. It is recommended that the SLPA not be supervised by more than three SLPs.

CONCLUSION

This document aims to provide guidance for the use of SLPAs in appropriate settings, thereby increasing access to timely and efficient speech-language services. The supervising SLP or SLPs are responsible for staying abreast of current guidelines (including state credentialing guidelines) and ensuring the quality of services rendered. Given that standards, state credentialing (e.g., licensure, etc.), and practice issues vary from state to state, this document's purpose is to provide information regarding ASHA's guidelines for the use of SLPAs for the treatment of communication disorders across practice settings.

DEFINITIONS

Accountability—refers to being legally responsible and answerable for actions and inactions of self or others during the performance of a task by the SLPA.

Aide/technician—individual who has completed on-the-job training, workshops, and other related tasks and who works under the direct supervision of an ASHA-certified SLP. See also *speech-language pathology aide/technician*.

Assessment—procedures implemented by the SLP for the differential diagnosis of communication and swallowing disorders, which may include, per the *ASHA Speech-Language Pathology Scope of Practice* [PDF], "culturally and linguistically appropriate behavioral observation and standardized and/or criterion-referenced tools; use of instrumentation; review of records, case history, and prior test results; and interview of the individual and/or family to guide decision making" (ASHA, 2016b, p. 11).
Assessments may also be referred to as *evaluations*, *tests*, and so forth.

Cultural responsiveness—provides individuals with "a broader perspective from which to view our behaviors as they relate to our actions with individuals across a variety of cultures that are different from our own". (Hyter & Salas-Provance, 2019, p. 7)

Culturally responsive practices—Care that takes the client's cultural perspectives, beliefs, and values into consideration in all aspects of education and/or service provision. Leininger (2002) defines this term as "the explicit use of culturally based care and health knowledge in sensitive, creative, and meaningful ways."

Direct supervision—in-view observation and guidance by an SLP while the SLPA performs an assigned activity. Direct supervision activities performed by the supervising SLP may include, but are not limited to, the following: observing a portion of the screening or treatment procedures performed by the SLPA, coaching the SLPA, and modeling for the SLPA. The supervising SLP must be present during all services provided to a medically fragile client by the SLPA (e.g., on-site or via synchronous telesupervision). The SLP can view and communicate with the student, patient, or client and SLPA via "real-time" telecommunication technology to supervise the SLPA, giving the SLP the opportunity to provide immediate feedback. This does not include reviewing a recorded session later.

Indirect supervision—the monitoring or reviewing of an SLPA's activities outside of observation and guidance during direct services provided to a student, patient, or client. Indirect supervision activities performed by the supervising SLP may include, but are not limited to, demonstration, records review, review and evaluation of audio- or video-recorded sessions, and interactive conferences that may be conducted by telephone, email, or other forms of telecommunication (e.g., virtual platforms).

Interpretation—summarizing, integrating, and using of data for the purpose of clinical decision making, which may only be done by SLPs. SLPAs may summarize objective data from a session to the family or team members.

Medically fragile—a term used to describe an individual who is acutely ill and in an unstable health condition. If an SLPA treats such an individual that treatment requires 100% direct supervision by an SLP.

Plan of care—a written service plan developed and monitored by the supervising SLP to meet the needs of an individual student, patient, or client. The plan may address needs for screening, observation, monitoring, assessment, treatment, and other services. Examples of care plans include Individualized Education Plans (IEPs), Individualized Family Service Plans (IFSPs), rehabilitation services plans, and so forth.

Progress monitoring—a process of collecting, graphing, and reviewing data on an individual's target skills to assess their response to treatment and then comparing their growth to a target trend line or goal to determine whether sufficient progress is being made. Definition adapted from Progress Monitoring webpage. (*National Center on Intensive Intervention*, n.d.)

Screening—a pass-fail procedure to identify, without interpretation, students, patients, or clients who may require further assessment following specified screening protocols developed by and/or approved by the supervising SLP.

Social Determinants of Health—the conditions in which people are born, grow, live, work, and age, including the health system. These circumstances are shaped by the distribution of money, power, and resources at global, national, and local levels, which are themselves influenced by policy choices. The social determinants of health are mostly responsible for health inequities-the unfair and avoidable differences in health status seen within and between countries. (World Health Organization, n.d.)

Speech-Language Pathology Aides/Technician—an individual who has completed on-the-job training, workshops, and other related tasks and who works under the direct supervision of an ASHA-certified SLP; this is another type of support personnel that may not meet the requirements as an ASHA certified SLPA. See also aide/technician

Speech-Language Pathology Assistant—an individual who, following academic coursework, clinical practicum, and credentialing can perform tasks prescribed, directed, and supervised by ASHA-certified SLPs.

Supervising Speech-Language Pathologist—an SLP who holds a Certificate of Clinical Competence in Speech-Language Pathology (CCC-SLP) from ASHA and/or a state licensure (where applicable), has an active interest and desire to collaborate with support personnel, has a minimum of 9 months of experience after being awarded ASHA certification, has completed the 2-hour supervision requirement per the *ASHA Certification Standards* (ASHA, 2020a) and adheres to state credentialing guidelines for supervision of the SLPA, and who is licensed and/or credentialed by the state (where applicable).

Supervision—the provision of direction and evaluation of the tasks assigned to an SLPA. Methods for providing supervision include direct supervision, indirect supervision, and telesupervision.

Support Personnel—these individuals perform speech-language tasks as prescribed, directed, and supervised by ASHA-certified SLPs. There are different levels of support personnel based on training and scope of responsibilities. The term support personnel includes SLPAs and speech-language pathology aides/technicians. ASHA is operationally defining these terms for ASHA resources. Some states use different terms and definitions for support personnel (e.g., *assistant speech-language pathologist, speech-language pathologist paraprofessional*, and *SLP assistant*, among others).

Telepractice—applying telecommunications technology to the delivery of professional services at a distance by linking clinician to client, or clinician to clinician, for assessment, intervention, and/or consultation (ASHA, n.d.-c).

Telesupervision—the SLP can view and communicate with the patient and SLPA in real time via telecommunication software (e.g., virtual platforms), webcam, telephone, and similar devices and services to supervise the SLPA. This enables the SLP to give immediate feedback. Telesupervision does not include reviewing a recorded session later.

REFERENCES

American Speech-Language-Hearing Association. (n.d.-a). *Bilingual service delivery* [Practice portal]. https://www.asha.org/practice-portal/professional-issues/bilingual-service-delivery/

American Speech-Language-Hearing Association. (n.d.-b). *Cultural competence* [Practice portal]. https://www.asha.org/practice-portal/professional-issues/cultural-competence/

American Speech-Language-Hearing Association. (n.d.-c). *Telepractice* [Practice portal]. https://www.asha.org/PracticePortal/Professional-Issues/Telepractice/

American Speech-Language-Hearing Association. (2016a). *Code of ethics* [Ethics]. https://www.asha.org/policy/et2016-00342/

American Speech-Language-Hearing Association. (2016b). *Scope of practice in speech-language pathology* [Scope of practice]. https://www.asha.org/policy

American Speech-Language-Hearing Association (2017). *Issues in ethics: Cultural and linguistic competence.* https://www.asha.org/Practice/ethics/Cultural-and-Linguistic-Competence

American Speech-Language-Hearing Association. (2020a). *2020 Standards and implementation procedures for the Certificate of Clinical Competence in Speech-Language Pathology.* https://www.asha.org/certification/2020-slp-certification-standards/

American Speech-Language-Hearing Association. (2020b). *Assistants code of conduct.* https://www.asha.org/policy/assistants-code-of-conduct/

Hyter, Y., & Salas-Provance, M. (2019). *Culturally responsive practices in speech, language, and hearing sciences.* Plural Publishing.

Ladson Billings, G. (1994). *The dreamkeepers.* Josey Bass.

Leininger, M. (2002). Theory of culture care and the ethnonursing research method. In M. Leininger & M. R. McFarland (Eds.), *Transcultural nursing: Concepts, theories, research and practice* (pp. 71–98). McGraw-Hill.

National Center on Intensive Intervention (n.d.). *Progress monitoring.* https://intensiveintervention.org/data-based-individualization/progress-monitoring

Vose AK, Kesneck S, Sunday K, Plowman E, & Humbert I. (2018). A survey of clinician decision making when identifying swallowing impairments and determining treatment. *Journal of Speech, Language, and Hearing Research, 61*(11), 2735–2756.

World Health Organization. (n.d.). *Social determinants of health.* https://www.who.int/health-topics/

APPENDIX 1–B
A Day in the Life of an SLPA:
Interviews and Advice from SLPAs

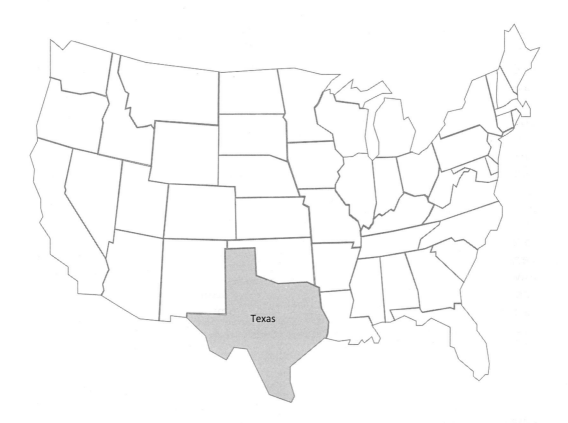

Texas

A DAY IN THE LIFE OF SARA

A Traveling SLPA

Sara is a licensed SLPA in the state of Texas. According to the ASHA (n.d., Statutory and Regulatory Requirements, para. 1), obtaining an SLPA license in Texas requires the following:

- a baccalaureate degree with an emphasis in communicative sciences and disorders,

- Show proof of completion of no fewer than 24 semester hours in speech-language pathology/ audiology, and
- No fewer than 25 hours of clinical observation in the area of speech-language pathology and 25 hours of clinical assisting experience in speech-language pathology (note: if the applicant has a bachelor's degree in another major, the Board of Examiners shall evaluate on a case-by-case basis).

SLPAs in Texas must be supervised by a licensed SLP at least 2 hours per week, of which at least 1 hour must be face-to-face supervision at the location where the SLPA is employed.

Sara earned a bachelor's degree in communicative disorders. She feels fortunate to have attended a bachelor's program that also offered her the opportunity to obtain 100 hours of clinical practicum as an SLPA.

Sara is currently employed as an SLPA for a company that provides services to individuals in home settings, head start programs, and daycares. A typical day for Sara consists of traveling to these different locations to provide treatment services. Sara typically sees clients for 30-minute treatment sessions and makes about 125 to 200 visits per month. Her clients are very diverse, many of whom come from low-income households. They range in age from as young as 18 months to as old as 17 years. They have a wide spectrum of disorders, including a variety of speech and language impairments.

Rewards

Sara enjoys building rapport with her clients and their families. She finds the most rewarding aspect of her job the positive impact that she can make on her clients'

lives and in seeing the joy of the children she works with when she travels to their homes to provide services. She reports that in some cases, her clients and their families tell her that her services are the highlight of their day/week.

Challenges

One of the challenges of Sara's job is moving from home to home, hauling her equipment in and out of her car. She feels though, that being in a client's home is also a big advantage, as she is able to get to know the parents and families of her clients.

Words of Wisdom

Sara reports that being an SLPA is "highly rewarding." To individuals interested in pursuing a career as an SLPA, Sara recommends attending a school that offers an opportunity to complete your degree in communicative disorders, as well as obtain the observation and clinical hours required to become an SLPA.

Reference

American Speech-Language-Hearing Association (ASHA). (n.d.). *ASHA state-by-state.* https://www.www.asha.org/advocacy/state/info/tx/texas-support-personnel-requirements/

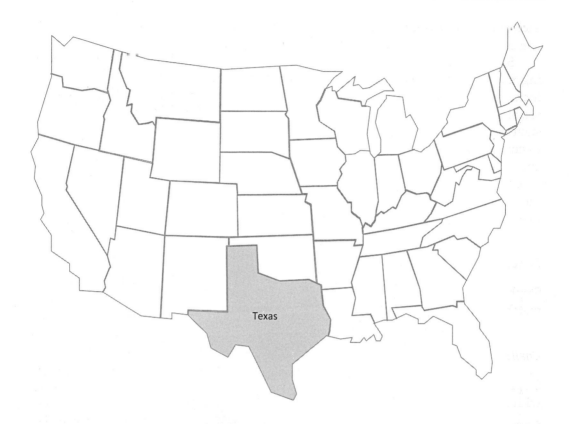

A DAY IN THE LIFE OF STEPHANIE

Never Give Up!

Stephanie is been a licensed SLPA in the state of Texas for 5 years. She has a bachelor's degree in communicative disorders and completed 50 hours of clinical practicum as part of her training to become an SLPA.

Stephanie currently works in a private practice, providing treatment services to individuals who range in age from 2 to 11 years, including individuals with ASD, speech sound disorder (SSD), stuttering, Down syndrome, and cleft lip/palate.

A typical day for Stephanie starts at 8:30 AM. First, she retrieves the speech folders for each client on her treatment schedule. These folders contain an initial evaluation, testing, monthly summary reports, a calendar, and speech notes (which include each client's individual goals). Next, Stephanie plans her sessions, writing out the goals developed by her supervising SLP and possible activities for each. She then decides which activities work best for each client's goals and collects her materials.

Stephanie sees three to five clients every morning and then an additional three to four clients in the afternoon. Treatment is provided on a one-to-one basis, although sometimes social skills are targeted in group sessions. During her sessions, she tallies the client's responses on a blank sheet of paper, where she has written each client's goals for that session. After each of her sessions, Stephanie writes a formal Subjective Objective Assessment and Plan (SOAP) note for each client. Her supervising SLP reviews these notes at the end of each day.

Stephanie is also charged with keeping the treatment rooms orderly, which includes cleaning and sanitizing materials. She assists with administrative duties, such as auditing therapy folders quarterly to ensure all needed information is present and up to date. Stephanie participates twice weekly in team meetings, one with the entire staff and the other with her fellow SLPAs and SLP supervisor.

Rewards

Stephanie's greatest reward as an SLPA is watching her clients make progress.

Challenges

Stephanie's biggest challenge is working with children who have behavioral issues, such as children who are not compliant with requests during the session. She also has clients who can exhibit aggressive behavior during treatment sessions when they become frustrated or are asked to complete nondesired tasks.

Words of Wisdom

Stephanie's words of wisdom to new SLPAs are: (a) take the time to do research about different diagnoses and disabilities and (b) "Don't give up!" When Stephanie first started working as an SLPA, she worked primarily with individuals with ASD. She recalls this was very challenging because many of her clients did not interact with her. As Stephanie put it, they seemed to be "in their own world." She also recalls they often cried, screamed, hit, or bit themselves.

In these early days of her career, Stephanie remembers sitting in her car during lunch one day, crying and thinking, "I can't do this. I don't know what I am doing!" Her supervising SLP told her that once she understands autism, working with these clients will not be so hard. For Stephanie, this advice was absolutely correct. With perseverance, research, and a knowledgeable supervising SLP, Stephanie now has the techniques needed to help her clients succeed (those with ASD and all her clients). Now, she remembers to take it one day at a time and she realizes, "I can do this!"

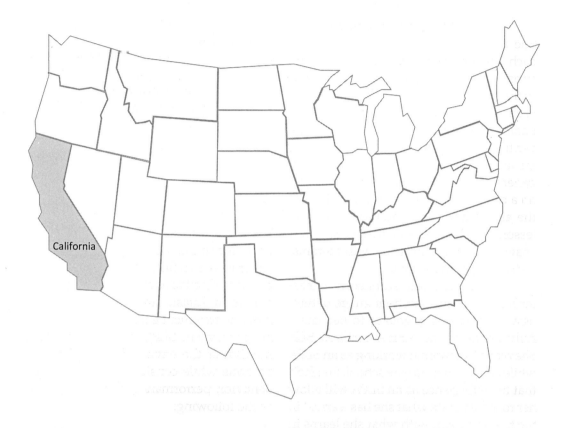

California

A DAY IN THE LIFE OF MIKA

Training to be an SLP

Mika is a licensed SLPA in the state of California. According to ASHA (n.d., Statutory and Regulatory Requirements, para. 1), to obtain an SLPA license in California requires at least one of the following qualifications:

- an associate of arts or sciences degree from an SLPA-accredited and board-approved program, or
- a bachelor's degree in speech-language pathology or communicative disorders from an accredited and board-approved program, and

completion of 70 hours of fieldwork/clinical experience.

Mika has a bachelor's degree in communicative disorders and completed 100 hours of clinical practicum as an SLPA.

Mika currently works as an SLPA in a private practice, providing treatment services to children, mostly ages 2 to 5 years, who have a variety of impairments including expressive/receptive language delay and ASD. She also provides treatment to older children as part of a social skills group focused on pragmatic skills, such as problem solving, perspective taking, appropriate/inappropriate conversation topics, and understanding nonverbal cues. These groups comprise three to five children, with similar ages and abilities, all who have been diagnosed with ASD.

Mika's typical day is roughly 8 hours. She arrives 30 minutes early to review each client's file and any notes from her supervising SLP. In the mornings, she also gathers the toys and materials needed for each session. She carries out treatment goals, mostly through play-based intervention. Her treatment sessions occur throughout the course of her day and are generally 50-minute sessions, provided on a one-on-one basis with each client. In the afternoons, Mika prepares files and lesson plans for the next day. She also answers phones and helps with administrative duties as needed.

Mika is currently enrolled in a master's program in speech-language pathology. Her long-term goal is to become a fully licensed and ASHA-certified SLP. She plans to continue working as an SLPA while attending graduate school. She feels that her experience as an SLPA will allow her to incorporate what she has learned in the therapy room with what she learns in the classroom. She is very eager to learn more, including procedures for assessment and diagnosis and an expanded range of treatment procedures. She is particularly excited to participate in internships and clinical practica with individuals she has not yet worked with as an SLPA, such as individuals with swallowing disorders and aphasia.

Rewards

Mika feels extremely lucky to be working with a supervising SLP and fellow clinicians who view her as a full member of a team. Her greatest reward is in having an opportunity to provide services to clients on a one-on-one basis for 50-minute sessions. She believes this provides truly individualized treatment, which leads to dramatic progression over time. She says that "watching her clients inch closer and closer to their goals is an amazing feeling." As an SLPA, she has been able to make a connection with her clients and share in their feeling of excitement when they progress, make changes, and overcome challenges.

Challenges

Mika finds controlling the environment, addressing behavior, and building rapport among the most challenging aspects of her role as an SLPA. She believes that to be truly effective as an SLPA, she must be able to multitask, simultaneously implementing treatment goals (as developed by her supervising SLP), collecting data, and modifying the environment. This must be done while considering each client's behavior, performance, and needs, such as the following:

- Will this client cry?
- Is this the first time away from mom or dad?
- How do I keep the client on task while I take notes?
- What encourages good behavior?
- How do I make therapy fun but still task driven?

Words of Wisdom

First and foremost, Mika recommends that all SLPAs thoroughly understand their scope of practice. Mika also stresses that as an SLPA, you must be knowledgeable and passionate about what you do. Mika has learned that it is important to know pertinent information in the field, but it is equally important to deliver what you know in a motivating and fun environment that is geared to each client's individual needs. She recommends that SLPAs take advantage of their environment and be willing to learn. She has found it very helpful to observe other clinicians and brainstorm ways she can improve her performance as an SLPA.

Reference

American Speech-Language-Hearing Association (ASHA). (n.d.). *ASHA state-by-state*. https://www.asha.org/advocacy/state/info/ca/california-support-personnel-requirements/

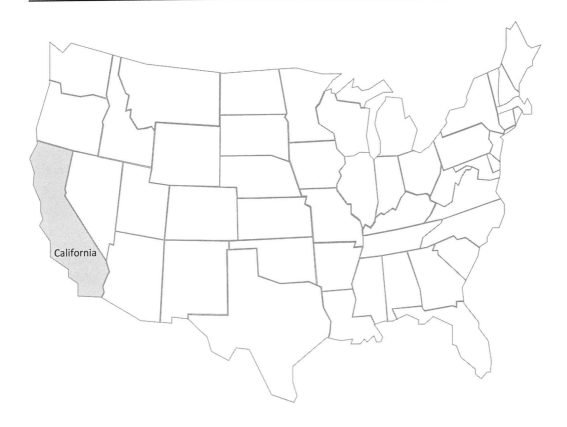

California

A DAY IN THE LIFE OF JACKIE

Set Yourself Apart

Jackie is a licensed SLPA in the state of California. Jackie became an SLPA by completing an associate's degree in speech-language pathology assisting. Jackie currently works in a public school setting, with children in kindergarten through eighth grade. She works at two separate elementary school campuses, providing treatment to students with a variety of impairments, including individuals with SSD and ASD. Between her two campuses, Jackie works in self-contained, functional skills classrooms and ASD-specific classrooms.

A typical day for Jackie consists of language and articulation "pull-out" treatment, when she works with students on a one-on-one basis or in small groups, and "push-in" treatment, provided to students in self-contained classrooms. A big part of Jackie's job includes scheduling treatment sessions, data collection, and recordkeeping. When needed, she also assists her supervising SLP with in-class observations and screenings.

Rewards

For Jackie, her greatest reward as an SLPA is developing relationships with students and observing their progress. She believes this comes from providing ongoing services and keeping accurate records.

Challenges

Jackie finds scheduling treatment for students in multiple grade levels, each with individual needs, to be one of the most challenging aspects of her job.

Words of Wisdom

Jackie's words of wisdom for a new SLPA are to "set yourself apart by having an area of specialty (e.g., autism, augmentative and alternative communication [AAC], sign language)." She believes that to be a successful SLPA, you must learn as much as you can during and after your training. Jackie attends professional development workshops on a regular basis to enhance her skills. In California, SLPAs are required to complete 12 hours of continuing professional development (CPD) every 2 years (ASHA, n.d.). Jackie accrues well over this minimum and feels it has been the secret to her success. She also believes being a team player is critical and recommends that new SLPAs be open to completing any and all tasks within their scope of practice.

Reference

American Speech-Language-Hearing Association (ASHA). (n.d.). *ASHA state-by-state.* https://www.asha.org/advocacy/state/info/ca/california-support-personnel-requirements/

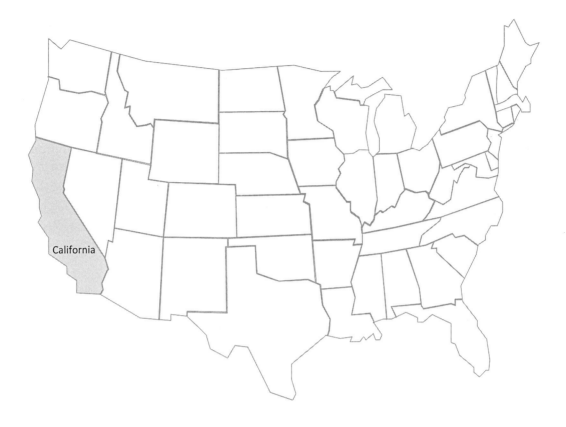

California

A DAY IN THE LIFE OF SUSAN

A Bilingual SLPA

Susan is a licensed SLPA in the state of California. Susan has an associate's degree in speech-language pathology assisting and completed 216 hours of clinical practicum with both children and adults as part of her training.

Susan works in a public school setting in California with children ages 3 to 12 years, many of who have articulation problems, language delays, or both. She also works with individuals with Down syndrome, ASD, and other disabilities. The students at her school have diverse cultural and linguistic back-grounds. Many come from low-income households.

Susan works an 8-hour day. She spends 2 hours per day completing paperwork, preparing materials for therapy sessions, performing recordkeeping, and working with the office manager to contact parents, teachers, and representatives from other disciplines to schedule individualized educational plan (IEP) meetings, and preparing notices and documents for IEP meetings. She also assists her supervisor in preparing materials to share with parents. Often these materials go beyond solely speech and language domains, such as activities for parents to do with their children outside of school and resources for affordable clothing and low-cost medical and dental services. The remainder of her day is spent providing therapy to students in small groups or one-on-one. She also assists her supervising SLP with screenings and assessment of Spanish-speaking students.

Susan is an English-Spanish bilingual SLPA. According to ASHA's (2022) scope-of-practice document, SLPAs who use multiple languages may engage in the following tasks (Responsibilities for Practitioners who use Multiple Languages, para 1.):

- Assist the SLP with interpretation and translation in the student's, patient's, or client's first language during screening and assessment activities exclusive of clinical interpretation of results.
- Interpret for students, patients, clients, and families who communicate using a language other than English, when the provider has received specialized training with interpreting skills in the student's, patient's, or client's first language.
- Provide services in another language for individuals who communicate using a language other than English or for those who are developing English language skills. Such services are based on the provider's skills and knowledge of the language spoken by the student, patient, or client.

Susan performs each of these tasks at her school sites on a regular basis. She is also called to assist with bilingual assessment at the eight other schools within her district and received training as a district translator. She has learned to be flexible in her role as a bilingual SLPA and notes

that "one size does fit all." She has noticed that often materials are not available in other languages and in these cases, she works with her supervising SLP to translate information for her clients and their families. She feels that this is critical to connecting with her client's families and granting them equal access to resources. She also conducts the majority of her treatment sessions in Spanish.

Rewards

According to Susan, the most rewarding part of her job is seeing growth in the students she works with and helping them successfully exit the speech program. She looks forward to hearing about their achievements as they transition from middle school to high school.

Challenges

Susan's greatest challenge is not always having the right or current tools to work with her students, such as computer programs, iPads, or materials in general. She has at times spent her own money on materials, supplies, and reinforcements for her students, as her school district does not consistently provide these items.

Words of Wisdom

Susan thinks those training to be an SLPA should have a realistic picture of what it means to be an SLPA. She says it is not always like textbooks and classes make it seem. There are real challenges, such as when you may not have the resources or tools you need to do your job effectively. Susan's advice is not to become an SLPA for the money but because you love working with children, especially those with disabilities and behavioral challenges.

She has also found it very valuable to get to know as much as she can about the clients she works with. She reads their reports carefully and tries to get a sense of their family life and circumstances, such as who they live with, whether they are immigrants and which country they are from, their economic background, whether multiple families live in the home, and whether they live in a house, apartment, or motel. She finds this helps her to understand her clients better and to find ways to motivate them to do their best and be successful.

Reference

American Speech-Language-Hearing Association (ASHA). (2022). *Speech-language pathology assistant scope of practice.* https://www.asha .org/policy/slpa-scope-of-practice/

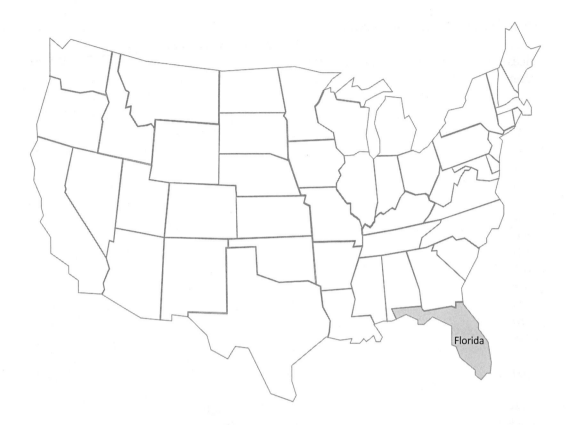

A DAY IN THE LIFE OF LAURE

An Amazing Field

Laure is a licensed SLPA in Florida. In Florida, to be certified as an SLPA, among other requirements, one must complete the following:

A bachelor's degree from a regionally accredited college or university, including completion of 24 semester hours as specified by the board from a Council for Higher Education–accredited institution

SLPAs also receive on-the-job training by a licensed SLP who maintains responsibility for all services performed by the SLPA (ASHA, n.d.). SLPAs in Flor-

ida must complete 20 CEU per biennium certificate renewal (two of these hours must be in an approved course related to the prevention of medical errors; ASHA, n.d., para. 1).

Laure has a bachelor's degree in management information systems. She also completed more than 200 hours of practicum (24 semester hours) to obtain her license as an SLPA. Laure is currently enrolled in a master's program in communication science and disorders. She has three semesters left in completing her master's degree.

She currently works in a private practice setting with children ranging in age from 3 to 13 years. Half of her caseload consists of individuals with SSD and specifically, those with articulation goals. She also works with individuals who have delays in receptive and/or expressive language skills. A typical day for Laure consists of providing therapy services as directed by her supervising SLP, often using play-based, child-directed approaches. For the most part, Laure sees clients individually, but there are times when she also works with small groups of students.

Rewards

Laure really enjoys the relationship she has been developing with her supervising SLP. She has also been able to develop an excellent rapport with her clients, their parents, and school personnel. She loves seeing her clients' progress and watching them grow and develop both personally and academically.

Challenges

Laure finds that the most challenging aspect of her job is managing client behavior, especially for students with severe developmental delays who may exhibit high levels of frustration, and for younger children who need consistent structure and redirection. She has noticed that sometimes helping a client participate and remain on task may be as simple as discovering the client's likes and dislikes and determining what learning modality works best for the client. For example, she has found that some children do not respond well to auditory-visual stimulation, and in that case, they may need a more kinesthetic approach where they are allowed to touch and do things themselves. Other children may just need positive, visual reinforcement, which gives them instant reward for small successes.

Words of Wisdom

Laure's advice to new SLPAs is to "hang in there because this is an amazing field." Laure recalls that when she first started, she was "so green," with little experience. However, after working as an SLPA for the past year, she has found it to be truly rewarding and cannot help but tell others who are considering going into this field, especially those who may be struggling to get through their training, that it is well worth it!

Reference

American Speech-Language-Hearing Association (ASHA). (n.d.). *ASHA state-by-state*. https://www.asha.org/advocacy/state/info/fl/florida-support-personnel-requirements/

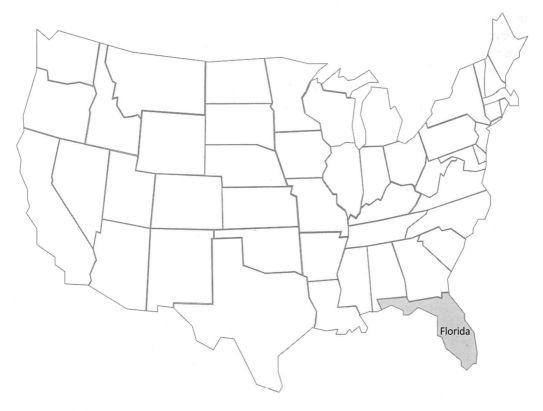

Florida

A DAY IN THE LIFE OF ALYSON

There Are No Wrong Questions

Alyson is a licensed SLPA in the state of Florida. She has a bachelor's degree in communicative disorders and completed 20 hours of clinical practicum as part of her training to become an SLPA. Alyson works part-time for a private practice, providing services to individuals ages 3 to 12 years with primarily SSD and language impairments. She is currently working and applying to graduate schools as she hopes to complete her master's degree and become a fully certified SLP.

Rewards

Alyson says the most rewarding aspect of her job as an SLPA is seeing the prog-

ress her clients make, whether they make small or big gains.

Challenges

For Alyson, the most challenging aspects of working as an SLPA are finding the right activities and materials to work effectively with each client. She feels that without the clinical and educational background that comes with a master's degree, she does not always know where to begin.

Words of Wisdom

Alyson recommends that SLPAs, regardless of their experience, should "ask lots of questions." She often faces problems or situations that she is not sure how to address, but she feels fortunate to work in a friendly and safe environment where everyone is willing to help one another. She regularly seeks the guidance of her supervising SLP. She feels there are no wrong questions, but the important thing is to ask.

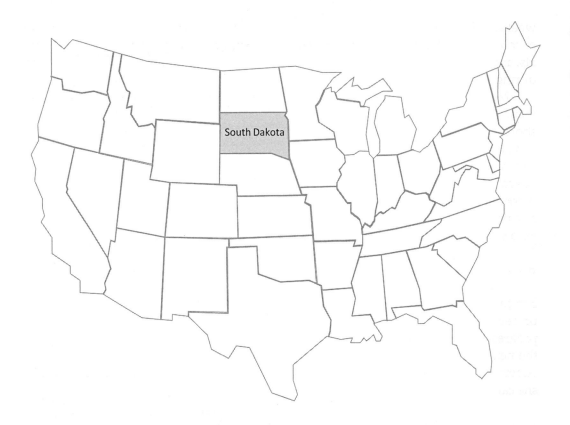

Two Sites and Two Supervisors

Jennifer is a licensed SLPA in the state of South Dakota. To obtain a license in South Dakota, individuals must (ASHA, n.d.):

■ Hold an associate's degree in SLPA or a bachelor's degree with major emphasis in speech-language pathology or communication disorders from an accredited academic institution;

■ Complete a minimum of 100 clock hours of supervised clinical practicum as an SLPA, while either on the job or during academic preparation; and

■ have committed no act for which disciplinary action is justified.

SLPAs in South Dakota must be supervised by a licensed SLP with at least 3 years of experience (ASHA, n.d.). Jennifer has an associate's degree in speech-language pathology assisting, which included both observation and 100 hours of clinical experience as an SLPA.

Jennifer works in an elementary school setting, with children in kindergarten through third grade. She primarily works with individuals with SSD, and in particular, students with goals targeting articulation. She also provides services to students with fluency and language disorders. Jennifer's time is split between two different school sites, each with a designated supervising SLP. Her supervising SLPs see the clients she treats once per week. She meets with both supervisors once per week to discuss clients, materials, and anything else that might come up during the week.

Most days, Jennifer provides treatment to students back to back, with a short break in her day for lunch and to travel between sites. She plans for her treatment sessions after school or one afternoon a week designated for paperwork and planning. Her treatment is usually provided to small groups of students who share similar goals.

Rewards

For Jennifer, the most rewarding aspect of being an SLPA is getting to see the progress students make from one year to the next. She also feels fortunate to have supervisors who have different styles so she can learn from both.

Challenges

Jennifer finds that the most challenging aspect of her job as an SLPA is working with students who have challenging behaviors. She says you never know what type of day a student is having and need to be prepared.

Words of Wisdom

Jennifer's words of wisdom for new SLPAs are to remember that each student is unique. She believes you can find the right way to help each student if you keep in mind that every little thing is a learning experience for that student. If you do not feel like they accomplished enough during a specific session, Jennifer encourages new SLPAs to remember that more sessions are ahead (and to try again).

Reference

American Speech-Language-Hearing Association (ASHA). (n.d.). *ASHA state-by-state.* https://www.asha.org/advocacy/state/info/sd/south-dakota-support-personnel-requirements/

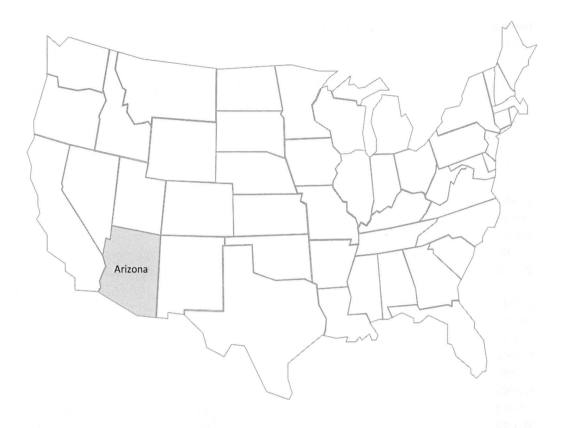

A DAY IN THE LIFE OF ELISE

Making It Work, Even in Less-Than-Ideal Circumstances

Elise has a bachelor's degree in speech and hearing science and is attending school to complete her master's degree in speech-language pathology. Elise holds licensure as an SLPA in Arizona. In Arizona, for all settings, SLPAs must be licensed with the state's Department of Health Services (ASHA, n.d.). To be eligible for licensure, SLPAs must complete an approved training program (or the equivalent) from a nationally or regionally accredited college or university. Requirements include

- A minimum of 100 hours of clinical interaction under

the supervision of a licensed master's level speech-language pathologist (ASHA, n.d., Statutory and Regulatory Requirements)

Elise received her training as an SLPA while completing her bachelor's degree in speech and hearing science, including 25 observation hours and 100 supervised clinical interaction hours as an SLPA. She currently works in an elementary school.

A typical day for Elise starts at 7:00 AM and ends at 2:30 PM. Elise works with individuals or small groups of students (two to four), providing therapy for articulation, language, and pragmatic disorders. Under the direction of her supervising SLP, she plans the groups and records data on student performance. She also attends parent or IEP meetings with her supervising SLP for the children on her caseload.

Rewards

What Elise finds most rewarding is working with students.

Challenges

Elise's supervisor makes her schedule. She sometimes wishes the children were grouped differently, but there are constraints on when students are available. She often has groups of students with mixed goals; some with articulations goals, some with language, and so forth. She finds this challenging at times and wishes she could work with certain students in one-on-one sessions. She is also at two different schools, one of which does not have a dedicated speech room. This means she must provide services in grade level pods where there are distractions from other small groups and people walking by while she is working with her students.

Words of Wisdom

Elise's words of wisdom for future SLPAs is to establish clear expectations for students. Elise carries a laminated page that says "speech expectations." Her students love reciting the expectations to her at the beginning of the group. Elise also always has at least three activities planned for each session. This way if one is not working well, she can easily move on to another activity. Elise also recommends that SLPAs try to observe many different SLPs. She encourages other SLPAs not to be afraid to contact SLPs in their specialty area and ask to observe their sessions. She cold called several SLPs and found it to be a great learning experience.

Reference

American Speech-Language-Hearing Association (ASHA). (n.d.). *ASHA state-by-state.* https://www.asha.org/advocacy/state/info/az/arizona-support-personnel-requirements/

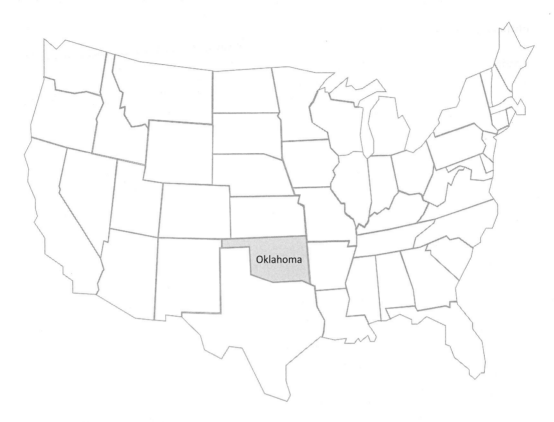

A DAY IN THE LIFE OF BEATRICE

Being Open to Advice Is Key

Beatrice has an associate's degree in speech-language pathology assisting from a community college and a license in Oklahoma as an SLPA. Beatrice works in a secondary school. A typical day for her consists of helping to schedule and attend IEP meetings with her supervisor, scheduling sessions, creating therapy activities, providing one-on-one and group therapy sessions, co-leading social skills groups for students not on IEPs, and attending professional development trainings.

Rewards

Beatrice says the most rewarding part of her job is "helping kids, especially in the secondary grades, find their voice [because] they are past the age where articulation issues are cute." She notes that her students use figurative language and slang to communicate so giving them the confidence they need through communication skills training helps to shape the adults they will become.

Challenges

Beatrice finds scheduling session times very challenging. She also finds that paperwork demands more of my attention than she initially thought it would.

Words of Wisdom

Beatrice recommends that SLPAs take advantage of their clinical hours. She encourages all SLPAs to not just observe during these hours, but to work with their clinical supervisor to try new things and importantly, to be open to any and all advice. Beatrice also recommends that SLPAs take advantage of free trainings, webinars, and other avenues for developing their skills as SLPAs.

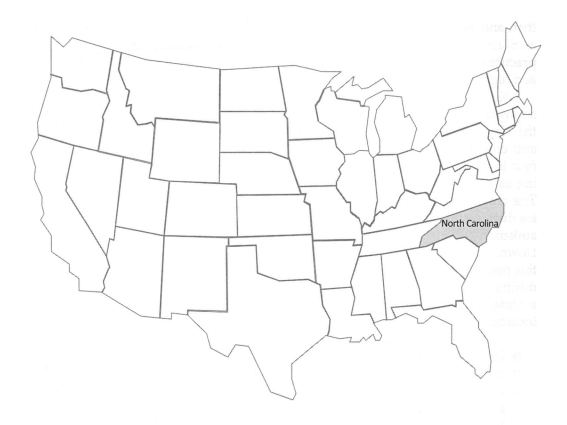

North Carolina

Changing Perceptions: ASHA Certification for SLPAs

Kelly has a bachelor's degree in early childhood education and associate's degree in speech-language pathology assisting from a community college. She is currently working in North Carolina (NC) with registration from NC Board of Examiners for SLPA. In North Carolina, SLPA must register with the North Carolina Board of Examiners for Speech and Language Pathologists and Audiologists (ASHA, n.d.). Qualifications to do so include (ASHA, n.d., Statutory and Regulatory Requirements):

■ An associate's degree in speech-language pathology assisting

from an accredited institution of higher learning, community college, or equivalent program; or

■ Successful completion of a bachelor's degree from an accredited institution as well as evidence of successful completion of courses in speech-language assisting developed by the N. C. Department of Community Colleges and a passing score on a competency test approved by the Board.

For the past 3 years, Kelly has worked primarily in early intervention settings with children birth to 3 years of age. Prior to that, she was employed for 8 years in a private practice setting with a caseload of children 0 to 18 years of age. Prior to that, and in her first 3 years of work as an SLPA, she was employed by a private practice that contracted with elementary and high schools.

Kelly's work as an SLPA consists of seeing children in daycares, homes, and in the clinic. She begins work around 8:30 AM and ends somewhere between two and four in the afternoon (later if she is serving as an interpreter for an evaluation). The children she serves at the moment are dual language learners and those with autism, speech and language delays, and Down syndrome. Kelly reports that at this point, she sets and manages her time during the day independently, juggling a wide ranges of duties and activities, including

- Creating client files,
- Maintaining daily notes,
- Creating activities to address goals provided by her supervisor,
- Maintaining communication with her supervisor regarding clients,
- Making calls to families as necessary to schedule sessions,
- Collecting data, and
- Serving as an interpreter for evaluations.

Rewards

Kelly states that the most rewarding part of her work is having the opportunity to work one-on-one with children, and knowing that for some, she may be the only bright spot in their day.

Challenges

Kelly finds it challenging that as an SLPA she is not as well respected or as independent as certified occupational therapy assistants (COTAs) and physical therapy assistants (PTAs). She believes that not having an ASHA certification behind her (and supporting the work of all SLPAs) is a barrier to advancing the standing of assistants in the field of speech-language pathology. She is hopeful this will change when ASHA pursues formal certification for SLPAs.*

Words of Wisdom

Kelly's words of wisdom to future SLPAs is to love what you do and make sure that you like children if you plan to work with them as an SLPA.

Reference

American Speech-Language-Hearing Association (ASHA). (n.d.). *ASHA state-by-state.* https://www.asha.org/advocacy/state/info/nc/north-carolinasupport-personnel-requirements/

Council for Clinical Certification in Audiology and Speech-Language Pathology of the American Speech-Language-Hearing Association. (2020). *2020 Standards for ASHA Speech-Language Pathology Assistants Certification.* https://www.asha.org/certification/2020-slpa-certification-standards/

---

*NOTE: When this story was originally collected, Kelly did not have an ASHA C-SLPA, nor was one offered by ASHA. However, in 2020 ASHA began offering formal certification for SLPAs (Council for Clinical Certification in Audiology and Speech-Language Pathology of the American Speech-Language-Hearing Association, 2020). Also effective in 2020, North Carolina began accepting ASHA Assistant Certification in lieu of the North Carolina Jurisprudence exam and the North Carolina SLP-A administered exam. They are also still accepting passing scores on both exams for those who do not have an ASHA C-SLPA (ASHA, n.d., Statutory and Regulatory Requirements).

APPENDIX 1–C
Sample Job Description—Medical Setting

SPLA JOB DESCRIPTION

Medical Facility Example

General Summary

The speech-language pathology assistant, as a member of an interdisciplinary team, works under the supervision of a certified speech-language pathologist in implementation of services for the rehabilitation of patients with speech, language, cognitive, swallowing, oral muscular, and augmentative alternative communication disorders, and hearing impairments.

Essential Duties and Responsibilities

1. Prepares patients for treatment.
2. Prepares treatment areas and equipment for use.
3. Implements documented treatment plans developed by speech-language pathologists.
4. Accurately collects and records subjective and objective data.
5. Records patient status with regard to established objectives as stated in the treatment plan and reports this information to the supervising speech-language pathologist.
6. Assists the speech-language pathologist in the assessment of patients.
7. Orders supplies and equipment.
8. Engages in various clerical tasks including entry of orders for patient care, filing, billing, and ordering equipment and supplies.

9. Maintains and cleans equipment, adhering to infection control protocol.
10. Maintains the confidentiality of information pertaining to patients and their families.
11. Behaves in accordance with the mission and values of the organization.
12. Participates in quality improvement initiatives as directed by the speech-language pathologist.
13. Respects and appropriately considers age, gender, cultural background, and related factors when providing services.

Supplemental Duties and Responsibilities

1. Participates in educational activities for patients, families, and other health professionals.
2. Participates in organizational committees as time, interest, and necessity permits and dictates.

Required Education, Experience, and Licensure

1. The SLPA must meet state requirements for health.
2. The SLPA must have one of the following:
   - Associate's degree from a speech-language pathology assistant program;
   - Bachelor's degree in speech-language pathology;
   - Completion of a college-based speech-language pathology assistant certificate program; or

■ Required education as designated by the state licensing board or other regulatory agency.

Required Skills and Abilities

1. Knowledge of speech-language pathology treatment and equipment.
2. Ability to follow oral and written directions, including treatment plans.
3. Ability to work under direct and indirect supervision.
4. Ability to show excellent judgment for continuation or discontinuation of a patient's treatment under conditions of pain or discomfort.
5. Analytical skills necessary to identify and report changes in the patient and equipment.
6. Flexibility and adaptability, as the job combines patient care, clinic/equipment maintenance, and clerical responsibilities.
7. Ability to pay close attention to visual and auditory detail.
8. Ability to use a variety of computer programs for documentation and patient treatment.
9. Ability to push wheelchair-bound patients and assist ambulatory patients.
10. Ability to walk and stand up for 90% of the work day.

Working Conditions

1. Work is a combination of sedentary and physical activities completed in a normal patient care and office environment.
2. Travel in a company or personal vehicle may be required.
3. Exposure to body fluids is frequent. Exposure to blood-borne pathogens and other infectious material is possible.
4. Exposure to verbally and/or physically aggressive patients is possible.

Reporting Relationships

The SLPA is directly and indirectly supervised by a certified speech-language pathologist. The supervising SLP maintains legal and moral responsibility for all services provided by the SLPA and ensures that such services are in compliance with the ASHA Code of Ethics, ASHA Guidelines for Speech-Language Pathology Assistants, and state licensure laws.

APPENDIX 1–D
Sample Job Description—Educational Setting

SLPA JOB DESCRIPTION

Educational Facility Example

General Summary

The speech-language pathology assistant, as a member of an educational team, works under the supervision of a certified speech-language pathologist in implementation of services for children/students with speech, language, cognitive, voice, swallowing, oral muscular, and augmentative/alternative communication disorders, and hearing impairments.

Essential Duties and Responsibilities

1. Prepares work area and materials for use.
2. Accompanies the student from the classroom to the service area or prepares classroom for service delivery.
3. Implements documented treatment/intervention plans developed by the speech-language pathologist.
4. Accurately collects and records subjective and objective data.
5. Records student's status with regard to established objectives as stated in the treatment plan and reports this information to the supervising speech-language pathologist.
6. Assists the speech-language pathologist in the assessment of students.
7. Orders supplies and equipment.
8. Engages in various clerical tasks, including filing and copying.
9. Maintains and cleans equipment, adhering to infection control protocol.
10. Maintains the confidentiality of information pertaining to students and their families.
11. Behaves in accordance with the educational facility guidelines.
12. Respects and appropriately considers age, gender, cultural/linguistic background, and related factors when providing services.

Supplemental Duties and Responsibilities

1. Participates in educational facility activities and committees as requested by the speech-language pathologist.
2. Participates in classroom activities as requested by the speech-language pathologist.
3. Participates in conferences as requested by the speech-language pathologist.

Required Education, Experience, and Licensure

1. The SLPA must meet state and facility requirements for health.
2. The SLPA must have one of the following:
   - Associate's degree from a speech-language pathology assistant program;
   - Bachelor's degree in speech-language pathology;
   - Completion of a college-based speech-language pathology assistant certificate program; or

- Required education as designated by the state licensing board or other regulatory agency.

Required Skills and Abilities

1. Knowledge of speech-language pathology equipment, materials, and procedures.
2. Ability to follow oral and written directions, including intervention plans.
3. Ability to work with students individually and in groups.
4. Ability to interact appropriately with others involved in the student's program, including the teacher, parent, and other personnel.
5. Analytical skills necessary to identify and report changes in the student or equipment.
6. Flexibility and adaptability, as the job combines direct intervention, classroom work, equipment/materials maintenance, and clerical responsibilities.
7. Ability to pay close attention to visual and auditory detail.
8. Ability to use a variety of computer programs for intervention and documentation.

9. Ability to walk and stand up for 90% of the work day.

Working Conditions

1. Work is a combination of sedentary and physical activities completed in a normal educational environment.
2. Travel between educational facilities in a personal vehicle may be required.
3. Exposure to body fluids and other infectious material is possible.
4. Exposure to verbally and/or physically aggressive students is possible.

Reporting Relationships

The SLPA is directly and indirectly supervised by a certified speech-language pathologist. The supervising SLP maintains legal and moral responsibility for all services provided by the SLPA, and ensures that such services are in compliance with the ASHA Code of Ethics, ASHA Guidelines for Speech-Language Pathology Assistants, state regulatory and licensure laws, and educational facility guidelines.

APPENDIX 1–E

Example of Competency-Based Assessment

SLPA SCOPE OF RESPONSIBILITIES COMPETENCY ASSESSMENT*						
Competency*	Does Not Meet	Needs Improvement	Meets Requirements	Exceeds Requirements	Far Exceeds Requirements	Comments
Self-identifying (e.g., verbally, in writing, signage, titles on name badges) as an SLPA to students, patients, clients, families, staff, and others.						
Exhibiting compliance with federal, state, and local regulations, including the Health Insurance Portability and Accountability Act (HIPAA), the Family Educational Rights and Privacy Act (FERPA), reimbursement requirements, and state statutes and rules regarding SLPA education, training, and scope of practice.						
Administering and scoring screenings for clinical interpretation by the SLP.						

Competency*	Does Not Meet	Needs Improvement	Meets Requirements	Exceeds Requirements	Far Exceeds Requirements	Comments
Assisting the SLP during assessment of students, patients, and clients (e.g., setting up the testing environment, gathering and prepping materials, taking notes as advised by the SLP).						
Administering and scoring assessment tools that (a) the SLPA meets the examiner requirements specified in the examiner's manual and (b) the supervising SLP uses to verify the SLPA's competence in administration, exclusive of clinical interpretation.						
Administering and scoring progress monitoring tools exclusive of clinical interpretation if (a) the SLPA meets the examiner requirements specified in the examiner's manual and (b) the supervisor has verified the SLPA's competence in administration.						
Implementing documented care plans or protocols (e.g., individualized education plan [IEP], individualized family service plan [IFSP], treatment plan) developed and directed by the supervising SLP.						

continues

Appendix 1–E. *continued*

Competency*	Does Not Meet	Needs Improvement	Meets Requirements	Exceeds Requirements	Far Exceeds Requirements	Comments
Providing direct therapy services addressing treatment goals developed by the supervising SLP to meet the needs of the student, patient, client, and family.						
Adjusting and documenting the amount and type of support or scaffolding provided to the student, patient, or client in treatment to facilitate progress.						
Developing and implementing activities and materials for teaching and practice of skills to address the goals of the student, patient, client, and family per the plan of care developed by the supervising SLP.						
Providing treatment through a variety of service delivery models (e.g., individual, group, classroom based, home based, cotreatment with other disciplines) as directed by the supervising SLP.						
Providing services via telepractice to students, patients, and clients who are selected by the supervising SLP.						

Competency*	Does Not Meet	Needs Improvement	Meets Requirements	Exceeds Requirements	Far Exceeds Requirements	Comments
Documenting student, patient, or client performance (e.g., collecting data and calculating percentages for the SLP to use; preparing charts, records, and graphs) and report this information to the supervising SLP in a timely manner.						
Providing caregiver coaching (e.g., model and teach communication strategies, provide feedback regarding caregiver-child interactions) for facilitation and carryover of skills.						
Sharing objective information (e.g., accuracy in speech and language skills addressed, participation in treatment, response to treatment) regarding student, patient, and client performance to students, patients, clients, caregivers, families, and other service providers without interpretation or recommendations as directed by the SLP.						
Programming augmentative and alternative communication (AAC) devices.						

continues

Appendix 1–E. *continued*

Competency*	Does Not Meet	Needs Improvement	Meets Requirements	Exceeds Requirements	Far Exceeds Requirements	Comments
Providing training and technical assistance to students, patients, clients, and families in the use of AAC devices.						
Developing low-tech AAC materials for students, patients, and clients.						
Demonstrating strategies included in the feeding and swallowing plan developed by the SLP and sharing information with students, patients, clients, families, staff, and caregivers.						
Assisting students, patients, and clients with feeding and swallowing skills developed and directed by the SLP when consuming food textures and liquid consistencies.						
SLPAs Who Use Multiple Languages (as applicable)						
Assist the SLP with interpretation and translation in the student's, patient's, or client's first language during screening and assessment activities exclusive of clinical interpretation of results.						

Competency*	Does Not Meet	Needs Improvement	Meets Requirements	Exceeds Requirements	Far Exceeds Requirements	Comments
Interpret for students, patients, clients, and families who communicate using a language other than English, when the provider has received specialized training with interpreting skills in the student's, patient's, or client's first language.						
Provide services in another language for individuals who communicate using a language other than English or for those who are developing English-language skills. Such services are based on the provider's skills and knowledge of the language spoken by the student, patient, or client.						
Administrative Support						
Assist with clerical duties and site operations (e.g., scheduling, recordkeeping, maintaining inventory of supplies and equipment).						
Perform safety checks and maintenance of equipment.						

continues

Appendix 1–E. *continued*

Competency*	Does Not Meet	Needs Improvement	Meets Requirements	Exceeds Requirements	Far Exceeds Requirements	Comments
Prepare materials for screening, assessment, and treatment services.						
Prevention and Advocacy						
Present primary prevention information to individuals and groups known to be at risk for communication and swallowing disorders.						
Promote early identification and early intervention activities.						
Advocate for individuals and families through community awareness, health literacy, education, and training programs to promote and facilitate access to full participation in communication—including addressing the social determinants of health and health disparities.						

Competency*	Does Not Meet	Needs Improvement	Meets Requirements	Exceeds Requirements	Far Exceeds Requirements	Comments
Provide information to emergency response agencies for individuals who have communication, swallowing, and/or related disorders.						
Advocate at the local, state, and national levels for improved public policies affecting access to services and research funding.						
Support the supervising SLP in research projects, in-service training, marketing, and public relations programs.						
Participate actively in professional organizations.						

Note: Competencies based on American Speech-Language-Hearing Association (ASHA). (2022). *Speech-language pathology assistant scope of practice.* http://www.asha.org/policy. Copyright 2022 American Speech-Language-Hearing Association. All rights reserved.

Recommendations for Additional Training/Education

_____

_____

_____

APPENDIX 1–F
Technical Proficiency Checklist

Verification of Technical Proficiency of a Speech-Language Pathology Assistant

Speech-Language Pathology Assistant Name: _____

Supervisor(s) Name: _____

Program/Facility Name: _____

Skills	Achievement of Skill Yes	No
Clerical/Administrative Skills		
Assists with clerical skills and departmental operations (e.g., preparing materials, scheduling activities, keeping records)		
Participates in in-service training		
Performs checks, maintenance, and calibration of equipment		
Supports supervising SLP in research projects and public relations programs		
Collects data for quality improvement		
Prepares and maintains patient/client charts, records, graphs for displaying data		
Interpersonal Skills		
Uses appropriate forms of address with patient/client, family, caregivers, and professionals (e.g., Dr., Mr., Mrs., Ms.)		
Greets patient/client, family, and caregiver and identifies self as a speech-language pathology assistant		
Restates information/concerns to supervising SLP as expressed by patient/client, family, and caregivers, as appropriate		
Directs patient/client, family, and caregivers to supervisor for clinical information		
Is courteous and respectful in various communication situations		
Uses language appropriate to a patient/client, family, or caregiver's education level, communication style, developmental age, communication disorder, and emotional state		
Demonstrates awareness of patient/client needs and cultural values		
Conduct in Work Setting		
Recognizes own limitations within the ASHA SLPA Scope of Practice		
Upholds ethical behavior and maintains confidentiality as described in the ASHA SLPA Scope of Practice		

Skills	Achievement of Skill	
	Yes	No
Maintains client records in accordance with confidentiality regulations/laws as prescribed by supervising SLPs		
Discusses confidential patient/client information only at the direction of supervising SLP		
Identifies self as an assistant in all written and oral communication with the client/patient, family, caregivers, and staff		
Demonstrates ability to explain to supervising SLP the scope of information that should be discussed with the patient/client, family, caregivers, and professionals		
Arrives punctually and prepared for work-related activities		
Completes documentation and other tasks in a timely manner		
Maintains personal appearance and language expected for the specific work setting		
Evaluates own performance		
Uses screening instruments and implements treatment protocols only after appropriate training and only as prescribed by supervising SLP		
Seeks clarification from supervising SLP as needed to follow the prescribed treatment or screening protocols		
Actively participates in interaction with supervisor demonstrating use of supervisor's feedback		
Maintains accurate records representing assigned work time with patients/clients		
Implements appropriate infection control procedures and universal precautions consistent with the employer's standards and guidelines		
Implements injury prevention strategies consistent with employer's standards and guidelines		
Uses appropriate procedures for physical management of clients according to employer's standards and guidelines and state regulations		
Technical Skills as Prescribed by Supervising SLP		
Accurately administers screening instruments, calculates and reports the results of screening procedures to supervising SLP		
Provides instructions that are clear, concise, and appropriate to the client's developmental age, level of understanding, language use, and communication style		
Follows treatment protocol as developed and prescribed by supervising SLP		
Provides appropriate feedback to patients/clients as to accuracy of their responses		
Identifies and describes relevant patient/client responses to supervising SLP		
Identifies and describes relevant patient/client, family, and caregiver behaviors to supervising SLP		
Uses appropriate stimuli, cues/prompts with the patient/client to elicit target behaviors as defined in the treatment protocol		

continues

Skills	Achievement of Skill	
	Yes	No
Maintains on-task or redirects off-task behavior of patients/clients in individual or group treatment, consistent with the patient/client's developmental age, communication style, and disorder		
Provides culturally appropriate behavioral reinforcement consistent with the patient/client's developmental age and communication disorder		
Accurately reviews and summarizes patient/client performance		
Uses treatment materials that are appropriate to the developmental age and communication disorder of the patient/client and the culture of the patient/client/family		
Starts and ends the treatment session on time		
Obtains cosignature of supervising SLP on documentation		
Accurately records target behaviors as prescribed by supervising SLP		
Accurately calculates chronological age of the patient/client		
Correctly calculates and determines percentages, frequencies, averages, and standard scores		
Uses professional terminology correctly in communication with supervising SLP		
Maintains eligible records, log notes, and written communication		
Appropriately paces treatment session to ensure maximum patient/client response		
Implements designated treatment objectives/goals in specific appropriate sequence		

APPENDIX 1–G
Direct Observation of Skills Brief Checklist—Medical Setting

Speech-Language Pathology Assistant: _____

Supervising SLP: _____

Patient/Client Observed: _____

Date/Time of Observation: _____

Rate the following on a scale of 1 (disagree) to 5 (agree).

Interpersonal Skills

1. Maintains appropriate patient/client relationship.   ○1 ○2 ○3 ○4 ○5
2. Demonstrates appropriate level of self-confidence.   ○1 ○2 ○3 ○4 ○5
3. Considers patient's needs.   ○1 ○2 ○3 ○4 ○5
4. Considers patient's cultural values.   ○1 ○2 ○3 ○4 ○5
5. Uses language appropriate for patient's age and education.   ○1 ○2 ○3 ○4 ○5
6. Is courteous and respectful at all times.   ○1 ○2 ○3 ○4 ○5

Personal Qualities

1. Arrives punctually for treatment sessions.   ○1 ○2 ○3 ○4 ○5
2. Arrives prepared for treatment sessions.   ○1 ○2 ○3 ○4 ○5
3. Appearance is appropriate for treatment sessions.   ○1 ○2 ○3 ○4 ○5
4. Recognizes professional boundaries during treatment sessions.   ○1 ○2 ○3 ○4 ○5
5. Stays within professional boundaries during treatment sessions. ○1 ○2 ○3 ○4 ○5

Technical and Treatment Skills

1. Completes assigned tasks within designated treatment sessions. ○1 ○2 ○3 ○4 ○5
2. Uses appropriate materials based on treatment plan.   ○1 ○2 ○3 ○4 ○5
3. Uses materials that are age and culturally appropriate.   ○1 ○2 ○3 ○4 ○5
4. Uses materials that are motivating.   ○1 ○2 ○3 ○4 ○5
5. Prepares the treatment/intervention settings to meet the   ○1 ○2 ○3 ○4 ○5
   needs of the patient/client.
6. Accurately determines correct vs. incorrect responses.   ○1 ○2 ○3 ○4 ○5
7. Provides appropriate feedback as to the response accuracy.   ○1 ○2 ○3 ○4 ○5
8. Verbally reports the session.   ○1 ○2 ○3 ○4 ○5
9. Provides appropriate documentation of the session.   ○1 ○2 ○3 ○4 ○5

Comments:

APPENDIX 1–H
Direct Observation Skills Brief Checklist—Educational Setting

Speech-Language Pathology Assistant: _____

Supervising SLP: _____

Student Observed: _____

Date/Time of Observation: _____

Rate the following on a scale of 1 (disagree) to 5 (agree).

Interpersonal Skills

1. Maintains appropriate relationship with student   ○1 ○2 ○3 ○4 ○5
2. Demonstrates appropriate level of self-confidence.   ○1 ○2 ○3 ○4 ○5
3. Considers the student's cultural/linguistic needs.   ○1 ○2 ○3 ○4 ○5
4. Uses language appropriate for student's age and education.   ○1 ○2 ○3 ○4 ○5
5. Is courteous and respectful at all times.   ○1 ○2 ○3 ○4 ○5

Personal Qualities

1. Arrives punctually for the intervention session.   ○1 ○2 ○3 ○4 ○5
2. Arrives prepared for the intervention session.   ○1 ○2 ○3 ○4 ○5
3. Appearance is appropriate for the intervention session.   ○1 ○2 ○3 ○4 ○5
4. Recognizes professional boundaries during the intervention session.   ○1 ○2 ○3 ○4 ○5
5. Stays within professional boundaries during the intervention session.   ○1 ○2 ○3 ○4 ○5

Technical and Intervention Skills

1. Completes assigned tasks within the designated session.   ○1 ○2 ○3 ○4 ○5
2. Uses appropriate materials based on treatment plan.   ○1 ○2 ○3 ○4 ○5
3. Uses materials that are age and culturally appropriate.   ○1 ○2 ○3 ○4 ○5
4. Uses materials that are motivating.   ○1 ○2 ○3 ○4 ○5
5. Prepares the intervention setting to meet the needs of the student.   ○1 ○2 ○3 ○4 ○5
6. Accurately determines correct vs. incorrect responses.   ○1 ○2 ○3 ○4 ○5
7. Provides appropriate feedback as to the response accuracy.   ○1 ○2 ○3 ○4 ○5
8. Verbally reports the session.   ○1 ○2 ○3 ○4 ○5
9. Provides appropriate documentation of the session.   ○1 ○2 ○3 ○4 ○5

Comments:

APPENDIX 1–I
Skills Proficiency Checklist

SLPA: _____ Supervising SLP: _____

Skills or Proficiency	Self-Rating			Supervising SLP Rating			
	Date	Proficiency Level		Date	Proficiency Level	How Learned	Demonstrated

Competence Levels
1. *Little or no experience*
2. *Some experience, requires practice/assist.*
3. *Proficient with occasional supervision*
4. *Proficient with independent performance*

How Learned
Observation
On-the-job training
Class
Video
Policy/procedure

Demonstrated
Direct observation
Test (written/verbal)
Certificate/license
Discussion
Other

CHAPTER 2

Defining Roles:
Supervision and Mentoring

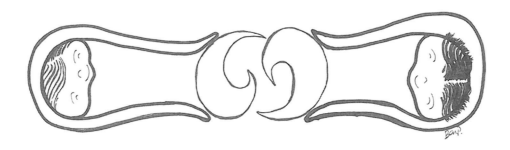

People seldom improve when they have no other model but themselves to copy.
—Oliver Goldsmith (Irish poet and playwright)

SUPERVISION

Role of Your Supervisor

Speech-language pathology assistants (SLPAs) operate under the supervision of a qualified speech-language pathologist (SLP). As an SLPA, an important question to ask is, "What is the role of my supervisor?" Understanding the role of your supervisor allows you to practice as an SLPA given prescribed regulations. The American Speech-Language-Hearing Association (ASHA) has recommended guidelines for supervising SLPAs and the roles and responsibilities of those who supervise them (ASHA, 2022). The overarching theme in these recommendations casts the primary role of the supervisor as the decision maker in directing the nature of services provided and as the individual responsible for providing oversight to protect the patient's or client's safety and ensure the highest quality of care. The SLPA's goal is also to maintain the highest quality care for the individuals she or he serves. In this context, as the image at the start of the chapter suggests, the supervisor and SLPA are partners in bringing excellent care to individuals with communicative disorders. Ultimately, though, "diagnosis and treatment for the students, patients, and clients served remains the legal and ethical responsibility of the supervisor" (ASHA, 2022, Supervision of SLPAs, para. 2). The responsibility for patient care cannot be delegated to an SLPA. The SLPA's services should be viewed as an extension of the SLP, not an alternative to services provided by the SLP. The purpose of SLPA services should not be to significantly increase the caseload size of the SLP (ASHA, 2022). This means that SLPAs should be used to deliver services only to those individuals on the supervising SLP's caseload. Importantly, as discussed in Chapter 1, ASHA details that "under no circumstances should an assistant have his or her own caseload" (ASHA, 2022, Supervision of SLPAs, para. 1).

Just as you are expected to be very familiar with your roles and responsibilities, you should also be familiar with those of your supervisor. ASHA expects that SLPA supervisors will do the following (ASHA, 2022, Expectations for the Supervising SLP, para. 21):[1]

- Adhere to the principles and rules of the ASHA Code of Ethics (ASHA, 2016).
- Adhere to applicable licensure laws and rules regulating the practice of speech-language pathology.
- Conduct ongoing competency evaluations of the SLPAs.
- Provide and encourage ongoing education and training opportunities for the SLPA consistent with competency and skills required to meet the needs of the students, patients, and clients served.
- Develop, review, and modify treatment plans for students,

patients, and clients that the SLPA implements under the supervision of the SLP.
- Make all case management decisions.
- Adhere to the supervisory responsibilities for SLPs.
- Retain legal and ethical responsibility for all students, patients, and clients served.
- Maintain an active interest in collaborating with SLPAs.

Amount and Type of Supervision

Another question asked is, "How much will I be supervised?" or "How much supervision is required?" ASHA categorizes supervision as either direct supervision or indirect supervision (ASHA, 2022). Direct supervision is in-person and in-view observation and guidance *while* the SLPA is performing clinical activities. Direct supervision can also occur via telecommunication while the SLPA is performing clinical activities. Indirect supervision consists of activities in which the SLP is not physically present or observing the SLPA during clinical activities, such as reviewing audio- or video-recorded sessions, reviewing data and information submitted by the SLPA, and conducting supervisory conferences.

ASHA states that the supervisor must make herself or himself available to the SLPA for immediate contact while SLPAs are performing their duties. SLPAs may not perform tasks when "supervising SLP cannot be reached by personal contact, that is, phone, pager, or other immediate or electronic means" (ASHA, 2022, Requirements for the Frequency and Amount of Supervision, para. 10). This means that if your supervising SLP is not available, your service provision to clients must be discontinued until adequate supervision can be obtained, including things like extended absences due to maternity leave, illness, or if your supervisor leaves that site to accept employment elsewhere (ASHA, 2022).

Relative to the amount and frequency of ongoing supervision, 100% *direct* supervision is required for medically fragile individuals (ASHA, 2022). The level of supervision for non–medically fragile individuals will vary based on a variety of factors, including your experience, the clients served, the setting, and the tasks assigned (ASHA, 2022). For example, it is anticipated that more supervision will be needed when you begin a position, when you are working with a new client, and when you are performing tasks that are new to you. Each supervisor will be responsible for determining the amount and nature of your supervision in order to ensure the highest quality of care for all individuals you serve. For example, before an SLPA engages in services with any client, ASHA states that the supervising SLP should have "first contact" with that individual in order to establish a plan of care (ASHA, 2002). Thereafter, ASHA minimums for ongoing supervision include documentation of *direct* supervision provided by the SLP for each student, patient, or client at least every 30 to 60 days (depending on frequency of visits/sessions and setting) (ASHA, 2022, Requirements for the Frequency and Amount of Supervision, para. 2).

ASHA's SLPA scope of practice also outlines that supervising SLPs should review data on individuals served by an SLPA and document the level of supervision provided to an SLPA at regular intervals (ASHA, 2022). How this supervision is documented will vary across settings and supervisors. Appendices 2–A to 2–C have examples of forms used for recording supervision. Chapter 1 contains additional details on common evaluation practices, such as competency-based assessment and samples of ASHA-recommended proficiency checklists and observation forms. Lastly, ASHA states that supervisors should arrange designated days and times of day (morning or afternoon) in such a way that all students, patients, and clients receive direct contact with the supervising SLP (ASHA, 2022).

Each of these details above should be included in a supervisory plan, developed by your supervising SLP. You should familiarize yourself with this plan and be proactive in discussing the levels and types of supervision you are receiving. Remember, too, that individual state regulating agencies may differ in the minimal levels of supervision required and therefore the nature of your supervision. You should also familiarize yourself with all local and state regulations regarding the amount and nature of supervision required in your setting for SLPAs.

Supervisor Training and Credentials

ASHA's SLPA scope of practice outlines supervisor qualifications. These are outlined in Box 2–1. Beyond qualifications, a supervisor also has to have a desire to supervise SLPAs and the time and resources needed to do so. Think about this when interviewing for employment as an SLPA. Don't be hesitant to ask questions in this area. You want to make sure as an SLPA that you are in a setting in which the supervision you receive is effective in allowing you to provide the highest quality of care for the individuals you serve.

Box 2–1. Qualifications of a Supervising SLP
(ASHA, 2022, Qualifications for Supervising SLP, para. 1)[1]

- Hold the Certificate of Clinical Competence in Speech-Language Pathology (CCC-SLP) from ASHA and/or possess the necessary state credentials
- Completion of a minimum of 9 months of experience after being awarded ASHA certification (i.e., completion of the 9-month clinical fellowship followed by 9 months of experience)
- Completion of a minimum of 2 hours of professional development in clinical instruction/supervision
- Adherence to state guidelines for supervision of the SLPA
- It is recommended that the professional development course taken in clinical instruction or supervision include content related to the supervision of SLPAs

---

Supervisory Relationship

Another factor to consider about supervision is your relationship with your supervisor. When discussing rules and regulations, often missed in the black and white of guidelines, is the importance of this relationship and the effort involved in establishing an effective working relationship. It is a two-way street. Creating an effective working relationship requires effort and commitment from both you and your supervisor. Keep in mind that the level of service you provide will depend heavily on the nature of the supervisory relationship you develop together. Ideally, the relationship is one of reciprocity or, as McCready (2007) described, a relationship in which both the SLPA and the supervisor give and take mutually and complement one another professionally. Active listening and good conflict resolution skills will be at the heart of this relationship (McCready, 2007). The sections that follow address expectations, supervisory

conferences, and feedback, each of which is important to fostering a good working relationship with your supervisor.

Expectations

Expectations set the stage for all workplace behaviors. Your supervisor will have expectations for you in the performance of your duties as an SLPA. You will also have expectations of your supervising SLP in the execution of her or his duties as your supervisor. These expectations will likely have multiple levels and change given specific circumstances. It is impossible to list everything that will be expected of you or what you can expect of your supervisor. As such, it is critical that you have an ongoing dialogue about these expectations. Many workplace conflicts occur between a supervisor and a supervisee because there is a misunderstanding about what is expected of each person. A good rule of thumb is to never assume you know what is expected. Rather, directly clarifying expectations is the best course of action.

Supervisory Conferences

Supervisory conferences are a critical part of supervision. A fair amount of research has been conducted on the nature of supervisory conferences in the field of speech-language pathology, most of it directed at supervisors in terms of their role in these conferences (e.g., supervisor training, communication, style; McCrea & Brasseur, 2003). From a supervisee's perspective, though, it is important that you also look closely at your role in shaping supervisory conferences. First, realize that a supervisory conference is not a static, once-per-year event, like a performance review. Rather, these conferences are an ongoing dialogue between you and your supervisor. These interactions can take many forms, depending on your setting, such as formal weekly or daily meetings or more informal discussions with your supervisor. These conferences are an opportunity to receive feedback, share and clarify expectations, address clinical issues and concerns, develop goals, seek avenues of skill development, and further shape the nature of the relationship between you and your supervisor. Some ways you can contribute to this process are as follows:

1. Work with your supervisor to establish a routine schedule for conferences. It is most effective to establish a routine schedule for conferences versus, for example, meeting as available or as needed (Dowling, 2001).
2. Help to develop the agenda for your conferences by providing questions and suggested items to discuss in advance of the next conference. Make a list of any pressing questions you may have for your supervisor. If possible, providing this to your supervisor in advance of the conference time will be helpful. As time is often limited, select your questions carefully to maximize the productivity of your conference time.
3. Take notes about items discussed and things that require follow-up. Keep a journal of conferences, recording questions, answers, to-do lists, and any other important aspects of this process; however, you should not record any personal information about your clients in this journal. If you want to make clinical notes, use initial or client pseudonyms.
4. Contribute actively to the discussion during the conference. Use this opportunity to ask questions and clarify information presented. This is also an opportunity for you to share your perspectives on related issues.
5. Employ good interpersonal communication and good listening skills.
6. After the conference, take time to reflect on the content as well as your contributions and ways to enhance conferences in future. Use your notes to reflect on the discussion and document any additional observations, questions, comments, or concerns to be addressed at the next conference.

Feedback

As may be evident at this point, feedback is a key component of the supervisory process (McCrea & Brasseur, 2003; Nelson, 2009). Box 2–2 highlights characteristics of effective feedback. Supervisees across all

---

Box 2–2. Characteristics of Effective Feedback

Effective feedback is

- Given for a good reason
- Specific and descriptive
- Relevant
- About behavior that can be changed
- Given at appropriate time (usually right after observation but in an appropriate setting)
- Open to discussion
- A balance of positive and negative

---

levels of training generally recognize the value of effective feedback (Moss, 2007). In two studies by Moss (2007), feedback was specifically highlighted by SLPAs and SLPAs in training as important to both clinical success and satisfaction with training and supervision (Ostergren, 2012; Ostergren & Aguilar, 2012). As an SLPA, you will receive feedback from your supervisor in a variety of ways. As discussed above, these may include formal feedback through competency assessments and performance evaluation tools. You will also receive feedback via informal methods, including verbal comments and discussion during supervisory conferences and/or informal written notes from your supervisor (McCrea & Brasseur, 2003). Feedback may occur after task completion or during, such as commenting and guiding your behavior if a supervisor participates in a therapy session with you. As an SLPA, you should seek both formal and informal feedback from your supervisor. Both will be important for helping develop your skills and providing the highest quality of care for the clients you serve.

It is critical that you receive this feedback in a way that is productive in shaping your skills but also in a manner that shapes the nature of future feedback. Providing and receiving feedback, especially negative feedback, is not always easy, particularly if the feedback involves aspects of the supervisory relationship or personal issues (Nelson, 2009). Some suggestions for ways you can enhance this process are the following:

- Don't take it personally! SLPAs who develop exceptional skills are those who realize that no matter what the task, there is always room for improvement, and effective feedback helps you improve. If your supervisor suggests areas to improve, view this as an opportunity to change and grow in your skills.
- Keep an open mind and to try to see your supervisor's perspective in the feedback provided.
- Use reflection when you receive feedback. Listen or read (in the case of written feedback) and

attempt to understand before you react or respond.

- Know yourself and let your supervisor know your preference for the method of feedback. Do you prefer feedback to be verbal, written, or a combination of both? It is okay to let your supervisor know your preference, but be careful to take into consideration the demands on your supervisor in this respect. For example, receiving extensive written feedback on every task performed is not realistic, but working with your supervisor to identify tasks where specific written feedback may be helpful to you is.

- Seek modifications to feedback, as needed. If you are receiving feedback that is overly critical or overly positive, discuss this with your supervisor. Similarly, if the feedback is not specific or descriptive, ask for clarification.

If the feedback is not given in time for you to implement changes, problem solve with your supervisor to change the timing of feedback in the future. Remember to employ good interpersonal communication skills and tact when requesting modifications to feedback.

Supervisory conferences are an excellent time to discuss the nature of the feedback you receive. As an SLPA, you will receive feedback, but you can also offer feedback to your supervisor about the supervisory process. In preparation for discussions about the feedback, it is helpful to reflect on the nature of effective feedback. Are you receiving positive and negative feedback? Is it given about

behaviors that you can change and at an appropriate time so that you can incorporate change into future performance? Is it specific, descriptive, and relevant? These are all areas that can be discussed with your supervisor to optimize feedback.

MENTORING

Mentoring is defined as "a developmental partnership through which one person shares knowledge, skills, information, and perspective to foster the personal and professional growth of someone else" (ASHA, n.d.-a, p. 3). SLPAs often view their supervisor as a mentor, but it is important to remember that supervisor and mentor are not synonymous roles (ASHA, 2008). The primary role of a supervisor, as discussed above, is to ensure client safety and the highest quality of care. This is done by providing oversight and accountability to the process, including, for example, "providing grades or conducting performance evaluations or documenting professional behavior and clinical performance" (ASHA, 2008, Mentoring in Supervision, para. 1). Mentors, on the other hand, are individuals who are not necessarily charged with this oversight but take an active role in fostering the development of your professional growth, personal growth, or both. Having a professional mentor is important and has been shown to be related to increases in work satisfaction and career-related motivation and involvement, as well as to a more positive self-image of the mentee and more positive attitudes toward workplace interpersonal relationships (Eby et al., 2008).

It may be that your supervisor views herself or himself as a mentor to you. If so, this is excellent. You can foster this relationship by taking into consideration the roles of a mentee (Box 2–3), as well as the roles of a mentor (Box 2–4). If your supervisor does not view her or his role as your mentor, this is okay too. In that case, this is an opportunity to develop a mentoring relationship with another individual. Ideally, as an SLPA, it is highly valuable to develop relationships with multiple mentors who each have a vested interest in shaping your professional and personal growth. Remember, too, that a mentor is not necessarily all purpose. Mentors can serve different roles, either personal, professional, or both, depending on their goals and yours.

Finding a mentor can seem like an intimidating and mysterious task. The truth is that some mentoring relationships develop naturally, and others require work on your part to identify and cultivate a suitable mentoring relationship. It is also true that a certain amount of chemistry, in terms of connecting personally with that person, is an important part of this process (ASHA, n.d.-a). There may also be failed attempts where a mentor-mentee relationship looks promising but does not expand to its fullest potential for a variety of reasons. Do not let this discourage you from seeking mentors.

The mentee is the driver of a mentoring relationship. As such, the first step in this process is for you to identify your personal and professional goals. That is, "What do you hope to accomplish from a mentoring relationship?" or "What skills or knowledge do you hope to gain?" Next, you can explore formal and informal channels for identifying individuals who may have an interest in helping you to accomplish your goals.

Professional organizations, such as ASHA, are often a good place to explore more formal channels of mentoring.

Box 2–3. Roles of a Mentee

- Driver of Relationship
  Identify the skills, knowledge, and goals that you want to achieve and communicate them to your mentor. Bring up new topics that are important to you at any point and give feedback to your mentor.
- Development Planner
  Maintain a mentoring plan and work with your mentor to set up goals, developmental activities, and time frames.
- Resource Partner
  Work with your mentor to seek resources for learning; identify people and information that might be helpful.
- Teacher
  Look for opportunities to give back to your mentor; share any information that you think might be valuable.
- Continuous Learner
  Take full advantage of this opportunity to learn.

Box 2–4. Roles of a Mentor

- **Coach and Adviser**
  Gives advice and guidance, shares ideas, and provides feedback. Shares information on "unwritten rules for success" within the environment and organization.
- **Source of Encouragement and Support**
  Acts as a sounding board for ideas and concerns about school and career choices, providing insight into possible opportunities. Provides support on personal issues if appropriate.
- **Resource Person**
  Identifies resources to help the mentee enhance personal development and career growth. Expands the mentee's network of contacts.
- **Champion**
  Serves as an advocate for the mentee whenever the opportunity presents itself. Seeks opportunities to increase visibility of the mentee.
- **Devil's Advocate**
  When appropriate, plays the devil's advocate to help the mentee think through important decisions and strategies.

Another avenue in identifying formal mentoring programs is through state speech, language, and hearing associations. You can explore their websites or contact your regional representative to see if formal mentoring programs are available to you. Similarly, if you are employed in a large company or school district, check with your human resources department to see if there are any formal mentoring programs offered to employees.

You can also seek mentors through more informal channels. Start by making a list of individuals in your professional and personal environments or those you have met at various points in your career or education who may be potential mentors. Compare this list to your personal and professional goals and see if there are any potential matches. If someone listed has not already reached out to you as a mentor, make first contact to initiate the relationship. Try first to develop an open line of communication and personal contact with the person before jumping into questions about mentoring (Hannon, n.d.). Getting to know each other's personal styles allows you and your potential mentor to see if your personalities are a good fit. The next step is to share your interests and related professional or personal goals with that person. Starting out with "Will you be my mentor?" can be too formal and may seem like a big commitment. You can begin instead by asking for advice on a single issue or problem and then build from there (Hannon, n.d.). If the person seems receptive to answering your questions and offering insight, keep the relationship going. Acknowledge the person's assistance and look for ways you can offer support or information to your mentor in turn. Try to establish regular contact with the person, keeping in mind the roles of mentor and mentee as you continue to foster the relationship.

Regardless of how you identify a mentor (formally or informally), be active in growing the relationship. Box 2–5 contains a few additional suggestions for maintaining a successful mentoring relationship. Lastly, once you have a mentor and have established a positive working relationship, it is important to set goals that you and your mentor can work to accomplish (ASHA, n.d.-b). You should write them down in a journal or calendar to keep track of your progress in achieving your goals. ASHA (n.d.-b) recommends the following tips for successful goal writing:

1. Be specific about your goals.
2. Set a goal for something you really want to accomplish.
3. Break up your goals into manageable subgoals.
4. Give yourself credit when you accomplish a goal.
5. Categorize your goals by the areas of your life that you would like to improve (e.g., financial, career, educational, social).
6. Review your goals daily.
7. Involve family, friends, and colleagues for support, motivation, and resources.

Box 2–5. Guidelines for Mentoring Success

- Be sure you are clear about how often you will communicate; whether it will be by phone, e-mail, or both; how quickly you will respond; and confidentiality.
- Make contact frequently, especially during the first few weeks, to build a trusting relationship.
- Respect your mentor's experience and views even if you don't agree.
- Follow up when you make a commitment to get information or take action.
- Don't ever leave your mentor hanging. If you don't respond, the mentor will feel that he or she wasn't helpful. You never want to leave someone who has volunteered to help with this kind of impression.
- Be appreciative of whatever you get from your mentor; learn his or her strengths and seek advice in those areas.
- Work hard to make the relationship a two-way street. This means you should always be on the lookout for information and resources that might be of interest to your mentor (e.g., articles you read or information you come across).
- Be flexible and enjoy the experience!

REFERENCES

American Speech-Language-Hearing Association. (n.d.-a). *The power of passionate mentoring: The ASHA gathering place mentoring manual.* http://asha.org/uploadedFiles/students/gatheringplace/MentoringManual.pdf

American Speech-Language-Hearing Association. (n.d.-b). *Writing mentoring goals and objectives.* http://www.asha.org/students/gatheringplace/step/goals/

American Speech-Language-Hearing Association. (2008). *Clinical supervision in speech-language pathology* [Technical report]. http://www.asha.org/policy

American Speech-Language-Hearing Association. (2016). *Code of ethics* [Ethics]. https://www.asha.org/policy/et2016-00342/

American Speech-Language-Hearing Association. (2022). *Speech-language pathology assistant scope of practice.* http://www.asha.org/policy

Dowling, S. (2001). *Supervision: Strategies for successful outcomes and productivity.* Allyn & Bacon.

Eby, L. T., Allen, T. D., Evans, S. C., Ng, T., & DuBois, D. L. (2008). Does mentoring matter? A multidisciplinary meta-analysis comparing mentored and non-mentored individuals. *Journal of Vocational Behavior, 72*(2), 254–267.

Hannon, K. (n.d.). How to find a mentor. *Forbes.* http://www.forbes.com/sites/kerryhannon/2011/10/31/how-to-find-amentor

McCrea, E., & Brasseur, J. (2003). *The supervisory process in speech-language pathology and audiology.* Pearson Education.

McCready, V. (2007). Supervision of speech-language pathology assistants: A reciprocal relationship. *ASHA Leader.* http://www.asha.org/Publications/leader/2007/070508/f070508b/

Moss, L. B. (2007). Supervisory feedback: A review of the literature. *Perspectives on Administration and Supervision, 17*(1), 10–12.

Nelson, L. (2009). Feedback in supervision. *Perspectives on Administration and Supervision, 19*(1), 19–24.

Ostergren, J. (2012). Bachelor's level speech-language pathology assistants (SLPAs) in California: A bachelor's level clinical practicum course. *Contemporary Issues in Communication Sciences and Disorders, 39*, 1–11.

Ostergren, J., & Aguilar, S. (2012). A survey of speech-language pathology assistants in California: Current trends in demographics, employment, supervision, and training. *Contemporary Issues in Communication Sciences and Disorders, 39*, 121–136.

CHAPTER ENDNOTES

1. American Speech-Language-Hearing Association. (2022). *Speech-language pathology assistant scope of practice.* Available from http://www.asha.org/policy © Copyright 2022 American Speech-Language-Hearing Association. All rights reserved. Reprinted with permission.

APPENDIX 2–A
Supervisor Log of Direct and Indirect Observations

Week ending: _____

SLPA: _____

Supervising SLP: _____

Patient	Mon.	Tues.	Wed.	Thurs.	Fri.	Sat./Sun.
Other Activities						
Billing						
Equipment Maintenance						
Documentation						
Conferences/Inservices						
Other Clerical						

Indicate DO for direct observation + time
Indicate IDO for indirect observation + time

Comments:

APPENDIX 2–B
SLPA Weekly Activity Log

Week ending: _____

SLPA: _____

Supervising SLP: _____

Patient	Mon.	Tues.	Wed.	Thur.	Fri.	Sat./Sun.
Total treatment time						
Total direct supervision						

	Mon.	Tues.	Wed.	Thur.	Fri.	Sat./Sun.
Documentation time						
Meeting with supervisor						
Other meetings/ conferences						
Observation of sessions						
Equipment maintenance						
Clerical tasks						

S *indicates* supervised session.

APPENDIX 2–C
SLPA Weekly Activity Record

SLPA: _____

Supervising SLP: _____

Week ending: _____

Total hours week: _____

Activity   Time Spent

1. Direct patient treatment/intervention   _____

2. Observation of other sessions   _____

3. Meeting with supervising SLP   _____

4. Other meetings/conferences (list)   _____

   _____

   _____

   _____

   _____

5. Equipment/materials maintenance   _____

6. Documentation   _____

7. Clerical activities   _____

        A. Total time directly observed by the SLP   _____

        B. Total treatment time provided this week   _____

Percent of time directly observed by the SLP (A/B)   _____

CHAPTER 3

Ethical Conduct

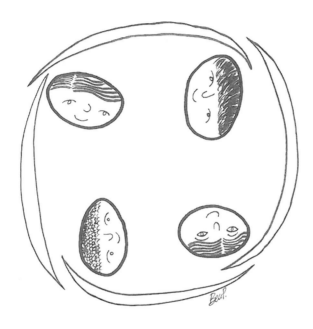

Action indeed is the sole medium of expression for ethics.
—Jane Addams (first American woman
to receive the Nobel Peace Prize)

ETHICS, MORALS, AND LAW

Webster's dictionary defines ethics as "the discipline dealing with what is good and bad and with moral duty and obligation" (Merriam-Webster, 2003). Hence, at its very core, ethics is the study of morality, or what is good and bad and right and wrong. Morals form the ground rules for society's laws. In contrast, laws are enforceable, written rules based on the concepts of justice and equality (Horner, 2003). In the simplest terms, laws dictate what we must do, whereas morals (and thereby ethics) address what we should do (Horner, 2003). A related term, *integrity*, refers to an adherence to high moral standards. As such, a person with professional integrity is someone who adheres to ethical principles in the execution of his or her professional duties.

Often, when students (and professionals) hear that what follows is a discussion of ethics, they brace themselves for a long, difficult discussion of these complex and intertwined terms. However, as Chabon and Morris (2004) highlight, "Ethics is really about helping one to make good decisions" (para. 2). In this light, the study of ethics and an understanding of ethical conduct can be a compass to navigate your professional obligations as a speech-language pathology assistant (SLPA).

ASHA CODE OF ETHICS

The concept of professional ethics refers to the "principles of conduct governing an individual or a group" (Merriam-Webster, 2003). The American Speech-Language-Hearing Association (ASHA) has a professional Code of Ethics (ASHA, 2016a), which can be considered one of the primary guiding documents of the field of speech-language pathology. According to ASHA, the purpose of this code is to "ensure the welfare of the consumer and protect the reputation and integrity of professions" (ASHA, 2016a, Preamble, para. 1). The code consists of four ethical principles and related rules of ethics that form the basic moral foundation of the code. The four ethical principles of this code are listed in Box 3–1. Appendix 3–A contains ASHA's complete Code of Ethics.

ASHA's Code of Ethics states that members, nonmember certificate holders, and individuals who are applying for membership or certification shall observe these principles as "affirmative

---

Box 3–1. ASHA's Four Ethical Principles (ASHA, 2016a)

Principle I (Responsibility to Persons Served Professionally and to Research Participants, Both Human and Animal)
Individuals shall honor their responsibility to hold paramount the welfare of persons they serve professionally or who are participants in research and scholarly activities, and they shall treat animals involved in research in a humane manner.

Principle II (Responsibility for One's Professional Competence)
Individuals shall honor their responsibility to achieve and maintain the highest level of professional competence and performance.

Principle III (Responsibility to the Public)
Individuals shall honor their responsibility to the public when advocating for the unmet communication and swallowing needs of the public and shall provide accurate information involving any aspect of the professions.

Principle IV (Responsibility for Professional Relationships)
Individuals shall uphold the dignity and autonomy of the professions, maintain collaborative and harmonious interprofessional and intraprofessional relationships, and accept the professions' self-imposed standards.

obligations under all conditions of professional activity" (ASHA, 2016a, Preamble, para. 5). ASHA maintains a Board of Ethics (BOE), charged with the responsibility of reviewing, publishing, and amending its Code of Ethics and developing educational programs and materials applicable to ethical conduct (ASHA, 2016b).

As discussed in Chapter 1, SLPAs can apply to receive ASHA certification as an SLPA (C-SLPA). This is an optional designation for qualified support personnel in speech-language pathology (Council for Clinical Certification in Audiology and Speech-Language Pathology of the American Speech-Language-Hearing Association, 2020). Individuals with this designation have met established criteria and standards of practice, which support effective clinical service. Further, individuals with this designation must agree to follow all ASHA policies regarding support personnel, working only under the supervision of a qualified CCC-SLP. These individuals can access ASHA resources and benefits related to their role as assistants.

ASSISTANTS CODE OF CONDUCT

In 2020, ASHA established a code of conduct to provide explicit guidance for assistants in their clinical practice that applies to the following:

- Audiology assistants holding the Certified Audiology Assistant (C-AA)
- Speech-language pathology assistants holding the Certified Speech-Language Pathology Assistant (C-SLPA)
- Applicants for assistants' certification

The code defines the SLPA role through a mix of obligatory and disciplinary measures, as well as through an aspirational and descriptive lens. This document was crafted with broad strokes that allow it to be applied across individuals, settings, and tasks. There are three principles that serve as the foundation for the Code of Conduct, and these parallel the principles found in ASHA's Code of Ethics, which involve responsibility to persons served professionally, to the public, and for professional relationships (ASHA, 2020, Preamble, para 4). The three principles of conduct of this code are listed in Box 3–2. Appendix 3–B contains the complete Assistants Code of Conduct.

Box 3–3 contains several conduct fundamentals that may be relevant to you as an SLPA:

Of note is that these two documents underscore the principle that the ethical responsibility for patient care cannot be delegated to the SLPA, and as such, the supervisor is responsible for the actions of the assistant during service provision. Furthermore, ASHA's Scope of Practice for SLPAs specifically states that "the supervising SLP retains full legal and ethical responsibility for students, patients, and clients served" (ASHA, 2022, Responsibilities Within the Scope of Practice for SLPAs, para. 1).

Analysis of the Assistants Code of Conduct is highly valuable for SLPAs and their supervising SLP as it functions as a protective measure for both the professionals and the clients served. Following the conduct fundamentals described supports responsible service delivery with high levels of integrity.

This next section provides a framework for how to use this information when making ethical decisions in your work as an SLPA.

Box 3–2. ASHA's Three Principles of Code of Conduct (ASHA, 2020)

Principle of Conduct I
Assistants shall honor their responsibility to hold paramount the welfare of persons they serve professionally.

Principle of Conduct II
Individuals shall honor their responsibility to the public by providing accurate information in all communications and by providing services with honesty, integrity, and compassion.

Principle of Conduct III (Responsibility to the Public)
Assistants shall maintain collaborative and harmonious interprofessional and intraprofessional relationships.

Box 3–3. Relevant Code of Conduct Fundamentals (ASHA, 2020)

- *Principle of Conduct I, Rule B:* Assistants who hold the C-AA or C-SLPA shall engage in only those work areas that are within the scope of their competence, considering their certification status, education, training, and experience.
- *Principle of Conduct I, Rule L:* Assistants shall not misrepresent their credentials and shall fully inform those they serve of their role and the role and professional credentials of their supervising audiologist or speech-language pathologist.
- *Principle of Conduct II, Rule F:* Assistants shall avoid engaging in conflicts of interest whereby personal, financial, or other considerations have the potential to influence or compromise judgement and objectivity.
- *Principle of Conduct III, Rule G:* Assistants shall not discriminate in their relationships with colleagues, and with members of other professions on the basis of factors including but not limited to age, disability, ethnicity, gender identity, national origin, race, religion, sex, sexual orientation, or socioeconomic or veteran status.
- *Principle of Conduct III, Rule N:* Assistants shall comply with local, state, and federal laws and regulations applicable to their practice.

ETHICAL DECISION-MAKING

Armed with a discussion of ethics in general and a review of ASHA's Code of Ethics and the Assistants Code of Conduct, we now revisit the concept of ethics as a compass that helps you navigate decisions about what you should do in the execution of your daily duties as an SLPA. Rarely do threats to ethical conduct in our professional (or personal) lives present themselves in conveniently identified and easily resolved scenarios. Careful and thoughtful reflection is often required, both in identifying the parameters of a conflict and in suggesting a potential course of action.

Several authors in the field of speech-language pathology have suggested ways of approaching this task using frameworks for ethical decision-making (Body & McAllister, 2009; Chabon & Morris, 2004; Irwin et al., 2007). One framework that appears particularly applicable is Chabon and Morris's (2004) discussion of consensus building is ethical decision-making. These concepts have been applied to represent the unique elements of service provision as an SLPA (Figure 3–1). The sample scenario described in Box 3–4 is a hypothetical one for the purpose of describing the use of Chabon and Morris's framework. A worksheet that can be used in addressing ethical principles using this framework is available on the companion website of this textbook.

A completed version of this worksheet for this case can be found in Appendix 3–C so you can follow along as you read the description below.

The initial phase of ethical decision-making is the information-gathering and clarification phase (see Figure 3–1). You can start by making sure that you understand the circumstances of a situation accurately and gather any additional facts needed to understand the situation fully. In our sample scenario, it is important to clarify if, in fact, the supervisor meant for Amber to perform the assessment on her own (i.e., collecting, summarizing, and interpreting the data) or if the supervisor realizes that Amber does not meet the requirements of the test manual. Alternatively, perhaps there had been some form of miscommunication and Amber's supervisor only meant to request that Amber help administer or prepare for testing (as Amber has done previously).

As Figure 3–1 indicates, in this phase, it is important to view the circumstances from all perspectives, carefully considering your own motives and role, as well as those of others involved. In the sample scenario, it is important to think about why the supervisor made the request and if there are extenuating circumstances surrounding it. It appears from the details that time and several impending IEP meetings and reports may be factors. The fact that Amber had assisted with tests previously may be relevant to the situation. Amber's role as the assistant and her relationship with her supervisor are also facts to consider further. Amber and her supervisor appear to have a good working relationship, and as such, Amber likely has a desire to help her supervisor, but Amber may also be concerned that telling her supervisor that she cannot do something may affect her job or this relationship. The sample scenario indicates that this is indeed a concern for Amber and that she wants to help her supervisor if she can. Of course, none of these factors necessarily makes the situation ethical, but they are nonetheless important to consider and may play a role in helping to identify a possible course of action.

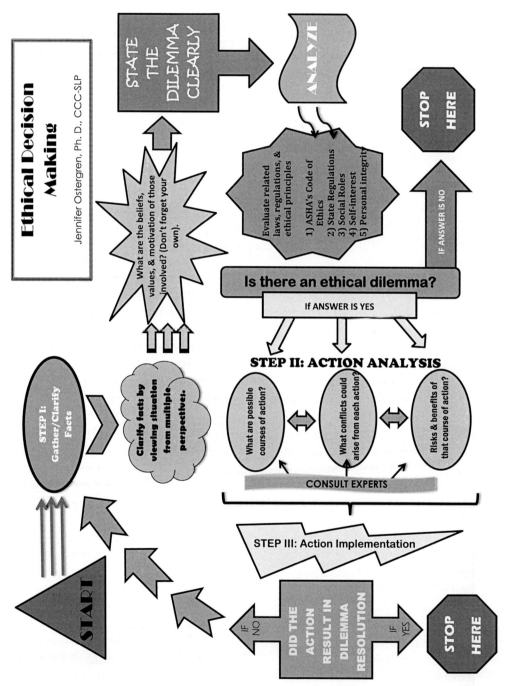

Figure 3–1. Ethical decision-making framework.

Box 3–4. Sample Scenario

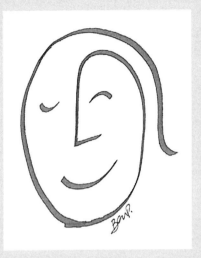

Amber is a C-SLPA employed in a large, urban elementary school setting. She has worked in this setting for more than a year. She is currently supervised by an experienced SLP, who has an ASHA Certificate of Clinical Competence (CCC). Amber herself is ASHA certified. Amber's supervisor has one of the highest caseloads in their district. Next week, her supervisor has several individualized educational plan (IEP) meetings scheduled. She has expressed to Amber that she is behind schedule in writing documentation for these meetings and in performing follow-up assessments. Amber's supervisor just asked her to perform and analyze a diagnostic assessment on a client in preparation for an upcoming IEP meeting. Amber has observed her supervisor administering assessments and has frequently taken part in assisting her supervisor during assessments, such as preparing materials and helping to record data during the assessment; however, consistent with her scope of duties, Amber has not administered these tests independently, nor has she interpreted or summarized the results. Further, based on the requirements of the assessor described in the test manual, Amber does not meet these requirements and thus is not qualified to administer the assessment. Amber and her supervisor have a good working relationship. Amber wants to help her supervisor, but Amber is concerned that this request violates her licensing regulations and ASHA's Code of Ethics. She is unsure how to address this situation.

Also in this phase, it is important to review any relevant rules, laws, and ethical principles (see Figure 3–1). As a general rule, some important documents for SLPAs to consider are ASHA's Code of Ethics (see Appendix 3–A; ASHA, 2016a), ASHA's Scope of Practice for SLPAs (see Appendix 1–A in Chapter 1; ASHA, 2022), and ASHA's Assistants Code of Conduct (see Appendix 3–B; ASHA, 2020), as well as applicable state regulations and laws governing SLPAs and their supervisors, and any employer documents regarding policies and procedures. In the sample scenario, the supervisor is an ASHA CCC-SLP. As such, the documents referred to above are important to consider and directly relate to the supervisor's actions in this matter. Several principles that apply to this situation include:

ASHA's Code of Ethics

- **Principle of Ethics I, Rule F:** Individuals who hold the Certificate of Clinical Competence shall not delegate tasks that require the unique skills, knowledge, judgment, or credentials that are within the scope of their profession to aides, assistants, technicians, support personnel, or any nonprofessionals over whom they have supervisory responsibility.
- **Principle of Ethics II, Rule E:** Individuals in administrative or supervisory roles shall not require or permit their professional staff to provide services or conduct research activities that exceed the staff

member's certification status, competence, education, training, or experience.
- **Principle of Ethics IV, Rule I:** Individuals shall not knowingly allow anyone under their supervision to engaged in any practice that violates the Code of Ethics.

Scope of Practice for SLPAs

- *Responsibilities Within the Scope of Practice for SLPAs:*
  - Administering and scoring assessment tools that (a) the SLPA meets the examiner requirements specified in the examiner's manual and (b) the supervising SLP uses to verify the SLPA's competence in administration, exclusive of clinical interpretation.
  - Administering and scoring progress monitoring tools exclusive of clinical interpretation if (a) the SLPA meets the examiner requirements specified in the examiner's manual and (b) the supervisor has verified the SLPA's competence in administration.

Assistants Code of Conduct

- **Principle of Conduct I, Rule A:** Assistants shall engage only in those activities delegated by the supervising audiologist or speech-language pathologist and permitted by local, state, or federal regulations.

■ **Principle of Conduct I, Rule B:**
Assistants who hold the C-AA
or C-SLPA shall engage in only
those work areas that are within
the scope of their competence,
considering their certification
status, education, training, and
experience.

■ **Principle of Conduct II, Rule D:**
Assistants shall not knowingly
make false financial or
nonfinancial statements and shall
complete all materials honestly
and without omission.

In Amber's case, she is a C-SLPA and
therefore has agreed to abide by ASHA
rules and regulations regarding SLPA
practices. From Amber's perspective as an
SLPA, the following two ethical principles
seem most related to this situation:

■ **Principle of Ethics I, Rule A:**
Individuals shall provide all
services and scientific activities
competently.

■ **Principle of Ethics II, Rule E:**
Individuals in administrative
or supervisory roles shall
not require or permit their
professional staff to provide
services or conduct research
activities that exceed the staff
member's certification status,
competence, education, training,
or experience.

Furthermore, Amber is registered as
an SLPA in her state, and her state regulations prohibit SLPAs from performing
diagnostic assessments.

At the end of the gather/clarify information phase, the next step is to ask
yourself, "Is this an ethical dilemma?"

(see Figure 3–1). If the answer is no, then
you are not facing an ethical dilemma. If
the answer is yes, then the next step is to
begin the action analysis phase by identifying a plausible course of action. Ask
yourself, "What actions can I take?" For
each course of action, think about the
following:

1. What does that course of action entail?
Is it feasible?
2. Who will be affected by that course of
action (either negatively or positively)?
3. What are the risks and benefits of that
course of action?
4. Will that action result in an ethical
resolution to the dilemma at hand?

Obviously, the final consideration in
this phase (whether action will result in
an ethical resolution) is the most important; however, sometimes it is helpful to
start with listing all courses of action.

Ideally, the action analysis phase
reveals a course of action that can resolve
the ethical dilemma (see Figure 3–1). If
not, then an additional branching step
may be required, which involves consulting with experts, supervisors, or colleagues. This in fact can occur at any step
in the process when additional assistance
or insight is needed, but it is important to
remember that self-analysis is key. You are
likely the person closest to this situation,
as it affects you personally or professionally. As such, you are the first expert to
analyze the situation, bringing in additional insight from outside perspectives
as needed.

A word of caution as well in seeking
additional opinions: SLPAs must maintain
confidentiality, particularly when discussing any situation that involves clients or
their families. Federal regulations prohibit

you from discussing personal information about the clients you serve (Annett, 2001). Furthermore, ASHA's Scope of Practice for the SLPA (2022) mandates compliance with the Health Insurance Portability and Accountable Act (HIPPA) and the Family Educational Rights and Privacy Act (FERPA). ASHA's Code of Ethics (2016a) also specifically addresses the matter of client confidentiality and confidentiality in relationships with colleagues. Appendix 3–D contains a copy of ASHA's statement on confidentiality. This topic is also given additional consideration at the end of this chapter.

In the sample scenario, as highlighted in Table 3–1, there are several potential courses of action.

The final stage in this process is the action implementation phase (see Figure 3–1). In this stage, you implement the course of action decided on in the action analysis phase. At the end of the action implementation phase, hopefully the situation is resolved and the ethical dilemma eliminated. If not, this process starts over again, as you restart the gather and clarify facts, action analysis, and action implementation phases until a satisfactory conclusion is reached. In the sample scenario, the action selected for implementation is bolded in Table 3–1. Amber plans to speak directly with her supervisor about her concerns regarding performing assessments for which she has not met the specified required qualifications, highlighting that this activity is outside the scope of responsibilities of an SLPA according to ASHA and state regulations. In light of this, Amber will rearrange her schedule so that she can assist her supervisor during administration of the assessment and offer to stay late to prepare test materials. Furthermore, Amber has identified a few clerical tasks she can perform to help decrease the demands on her supervisor's

Table 3–1. Potential Courses of Action for Sample Scenario

Possible Course of Action	Benefits	Risks	Ethical Resolution? (Yes/No)
Amber could assess the client (as requested) but not tell anyone and allow her supervisor to sign the report as if the speech-language pathologist (SLP) conducted this assessment.	• Amber avoids conflict with her supervisor by not having to tell her that assessment is outside Amber's scope of responsibilities.	• Violation of ethical principles for both Amber and her supervisor. • Negative impact on quality of care for the client. • Potential for sanctions from state licensing board, for both Amber and her supervisor. • Potential for sanctions from the American Speech-Language-Hearing Association's (ASHA's) Board of Ethics for Amber's supervisor.	No

Table 3–1. *continued*

Possible Course of Action	Benefits	Risks	Ethical Resolution? (Yes/No)
Amber can tell her supervisor that she does not meet the required qualifications for this assessment as stated in the test manual, and as such, Amber is not able to assess the client as requested. She can, however, offer to assist in the assessment and in any other duties within Amber's scope of responsibilities so that the supervisor has additional time to assess the client.	• No violation of ethical principles. • Quality of client care is maintained, as Amber has reduced the supervisor's workload in other ways; the client can be assessed by the SLP, who is qualified to do so.	• Amber's supervisor may disagree or may be upset that Amber has refused to do something requested. If good interpersonal skills are used in addressing this situation, this risk may be mitigated.	Yes
Amber could assess the client (as requested) but report her supervisor's conduct to the state licensing board, ASHA's Board of Ethics, and their employer.	• Amber avoids direct conflict with her supervisor by not having to tell the supervisor that assessment is outside Amber's scope of responsibilities.	• Violation in ethical principles for both Amber and her supervisor.* • Negative impact on quality of care for the client. • Potential for sanctions from state licensing board for both Amber and her supervisor. *NOTE: Although Amber reported her supervisor to ASHA's Board of Ethics, Amber would still be engaging in unethical conduct by performing the assessment, which was not in the best interest of the client.	No
Amber could avoid mentioning this conflict to her supervisor and call in sick the day the assessment is scheduled so she does not have to do it.	• Amber avoids direct conflict with her supervisor by not having to tell her that assessment is outside Amber's scope of responsibilities. • No sanctions from state licensing board for either Amber or her supervisor as the assessment is not performed by Amber.	• Potential negative impact on quality of care as the assessment may not be performed as needed, which isn't in the best interest of the client. Alternatively, the supervisor may simply reschedule the assessment for another day when Amber is available, and in that case, the issue has not been resolved and will resurface when Amber returns.	No

schedule so that the supervisor has time to complete the assessment.

As this case illustrates, ethical decision-making requires careful consideration from multiple perspectives. Making decisions based on ethics takes practice. Using a structured framework like the one discussed in this chapter is a first step in developing your skills in this area. Appendix 3–E contains additional ethical scenarios samples applicable to SLPAs. Use the worksheet and framework provided to practice your skills in this area. Taking it a step further by discussing your conclusions with others in the profession is also an excellent way to hone your skills in this area.

Finally, a discussion of ethical conduct would not be complete without highlighting the role of good interpersonal skills and conflict resolution in resolving ethical dilemmas professionally. Chapter 4 addresses this topic in greater detail, including several guiding principles for resolving conflict effectively.

CONFIDENTIALITY

Before we close the chapter on ethics, let's take a closer look at the topic of confidentiality. As highlighted above, when discussing ethical matters, you should maintain confidentiality of client information, confidentiality in your relationships with colleagues, and confidentiality regarding every other aspect of your role as an SLPA. This issue of confidentiality, however, goes beyond discussing an ethical dilemma (Annett, 2001; ASHA, 2018; O'Neil-Pirozzi, 2001). Appendix 3–D presents ASHA's confidentiality statement, which includes confidentiality of client information and confidentiality in relationships with peers and colleagues.

Confidentiality of Client Information

Confidentiality of client information encompasses both verbal and written information. In addition, beyond ASHA's Code of Ethics, the privacy and security of documentation are governed by federal regulations outlined in HIPAA and FERPA (U.S. Department of Education, n.d.; U.S. Department of Health and Human Services, n.d.). HIPAA regulations outline rules pertaining to health care providers and health-related information. FERPA regulations outline rules applicable to school personnel and educational records. Both require specific and explicit consent for providers to use and disclose protected information. They also stipulate that individuals have a right to review and correct their official records, be notified of disclosure history, and receive notice of policies regarding disclosure of protected information. As such, it is critical that SLPAs maintain confidentiality of all client information, including all aspects of a client's care. This means that you must not share the details about any aspect of your services with anyone other than your supervising SLP, those specifically granted access to this information by your client (in writing), or as expressly required by law. This confidentiality includes verbal information, written materials, and audio and video recordings. Written documents and audio and visual recordings must be kept in a secure location and may not be stored, electronically or in hard-copy form, in locations where those without specific permission are able to view this information. It is crucial that you take confidentiality seriously. Some reminders to ensure your client's confidentiality include the following:

1. Do not share information about your client with anyone not specifically granted access to this information. This includes sharing information about your client with your family or friends, as they are not specifically authorized service providers.
2. Do not speak in public locations about your client.
3. Do not remove any documents (written, audio, or visual) from clinical or educational locations.
4. Get specific permission to forward or copy any information about your client.
5. If you are given passwords or access codes to confidential information, do not share this information with others and do not store this information in a public location.
6. Do not dispose of client information without first adequately destroying or removing all confidential information. Your employer should have specific procedures for doing so.

Confidentiality in Relationships With Peers and Colleagues

Confidentiality in relationships with colleagues, peers, and other professionals takes on several meanings (ASHA, 2016a, 2018). First, you should be careful not to misrepresent yourself or others in your verbal or written communications. In addition, when conflicts arise, you should limit discussion of these matters to those involved. This means you should not discuss conflict with colleagues and peers in public locations. If you must seek additional guidance, do so with discretion and confidentiality. Chapter 4 provides additional details about confidentiality in written communications.

REFERENCES

American Speech-Language-Hearing Association. (2016a). *Code of ethics* [Ethics]. https://www.asha.org/Code-of-Ethics/

American Speech-Language-Hearing Association. (2016b). *Practices and procedures of the board of ethics.* https://www.asha.org/policy/et2017-00348/

American Speech-Language-Hearing Association. (2018). *Issues in ethics: Confidentiality.* https://www.asha.org/practice/ethics/confidentiality/

American Speech-Language-Hearing Association. (2020). *Assistants code of conduct.* https://www.asha.org/policy/assistants-code-of-conduct/

American Speech-Language-Hearing Association. (2022). *Speech-language pathology assistant scope of practice* [Scope of practice]. www.asha.org/policy/

Annett, M. M. (2001). Law concerns privacy, transfer of patient data: New regulations will affect SLPs, audiologists across settings. *ASHA Leader, 6*(3). https://leader.pubs.asha.org/doi/10.1044/leader.PA.06032001.1

Body, R., & McAllister, L. (2009). *Ethics in speech and language therapy.* John Wiley.

Chabon, S. S., & Morris, J. F. (2004). A consensus model for making ethical decisions in a less-than-ideal world. *ASHA Leader.* http://www.asha.org/Publications/leader/2004/040217/040217e.htm

Council for Clinical Certification in Audiology and Speech-Language Pathology of the American Speech-Language-Hearing Association. (2020). *2020 Standards for ASHA speech-language pathology assistants certification.* https://www.asha.org/certification/2020-slpa-certification-standards/

Horner, J. (2003). Mortality, ethics, and law: Introductory concepts. *Seminars in Speech and Language, 24,* 263–274. https://doi.org/10.1055/s-2004-815580

Irwin, D., Pannbacker, M., Powell, W., & Vekovius, G. (2007). *Ethics for speech-language pathologists and audiologists: An illustrative casebook.* Thomson Delmar Learning.

Merriam-Webster. (2003). *Merriam-Webster's collegiate dictionary* (11th ed.).

O'Neil-Pirozzi, T. M. (2001). Please respect patient confidentiality. *Contemporary Issues in Communication Sciences and Disorders, 28,* 48–51.

U.S. Department of Education. (n.d.). *Family Educational Rights and Privacy Act (FERPA): General information.* http://www2.ed.gov/policy/gen/guid/fpco/ferpa/index.html

U.S. Department of Health and Human Services. (n.d.). *Summary of HIPPA security rules.* https://www.hhs.gov/hipaa/for-professionals/security/laws-regulations/index.html

CHAPTER ENDNOTES

1. American Speech-Language-Hearing Association. (2016). *Code of ethics* [Ethics]. Available from http://www.asha.org/policy Copyright 2016 American Speech-Language-Hearing Association. All rights reserved. Reprinted with permission.

2. American Speech-Language-Hearing Association. (2020). *Assistants code of conduct.* https://www.asha.org/policy/assistants-code-of-conduct/ Copyright 2020 American Speech-Language-Hearing Association. All rights reserved. Reprinted with permission.

APPENDIX 3–A
ASHA Code of Ethics

PREAMBLE

The American Speech-Language-Hearing Association (ASHA; hereafter, also known as "The Association") has been committed to a framework of common principles and standards of practice since ASHA's inception in 1925. This commitment was formalized in 1952 as the Association's first Code of Ethics. This code has been modified and adapted as society and the professions have changed. The Code of Ethics reflects what we value as professionals and establishes expectations for our scientific and clinical practice based on principles of duty, accountability, fairness, and responsibility. The ASHA Code of Ethics is intended to ensure the welfare of the consumer and to protect the reputation and integrity of the professions.

The ASHA Code of Ethics is a framework and focused guide for professionals in support of day-to-day decision making related to professional conduct. The code is partly obligatory and disciplinary and partly aspirational and descriptive in that it defines the professional's role. The code educates professionals in the discipline, as well as students, other professionals, and the public, regarding ethical principles and standards that direct professional conduct.

The preservation of the highest standards of integrity and ethical principles is vital to the responsible discharge of obligations by audiologists, speech-language pathologists, and speech, language, and hearing scientists who serve as clinicians, educators, mentors, researchers, supervisors, and administrators. This Code of Ethics sets forth the fundamental principles and rules considered essential to this purpose and is applicable to the following individuals:

- a member of the American Speech-Language-Hearing Association holding the Certificate of Clinical Competence (CCC)
- a member of the Association not holding the Certificate of Clinical Competence (CCC)
- a nonmember of the Association not holding the Certificate of Clinical Competence (CCC)
- an applicant for certification, or for membership and certification

By holding ASHA certification or membership, or through application for such, all individuals are automatically subject to the jurisdiction of the Board of Ethics for ethics complaint adjudication. Individuals who provide clinical services and who also desire membership in the Association must hold the CCC.

The fundamentals of ethical conduct are described by Principles of Ethics and by Rules of Ethics. The four Principles of Ethics form the underlying philosophical basis for the Code of Ethics and are reflected in the following areas: (I) responsibility to persons served professionally and to research participants, both human and animal; (II) responsibility for one's professional competence; (III) responsibility to the public; and (IV) responsibility for professional relationships. Individuals shall honor and abide by these Principles as affirmative obligations under all conditions of applicable professional activity. Rules of Ethics are specific statements of minimally acceptable as well as unacceptable professional conduct.

The code is designed to provide guidance to members, applicants, and certified individuals as they make professional decisions. Because the code is not intended to address specific situations and is not inclusive of all possible ethical dilemmas, professionals are expected to follow the written provisions and to uphold the spirit and purpose of the code. Adherence to the Code of Ethics and its enforcement results in respect for the professions and positive outcomes for individuals who benefit from the work of audiologists, speech-language pathologists, and speech, language, and hearing scientists.

TERMINOLOGY

ASHA Standards and Ethics: The mailing address for self-reporting in writing is American Speech-Language-Hearing Association, Standards and Ethics, 2200 Research Blvd., #313, Rockville, MD 20850.

Advertising: Any form of communication with the public about services, therapies, products, or publications.

Conflict of interest: An opposition between the private interests and the official or professional responsibilities of a person in a position of trust, power, and/or authority.

Crime: Any felony; or any misdemeanor involving dishonesty, physical harm to the person or property of another, or a threat of physical harm to the person or property of another. For more details, see the "Disclosure Information" section of applications for ASHA certification found on www.asha.org/certification/AudCertification/ and www.asha.org/certification/SLPCertification/

Diminished decision-making ability: Any condition that renders a person unable to form the specific intent necessary to determine a reasonable course of action.

Fraud: Any act, expression, omission, or concealment—the intent of which is either actual or constructive—calculated to deceive others to their disadvantage.

Impaired practitioner: An individual whose professional practice is adversely affected by addiction, substance abuse, or health-related and/or mental health related conditions.

Individuals: Members and/or certificate holders, including applicants for certification.

Informed consent: May be verbal, unless written consent is required; constitutes consent by persons served, research participants engaged, or parents and/or guardians of persons served to a proposed course of action after the communication of adequate information regarding expected outcomes and potential risks.

Jurisdiction: The "personal jurisdiction" and authority of the ASHA Board of Ethics over an individual holding ASHA certification and/or membership, regardless of the individual's geographic location.

Know, known, or knowingly: Having or reflecting knowledge.

May vs. shall: May denotes an allowance for discretion; shall denotes no discretion.

Misrepresentation: Any statement by words or other conduct that, under the circumstances, amounts to an assertion that is false or erroneous (i.e., not in accordance with the facts); any statement made with conscious ignorance or a reckless disregard for the truth.

Negligence: Breaching of a duty owed to another, which occurs because of a failure to conform to a requirement, and this failure has caused harm to another individual, which led to damages to this person(s); failure to exercise the care toward others that a reasonable or prudent person would take in the circumstances or taking actions that such a reasonable person would not.

PRINCIPLES OF ETHICS I

Individuals shall honor their responsibility to hold paramount the welfare of persons they serve professionally or who are participants in research and scholarly activities, and they shall treat animals involved in research in a humane manner.

Rules of Ethics

A. Individuals shall provide all services and scientific activities competently.

B. Individuals shall use every resource, including referral and/or interprofessional collaboration when appropriate, to ensure that quality service is provided.

C. Individuals shall not discriminate in the delivery of professional services or the conduct of research and scholarly activities on the basis of race or ethnicity, gender, gender identity/gender expression, sexual orientation, age, religion, national origin, disability, culture, language, or dialect.

D. Individuals shall not misrepresent the credentials of aides, assistants, technicians, support personnel, students, research interns, Clinical Fellows, or any others under their supervision, and they shall inform those they serve professionally of the name, role, and professional credentials of persons providing services.

E. Individuals who hold the Certificate of Clinical Competence may delegate tasks related to provision of clinical services to aides, assistants, technicians, support personnel, or any other persons only if those persons are adequately prepared and are appropriately supervised. The responsibility for the welfare of those being served remains with the certified individual.

F. Individuals who hold the Certificate of Clinical Competence shall not delegate tasks that require the unique skills, knowledge, judgment, or credentials that are within the scope of their profession to aids, assistants, technicians, support personnel, or any nonprofessionals over whom they have supervisory responsibility.

G. Individuals who hold the Certificate of Clinical Competence may delegate tasks related to provision of clinical services that require the unique skills, knowledge, and judgment that are within the scope of practice of their profession only if those students are adequately prepared and are appropriately supervised. The responsibility for the welfare of those being served remains with the certified individual.

H. Individuals shall obtain informed consent from the persons they serve about the nature and possible risks and effects of services provided, technology employed, and products dispensed. This obligation also includes informing persons served about possible effects of not engaging in treatment or not following clinical recommendations. If diminished decision-making ability of persons served is suspected, individuals should seek appropriate authorization for services, such as authorization from a spouse, other family member, or legally authorized/appointed representative.

I. Individuals shall enroll and include persons as participants in research or teaching demonstrations only if participation is voluntary, without coercion, and with informed consent.

J. Individuals shall accurately represent the intended purpose of a service, product, or research endeavor and shall abide by established guidelines for clinical practice and the responsible conduct of research.

K. Individuals who hold the Certificate of Clinical Competence shall evaluate the effectiveness of services provided, technology employed, and products dispensed, and they shall provide services or dispense products only when benefit can reasonably be expected.

L. Individuals may make a reasonable statement of prognosis, but they shall not guarantee—directly or by implication—the results of any treatment or procedure.

M. Individuals who hold the Certificate of Clinical Competence shall use independent and evidence-based clinical judgment, keeping paramount the best interests of those being served.

N. Individuals who hold the Certificate of Clinical Competence shall not provide clinical services solely by correspondence, but may provide services via telepractice consistent with professional standards and state and federal regulations.

O. Individuals shall protect the confidentiality and security of records of professional services provided, research and scholarly activities conducted, and products dispensed. Access to these records shall be allowed only when doing so is necessary to protect the welfare of the person or of the community, is legally authorized, or is otherwise required by law.

P. Individuals shall protect the confidentiality of any professional or personal information about persons served professionally or participants involved in research and scholarly activities and may disclose confidential information only when doing so is necessary to protect the welfare of the person or of the community, is legally authorized, or is otherwise required by law.

Q. Individuals shall maintain timely records and accurately record and bill for services provided and products dispensed and shall not misrepresent services provided, products dispensed, or research and scholarly activities conducted.

R. Individuals whose professional practice is adversely affected by substance abuse, addiction, or other health related conditions are impaired practitioners and shall seek professional assistance and, where appropriate, withdraw from the affected areas of practice.

S. Individuals who have knowledge that a colleague is unable to provide professional services with reasonable skill and safety shall report this information to the appropriate authority, internally if a mechanism exists and, otherwise, externally.

T. Individuals shall provide reasonable notice and information about alternatives for obtaining care in the event that they can no longer provide professional services.

PRINCIPLE OF ETHICS II

Individuals shall honor their responsibility to achieve and maintain the highest level of professional competence and performance.

Rules of Ethics

A. Individuals who hold the Certificate of Clinical Competence shall engage in only those aspects of the professions that are within the scope of their professional practice and competence, considering their certification status, education, training, and experience.

B. Members who do not hold the Certificate of Clinical Competence may not engage in the provision of clinical services; however, individuals who are in the certification application process may engage in the provision of clinical services consistent with current local and state laws and regulations and with ASHA certification requirements.

C. Individuals who engage in research shall comply with all institutional, state, and federal regulations that address any aspects of research, including those that involve human participants and animals.

D. Individuals shall enhance and refine their professional competence and expertise through engagement in lifelong learning applicable to their professional activities and skills.

E. Individuals in administrative or supervisory roles shall not require or permit their professional staff to provide services or conduct research activities that exceed the staff member's certification status, competence, education, training, and experience.

F. Individuals in administrative or supervisory roles shall not require or permit their professional staff to provide services or conduct clinical activities that compromise the staff member's independent and objective professional judgment.

G. Individuals shall make use of technology and instrumentation consistent with accepted professional guidelines in their areas of practice. When such technology is not available, an appropriate referral may be made.

H. Individuals shall ensure that all technology and instrumentation used to provide services or to conduct research and scholarly activities are in proper working order and are properly calibrated.

PRINCIPLE OF ETHICS III

Individuals shall honor their responsibility to the public when advocating for the unmet communication and swallowing needs of the public and shall provide accurate information involving any aspect of the professions.

Rules of Ethics

A. Individuals shall not misrepresent their credentials, competence, education, training, experience, and scholarly contributions.
B. Individuals shall avoid engaging in conflicts of interest whereby personal, financial, or other considerations have the potential to influence or compromise professional judgment and objectivity.
C. Individuals shall not misrepresent research and scholarly activities, diagnostic information, services provided, results of services provided, products dispensed, or the effects of products dispensed.
D. Individuals shall not defraud through intent, ignorance, or negligence or engage in any scheme to defraud in connection with obtaining payment, reimbursement, or grants and contracts for services provided, research conducted, or products dispensed.
E. Individuals' statements to the public shall provide accurate and complete information about the nature and management of communication disorders, about the professions, about professional services, about products for sale, and about research and scholarly activities.
F. Individuals' statements to the public shall adhere to prevailing professional norms and shall not contain misrepresentations when advertising, announcing, and promoting their professional services and products and when reporting research results.
G. Individuals shall not knowingly make false financial or nonfinancial statements and shall complete all materials honestly and without omission.

PRINCIPLES OF ETHICS IV

Individuals shall uphold the dignity and autonomy of the professions, maintain collaborative and harmonious interprofessional and intraprofessional relationships, and accept the professions' self-imposed standards.

Rules of Ethics

A. Individuals shall work collaboratively, when appropriate, with members of one's own profession and/or members of other professions to deliver the highest quality of care.
B. Individuals shall exercise independent professional judgment in recommending and providing professional services when an administrative mandate, referral source, or prescription prevents keeping the welfare of persons served paramount.
C. Individuals' statements to colleagues about professional services, research results, and products shall adhere to prevailing professional standards and shall contain no misrepresentations.
D. Individuals shall not engage in any form of conduct that adversely reflects on the professions or on the individual's fitness to serve persons professionally.

E. Individuals shall not engage in dishonesty, negligence, fraud, deceit, or misrepresentation.

F. Applicants for certification or membership, and individuals making disclosures, shall not knowingly make false statements and shall complete all application and disclosure materials honestly and without omission.

G. Individuals shall not engage in any form of harassment, power abuse, or sexual harassment.

H. Individuals shall not engage in sexual activities with individuals (other than a spouse or other individual with whom a prior consensual relationship exists) over whom they exercise professional authority or power, including persons receiving services, assistants, students, or research participants.

I. Individuals shall not knowingly allow anyone under their supervision to engage in any practice that violates the Code of Ethics.

J. Individuals shall assign credit only to those who have contributed to a publication, presentation, process, or product. Credit shall be assigned in proportion to the contribution and only with the contributor's consent.

K. Individuals shall reference the source when using other persons' ideas, research, presentations, results, or products in written, oral, or any other media presentation or summary. To do otherwise constitutes plagiarism.

L. Individuals shall not discriminate in their relationships with colleagues, assistants, students, support personnel, and members of other professions and disciplines on the basis of race, ethnicity, sex, gender identity/gender expression, sexual orientation, age, religion, national origin, disability, culture, language, dialect, or socioeconomic status.

M. Individuals with evidence that the Code of Ethics may have been violated have the responsibility to work collaboratively to resolve the situation where possible or to inform the Board of Ethics through its established procedures.

N. Individuals shall report members of other professions who they know have violated standards of care to the appropriate professional licensing authority or board, other professional regulatory body, or professional association when such violation compromises the welfare of persons served and/or research participants.

O. Individuals shall not file or encourage others to file complaints that disregard or ignore facts that would disprove the allegation; the Code of Ethics shall not be used for personal reprisal, as a means of addressing personal animosity, or as a vehicle for retaliation.

P. Individuals making and responding to complaints shall comply fully with the policies of the Board of Ethics in its consideration, adjudication, and resolution of complaints of alleged violations of the Code of Ethics.

Q. Individuals involved in ethics complaints shall not knowingly make false statements of fact or withhold relevant facts necessary to fairly adjudicate the complaints.

R. Individuals shall comply with local, state, and federal laws and regulations applicable to professional practice, research ethics, and the responsible conduct of research.

S. Individuals who have been convicted; been found guilty; or entered a plea of guilty or nolo contendere to (1) any misdemeanor involving dishonesty, physical harm—or the threat of physical harm—to the person or property of another, or (2) any felony, shall self-report by notifying ASHA Standards and Ethics (see Terminology for mailing address) in writing within 30 days of the conviction, plea, or finding of guilt. Individuals shall also provide a certified copy of the conviction, plea, nolo contendere record, or docket entry to ASHA Standards and Ethics within 30 days of self-reporting.

T. Individuals who have been publicly sanctioned or denied a license or a professional credential by any professional association, professional licensing authority or board, or other professional regulatory body shall self-report by notifying ASHA Standards and Ethics (see Terminology for mailing address) in writing within 30 days of the final action or disposition. Individuals shall also provide a certified copy of the final action, sanction, or disposition to ASHA Standards and Ethics within 30 days of self-reporting.

APPENDIX 3-B
Assistants Code of Conduct

PREAMBLE

The American Speech-Language-Hearing Association (ASHA; hereafter, also known as "The Association") has been committed to a framework of common principles and standards of practice since ASHA's inception in 1925. This commitment was formalized in 1952 as the Association's first Code of Ethics for audiologists, speech-language pathologists, and speech, language, and hearing scientists.

Now that ASHA has established the Assistants Certification Program, a code of conduct was created to guide certified assistants in their clinical practice. Preservation of the highest standards of integrity and ethical conduct is vital to the responsible practice of audiology and speech-language pathology assistants. The Assistants Code of Conduct (hereafter, "Code of Conduct") is intended to ensure the welfare of the consumer and to protect the reputation and integrity of the professions.

The Code of Conduct is a framework and focused guide in support of day-to-day decision making related to assistants'

conduct. The Code of Conduct is partly obligatory and disciplinary, and partly aspirational and descriptive, in that it defines the assistant's role. This Code of Conduct sets forth the fundamental principles and rules and is applicable to the following individuals:

- Audiology assistants holding the Certified Audiology Assistant (C-AA)
- Speech-language pathology assistants holding the Certified Speech-Language Pathology Assistant (C-SLPA)
- Applicants for assistants certification

The Code of Conduct is designed to provide guidance to assistants certification applicants and certified assistants in their roles as assistants. The three principles underlying the Code of Conduct are in the following areas: (1) responsibility to persons served professionally, (2) responsibility to the public, and (3) responsibility for professional relationships.

Because the Code of Conduct is not intended to address specific situations and is not inclusive of all possible conduct-related ethical dilemmas, assistants are expected to follow the written provisions and to uphold the spirit and purpose of the Code of Conduct. Audiology and speech-language pathology assistants are encouraged to seek additional advice or consultation in instances where the guidance of the Code of Conduct may not be definitive.

The Code of Conduct establishes that assistants are not independent practitioners. Accordingly, assistants must be supervised by appropriately-credentialed audiologists or speech-language pathologists consistent with state licensing laws and/or with ASHA's Code of Ethics.

By holding ASHA assistants certification, or through application for such, all individuals are automatically subject to the jurisdiction of the ASHA Board of Ethics for Code of Conduct complaint adjudication. Adherence to the Code of Conduct and its enforcement results in respect for the discipline and positive outcomes for individuals who benefit from the work of audiology and speech-language pathology assistants, audiologists, speech-language pathologists, and speech, language, and hearing scientists.

TERMINOLOGY

ASHA Standards and Ethics: The mailing address for self-reporting in writing is American Speech-Language-Hearing Association, Standards and Ethics, 2200 Research Blvd., #313, Rockville, MD 20850.

Advertising: Any form of communication across a variety of platforms, including social media, with the public about services, therapies, products, or publications.

Confidentiality: The duty of an individual to refrain from sharing confidential information with others through any verbal, written, or electronic means, including social media platforms, except with the express written consent of the other party or as required by law.

Conflict of Interest: An opposition between the private interests and the official or professional responsibilities of a person in a position of trust, power, and/or authority.

Crime: Any felony; or any misdemeanor involving dishonesty, physical harm to the person or property of another, or a threat of physical harm to the person or property of another (for more details, see the "Disclosure Information" on http://www.ashaassistants.org).

Fraud: Any act, expression, omission, or concealment—the intent of which is either actual or constructive—calculated to deceive others to their disadvantage.

Gender Identity: One's innermost concept of self as male, female, a blend of both, or neither—how individuals perceive themselves and what they call themselves. One's gender identity can be the same or different from their sex assigned at birth.

Jurisdiction: The "personal jurisdiction" and authority of the ASHA Board of Ethics over an individual holding ASHA assistants certification, or an applicant for assistants certification, regardless of the individual's geographic location.

Know, known, or knowingly: Having or reflecting knowledge.

May vs. shall: *May* denotes an allowance for discretion; *shall* denotes no discretion.

Misrepresentation: Any statement by words or other conduct that, under the circumstances, amounts to an assertion that is false or erroneous (i.e., not in accordance with the facts); any statement made with conscious ignorance or a reckless disregard for the truth.

National origin: Encompasses related aspects, including ancestry, culture, language, dialect, citizenship, and immigration status.

Negligence: Breaching of a duty owed to another, which occurs because of a failure to conform to a requirement, and this failure has caused harm to another individual, which led to damages to this person(s); failure to exercise the care toward others that a reasonable or prudent person would take in the circumstances, or taking actions that such a reasonable person would not.

Nolo contendere: No contest.

Plagiarism: False representation of another person's idea, research, presentation, result, or product as one's own through irresponsible citation, attribution, or paraphrasing; ethical misconduct does not include honest error or differences of opinion.

Publicly sanctioned: A formal disciplinary action of public record, excluding actions due to insufficient continuing education, checks returned for insufficient funds, or late payment of fees not resulting in unlicensed practice.

Reasonable or reasonably: Supported or justified by fact or circumstance and being in accordance with reason, fairness, duty, or prudence.

Self-report: A professional obligation of self-disclosure that requires (a) notifying ASHA Standards and Ethics and (b) mailing a hard copy of a certified document to ASHA Standards and Ethics (address for self-reporting is provided in the second item of this Terminology section, above). All self-reports are subject to a separate ASHA Certification review process, which, depending on the seriousness of the self-reported information, takes additional processing time.

Shall vs. may: *Shall* denotes no discretion; *may* denotes an allowance for discretion.

Written: Encompasses electronic and hard-copy writings or communications, including communication through websites and other online networking platforms.

PRINCIPLE OF CONDUCT I

Assistants shall honor their responsibility to hold paramount the welfare of persons they serve professionally.

Conduct Fundamentals

A. Assistants shall engage only in those activities delegated by the supervising audiologist or speech-language pathologist and permitted by local, state, or federal regulations.

B. Assistants who hold the C-AA or C-SLPA shall engage in only those work areas that are within the scope of their competence, considering their certification status, education, training, and experience.

C. Assistants shall not discriminate in the delivery of their services on the basis of the following characteristics, which include but are not limited to age, disability, ethnicity, gender identity, national origin, race, religion, sex, sexual orientation, or socioeconomic or veteran status.

D. Assistants shall accurately represent the intended purpose of a service or product and shall abide by established guidelines for the clinical practice of assistants.

E. Assistants shall protect the confidentiality and security of records of professional services provided and products dispensed as directed by the supervising audiologist or speech-language pathologist. In consultation with the supervising audiologist or speech-language pathologist, access to these records shall be allowed only when doing so is necessary to protect the welfare of the person or of the community, is legally authorized, or is otherwise required by law.

F. Assistants shall maintain timely and accurate records about services provided and products dispensed as directed by the supervising audiologist or speech-language pathologist.

G. Assistants whose practice is adversely affected by substance abuse, addiction, or other health-related conditions shall seek professional assistance and, where appropriate, withdraw from the affected areas of practice.

H. Assistants who have knowledge that a colleague is unable to provide professional services with reasonable skill and safety shall report this information to the appropriate authority, internally if a mechanism exists and, otherwise, externally.

I. Assistants shall provide reasonable notice to the supervising audiologist or speech-language pathologist in the event that they can no longer provide clinical services.

J. Assistants shall enhance and refine their professional competence and expertise through engagement in lifelong learning applicable to their professional activities and skills.

K. Assistants shall make use of technology and instrumentation consistent with accepted professional guidelines in their areas of practice under the direction of the supervising audiologist or speech-language pathologist.

L. Assistants shall not misrepresent their credentials and shall fully inform those they serve of their role and the role and professional credentials of their supervising audiologist or speech-language pathologist.

PRINCIPLE OF CONDUCT II

Individuals shall honor their responsibility to the public by providing accurate information in all communications and by providing services with honesty, integrity, and compassion.

Conduct Fundamentals

A. Assistants shall not misrepresent services provided.

B. Assistants shall not defraud, or participate in fraud, through intent, ignorance, or negligence or engage in any scheme to defraud in connection with obtaining payment, reimbursement, or grants and contracts for services provided, research conducted, or products dispensed.

C. Assistants' statements to the public shall not contain misrepresentations when advertising, announcing, and promoting their services.

D. Assistants shall not knowingly make false financial or nonfinancial statements and shall complete all materials honestly and without omission.

E. Assistants shall not engage in dishonesty, negligence, fraud, deceit, or misrepresentation.

F. Assistants shall avoid engaging in conflicts of interest whereby personal, financial, or other considerations have the potential to influence or compromise judgment and objectivity.

PRINCIPLE OF CONDUCT III

Assistants shall maintain collaborative and harmonious interprofessional and intraprofessional relationships.

Conduct Fundamentals

A. Assistants shall work collaboratively with audiologists and speech-language pathologists and/or members of other professions to deliver the highest quality of care.

B. Assistants shall not engage in any form of conduct that adversely reflects on assistants or on the assistant's fitness to provide services.

C. Applicants for assistants certification shall not knowingly make false statements and shall complete all application and disclosure materials honestly and without omission.

D. Assistants shall not engage in any form of harassment, power abuse, or sexual harassment.

E. Assistants shall not engage in sexual activities with individuals served (other than a spouse or other individual with whom a prior consensual relationship exists).

F. Assistants shall reference the source when using other persons' ideas, research, presentations, results, or products in written, oral, or any other media presentation or summary. To do otherwise constitutes plagiarism.

G. Assistants shall not discriminate in their relationships with colleagues, and with members of other professions on the basis of factors including but not limited to age, disability, ethnicity, gender identity, national origin, race, religion, sex, sexual orientation, or socioeconomic or veteran status.

H. Assistants with evidence that the Assistants Code of Conduct may have been violated by a certified assistant(s) have the responsibility to work collaboratively to resolve the situation where possible and, where that fails or is not feasible, shall inform the Board of Ethics through its established procedures.

I. Assistants with evidence that the ASHA Code of Ethics may have been violated by an ASHA member or by an ASHA-certified audiologist or speech-language pathologist have the responsibility to work collaboratively to resolve the situation where possible and, where that fails or is not feasible, shall inform the Board of Ethics through its established procedures.

J. Assistants shall report members of other professions who they know have violated standards of care to the appropriate professional licensing authority or board, other professional regulatory body, or professional association when such violation compromises the welfare of persons served.

K. Assistants shall not file or encourage others to file complaints that disregard or ignore facts that would disprove the allegation; the Code of Conduct and the Code of Ethics shall not be used for personal reprisal, as a means of addressing personal animosity, or as a vehicle for retaliation.

L. Assistants making and responding to complaints shall comply fully with the policies of the Board of Ethics in its consideration, adjudication, and resolution of complaints of alleged violations of the Code of Conduct and the Code of Ethics.

M. Assistants involved in Code of Ethics and Code of Conduct complaints shall not knowingly make false statements of fact or withhold relevant facts necessary to fairly adjudicate the complaints.

N. Assistants shall comply with local, state, and federal laws and regulations applicable to their practice.

O. Assistants who have been convicted; been found guilty; or entered a plea of guilty or nolo contendere to (1) any misdemeanor involving dishonesty, physical harm—or the threat of physical harm—to the person or property of another, or (2) any felony, shall self-report by notifying ASHA Standards and Ethics (see Terminology section for mailing address) in writing within 30 days of the conviction, plea, or finding of guilt. Individuals shall also provide a certified copy of the conviction, plea, nolo contendere record, or docket entry to ASHA Standards and Ethics within 30 days of self-reporting.

P. Assistants who have been publicly sanctioned or denied a license or a professional credential by any professional association, professional licensing authority or board, or other professional regulatory body shall self-report by notifying ASHA Standards and Ethics (see Terminology section for mailing address) in writing within 30 days of the final action or disposition. Individuals shall also provide a certified copy of the final action, sanction, or disposition to ASHA Standards and Ethics within 30 days of self-reporting.

APPENDIX 3-C
Sample SLPA Ethical Decision-Making Worksheet

■ Who is involved in this situation?
Amber and her supervisor.

■ Who is affected by this situation?
Amber, her supervisor, and the client and his or her family (if Amber performs the assessment).

■ What are the motives and roles of others involved in this situation?
Amber's supervisor appears to be motivated by currently pressing issues in terms of a large number of reports and assessments that need to be done soon. Additional clarification may be needed as to why this particular client was highlighted as a person Amber should be involved in assessing. Perhaps Amber and this client have a positive relationship or there is some input Amber's supervisor feels will be valuable from Amber in terms of assessment or the client's progress report. Related to this, Amber can also clarify her supervisor's intent with this request. Was the request that Amber assist in this assessment or that Amber perform this assessment independently? The role of Amber's supervisor is that of Amber's superior, which is a position of power in terms of Amber's employment and performance evaluation, as well as potential future supervision.

■ What is your own motive (role) in the situation?
Amber's role is that of an assistant who works under the direction of her supervisor.

Amber may be concerned how her supervisor will react if she tells her she cannot do something, both personally because they appear to have a good relationship, but also from an employment and supervision standpoint. Amber may be concerned she will lose her job or be rated poorly on evaluations if she tells her supervisor that assessment is outside of her scope of practice.

■ Describe applicable state regulations and laws (if any).
Regulations for Amber's state licensure specifically state she may not independently assess a client. They do state she can assist with assessment. Similarly, state regulations governing Amber's supervisor also specifically state that she may not delegate tasks such as assessment to support personnel.

- Describe applicable employer policies and/or procedures (if any).
  No specific employer-related policies or procedures on this matter were identified.

- List applicable ASHA ethical principles and rules of ethics (if any):

Ethical Principle	Ethical Rule
Applicable to Amber	
Principle of Ethics I	*Rule A: Individuals shall provide all services and scientific activities competently.*
Principle of Ethics II	*Rule E: Individuals in administrative or supervisory roles shall not require or permit their professional staff to provide services or conduct research activities that exceed the staff member's certification status, competence, education, training, and experience.*
Applicable to Amber's Supervisor	
Principle of Ethics I	*Rule F: Individuals who hold the Certificate of Clinical Competence shall not delegate tasks that require the unique skills, knowledge, judgment, or credentials that are within the scope of their profession to aides, assistants, technicians, support personnel, or any nonprofessionals over whom they have supervisory responsibility.*
Principle of Ethics II	*Rule E: Individuals in administrative or supervisory roles shall not require or permit their professional staff to provide services or conduct research activities that exceed the staff member's certification status, competence, level of education, training, and experience.*
Principle of Ethics IV	*Rule I: Individuals shall not knowingly allow anyone under their supervision to engage in any practice that violates the Code of Ethics.*

*Note: At the end of Step 1 (gather/clarify facts), you should be able to describe the nature of the problem accurately and in depth, factoring in each of the facts in Step 1. If not, continue to gather additional information. If by clarifying the facts, the ethical dilemma no longer exists, stop here. If not, proceed to Step 2 (action analysis).

STEP 2: ACTION ANALYSIS

Possible Course of Action	Benefits	Risks
Amber could assess the client (as requested) but not tell anyone and allow her supervisor to sign the report as if the speech-language pathologist (SLP) was the one who conducted this assessment.	▪ Amber avoids conflict with her supervisor by not having to tell the supervisor that assessment is outside Amber's scope of responsibilities.	▪ Violation of ethical principles, for both Amber and her supervisor. ▪ Negative impact on quality of care for the client. ▪ Potential for sanctions from state licensing board, for both Amber and her supervisor. ▪ Potential for sanctions from the American Speech-Language-Hearing Association (ASHA's) Board of Ethics for Amber's supervisor.
Amber can tell her supervisor that assessment is not within her scope of responsibilities, and as such, she is not able to assess the client (as requested). She can offer to assist in the assessment and in any other duties within Amber's scope of responsibilities so that the supervisor has additional time to assess the client.	▪ No violation in ethical principles. ▪ Quality in client care is maintained, as Amber has reduced the supervisor's workload in other ways so that the client can be assessed by the SLP, who is qualified to do so.	▪ Amber's supervisor may disagree or may be upset that Amber has refused to do something requested. If good interpersonal skills are utilized in addressing this situation, this risk may be mitigated.

Possible Course of Action	Benefits	Risks
Amber could assess the client (as requested) but report her supervisor's conduct to the state licensing board, ASHA's Board of Ethics, and their employer.	■ Amber avoids direct conflict with her supervisor by not having to tell the supervisor that assessment is outside Amber's scope of responsibilities.	■ Violation of ethical principles for both Amber and her supervisor.* ■ Negative impact on quality of care for the client. ■ Potential for sanctions from state licensing board, for both Amber and her supervisor. *Note:* Although Amber reported her supervisor to ASHA's Board of Ethics, Amber would still be engaging in unethical conduct as she performed the assessment, which was not in the best interest of the client.
Amber could not mention this conflict to her supervisor but call in sick the day the assessment is scheduled, so she does not have to assess the client.	■ Amber avoids direct conflict with her supervisor by not having to tell her supervisor that assessment is outside Amber's scope of responsibilities. ■ No sanctions from the state licensing board for either Amber or her supervisor as the assessment is not performed by Amber.	■ Potential negative impact on quality of care as the assessment may not be performed as needed, which isn't in the best interest of the client. Alternatively, the supervisor may simply reschedule the assessment for another day when Amber is available. and in that case, the issue has not been resolved and will resurface when Amber returns.

Consult Experts**

- Who are sources of assistance in problem solving this matter (e.g., supervisor, employer, coworker, etc.)?
  Amber has another SLP she has worked closely with in the same district. She may be an additional resource on the matter, given of course that Amber discusses this issue in confidence.

- What are the opinions of experts on your course(s) of action?
  After evaluating the possible course of actions, Amber decided there was only one that resulted in an ethical resolution. She decided not to involve her former supervisor in the matter at this time. For this particular issue, Amber felt she could resolve it without consulting others.

**Note: In consulting with others about the situation, you must do so with discretion and complete confidentiality. This is particularly true when the conflict involves a client. Federal law prohibits you from discussing any personal information about your client with anyone other than the SLP responsible for that client's care and those specifically authorized (typically in writing). When consulting, use only generic descriptions, without any names or personal information specifically identifying the individuals involved. Have this discussion in a private location where others cannot overhear your conversation.

STEP 3: ACTION IMPLEMENTATION***

- What action did you implement?
  Amber expressed to her supervisor that assessment was not within her scope of responsibilities, and as such, she was not able to assess the client, as requested. She offered to assist in the assessment by preparing the materials. Amber also indicated that she would be willing to stay late to assist with other scheduling and clerical duties needed in preparation for the upcoming IEPs.

- What was the outcome of your action?
  Amber's supervisor assessed the client and, with the additional help that Amber provided, was able to meet all her obligations in terms of upcoming IEPs. Amber's professional approach and good interpersonal skills preserved their relationship and helped Amber feel confident in addressing conflict in the future ethically.

***Note: The outcome of your action should resolve the ethical dilemma. If not, restart this process at Step 1 (gather/clarify facts) and proceed to Step 2 (action analysis) and Step 3 (action implementation) until an ethical resolution is achieved.

APPENDIX 3–D
ASHA Issues in Ethics: Confidentiality Statement (ASHA, 2018)

TABLE OF CONTENTS

ABOUT THIS DOCUMENT

Published 2018. This Issues in Ethics statement is a revision of *Confidentiality* (originally published in 2001 and revised in 2004 and 2013). It has been updated to make any references to the Code of Ethics consistent with the Code of Ethics (2016). The Board of Ethics reviews Issues in Ethics statements periodically to ensure that they meet the needs of the professions and are consistent with ASHA policies.

ISSUES IN ETHICS STATEMENTS: DEFINITION

From time to time, the Board of Ethics (hereinafter, the "Board") determines that members and certificate holders can benefit from additional analysis and instruction concerning a specific issue of ethical conduct. Issues in Ethics statements are intended to heighten sensitivity and increase awareness. They are illustrative of the Code of Ethics (2016) (hereinafter, the "Code") and are intended to promote thoughtful consideration of ethical issues. They may assist members and certificate holders in engaging in self-guided ethical decision making. These statements do not absolutely prohibit or require specified activity. The facts and circumstances surrounding a matter of concern will determine whether the activity is ethical.

INTRODUCTION

Professional persons in health care delivery fields (including those working in the public schools) have legal and ethical responsibilities to safeguard the confidentiality of information regarding the clients in their care. Scholars and those involved in human research have legal and ethical obligations to protect the privacy of persons who agree to participate in clinical studies and other research projects. Children and adults who are legally incompetent have the same right to privacy enjoyed by adults who are competent, although their rights will be mediated by a designated family member or a legal guardian.

There are federal statutes binding on all ASHA members who treat clients or patients, whether they work in health care facilities (where the Health Insurance Portability and Accountability Act [HIPAA] privacy and security rules apply), schools (which operate under the Family Educational Rights and Privacy Act [FERPA] as well as HIPAA), or private practice. There are also stringent federal statutes governing the treatment of human subjects in medical and other forms of scientific research. Individual states also have statutes governing the confidentiality of patient and client information, the protection of data gathered in research, and the privacy of students. It is the responsibility of all members of the audiology and speech-language pathology professions to know these laws and to honor them. Because state laws may vary, professionals moving from one state to another should take special care to familiarize themselves with the legal requirements of the new place of practice or residence. Educational institutions preparing professionals in the Communication Sciences and Disorders (CSD) discipline should give significant attention to informing all those entering the discipline about these legal requirements and should model good practice in their handling of confidential information concerning the students enrolled in their programs. Owners of businesses and managers of facilities should regularly review these legal requirements with the professionals and the staff whom they employ.

Institutions and facilities within which professionals see clients or pursue research may have their own policies concerning safeguarding privacy and maintaining confidential records. It is incumbent on the professionals in such settings to familiarize themselves with such workplace policies and regulations and to perform their work in conformity with these requirements. Owners and managers should make sure that such policies are readily available to their employees. Workplace training is desirable, and periodic reviews are recommended.

The Code identifies the confidentiality of information pertaining to clients, patients, students, and research subjects as a matter of ethical obligation, not just as a matter of legal or workplace requirements. Respect for privacy is implicitly addressed in Principle of Ethics I because to hold paramount the welfare of persons served is to honor and respect their privacy and the confidential nature of the information with which they entrust members of the professions. This broad, general obligation is further specified in both Rule O and Rule P.

Principle I, Rule O: Individuals shall protect the confidentiality and security of records of professional services provided, research and scholarly activities conducted, and products dispensed. Access to these records shall be allowed only when doing so is necessary to protect the welfare of the person or of the community, is legally authorized, or is otherwise required by law.

Principle I, Rule P: Individuals shall protect the confidentiality of any professional or personal information about persons served professionally or participants involved in research and scholarly activities and may disclose confidential information only when doing so is necessary to protect the welfare of the person or of the community, is legally authorized, or is otherwise required by law.

If there is variation among the different sources of rules on privacy, the professional should follow the most restrictive rule; for example, if the law seems to allow an action that the Code seems to prohibit, follow the Code. If there is conflict between sources, do what the law requires; for example, if workplace policies conflict on some point with legal requirements for confidential handling of records, the law takes precedence.

CONFIDENTIALITY ISSUES IN RESEARCH

Discussion

Attention to the protection of privacy begins with the planning of a research project, is crucial to the way research on human subjects is conducted, and extends through the review of research results (on both human and animal subjects) for publication and the sharing of data sets. Everyone involved—researchers, human subjects, support personnel, editors, reviewers, and data managers—should be aware of the ethical and legal requirements regarding privacy and should not compromise confidentiality for any reason.

Institutional review boards must be consulted about any research involving human subjects, and informed consent forms must be obtained and honored. Human subjects have a right to expect that their personal information will not be divulged when the results of a study are published or when data sets from a research project are shared with other investigators. Protecting the privacy of research subjects is an obligation for all those who are involved in the research.

Guidance

Data and the personal identities of individual participants in research studies must be kept confidential. There should be careful supervision of staff to make sure that they, too, are adhering to best practices in protecting the confidentiality of all participant data. Some reasonable precautions that should be taken to protect and respect participants' confidentiality include

- disseminating research findings without disclosing personal identifying information;
- storing research records securely and limiting access (i.e., records may be accessed only by authorized personnel);
- removing, disguising, or coding personal identifying information; and
- obtaining written informed consent from the participant (or, in the case of a child, the parent or guardian) to disseminate findings that include photographic/video images or audio voice recordings that might reveal personal identifying information.

Because legal requirements in this area are very strict and because institutions monitor research on human subjects carefully, professionals should seek further guidance directly from the appropriate personnel in their home institutions.

During the peer review of submitted manuscripts, all findings, information, and graphics in the manuscripts must be treated as highly confidential, and reviewers and editors alike have an obligation to protect findings from any form of premature disclosure. In a blind-review process, researchers' identities must be protected. In a double-blind review process, the anonymity of authors and reviewers alike must be scrupulously preserved. Editors and reviewers should make no prepublication use of information that they learn from submitted manuscripts.

CONFIDENTIALITY OF CLIENT INFORMATION

Discussion

Clients must be assured that all aspects of their communication with an audiologist or speech-language pathologist regarding themselves or their family members will be held in the strictest confidence. Clients who cannot trust professionals to treat information as confidential may withhold information that is important to assessment and treatment. When professionals disregard the privacy of their clients, the clients are injured in obvious and/or subtle ways. Evaluations, treatment plans and therapy, discussions with the client or the client's relatives, consultations with the family or with other professionals, treatment records, and payment negotiations should all be treated as confidential. All persons who come into possession of client information are equally bound by this requirement. Therapists, supervisors, assistants, and support staff in schools, facilities, and firms overseeing billing services are all prohibited from revealing client information to unauthorized third parties. ASHA members have a responsibility not only for monitoring their own conversations, securing records, and sharing client information, but also for ensuring that supervisees and support staff are

adhering to ethical requirements regarding privacy. ASHA members who oversee facilities delivering services should have in place policies and sanctions regarding violations of confidentiality by their employees or by students working under supervision.

Guidance with Respect to Verbal Communication

In the case of a competent adult, no one other than the client herself or himself has the right to authorize the release of information. In the case of a child, only the parent of record or guardian ad litem has this right. It should be noted that there will be cases (e.g., in custody disputes or under custody agreements) in which a biological or adoptive parent has neither the right to know client information nor the right to authorize disclosures. In the case of an incompetent adult, only the designated family member(s) or legal guardian has the right to authorize disclosure. Good practice suggests the following:

- In all treatment situations, a written form specifying disclosure of information should be provided to, and signed by, the client or client representative at the beginning of treatment.
- Every client record should contain a clear, specific, up-to-date, and easily located statement indicating who has the right of access to client information and who may authorize the release of such information to other parties.

For any release of information other than that specified in the preliminary privacy agreement or as required by law (e.g., a subpoena), audiologists and speech-language pathologists must obtain a release-of-information agreement from clients or their designated representatives. This includes obtaining permission to share information with another professional. It is prudent to obtain this permission in writing rather than rely on verbal assent.

In rare cases, courts or administrative bodies with subpoena power may legitimately require the disclosure of confidential information. When a court serves an organization or individual with a subpoena requiring records or other information as evidence in a legal proceeding, typically the professional complies with the request; however, it is often prudent for professionals to seek legal advice in such situations.

Professionals are prohibited from discussing clients in public places—such as elevators, cafeterias, staff lounges, restrooms, or clinical/business sites—with others, specifically including the practitioner's family members and friends. Practitioners sometimes think that if they do not use the client's name such discussions are acceptable, but this is not true. Any description of, or comment about, a client who is being served constitutes disclosure of confidential information.

The same restrictions that apply to face-to-face conversation also apply to digital and electronic forms of communication with professionals, colleagues, and friends.

Guidance With Respect to Written Records

Written records have a durability and reproducibility distinct from spoken information; therefore, additional concerns about the protection and handling of paper files or computerized records. These concerns and challenges have become more complex and intense as a result of the digitizing of information. Breaches of confidentiality can occur as a result of the way records are created, stored, or transmitted.

Ordinarily, professionals should not create, update, or store records on their personal electronic devices (e.g., computers, cell phones, and flash drives) or on personal online accounts. If a workplace is aware of and allows such off-site handling of records, then privacy safeguards, such as password protection and anonymized client identifications, should be meticulously observed. Records on portable devices should not be opened and read in public places such as coffee shops or on public transportation.

All therapists who practice independently and all businesses should have clear written policies concerning client records. Workplace policies concerning records management should typically address

- record accuracy and content;
- record storage, both electronic and paper;
- ownership of records;
- record access—both with respect to personnel who may read and manipulate the record and with respect to rights of access by clients;
- record review and retention and related statutes of limitation;
- transfer of information, including transfer by electronic means;
- procedures for handling requests for information by someone other than the client or the client's representative;

- use of client records for research; and

- destruction of material removed from records.

These policies should be observed without variance. Failure to comply with the requirements designed to protect client records not only puts client welfare at risk but also makes the practitioner vulnerable to ethics complaints and legal action.

It is particularly important for professionals serving clients in institutions and facilities to be aware of who owns the record. Usually, in a medical setting, the medical facility owns the record. In a private practice, the individual who is legally responsible for the practice owns the record. In a school setting, the school district owns the record. A report prepared by an audiologist or a speech-language pathologist in the course of employment in a particular setting is not owned by that audiologist or speech-language pathologist, and he or she may not remove or copy such confidential records while employed, upon termination of employment, or if the practice closes.

It is important for the professional to be aware of what information is necessary and appropriate for inclusion in the client's legal record and to exercise professional judgment in making notations in the client's record.

Appropriate steps must be taken to ensure the confidentiality and protection of electronic and computerized client records and information. All information should be password protected, and only authorized persons should have access to the records and information. Computerized records should be backed up routinely, and there should be plans for protecting computer systems in case of emergencies.

STUDENT PRIVACY ISSUES

Discussion

Many academic programs prepare audiologists and speech-language pathologists for entry into the CSD discipline. At all levels of professional education, students and student clinicians have privacy rights that educators must respect. Many of these rights are specifically protected by federal law (e.g., FERPA), and there may also be relevant state statutes. But, once again, safeguarding the privacy of information entrusted to a teacher, program administrator, or institution is an ethical and not just a legal obligation. Professional regard for students and student clinicians involves respecting each student as the arbiter of what personal information may be divulged and to whom it may be divulged.

Guidance With Respect to Students in Classes

Most academic institutions have very specific policies regarding access to, storage of, and release of confidential student academic and disciplinary records. Academic institutions are less likely to have written policies concerning appropriate conversations and communications among educators with respect to the students at that institution. Students do, however, have a right to assume that the knowledge that the faculty have of their academic achievements and personal situations will not be widely or carelessly shared. Verbal and electronically mediated discussion of a student's performance should be carefully restricted to those directly responsible for the student's education.

Student performance and personal disclosures should not be discussed in public places, such as elevators, hallways, cafeterias, coffee shops, restrooms, or campus transportation vehicles. Graded student work and records of student achievement must be carefully safeguarded; access to grades in electronic files stored on mobile devices should be password protected if the device is carried outside the faculty member's campus office. Sensitive personal information that a faculty member may possess should not be shared at all in the absence of a clear and compelling need to know on the part of the person making inquiries.

Guidance With Respect to Student Clinicians

Maintaining the confidentiality of information is a complex challenge in the case of student clinicians. Those who supervise student clinicians must ensure the privacy of client and student clinical records and should model high regard for client privacy and best practices in recording, securing, and storing client records. Supervisors and mentors must treat the performance, records, and evaluations of student clinicians as confidential.

Supervisors of student clinicians must be familiar with the rules for viewing and sharing client information in a teaching setting. For example, a student supervisor's discussion of a patient record for the purposes of education in a university clinic is not a violation of confidentiality, but a student's discussion of the same patient with other students or friends would constitute a violation of confidentiality.

When student clinicians work with clients, persons unrelated to the client may request information about the client's communication problem. Requests might come from an off-site clinic supervisor, clinical fellowship mentor, or a professional who supervises student teachers. Patient or client information cannot be disclosed without a signed release.

CONFIDENTIALITY IN RELATION TO PEERS AND COLLEAGUES

Discussion

Issues of confidentiality also arise for ASHA members and certificate holders in their relationships with colleagues as a result of information that they obtain as they serve in roles such as site visitor, consultant, supervisor, administrator, or reviewer of documents such as manuscripts, grant proposals, and fellowship applications. All of these roles allow access to peer information of a personal and confidential nature. These activities are covered broadly under Principle of Ethics IV, which states, "Individuals shall uphold the dignity and autonomy of the professions, maintain collaborative and harmonious interprofessional and intraprofessional relationships, and accept the professions' self-imposed standards."

Guidance

Information about colleagues and professional peers that is gathered or revealed in the course of evaluations, assessments, or reviews should be treated with the same care and respect that are appropriate to information about clients and research subjects.

When a colleague shares sensitive information or when one participates in committees or other groups that discuss sensitive or controversial matters, participants should clarify in a candid conversation what level of confidentiality is expected and scrupulously maintain the desired level. Records of such conversations should be appropriately secured with agreement as to their storage and disposal.

Matters that may result in disciplinary action by some body, board, or institution deserve special comment. Individuals reporting or responding to alleged violations of codes of ethics or professional codes of conduct are also dealing with confidential matters and acting in a confidential relationship with the adjudicating body. It would be prudent to consider all aspects of a matter confidential until a final decision is rendered. Once a final determination has been reached, it is important for the adjudicating body to clarify what information can now be shared and what information must remain confidential.

Adjudicating bodies themselves typically follow rules of confidentiality (some dictated by law and regulation, some dictated by the organization's internal governance policies and procedures) while the case is under consideration.

With respect to disclosure of decisions by adjudicating bodies, individuals need to inform themselves of pertinent laws and organizational policies. It would not be prudent simply to assume that the outcome can in all cases be made public. Even when the outcome can be made public, it is often the case that earlier filings, testimony, and deliberations must be maintained in confidence.

ASHA members who either place a complaint before the Board or find themselves responding to such a complaint have specific responsibilities to preserve the confidentiality of all materials relevant to the adjudication of complaints. Principle of Ethics IV, Rule P, is specific about this ethical obligation and states, "Individuals making and responding to complaints shall comply fully with the policies of the Board of Ethics in its consideration, adjudication, and resolution of complaints of alleged violations of the Code of Ethics."

APPENDIX 3–E
SLPA Ethical Dilemma Scenarios

Scenario 1: You are a newly hired SLPA in a public school setting. This is your first SLPA position and your first job in a public school. Your supervisor trained you for approximately 1 week, consisting of showing you paperwork and having you observe her providing services to students. She then became seriously ill and has taken an extended medical leave. The district supervisor has asked you to work until they can find a replacement supervisor for you, including providing treatment services to the students on the supervisor's caseload.

Scenario 2: You are an SLPA in a public school setting and attending graduate school for your master's degree in SLP. You have been employed as an SLPA for approximately 6 months under the supervision of an SLP. There is an opening for an SLP position at another school site, and the district supervisor tells you they would like to hire you for this position. She says that they will request a "waiver" for you to work in this position as an SLP, but in the meantime, she indicates that they need you to begin working in this position immediately, so until the paperwork is official, you will need to perform evaluation and treatment at the new school setting.

Scenario 3: You are an SLPA working in a medical setting that bills Medicare for services provided to patients. Your supervisor has trained you to work with individuals in this setting and you feel relatively competent in doing so, under her supervision. One day she mentions to you that SLPA services are not "billable" under Medicare, but she states that this setting allows you to provide services, as long as the paperwork indicates that the SLP provided the services. As such, your supervisor tells you not to document your services in official records but to let her know the status of the treatment sessions and she will enter that information into the system for you.

Scenario 4: You are an SLPA working in a private practice. Your supervisor has trained you to work with individuals in this setting and you feel competent doing so under her supervision. You are assigned a new client to work on treatment goals addressing memory and attention. When you read the client's chart, you see that she is HIV positive. You are pregnant and concerned that you will contract HIV/AIDS, so you tell your supervisor that you do not feel comfortable working with this client.

Scenario 5: You are an SLPA working in a public school setting. You have been working in this setting for 3 months. Thus far, you have received excellent training. You have a close relationship with one particular student and her family. The student's mother does not get along with your supervising SLP. As a result, the student's mom approaches you one afternoon and asks to speak with you about her child's goals, progress, and future recommendations for the student. She tells you that you "know her child best," and as such, she wants to know your opinion, not your supervisor's opinion, on the topic.

CHAPTER 4

Professional Conduct

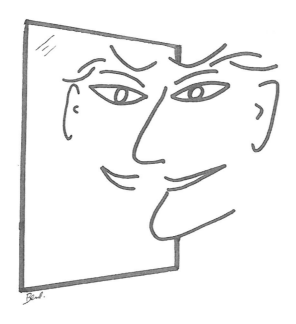

Learn from yesterday, live for today, hope for tomorrow.
The important thing is not to stop questioning.

—Albert Einstein (renowned physicist)

Being employed as a speech-language pathology assistant (SLPA) means that you enter a professional community in which you are expected to conform to community-accepted standards for professional conduct. Although your training provides you with the technical skills and competencies needed to perform your SLPA duties, there are still "soft skills" required to interface successfully within this professional community and to establish your credibility as an SLPA (American Speech-Language-Hearing Association [ASHA], n.d., para. 2). ASHA (n.d.) recommends five tips to establish your credibility as an SLPA, including the following:

1. Maintain a positive and pleasant attitude.
2. Project a professional image.
3. Convey a willingness to learn new things.
4. Demonstrate initiative.
5. Exhibit a sense of organization.

Broken down further, many of these skills have behaviors that fall under the categories of appearance, communication (verbal and written), self-assessment, and conflict resolution. Although you remain an individual with unique characteristics and contributions, as in any setting, there will be expectations of you in each of behavioral categories. Actively seeking to improve your skills in these areas will enhance your effectiveness, project professionalism, and increase your credibility as an SLPA. The sections that follow provide additional detail about each behavioral category.

APPEARANCE

Your appearance is one example of your ability to establish credibility (ASHA, n.d.; Piasecki, 2003). This does not mean that all SLPAs in all environments dress and look alike, but it does mean you should have a professional appearance. This includes wearing clean, neat, and suitable clothing (ASHA, n.d.; Piasecki, 2003). Wearing clothing that is clean and neat is a minimal requirement in any setting, but SLPAs often ask, "What is 'suitable' clothing?" For example, some questions you might ask are whether you must wear a suit and tie, whether jeans are acceptable, whether you can wear jewelry, and is perfume appropriate? What is suitable clothing varies across clinical settings, but generally, if you adhere to the following principles, you will be able to project a professional image and meet the appearance standards of your particular setting:

1. *Check the written professional attire policies in your setting.* Many settings have specific rules and regulations that require you to dress a certain way. Make sure you familiarize yourself with these rules and follow them in selecting suitable attire. In some cases, you may need to wear setting-specific attire (Piasecki, 2003). For example, in medical settings, you may be asked to wear a uniform, such as a lab coat or scrubs.

2. *Fit your clothing to your duties.* Think about what you will be expected to do and what physical positions that might entail. SLPAs may be in a variety of different positions throughout their day, from being seated behind a desk or table, to sitting and playing on the floor with young children, to working in playgroups or other community environments (e.g., grocery stores, parks, libraries), to walking on hospital floors, and many other possible positions. Match your clothing to the physical tasks you will be asked to perform. Consider safety and comfort in your decision. Generally, closed-toe and low-heeled shoes allow for the greatest safety in a variety of settings. Clothing that allows you to move freely in a variety of positions also optimizes safety.

3. *Blend into your environment and do not be a distraction.* Use those in your environment who are respected professionals as a general guideline. Look to your superiors for examples of what is expected. Importantly, do not wear clothing or accessories that will be distracting or draw attention to you. Remember that as an SLPA, you interact with a variety of individuals. Your attire should not be a distraction to your clients or others in your work environment. The emphasis should

be on what you do and not what you are wearing.

4. *Be conservative.* This aligns with not being a distraction (above) but also pertains to revealing and tight-fitting clothing. Cultural norms for what is acceptable vary (Piasecki, 2003). In all settings, you should err on the side of being more conservative, which usually translates to wearing clothing that reveals less skin and not wearing clothing that is excessively tight or form fitting.

In addition to attire, you should consider personal hygiene practices. Good personal hygiene is a minimum requirement (Piasecki, 2003), but consider carefully which personal hygiene products you might use. Because SLPAs work with a variety of individuals, you should limit the use of heavily scented personal products, such as perfumes, scented sprays, and body lotions. Some clients may be sensitive to these products or may have adverse medical reactions to them (Piasecki, 2003). Similarly, some clients may be sensitive to the scent of smoke (Piasecki, 2003). If you smoke, you should take steps to ensure no odor is present when you perform your duties as an SLPA.

You should also consider body jewelry (e.g., nose, brow, or lip rings) and exposed tattoos carefully. In some settings, they are acceptable, while in others, they may be a source of distraction and detract from the performance of your duties. Consult with your supervisor about what is appropriate in your setting and if it best to minimize or conceal tattoos and body jewelry (Piasecki, 2003).

Lastly, some employers may require you to wear a name tag or ID badge denoting your position and any other relevant employment information (e.g., your department; Piasecki, 2003). ASHA recommends that SLPAs identify themselves verbally, in writing or with titles on name badges (ASHA, 2022). Some state licensure standards for SLPAs have specific regulations about nametags and identifying yourself as an SLPA. Check with your supervisor about how to obtain an identification badge that meets those standards and make sure that you wear it visibly when you are performing your duties.

As with all aspects of your conduct, if you are unsure about the acceptable guidelines for appearance in your setting, contact your supervisor for suggestions and guidance.

COMMUNICATION

Verbal Communication

As professionals who specialize in speech and language, SLPAs are expected to communicate with a high level of proficiency. Verbal communication will be the cornerstone of your daily interactions with clients and coworkers in most settings (McNamara, 2007). Defining "professional" communication is not an easy task because the form and content of communication vary given the topic, communication partner(s), and setting (van Servellen, 1997). Generally, however, there are a few principles that guide communication in professional settings. First and foremost, remember that communication in employment settings is typically more formal, both in form and content, than in daily interactions, for example, with family and friends outside of work settings. A few tips to remember to enhance the effectiveness of your verbal communication and maintain the required level of formality are as follows:

1. Address individuals according to your environment. When working with adult clients, it is generally acceptable to address them as Mr., Mrs., Miss, Dr., and so on depending on their life role or title (Piasecki, 2003). With any age individual, client, or coworker, avoid pejorative terms such as *sweetie*, *honey*, and so forth (Piasecki, 2003). If you are unclear how someone prefers to be addressed, it is appropriate and courteous to ask.
2. If an individual has not revealed the appropriate pronoun to use, it is best to either avoid descriptive language that requires a pronoun or use gender-neutral terms when referring to that individual.
3. Speak clearly and at a rate appropriate for your communication partner(s). Match vocal loudness to the tone of the conversation (e.g., softer for personal, sensitive, or private matters; van Servellen, 1997).
4. Avoid using slang and profanity in work settings.
5. Be a good listener. Use active listening strategies, such as not interrupting people when they are speaking (van Servellen, 1997). Comment (as appropriate) on what speakers are saying to let them know that you understand and are paying attention to what they have to say.
6. Be mindful of your nonverbal communication and body language. Use welcoming body language, which includes smiling (as appropriate), maintaining good eye contact, not fidgeting when you are speaking or being spoken to, holding your arms and legs in an uncrossed position, and maintaining an appropriate distance in terms of personal space (Piasecki, 2003; van Servellen, 1997).
7. Be culturally sensitivity to differences in communication styles (van Servellen, 1997). Chapter 5 provides additional information about appropriate and effective communication.

In the context of service provision, effective verbal communication is critical (van Servellen, 1997). When working with clients and their families, be especially careful to reduce jargon usage in your verbal communication. Jargon refers to the technical terms used by a group of professionals. Avoiding jargon increases comprehension in communication with the individuals you serve and will ensure that you do not intimidate or offend the individuals you interact with by using words they do not have in common with you.

As an SLPA, service provision requires that you can comprehend specific aspects of spoken language and, in some cases, produce an accurate model of these structures. In terms of accents and nonstandard dialects used by speech-language pathology professionals, ASHA (1998) states that "there is no research to support the belief that audiologists and speech-language pathologists who speak a nonstandard dialect or who speak with an accent are unable to make appropriate diagnostic decisions or achieve appropriate treatment outcomes" (para. 8). Rather, ASHA says that if a professional speaks a nonstandard dialect or speaks with an accent, it will not affect treatment if the individual has the required level of knowledge about normal and disordered communication and the expected level of clinical case management skills. If modeling is necessary, the professional can model the target phoneme, grammatical feature, or other aspect of speech and language that targets the client's particular problem. If any of these factors affect your clinical services, speak with your supervisor about remediating these skills so that you can provide effective treatment.

Written Communication

Written communication is also an integral part of your daily interactions in the field of speech-language pathology (Goldfarb & Serpanos, 2009). Similar to the high expectations for verbal communication, as professionals specializing in speech and language, SLPAs are expected to be proficient in their written communication skills. These skills develop with time and training, but you should be vigilant in developing and enhancing them. Note that writing, as discussed in Chapter 9, is one of the primary modes of communication used by SLPAs. Chapter 9 contains helpful tips for ensuring accuracy of your written clinical notes. SLPAs may be required to write other documents as well. An important practice in ensuring excellent written communication is to proof your work, proof your work, and proof your work again. An advantage of written communication in that it is tangible and can be carefully reviewed and rewritten to achieve a high level of performance. This, of course, means that you must plan and allow time for careful proofing. Below are suggestions to help you have effective and professional written communication.

1. *Proof your written language carefully to ensure it is free of errors in grammar and spelling.* Using spell check and grammar check is a minimum step in proofing your written work, but realize that there is no substitute for careful review of any written documents you generate, for any purpose. If you are working in an electronic format, printing a hard copy version to proof may help you catch errors. Reading your written work aloud may also increase the accuracy of your proofing skills.

2. *Use formality in your written communication.* Generally, brief but complete sentences are required in most forms of written communication. Avoid using slang, colloquialisms (e.g., he is gonna' need, the clinician tried to get across the idea) and clichés (e.g., using tried-and-true methods, not the client's cup of tea; Hegde, 1998). In formal documents, spell out contractions (e.g., haven't should be written as have not, can't as cannot; Hegde, 1998).

3. *Ensure your written content is comprehensible to readers unfamiliar with your field.* Do not assume that readers of your written documents know what you know or share a similar background on a given topic. When you proof your written work, view it from the perspective of a new person reading new information. Does what you wrote make sense and have sufficient detail for a new person reading new information to understand it? If the answer is no, rewrite your document to ensure the content is understandable to all readers.

4. *Use standard forms of medical abbreviations and phonetic notation.* If you do not know the standard abbreviation for a word, spell out the entire word. Appendix 4–A contains a list of common medical abbreviations. Many online sources are also available to search for standard medical abbreviations. Appendix 4–B contains a list

of common International Phonetic Alphabet (IPA) symbols. More information about IPA symbols and their use is available in Chapter 13. Many word processors contain font libraries with IPA symbols, and you can also access digital IPA symbols through online keyboards, such as http://ipa.typeit.org/

5. *Learn from your mistakes.* You will receive feedback from your supervisor about the content and form of your written communication. You should save all comments and suggestions and incorporate these recommendations into all future documents. An excellent way to improve your writing is to make a list of the errors you have made and refer to that list when you proof new documents. Similarly, you can use lists of commonly misused (Appendix 4–C) and misspelled words (Appendix 4–D), textbooks, and online sources for common grammatical errors to help refine your writing skills over time.

One area that requires additional attention is electronic forms of written communication, including e-mails and social networking tools, such as Facebook, Twitter, and so on. As Chapter 3 discussed, all professional communication about the clients you serve is to be held in complete confidence. Appendix 3–D in Chapter 3 states ASHA's position on confidentiality. It is critical that you only communicate electronically to or about a client as specifically instructed by your supervisor. Many settings have specific rules and regulations about what type of written information can be sent electronically and how this information is to be transmitted. You should not use personal e-mail accounts for this purpose, nor should you ever post anything about your clients on social networking sites. Remember, too, that social networking tools, such as Facebook and Twitter, often serve as a source of information about you to those you interact with professionally, including your clients and their families, your coworkers, and current and prospective employers. Box 4–1 contains helpful tips regarding social media etiquette.

Disability–Sensitive Communication

Last, communication in all forms, whether verbal or written, must be sensitive to the needs and rights of people with disabilities. You should use person-first language when communicating with or referring to individuals with disabilities (Centers for Disease Control and Prevention, n.d.). This means referring to the person first and their disability second, such as the "person with aphasia" or "individuals with seizure disorders," not "the aphasic person" or "the epileptic." Similarly, you should not indicate that the person with a disability has suffered or is a victim in some way from their disability (Centers for Disease Control and Prevention, n.d.). This means not using phrases such as "the client suffers from a hearing loss," "the patient suffered a stroke," or "the client is afflicted with multiple sclerosis." Instead, you could say, "the client experienced a stroke," or "the patient has a diagnosis of multiple sclerosis." In addition, if you are referring to someone without a disability, do not refer to that person(s) as "normal" (Centers for Disease Control and Prevention, n.d.); it implies that the individual with a disability is not normal. Instead, state that the individual(s) is without a

---

Box 4–1. Social Media Etiquette

■ *Pick a professional screen name.*
■ *Create a professional profile and maintain a separate personal profile.*
  Keep your professional contacts separate from your personal
  contacts, and "do not send winks, pokes, virtual martinis, or
  invitations to your business contacts" (Ritch & McGary, n.d.,
  para. 3).
■ *Be careful with what you post online in any form.* Only post
  information that will portray you in a positive light to all who
  view it, including your supervisors, employers, and your clients
  and their families. Be sure to use privacy settings to limit who
  can view your personal information, but remember this is
  not an absolute fail-safe for keeping unflattering information
  private. The best course of action is to use restraint in posting
  anything online.
■ *Be respectful in all online communication.* In other words,
  "acknowledge people when they ask a question, apologize
  if you offend someone, and never ever spam, flame, or trash
  someone else online" (Ritch & McGary, n.d., para. 3).

---

specific disability, such as "individuals without aphasia," "individuals without visual impairments," and so on.

Using the correct terminology to refer to a disability is also important. According to the World Health Organization (WHO, n.d.), disability "is an umbrella term, covering impairments, activity limitations, and participation restrictions" (para. 2). Impairment is a problem in body function or structure, whereas an activity limitation is the difficulty an individual encounters in executing a task or action because of a specific impairment(s). Participation restriction refers to a problem experienced in life situations due to an impairment and activity limitation. Using these classifications, the WHO accounts for the role that personal and environmental factors (not just a person's impairment) play in participation restriction. Importantly, the WHO emphasizes that disability is a universal human experience, in that all human beings can experience a decrement in health and thereby some degree of disability.

In addition, as an SLPA, you need to be able to effectively communicate with individuals with a variety of disabilities. In doing so, it is critical that you view all individuals as unique in their needs, desires, and preferred methods of communication. For example, core principles in communicating with individuals with disabilities include the following (North Dakota Center for Persons With Disabilities, n.d., p. 7):

1. Communicate directly with the person with a disability (versus ignoring the

person and communicating instead with their caregiver or interpreter).

2. Offer to shake hands, even if the individual has limited hand movement.
3. Identify yourself when greeting someone who is visually impaired.
4. Wait until the assistance you offer is accepted before acting on behalf of an individual with a disability.
5. Treat adults with disabilities as adults.
6. Protect the personal space of individuals with a disability, including not leaning on their wheelchair or touching a service animal without permission.
7. Listen carefully and wait for an individual with a communication disability to finish speaking before you speak.
8. Position yourself at eye level when speaking with someone in a wheelchair.
9. Get the attention of people with a hearing disability by tapping on their shoulder or waving your hand.

Remember to relax when communicating with someone with a disability. Each time you meet someone with a disability, as with any person you meet, view it as an opportunity to get to know that person and to find out firsthand the preferred methods of communication.

SELF-ASSESSMENT AND SELF-IMPROVEMENT

Self-assessment, or self-evaluation as it is sometimes called, is the process of evaluating your own skills and abilities and then, importantly, seeking avenues for improvement (Moon-Meyer, 2004). This is critical to becoming a highly skilled

SLPA and is also part of professional conduct. SLPAs who seek self-improvement through self-assessment act in the best interest of their clients by ensuring the highest quality of care. SLPAs who engage in self-assessment and self-improvement will continue to grow in their skills over time and thereby reach high levels of proficiency. The evaluations of others, especially your supervisor, will be important in shaping this proficiency, but SLPAs who rely solely on others in their environment to improve their performance will ultimately be limited in their professional growth. Self-assessment and self-improvement can include any aspect of your performance as an SLPA, including your clinical skills and those skills outside the clinical realm, such as your interpersonal, written and verbal communication, and conflict resolution skills.

The first step in self-improvement is self-assessment. This requires that you carefully observe and reflect on your behaviors. If you are open to the fact that no one is perfect, observation and reflection about your own behaviors will usually reveal potential areas for improvement. Using audio or video recordings can be helpful in evaluating your own behaviors during clinical sessions (Moon-Meyer, 2004). Reflection and taking notes on a task immediately after completion can also be used. Remember, though, that if you are writing notes about what you do as an SLPA, as discussed in Chapter 3, you must do so in a way that protects the confidentiality of your clients. This generally means not recording any identifying information about clients in these written notes and using pseudonyms if you directly reference a client in your written notes. Largely, your notes for self-assessment should be about you, but in some cases, a confidential reference to a clinical interaction may be used to set the context for your narrative. Similarly, if you are recording a clinical session (audio or video), be sure to follow the policies in your setting for doing so, such as requesting permission, using required formats, and protecting the recordings as confidential information.

Individuals new to the process of self-assessment often struggle with what exactly to observe about their own performance or where to begin in the self-assessment process. ASHA forms are available for use as a starting point in the self-evaluation of intervention sessions (see Appendix 4–E and 4–F). Remember, though, that you can self-assess in any area of performance, not just service delivery.

In addition to rating yourself using predetermined categories and self-rating scales, another good way to focus your self-assessment is to observe and write down aspects of a task you performed that were (a) successful and (b) not successful (Crago, 1987). Once you do this, the next step is to identify what about your own behaviors and actions may have contributed to an area of success, an area of difficulty, or both. This is particularly applicable to clinical sessions but can be applied to any aspect of your professional duties as an SLPA. The topics discussed in Chapter 10 are an excellent starting point for areas to assess in the clinical realm.

A reflection journal can be used to record information about your successful and unsuccessful performance, as well as your own contributions to these outcomes. It can then be extended to reflect on how to improve or change your own behaviors for a more successful outcome, as well as a place to record goals and

progress in accomplishing self-improvement. Box 4–2 contains an example of an entry in a reflection journal. The companion website of this text contains a blank form for this.

In many ways, an entry in a reflection journal is like a note an SLPA may write about a client's performance. They both describe subjective and objective details about a given task or interaction, but an important distinction is that reflection journals focus on your own performance. There is often crossover, however, between discussion of the client's performance and discussion of your own performance. For example, the notes that SLPAs write about a client often include a section devoted to future plans from the SLPA's perspective. As such, observing and recording your own behaviors may help you generate ideas of things to modify in future sessions with a client. This concept is discussed in greater detail in Chapter 9.

Once you have reflected on areas to improve, do not stop there. Set a goal for improvement and continue to monitor your performance, adjusting until you achieve the desired outcome. Dating your reflection journal entries allows you to track overall patterns and change over time. You might also consider developing your own data collection methods for tracking specific behaviors over time. Chapter 9 discusses data collection methods for tracking client behaviors. Employing similar methods for your own performance is an excellent way to document progress and to improve over time. In addition, if there are more overarching goals that emerge from your self-reflection, such as additional education, training in a specific area, or both, write down these goals and work with your

---

Box 4–2. Sample Reflection Journal Entry

Date: 2/14/2018
Task(s): 10:00 a.m. Small Group Session (JL, AS, TM)

Successes:
JL and AS participated fully and had high levels of accuracy for target sounds. The session ended on time. The students appeared to enjoy the session and were eager to begin. I felt relaxed and was able to stay focused on each student's targets during the session.

Difficulties:
TM was distracted during the session. He left the table several times to look out the window. I wasn't sure how to shape this behavior other than reminding him that he needed to participate. I had difficulty keeping track of errors and the number and type of cues I gave for sound production. When I listened to the audio recording of the session, I provided many more models than I had noted on my data sheet. I also said "okay" twice when JL's target sound was not correct. The time spent explaining the session's activities took too long (10 minutes). The students argued about which activity to do first and who would go first in each activity.

Areas (Ways) to Improve:
1. *Increase structure of the session at the onset. Make sure to briefly instruct the students in the rules of the activity. Don't allow them to choose the order of the activities. Rotate who goes first per session or have them draw from a deck of cards and whoever gets the highest card goes first.*
2. *Improve data collection methods. Get additional examples of data collection sheets used for group sessions. Check with supervisor about her methods for effectively and quickly noting both errors and cues in group settings. Possibly, rearrange the data collection sheet in advance with a column to place an X under each type of cue. Place a sticky note reminder on my data collection sheet for next time reminding me not to say "okay." Listen to the audio recording from next week's session to record the number of "okays."*
3. *Close the blinds in the room or move the table so the students aren't distracted by the things happening outside the window.*

---

supervising speech-language pathologist (SLP) and/or mentor in developing a plan for improvement in these areas. Lastly, some additional ideas in the areas of self-assessment and self-improvement include the following:

■ Review setting-specific methods used to evaluate yourself (Dowling, 2001). Generally, there will be a set of standards by which you are evaluated for employment purposes, in many cases including a list of clinically related skills you are expected to perform. Chapter 1 contains several examples of SLPA performance measures. Look to these evaluation tools for ideas of specific areas to target in self-assessment and self-improvement.

■ Observe experienced clinicians (Dowling, 2001). For SLPAs, this usually means your supervising SLP. It may also mean observing other professionals, such as teachers, occupational therapists, and psychologists, who engage in activities with clients in your setting that are applicable to what you do. It could also mean observing more experienced SLPAs. This can be done once you have identified an area to improve, as a source of additional techniques in this area or as a source of ideas for areas of self-assessment.

■ Immerse yourself in the professional community of SLPs and related professionals. This means attending regional or national conferences and workshops in your clinical service area and participating in applicable training and workshops offered in your setting. This will provide you with state-of-the-art information applicable to the field of speech-language pathology and related topics that may stimulate ideas

for self-assessment or serve as a resource for self-improvement. In fact, as discussed in Chapter 1, one of ASHA's expectations is that SLPAs will "actively pursue continuing education and professional development activities" (ASHA, 2022, Expectations of an SLPA, para. 1). Some state regulating bodies also require formal or informal documentation regarding continuing education (CE) to maintain certification, licensure, or credentials as an SLPA.

As with any long-term goal, it is best to start small with a few attainable goals and work up from there. Similarly, do not attempt to reflect on every task you perform as an SLPA all at once. Start with tasks that are more structured or more in need of improvement and work up from there. Do not expect to achieve perfection overnight, or ever. The entire point of this process is to view self-improvement as a career-long goal, no matter your proficiency.

CONFLICT RESOLUTION

As an SLPA, no matter the setting, you will be required to work collaboratively with a variety of individuals, including your supervising SLP, as well as other SLPAs and SLPs in your specific setting. You will also collaborate with individuals from other disciplines. Table 4–1 contains a listing of some types of professions that SLPAs may work with across a variety of settings (Cascella et al., 2007).

Conflict occurs when individuals or groups disagree. Conflict is inevitable in any workplace setting (Victor, 2009).

Table 4–1. Professional Colleagues Across Settings

	Birth to 3 Years Settings	Educational Settings	Medical Settings
Audiologist	X	X	X
Chaplain			X
Childcare worker	X		
Dietician			X
Neuropsychologist			X
Nurse	X	X	X
Nurse's aide			X
Occupational therapist	X	X	X
Pediatric development specialist	X	X	
Physical therapist	X	X	X
Physician	X	X	X
Recreational therapist			X
Rehabilitation therapist			X
School counselor		X	
Social worker	X	X	X
Special education teacher	X	X	
Teacher (general education)	X	X	X

Source: Cascella, Purdy, and Dempsey, 2007, p. 263.

How conflicts are addressed will have a dramatic impact on their outcome (Culbertson, 2008). There are four possible outcomes of conflict, as listed in Figure 4–1. The most desirable outcome, when possible, is a win-win outcome for all involved. The best way to accomplish this outcome is to first set aside personal feelings and view the conflict objectively from the perspective of everyone involved.

Good interpersonal skills are also at the heart of positive conflict resolution (Gerrard et al., 1980). Interpersonal skills are "those skills that promote good relationships between individuals" (p. 2).

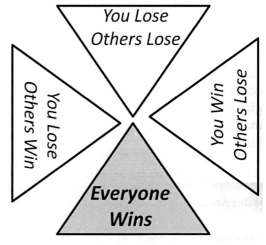

Figure 4–1. Possible outcomes of conflict.

Several guiding principles to resolving conflict effectively include the following:

1. *Employ active listening and good communication skills.* Communicate openly, clearly, and directly about the conflict to express your feelings, but do so in a way that respects the feelings of others. Using the communication tips discussed previously will help.

2. *When possible, seek resolutions to conflict that result in a positive outcome for all involved.* Let go of the need to be right or an attachment to a specific outcome (McCready, 2007). Place the conflict in perspective. Do not trivialize or avoid conflict, but also do not make conflict out of trivial matters (Culbertson, 2008).

3. *Be sensitive to the feelings of others and be ready to move on and work collaboratively once a conflict has been resolved.* Do not make the conflict personal. From the outset, separate facts from feelings and opinions and avoid placing blame for conflict (McCready, 2007). At all stages, consider the feelings of everyone involved and do not hold a grudge (Hull, 2003). This means being willing to admit if you are wrong and apologizing and forgiving others who err or have done something wrong.

In addition, Chapter 3 addresses ethical dilemmas and offers suggestions for addressing ethical conflict. These strategies are helpful in problem solving and making decisions during any conflict, not just those that pose an ethical dilemma.

REFERENCES

American Speech-Language-Hearing Association. (n.d.). *Five tips to become a more credible assistant.* http://www.asha.org/associates/Five-Tips-to-Become-a-MoreCredible-Assistant/

American Speech-Language-Hearing Association. (1998). *Students and professionals who speak English with accents and nonstandard dialects: Issues and recommendations* [Technical report]. http://www.asha.org/policy

American Speech-Language-Hearing Association. (2022). *Speech-language pathology assistant scope of practice.* http://www.asha.org/policy

Cascella, R., Purdy, M. H., & Dempsey, J. J. (2007). Clinical service delivery and work settings. In R. Paul & P. Cascella (Eds.), *Introduction to clinical methods in communication disorders* (pp. 259–302). Paul H. Brookes.

Centers for Disease Control and Prevention. (n.d.). *Communicating with and about people with disabilities.* http://www.cdc.gov/ncbddd/disabilityandhealth/pdf/DisabilityPoster_Photos.pdf

Crago, M. (1987). Supervision and self-exploration. In M. Crago & M. Pickering (Eds.), *Supervision in human communication disorders: Perspective on a process* (pp. 137–167). Singular Publishing.

Culbertson, R. (2008). Conflict: Your role in how it ends. *Perspectives on Administration and Supervision, 18*(3), 99–104. https://doi.org/10.1044/aas18.3.99

Dowling, S. (2001). *Supervision: Strategies for successful outcomes and productivity.* Allyn & Bacon.

Gerrard, B. A., Boniface, W. J., & Love, B. H. (1980). *Interpersonal skills for health professionals.* Reston Publishing.

Goldfarb, R., & Serpanos, Y. C. (2009). *Professional writing in speech-language pathology and audiology.* Plural Publishing.

Hegde, M. N. (1998). *A coursebook on scientific and professional writing for speech-language pathologists.* Singular Publishing.

Hull, R. H. (2003). The art of interpersonal persuasion. *ASHA Leader.* http://www.asha.org/Publications/leader/2003/031007/031007f.htm

McCready, V. (2007). Supervision of speech-language pathology assistants: A reciprocal relationship. *ASHA Leader.* http://www.asha.org/Publications/leader/2007/070508/f070508b/

McNamara, K. (2007). Interviewing, counseling, and clinical communication. In R. Paul & P. Cascella (Eds.), *Introduction to clinical methods in communication disorders* (pp. 203–236). Paul H. Brookes.

Moon-Meyer, S. (2004). *Survival guide for the beginning speech-language clinician*. Pro-Ed.

North Dakota Center for Persons With Disabilities. (n.d.). *Communicating effectively with people who have a disability*. http://www.labor.state.ny.us/workforcenypartners/forms/communication.pdf

Piasecki, M. (2003). *Clinical communication handbook*. Blackwell.

Ritch, S., & McGary, M. (n.d.). *Social media etiquette for professionals*. http://www.asha.org/associates/Social-Media-Etiquette-for-Professionals/

van Servellen, G. (1997). *Communication skills for health care professionals*. Aspen.

Victor, S. (2009, November). *Supervision and conflict resolution*. Paper presented at ASHA 2009 Annual Convention. file:///C:/Users/000666547/Downloads/1030_Victor_Shelley.pdf

World Health Organization. (n.d.). *Health topics: Disabilities*. http://www.who.int/topics/disabilities/en/

APPENDIX 4–A
Common Medical Abbreviations (ASHA, n.d.)

Aa
ADL: activities of daily living
A&O: alert and oriented
A/P: anterior-posterior
AROM: active range of motion
ASAP: as soon as possible

Bb
b.i.d.: twice a day
BP: blood pressure
BR: bed rest
BS: breath sounds
B/S: bedside
Bx: biopsy

Cc
With: (c with bar above it)
CA: cardiac arrest
ca: carcinoma
CAD: coronary artery disease
CBC: complete blood count
CC: chief complaint
CHI: closed head injury
c/o: complains of
CPR: cardiopulmonary resuscitation
CT: computerized tomography
CV: cardiovascular
CVA: cerebral vascular accident
CXR: chest x-ray

Dd
d/c: discontinue
DC: discharge

DNK: do not know
DNT: did not test
DOB: date of birth
d/t: due to
Dx: diagnosis

Ee
EENT: eye, ear, nose, throat
ENT: ear, nose, throat
ETOH: ethanol (alcohol)
exam: examination

Ff
FH: family history
f/u: follow-up

Gg
GCS: Glasgow Coma Scale
GERD: gastroesophageal reflux disease
GSW: gunshot wound

Hh
H/A: headache
HBP: high blood pressure
HEENT: head, eyes, ear, nose, throat
H_2O: water
h/o: history of
H&P: history and physical
HR: heart rate
HTN: hypertension
Hx: history

Ii
ICCU: intensive coronary care unit

ICU: intensive care unit

imp.: impression

Ll

LBW: low birth rate

LE: lower extremities

LOC: loss of consciousness, level of consciousness

LOS: length of stay

LUE: left upper extremity

Mm

MBSS: modified barium swallow study

MCA: middle cerebral artery

MRI: magnetic resonance imaging

MVA: motor vehicle accident

Nn

NG: nasogastric

NICU: neonatal intensive care unit

NKA: no known allergies

NPO: nothing by mouth

Oo

O_2: oxygen

OM: otitis media

OME: otitis media with effusion

ot.: ear

Pp

PE: physical examination

Ped.: Pediatrics

PEG: percutaneous endoscopic gastrostomy

PET: positron emission tomography

PH: past history

PMH: past medical history

p.o.: by mouth

PRN: as often as necessary, as needed

Qq

Q: every

q.h.: every hour

q.i.d.: four times a day

Rr

rehab.: rehabilitation

RLA: Rancho Los Amigo Scale

R/O: rule out

ROM: range of motion

RUE: right upper extremity

Ss

SCI: spinal cord injury

SH: social history

SOAP: subjective, objective, assessment, and plan

SOB: shortness of breath

s/s: signs and symptoms

Tt

TB: tuberculosis

TBI: traumatic brain injury

TIA: transient ischemic attack

TKR: total knee replacement

Tx: treatment, traction

Uu

UCD: usual childhood diseases

UCHD: usual childhood diseases

APPENDIX 4–B
Common International Phonetic Alphabet (IPA) Symbols

CONSONANTS:

IPA SYMBOL	EXAMPLE
/p/	Happy
/m/	Mother
/h/	Hello
/n/	Never
/w/	Wednesday
/b/	Baseball
/k/	Kite
/g/	Golf
/d/	Deliver
/t/	Tuesday
/ŋ/	Pink
/f/	Fall
/j/	Yellow
/r/	Carrot
/l/	Balloon
/s/	Saturday
/tʃ/	Church
/ʃ/	Shoe
/z/	Zoo
/dʒ/	Jewel
/v/	Volcano
/θ/	Thumb
/ð/	That
/ʒ/	Vision

VOWELS:

IPA SYMBOL	EXAMPLE
/i/	See
/ɪ/	Insect
/ʊ/	Foot
/u/	Boot
/e/	Bed
/ə/ Unstressed	Around
/ɜ/	Turn
/ɔ/	Lawn
/æ/	Apple
/ʌ/ Stressed	hut
/ɑ/	Father

R-COLORED VOWELS:

IPA SYMBOL	EXAMPLE
/ɝ/	Her
/ɚ/	Color

DIPHTHONGS:

IPA SYMBOL	EXAMPLE
/eɪ/	Play
/eə/	Their
/əʊ/	Boat
/ɪə/	Here
/ɔɪ/	Coin
/ʊə/	Tour
/aɪ/	Sky
/aʊ/	House

APPENDIX 4–C
Examples of Commonly Misused Words and Phrases

Effect ■ *a distinctive impression* <*the color gives the* effect *of being warm*> ■ *the creation of a desired impression* <*her tears were purely for* effect> ■ *the conscious subjective aspect of an emotion considered apart from bodily change* **Affect** ■ *something that inevitably follows an antecedent (as a cause or agent)* ■ *an outward sign* ■ *a set of observable manifestations of a subjectively experienced emotion* <*patients . . . showed perfectly normal reactions and* affects>	**Alternate** ■ *occurring or succeeding by turns* <*a day of* alternate *sunshine and rain*> ■ *arranged one above or alongside the other* ■ *every other: every second* <*he works on* alternate *days*> **Alternative** ■ *offering or expressing a choice* <*several* alternative *plans*> ■ *different from the usual or conventional* <alternative *lifestyle*>	**Incidence** ■ *rate of occurrence or influence* <*a high* incidence *of crime*> **Prevalence** ■ *the degree to which something is prevalent; especially: the percentage of a population that is affected with a particular disease at a given time*
Were ■ *past 2nd person singular, past plural, or past subjunctive of* BE **We're** ■ *we are* **Where** ■ *at, in, or to what place* <where *is the house*> <where *are we going*>	**Farther** ■ *at or to a greater distance or more advanced point* <*got no* farther *than the first page*> <*nothing could be* farther *from the truth*> ■ *to a greater degree or extent* <*see to it that I do not have to act any* farther *in the matter*> **Further** ■ *in addition:* MOREOVER ■ *to a greater degree or extent* <further *annoyed by a second intrusion*> <*my ponies are tired, and I have* further *to go*>	**Their** ■ *of or relating to them or themselves especially as possessors, agents, or objects of an action* <their *furniture*> <their *verses*> <their *being seen*> **They're** ■ *they are* **There** ■ *in or at that place* <*stand over* there> ■ *to or into that place* <*went* there *after church*> ■ *at that point or stage* <*stop right* there *before you say something you'll regret*>

continues

Abduct	**Elicit**	**Its**
■ *to draw or spread away (as a limb or the fingers) from a position near or parallel to the median axis of the body or from the axis of a limb*	■ *to draw forth or bring out <hypnotism elicited his hidden fears>* ■ *to call forth or draw out (as information or a response) <her remarks elicited cheers>*	■ *of or relating to it or itself, especially as possessor, agent, or object of an action <going to its kennel> <a child proud of its first drawings> <its final enactment into law>*
Adduct	**Evoke**	**It's**
■ *to draw (as a limb) toward or past the median axis of the body* ■ *to bring together (similar parts) <adduct the fingers>*	■ *to call forth or up: <evoke evil spirits>* ■ *to bring to mind or recollection <this place evokes memories>* ■ *to re-create imaginatively*	■ *it is*
Except	**You're**	**Principal**
■ *with the exclusion or exception of <daily except Sundays>*	■ *you are*	■ *most important, consequential, or influential: CHIEF <the principal ingredient> <the region's principal city>*
Accept	**Your**	
■ *to receive willingly <accept a gift>* ■ *to be able or designed to take or hold (something applied or added) <a surface that will not accept ink>* ■ *to give admittance or approval to <accept her as one of the group>* ■ *to endure without protest or reaction <accept poor living conditions>* ■ *to recognize as true: BELIEVE <refused to accept the explanation>* ■ *to make a favorable response to <accept an offer>* ■ *to agree to undertake (a responsibility) <accept a job>* ■ *to assume an obligation to pay; also: to take in payment <we don't accept personal checks>*	■ *of or relating to you or yourself or yourselves, especially as possessor or possessors <your bodies>, agent or agents <your contributions>, or object of an action <your discharge>* ■ *of or relating to one or oneself <when you face the north, east is at your right>*	*NOTE: This can also be a title, such as <Mr. Thomas is Principal of Thomas Jefferson Elementary School.>* **Principle** ■ *a comprehensive and fundamental law, doctrine, or assumption* ■ *a rule or code of conduct* ■ *habitual devotion to right principles <a man of principle>*

Personnel

- *a body of persons usually employed (as in a factory or organization)*
- *a division of an organization concerned with personnel*

Personal

- *of, relating to, or affecting a particular person: PRIVATE, INDIVIDUAL <personal ambition> <personal financial gain>*
- *done in person without the intervention of another; also: proceeding from a single person*
- *carried on between individuals directly <a personal interview>*
- *relating to the person or body*
- *relating to an individual or an individual's character, conduct, motives, or private affairs often in an offensive manner <a personal insult>*
- *intended for private use or use by one person <a personal stereo>*

Then

- *at that time*
- *soon after that: next in order of time <walked to the door, then turned>*
- *following next after in order of position, narration, or enumeration*
- *being next in a series <first came the clowns, and then came the elephants>*
- *in addition: BESIDES <then there is the interest to be paid>*

Than

- *used as a function word to indicate the second member or the member taken as the point of departure in a comparison expressive of inequality; used with comparative adjectives and comparative adverbs <older than I am> <easier said than done>*
- *used as a function word to indicate difference of kind, manner, or identity; used especially with some adjectives and adverbs that express diversity <anywhere else than at home>*
- *rather than—usually used only after prefer, preferable, and preferably*
- *other than*

Too

- *BESIDES, ALSO <sell the house and furniture too>*
- *to an excessive degree: EXCESSIVELY <too large a house for us>*
- *to such a degree as to be regrettable <this time he has gone too far>: VERY <didn't seem too interested>*

Two

- *being one more than one in number*
- *being the second—used postpositively <section two of the instructions>*

To

- *used as a function word to indicate movement or an action or condition suggestive of movement toward a place, person, or thing reached <drove to the city> <went to lunch>*
- *used as a function word to indicate direction <a mile to the south>*
- *used as a function word to indicate contact or proximity <applied polish to the table> <put her hand to her heart>*
- *used as a function word to indicate the place or point that is the far limit <100 miles to the nearest town>*
- *used as a function word to indicate relative position <perpendicular to the floor>*
- *used as a function word to indicate purpose, intention, tendency, result, or end <came to our aid> <drink to his health>*

continues

		To *(continued)*
		■ *used as a function word to indicate the result of an action or a process* <*broken all* to *pieces*> <*go* to *seed*> <to *their surprise, the train left on time*>
		■ *used as a function word to indicate position or relation in time: BEFORE* <*five minutes* to *five*>: *TILL* <*from eight* to *five*>
		■ *used as a function word: (1) to indicate a relation to one that serves as a standard* <*inferior* to *her earlier works*> *(2) to indicate similarity, correspondence, dissimilarity, or proportion* <*compared him* to *a god*>
		■ *used as a function word to indicate agreement or conformity* <*add salt* to *taste*> <to *my knowledge*>
		■ *used as a function word to indicate a proportion in terms of numbers or quantities* <*400* to *the box*> <*odds of ten* to *one*>
		■ *used as a function word to indicate that the following verb is an infinitive* <*wants* to *go*> *and often used by itself at the end of a clause in place of an infinitive suggested by the preceding context* <*knows more than she seems* to>

Medical Prefix	Medical Prefix	Medical Prefix
Inter- ■ *Among* <inter*dental*> ■ *In the midst of; within* <inter*oceptor*> Intra- ■ *within* <intra*galactic*> ■ *during* <intra*day*> ■ *between layers of* <intra*dermal*>	A-/An- ■ *Not, without, or less* <a*lexia*> <a*phonia*> <an*emia*> <an*oxia*> Dys- ■ *abnormal, difficult, or impaired* <dys*chromia*> <dys*pnea*> <dys*function*>	Hypo- ■ *under* ■ *beneath* ■ *down* <hypo*blast*> <hypo*dermic*> ■ *less than normal or normally* <hyp*esthesia*> <hypo*tension*> Hyper- ■ *excessively* <hyper*sensitive*> ■ *excessive* <hyper*emia*> <hyper*tension*>

Definitions provided from Merriam-Webster. (2003). *Merriam-Webster's collegiate dictionary* (11th ed.).

APPENDIX 4–D
Commonly Misspelled Words in English

A
acceptable
accidentally
accommodate
acquire
acquit
amateur
apparent
argument

B
believe

C
calendar
category
changeable
column
committed
conscience
conscientious
conscious
consensus

D
definite (ly)
discipline

E
embarrass (ment)
equipment

exceed
existence
experience

F
foreign

G
gauge
guarantee

H
harass
height
hierarchy
humorous

I
ignorance
immediate
independent
indispensable
inoculate
intelligence

J
judgment

L
leisure
liaison

library
license

M
maintenance
maneuver
millennium
minuscule
mischievous
misspell

N
neighbor
noticeable

O
occasionally
occurrence

P
pastime
perseverance
personnel
possession
precede
privilege
pronunciation
publicly

Q
questionnaire

R
receive/receipt
recommend
referred
reference
relevant
restaurant
rhyme
rhythm

S
schedule
separate
supersede

T
threshold
twelfth

U
until

Source: 100 Most Often ~~Mispelled~~ Misspelled Words in English. (2003). In YourDictionary.com. http:// grammar.yourdictionary.com/spelling-and-word-lists/misspelled.html

Self-Evaluation of Intervention Sessions—Educational Setting

Note: This form may be used in conjunction with the Direct Observation Skills Brief Checklist.

Date/Time of Session:

_____

Rate the following on a scale of 1 (disagree) to 5 (agree).

1. I maintained an appropriate relationship with the student throughout the session.   ○ 1 ○ 2 ○ 3 ○ 4 ○ 5

2. I was self-confident in this session.   ○ 1 ○ 2 ○ 3 ○ 4 ○ 5

3. I considered the student's needs in selecting my materials and interacting with this student.   ○ 1 ○ 2 ○ 3 ○ 4 ○ 5

4. I considered the student's cultural/linguistic needs in selecting my materials and interacting with this student.   ○ 1 ○ 2 ○ 3 ○ 4 ○ 5

5. I used language appropriate for the student's age and education.   ○ 1 ○ 2 ○ 3 ○ 4 ○ 5

6. I was courteous and respectful with this student.   ○ 1 ○ 2 ○ 3 ○ 4 ○ 5

7. I was punctual for the session.   ○ 1 ○ 2 ○ 3 ○ 4 ○ 5

8. I was prepared for the session.   ○ 1 ○ 2 ○ 3 ○ 4 ○ 5

9. I was dressed appropriately for this session.   ○ 1 ○ 2 ○ 3 ○ 4 ○ 5

10. I used time efficiently during this session.   ○ 1 ○ 2 ○ 3 ○ 4 ○ 5

11. I completed the assigned tasks during this session.   ○ 1 ○ 2 ○ 3 ○ 4 ○ 5

12. I accurately determined correct versus incorrect responses.   ○ 1 ○ 2 ○ 3 ○ 4 ○ 5

13. I provided appropriate feedback to the student.   ○ 1 ○ 2 ○ 3 ○ 4 ○ 5

14. The work area was appropriate for this student.   ○ 1 ○ 2 ○ 3 ○ 4 ○ 5

15. I was aware of my professional boundaries during this session.   ○ 1 ○ 2 ○ 3 ○ 4 ○ 5

16. I documented the results of the session appropriately.   ○ 1 ○ 2 ○ 3 ○ 4 ○ 5

17. I shared the results with my supervision.   ○ 1 ○ 2 ○ 3 ○ 4 ○ 5

Comments:

SLPA Signature: _____

APPENDIX 4–F
Self-Evaluation of Intervention Sessions—Medical Setting

Note: This form may be used in conjunction with the Direct Observation Skills Brief Checklist.

Date/Time of Session:

_____

Rate the following on a scale of 1 (disagree) to 5 (agree).

1. I maintained an appropriate relationship with the patient throughout the session ○ 1 ○ 2 ○ 3 ○ 4 ○ 5

2. I was self-confident in this session. ○ 1 ○ 2 ○ 3 ○ 4 ○ 5

3. I considered the patient's needs in selecting my materials and interacting with this patient. ○ 1 ○ 2 ○ 3 ○ 4 ○ 5

4. I considered the patient's cultural and linguistic needs in selecting my materials and interacting with this patient. ○ 1 ○ 2 ○ 3 ○ 4 ○ 5

5. I used language appropriate for the patient's age and education. ○ 1 ○ 2 ○ 3 ○ 4 ○ 5

6. I was courteous and respectful with this patient. ○ 1 ○ 2 ○ 3 ○ 4 ○ 5

7. I was punctual for the session. ○ 1 ○ 2 ○ 3 ○ 4 ○ 5

8. I was prepared for the session. ○ 1 ○ 2 ○ 3 ○ 4 ○ 5

9. I was dressed appropriately for this session. ○ 1 ○ 2 ○ 3 ○ 4 ○ 5

10. I used time efficiently during this session. ○ 1 ○ 2 ○ 3 ○ 4 ○ 5

11. I completed the assigned tasks during this session. ○ 1 ○ 2 ○ 3 ○ 4 ○ 5

12. I accurately determined correct versus incorrect responses. ○ 1 ○ 2 ○ 3 ○ 4 ○ 5

13. I provided appropriate feedback to the patient. ○ 1 ○ 2 ○ 3 ○ 4 ○ 5

14. The treatment environment was appropriate for this patient. ○ 1 ○ 2 ○ 3 ○ 4 ○ 5

15. I was aware of my professional boundaries during this session. ○ 1 ○ 2 ○ 3 ○ 4 ○ 5

16. I documented the results of the session appropriately. ○ 1 ○ 2 ○ 3 ○ 4 ○ 5

17. I shared the results with my supervision. ○ 1 ○ 2 ○ 3 ○ 4 ○ 5

Comments:

SLPA Signature: _____

CHAPTER 5

Cultural and Linguistic Diversity

Carolyn Conway Madding

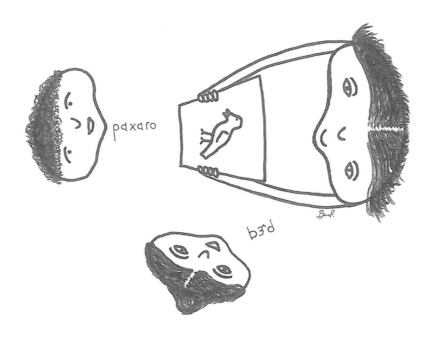

I know there is strength in the differences between us.
I know there is comfort where we overlap.

—Ani DiFranco (American singer, songwriter,
poet, and women's rights advocate)

DIVERSITY OVERVIEW: IMPORTANT STATISTICS

The United States has been a land of immigrants from its inception, resulting in a demographic collage that demonstrates great diversity. In fact, this coun- try is often referred to as the most diverse nation on earth. According to the U.S. Census National Population Projection Report (U.S. Census Bureau, 2021b), by 2044, more than half of all Americans are projected to belong to a minority group (any group other than non-Hispanic White alone), and by 2060, nearly one in five of the nation's total population is projected to be foreign born (Colby & Ortman, 2015). With diversity comes the challenge of integrating a multitude of cultures and languages into the tapestry of American life. As succinctly stated by Maya Angelou, "We should all know that diversity makes for a rich tapestry, and we must understand that all the threads of the tapestry are equal in value" (Angelou, 2021). Perhaps the most formidable tasks facing the United States in building the interwoven fabric of the United States lie in in the efforts to provide schooling and special education services to children, as well as health-related services to all who use myriad languages and come from a diversity of cultures.

According to Gambino (2017), the U.S. Census Bureau, American Community Survey is the most widely used source of language data in the country, and the 2019 survey revealed that more than 67 million persons (i.e., 67,802,345) in the United States older than 5 years use a language other than English in the home. The majority of those speaking a non-English language at home, however, are found within the Spanish-speaking community, numbering approximately 41 million individuals. Other non-English languages are represented by speakers of Indo-European languages, including dialects of French, Italian, Portuguese, German, Greek, Russian, and others (11,465,361); Asian and Pacific Island languages, including the Chinese macro-language, Japanese, Tagalog, Korean, Hmong, Vietnamese, Khmer, and others (10,973,317); and a variety of other languages, including Arabic (3,606,942). In total, 1,334 different languages are spoken in homes in the United States. According to the American Community Survey (2019), the percentage of individuals who spoke any language other than English as their primary language at home were highest in California (44.5%), followed by Texas (35.6%), New Mexico (34%), and New Jersey (32.2%). Those who spoke Spanish, the most widely used non-English home language, were most prevalent in California, Texas, New Mexico, and Florida.

Considering the vast number of languages spoken and the subsequent number of individuals who require services in those languages, capacity for appropriate speech-language services far exceeds the number of speech-language professionals available. According to ASHA (2021), of the 213,115 ASHA-certified individuals representing both audiologists and speech-language pathologists (SLPs), 8.2% self-identified as multilingual service providers. Of that group, SLPs numbered 15,728. There were 83 spoken languages used in service provision by the multilingual professionals. American Sign Language, Manually Coded English, and other *signed languages* were used by 934 audiologists and SLPs (ASHA, 2021). Of those multilingual ASHA-certified speech-language pathology service providers, nearly one half identified as of Hispanic or Latino descent and 10,807 spoke Spanish for assessment, therapy, and related services (ASHA, 2021).

The impact of language variations on municipalities, school districts, hospitals, and other community resources will continue to require adaptation in the foreseeable future. Many cities in the United States, as well as small towns and rural areas, must accommodate to provide best services for an everchanging demographic (ASHA, 2021). In our dynamic world that is subject to conflicts, wars, uprisings, and the need to flee for safety, there are, and will be, rising numbers of refugees and immigrants who speak languages such as

Ukrainian, Russian, Urdu, Pashto, Arabic, and a myriad of other world languages. Most communities will need to develop a concerted program to address cultural and linguistic diversity in order to provide appropriate speech-language services. To accomplish this goal, community members, interpreters, translators, transliterators, and other resources will be invaluable.

The challenges presented by immigrants and refugees, of course, serve to augment the existing need to provide appropriate services for those already within the American society. The United States is a patchwork of cultures, languages, and dialects, and although service providers cannot ever know the intricacies of such a multitude of languages and cultures, it is incumbent upon all to be dedicated to continuous and lifelong learning in this regard. The process begins by a self-examination of one's own culture, to be discussed later in this chapter.

Regardless of the professional service area covered by SLPs and speech-language pathology assistants (SLPAs), encountering language and cultural diversity is an existential certainty. In order to effectively compensate and adapt, all organizations and people within can develop awareness and subsequently strategize for positive outcomes. A preliminary step in the process is through intersectionality, which allows for the acknowledgment that everyone has their own experiences, which may include discrimination and oppression. Considerations of all the forces that can marginalize individuals, such as gender, race, class, sexual orientation, physical ability, country of origin, religion, or language used, should be examined as part of the pathway to cultural and linguistic understanding (Womankind, n.d.).

ASHA has therefore provided guidelines for assessment, intervention, and family interactions that embody the array of aforementioned factors. All speech-language professionals should follow ASHA's mandates for appropriate service provision to culturally and linguistically diverse (CLD) clients and students and avail themselves of continuing education opportunities related to CLD populations.

ASHA's commitment to diversity and inclusion dates back to 1969. According to ASHA, diversity encompasses the variety of experiences, skill, knowledge, and attributes that shape every individual, each of whom has a culture. As a professional organization, ASHA affirms the value of diversity and the importance of inclusion (D+I). Implicit in this affirmation is dedication by ASHA members, as well as to the people served, to practice and function in work environments where their clients are welcomed and valued, without discrimination or harassment. D+I is included in the ASHA Code of Ethics, and multicultural infusion is expected in all professional work (ASHA, 2016).

The sections of this chapter to follow, as well as the definitions at the end of this chapter, provide an overview of several important terms and concepts needed to serve CLD populations. Upon completion of the chapter, test your knowledge of this content with the questions in Appendix 5–A (answers provided).

DEFINITIONS, DISCUSSIONS, AND THE IMPORTANCE IN SERVICE PROVISION

According to Pappas and McKelvie (2021), culture is defined as the characteristics and knowledge of a particular group of people, encompassing language, religion, cuisine, social habits, music, and arts. It includes common patterns of behavior and establishes what is acceptable and not acceptable. Behaviors and beliefs of a culture are learned, and in the process of being passed from one generation to the next, changes are incorporated, incumbent with the times and with interactions among cultures. The latter can be seen in the influence of one culture upon another in language, the arts, and media.

Within the confines of the United States, myriad cultures exist, following their own ways of life. Cultural groups may not only be different from each other in their lifestyles and beliefs but may also speak languages and dialects specific to their groups, other than General American English (GAE). Note that GAE is in itself a dialect, often referred to in the literature as Mainstream American English. Note that failure to identify GAE as a dialect assigns it to a higher or more prestigious status than given to other dialects (Oetting, 2020). Due to the characteristics of life and language, groups differ both culturally and linguistically from other groups and from so-called mainstream culture. Mainstream culture is that which is widely recognized within a large number of people residing within a society and includes current modes of thought and expressions in media. In contrast to mainstream, some cultural enclaves may use GAE but may maintain a heritage language or dialect for in-group communication and may live within a blend of cultures, consisting of the mainstream and the specific group from which they arise. There are also diverse cultural groups, however, that use GAE, or another dialect of English, as their native or heritage language and differ only in their cultural attributes from so-called mainstream. They would be designated as culturally diverse but not necessarily linguistically diverse.

Dialects

In addition to numerous non-English languages spoken in the United States, dialectal variations of English abound. Dialects are rule-governed variations of a language. They may be spoken by a regional, ethnic, or socioeconomic group. Although dialects of a language are often intelligible to those outside the dialectal group, they may nevertheless vary in form, content, and use. Linguists often include 20 or more dialects of English used in the United States, including African American English, Appalachian English, Cajun English, Creole English, Rural Southern White English, and many others. ASHA's position statements have long recognized GAE as the prevalent term for the mainstream dialect of the United States. This is the dialect used in most educational settings and in the media. On the other hand, there are many other dialects used within the country. All dialects are rule governed and therefore do not represent a language deficit, nor should they be described as inferior or substandard. According to ASHA, all dialects represent a functional and effective tool of expression in English. Clinicians should be conscious of their individual attitudes toward certain dialects, whether they may seem prestigious or disparaged, as this can affect clinical services. Such an unconscious bias may be described as *linguicism*, or *accentism* (Grover et al., 2022).

It is ASHA's position, therefore, that no dialect of American English should be considered a speech or language disorder (ASHA, 2003). Speakers of English dialects do not present with language disorders but rather with language differences and dialectal differences. As such, they are not to be treated by SLPs or SLPAs. If an individual is referred for a screening or assessment and a culturally or linguistically appropriate assessment identifies only a dialectal difference from GAE, no further intervention is warranted. English dialect variation is neither invisible nor a *condition* (ASHA, 2003).

Similarly, if a referred client or student is bilingual or an English-language learner, influences of the individual's non-English language should not be construed as a deficit in English but as a language difference. As such, the client or student is not within the scope of treatment for the SLP or the SLPA. If the family or client wishes to produce English that is more consistent with GAE, an SLP with specialization in accent modification can assist by private arrangement, or other avenues can be explored by the individual or family. In schools, English-language learners should be enrolled in special courses to assist them in the development of English but should not be placed on the caseload of the SLP unless they present with a speech or language disorder in their native language, as well as in the emergence of English.

To differentiate between a language difference and a language disorder, the SLP must assess the client or student in all languages spoken. A true language disorder exists across languages as does a language-learning disability. If, however, assessment results identify variations in only one language, they are indicative of a language difference, not a language-learning disability. Box 5–1, as follows, contains helpful information as a knowledge base for use in addressing speech-language disorders in linguistically and culturally diverse populations.

Cultural Competence/Cultural Literacy/Cultural Humility

In any professional setting, a knowledge and understanding of linguistic and cultural diversity is mandatory for successful intervention. As stated by Lipson and Dibble (2005), "Health care professionals cannot provide good care without assessing both cultural group patterns and individual variation with a cultural group" (p. xi). Some ways to begin this process may be addressed through ethnographic methods; adept listening; an open, curious mind-set; and careful, considerate interviewing techniques (Agar, 1986). According to Westby et al. (2003), speech-language professionals "need to see the world through the eyes of the individuals they serve. Ethnographic interviewing provides a means of asking the right questions in the right ways to accomplish this." (p. 1) Ethnographic interviewing, through the clinician's open-ended questions, allows the client, student, or family to offer glimpses of their life and culture (Westby et al., 2003). To provide effective services, professionals must be attuned to all possible aspects of diversity, taking into consideration any issues related to racial or ethnic groups, language, dialect, religion, sexual orientation, age, and country of origin. Clinicians may collaborate with interpreters (oral language), translators (written language), transliterators (signed language), cultural informants, and cultural brokers to gain valuable knowledge leading to clinically appropriate services.

Professionals are not required to use the language of those referred for screening, assessment, or treatment, but understanding the basics of the culture is indeed important, even though the interactions may be through the use of an interpreter, a translator, or a transliterator.

Box 5–1. What Clinicians Should Know About Bilingualism and Speech–Language Disorders

- Most children, even those presenting with language disorders, have the capacity and facility to learn more than one language (ASHA, n.d.-a). Levels of function will vary between or among the languages, however, and one language will usually be dominant.
- Learning two languages will not confuse children, although dual-language development may be prolonged. Learning more than one language does not represent a cognitive overload so long as both languages are supported (Genesee, 2003).
- Bilingualism represents a positive effect and supports the acquisition of a second language (Uchikoshi & Maniates, 2010).
- Bilingual children develop an earlier understanding of taxonomic relations than their monolingual peers (e.g., *car* and *bus* are vehicles) (Marian et al., 2009).
- Bilingualism imposes costs to language processing but benefits to word learning (Bogulski et al., 2019).
- Empirical evidence suggests that bilingualism in children is associated with increased meta-cognitive skills (Marian et al., 2009).
- Bilingual and multilingual children must be assessed in each of their languages to differentiate between a language difference and a language disorder.
- Parents should be encouraged to maintain and model the home language, as this is their best language model. Suggesting the *English Only* home model not only limits overall language development but is also not ethical and does not have a research base. It also violates an ASHA mandate (ASHA, n.d.-a). Furthermore, it is both culturally and linguistically inappropriate, can be considered offensive, and may be construed as elitism, as well.

The ability to understand and relate effectively with individuals from different cultures and language groups has been frequently referred to as cultural competence (Hoodin, 2011) or cultural literacy (Haynes et al., 2012).

According to Khan (2021), the concept of cultural competence arose as part of the civil rights movement of the 1960s and 1970s. The term became widely used in health care and educational settings as a way to suggest that the more cultural knowledge one has, the more competent will be the professional service provided. Cultural competence terminology has evolved to cultural humility and sensitivity.

Cultural competence or cultural humility within a group other than one's own does not emerge spontaneously with the ability to produce, listen, comprehend, or read and write a nonnative language. A person must have experience within the community, often but not necessarily in tandem with language proficiency, to begin to develop a semblance of cultural understanding. Language ability in a nonnative language does not, therefore, equate to having cultural identity with the population. Community involvement, in tandem with language proficiency, will assist in the development of humility, sensitivity, and empathy, on the path to cultural competence. According to Khan (2021), the assumption that practitioners who are somehow culturally competent and can engage knowledgeably with people across cultures, and are therefore arbiters, is a false assumption. It can lead to bias and stereotyping, and it does not account for the lifelong learning required for so-called cultural competence through cultural humility and sensitivity.

The components of cultural humility consist of self-reflection, acknowledgment of one's own biases, ongoing curiosity, recognition that in sameness there are differences, and realization that there is never an end point in development of interpersonal knowledge. Cultural humility allows the clinician to genuinely attempt to comprehend a person's identities related to race and ethnicity, gender, sexual orientation, socioeconomic status, education, social needs, and others (Khan, 2021). In other words, cultural humility is a way of thinking, cultural competence is a way of becoming, and culturally responsive practice is a way of doing (That's Unheard of, n.d.).

When SLPAs decide to learn a second language to work more empathically and appropriately with individuals, their experience is restricted in some ways. Those who are nonnative language users differ from native or heritage language speakers in that language and culture may be learned linearly by nonnative users, that is, over considerable time. Conversely, native users learn the culture and language cohesively as a developmental process. Thus, they are often unaware of the enmeshing of language and culture. The professional who is learning the language and culture of another group must invest extensive time to approach being both linguistically and culturally competent (Madding, 2002). Cultural and linguistic knowledge is often appreciated by individuals and families being served but should not be construed as in-group acceptance.

In summary, language is the principal means through which the socialization process takes place. Culture and language are therefore inextricably intertwined during a child's development (Madding, 2002). Approaching cultural competence as a person outside the group requires time, attention to cues, and an intense interest in the culture and language. SLPAs, as part of the professional team addressing the needs of each client or student, should avail themselves of opportunities to learn as much as possible about the cultural and language background of every client (ASHA, 2022). Awareness is the first principle, followed by interest, investigation, and learning. SLPAs will be pleasantly surprised when clients react favorably to an interest in their culture, as well as when respect is shown for cultural values. Learning the language of the client, or being able to greet clients in their heritage language, represents a preliminary step in the continuum of cultural competence acquisition.

To learn more about a culture, we must first recognize the characteristics, values, and beliefs of our own culture. Then we can begin to ascertain the ways in which the behaviors and beliefs of others differ from each other and from the ones with which we are most familiar. Appendix 5–B contains cultural consciousness activities to help you explore your own cultural mores or rules. Acknowledging your own culture but respecting what is honored and cherished by others is of utmost importance in the practice of speech-language pathology.

We can learn about other cultures and languages through the Internet, from books and journal articles, through interpersonal relationships, and from cultural informants and cultural and linguistic brokers. The latter are those from the cultural community who can answer questions and provide information that will help the SLP and SLPA to approach and interact with clients, students, and families in a culturally appropriate manner. The cultural informant or broker must be knowledgeable about the specific client or student's culture and language community (ASHA, n.d.-b).

LANGUAGES OTHER THAN ENGLISH

As stated previously, according to the U.S. Census Bureau, American Community Survey (2019), there are more than 67 million individuals in the country, age 5 years and older, who speak a language other than English. Due to the free movement of populations within the United States, professionals in every state and territory may encounter clients or students who use any of these languages. It is therefore a priority to become acquainted with the basic characteristics of the language and related cultural distinctions of the student or client referred to the SLP and the SLPA.

Languages and Countries— A Guide for the Professional

SLPs and SLPAs can access phonemic inventories for many different languages and dialects at the following ASHA website: https://www.asha.org/practice/mul ticultural/phono/ (ASHA, n.d.-c). Cultural profiles and resources for service providers for a variety of groups are also included, as well as videos of assessment and treatment of bilingual individuals. The following languages are included in ASHA's phonemic inventory: Amharic, Arabic, Bosnian, Burmese, Chinese, English (including dialects), Haitian Creole, Hindi/Urdu, Hmong, Japanese, Korean, Pashto and Persian, Polish, Russian, Spanish (including regional dialects), Somali, Tagalog, Turkish, and Vietnamese. Information related to refugee populations is also presented at this website.

THE SLP AS AN INTERPRETER, A TRANSLATOR, OR A TRANSLITERATOR

As a solution to the relatively small corpus of bilingual SLPs to serve CLD populations, ASHA encourages the development of collaborative relationships with interpreters, translators, and transliterators (ASHA, n.d.-b; Langdon, 2002). Bilingual SLPAs may provide a valuable service to their supervising SLP and to the clients served, either as a direct service provider under supervision or as an interpreter (oral), translator (written), or transliterator (signed). See definitions at the end of the chapter for further differentiation among these roles. ASHA's 2022 SLPA Scope-of-Practice Document acknowledges these roles, stating that provided adequate training, planning, and supervision, SLPAs may perform the following tasks (ASHA, 2022):

- Assist the SLP with bilingual interpretation, translation, or transliteration during screening and assessment activities, exclusive of interpretation of results.
- Serve as interpreter, translator, or transliterator for patients, clients, students, and families who do not use English, or who use a signed language.

- Provide services under SLP supervision in another language for individuals who do not use English and for English-language learners.

Your Role as an Interpreter, a Translator, or a Transliterator

As an SLPA, to serve as a qualified interpreter, translator, or transliterator, you must carefully follow guidelines provided by ASHA (n.d.-d) and others who have written extensively in this area. Box 5–2 provides an overview of these requirements. Subsequent to gaining thorough background knowledge of your role as interpreter, translator, or transliterator, you may begin to work in this

---

Box 5–2. Basic Requirements for the SLPA to Serve as Interpreter, Translator, or Transliterator

1. Native or near-native high level of proficiency in the student's or client's native language or dialect, or signed method
2. Professional level of ability to provide accurate and complete oral interpretation or written translation
3. Familiarity with and respect for the student's or client's culture and language community
4. Knowledge of professional terminology
5. Maintenance of client, student, or family confidentiality of information
6. High-level oral and written or signing proficiency in both English and the non-English other language spoken or signed
7. Maintenance of neutrality between yourself and the client, student, or family
8. Ability to provide interpretation, translation, or transliteration without addition, subtraction, or commentary
9. Knowledge of assessment and therapeutic techniques, with special emphasis on those to be used with bilingual or non-English-speaking clients or students

capacity, under the guidance of your supervising SLP.

How to Prepare for Your Role as an Interpreter, a Translator, or a Transliterator

Box 5–3 outlines helpful tips in preparing to work as an interpreter, a translator, or a transliterator.

WORKING WITH AN INTERPRETER, A TRANSLATOR, OR A TRANSLITERATOR

When you are assigned to work with a client or student who is bilingual or whose language is not one you speak, your first step is to consult with your supervising SLP.

As your supervisor, the SLP is legally and ethically responsible for all clients and students on the caseload and delegates tasks to you, the SLPA (ASHA, 2022). You must have the compliance and permission of the SLP before you can seek the interpreter, translator, or transliterator you need for appropriate intervention (ASHA, 2020). Keeping in mind the ASHA mandates for service provision mentioned earlier in this chapter, be sure to express the importance of contacting a qualified interpreter, translator, or transliterator to assist in your interactions with the client or student. Legal and ethical standards (ASHA, 2020); Civil Rights Act of 1964, as amended; and the Individuals

---

Box 5–3. Helpful Tips for the SLPA in Preparation to Serve as an Interpreter, a Translator, or a Transliterator

1. Although you may be bilingual or are efficient in a signed language, do not volunteer or allow yourself to be solicited as an interpreter, a translator, or a transliterator, unless you meet all the minimum requirements listed in Box 5–2. SLPs and other team members may urge you to take on the role when they learn of your bilingual skills. Be honest about your abilities and maintain adherence to basic requirements listed in Box 5–2.

2. Do not serve as an interpreter, a translator, or a transliterator if you are not from the same language community or cultural background as the client or student. Examples of mismatches: You are Mexican American, and the client is from Spain or Argentina; you are Egyptian American, and your client is from Yemen; you are Mexican American, and your client is from a rural, indigenous community in Guatemala. Mismatches such as these may result in inaccurate interpretations, translations, and cultural misunderstandings. To avoid mismatches, seek the advice of cultural informants and cultural brokers.

With Disabilities Education Act of 1990, as amended, all require that services to individuals who speak a language other than spoken English must be delivered in the language most appropriate to the student, client, patient, or family.

Choosing an Interpreter, a Translator, or a Transliterator

Many school districts, hospitals, and other service sites maintain a bank of interpreters, translators, and transliterators. Inquire if such a list exists and whether the interpreters, translators, or transliterators meet the basic requirements listed in Box 5–2. In cases where no resources are available, it is incumbent upon the supervising SLP to locate and train an interpreter, a translator, or a transliterator. A cultural informant may assist in locating an appropriate person or one who is willing to be trained. Family members, and most especially children, should not be solicited for this task for many reasons. Among those may be a vested interest in the case of the client, difficulty in being impartial, and the tendency to cue the client. Children may be embarrassed, cannot be counted on to maintain confidentiality, and do not possess the maturity to follow the basic requirements to be an interpreter, a translator, or a transliterator. Whenever possible, choose a trained professional, or make arrangements for training.

Using an Interpreter, a Translator, or a Transliterator

Box 5–4 provides helpful tips for working with an interpreter, a translator, or a transliterator, including guidelines for before, during, and after treatment sessions.

Bilingual: A bilingual individual possesses the ability to use more than one language effectively (Bhatia & Ritchie, 2006). A bilingual person may be fully competent in oral languages (or sign and speech) without the ability to read or write in more than one language.

Bilingual service provider: Bilingual service providers are those individuals who "speak their primary language and speak (or sign) at least one other language with native or near-native proficiency in lexicon (vocabulary), semantics (meaning), phonology (pronunciation), morphology/syntax (grammar), and pragmatics (uses) during clinical management. In addition to linguistic proficiency, bilingual service providers must have the specific knowledge and skill sets necessary for the services to be delivered" (ASHA, n.d.-d, Bilingual Service Providers, para. 1).

Accentism: A term used to describe discriminatory or unfair behavior centered on someone's accent or language.

Biliterate: A biliterate person is one who speaks, reads, and writes effectively in more than one language.

BIPOC: A term specific to the United States that stands for Black, Indigenous, and People of Color. Demonstrates the solidarity between communities of color.

Cultural broker: A person knowledgeable about the client's/patient's culture and/or speech-language community. The broker passes cultural/community-related information between the client and the clinician in order to optimize services. The cultural broker overlaps with the services of a cultural informant.

Box 5–4. Helpful Tips in Working With an Interpreter, a Translator, or a Transliterator (ASHA, n.d.-d)

Before the Session

1. Meet with the interpreter, translator, or transliterator. Plan sufficient time to review the procedures, goals, and professional terminology and to develop rapport.
2. Remind the interpreter, translator, or transliterator to avoid nonverbal cues such as intonational changes or hand gestures.
3. Ensure that the interpreter, translator, or transliterator will maintain confidentiality.
4. Inquire about specific cultural or linguistic information that may assist you in working with the client.
5. Learn the appropriate greetings and hierarchy within the family and learn the proper pronunciation of names. Hierarchy within the family may have important implications for appropriate service delivery (e.g., person to be addressed as head of family, etc.).

During the Session

1. Define your role as the SLPA and introduce the interpreter, translator, or transliterator to the client.
2. Talk directly to the client and not to the interpreter, translator, or transliterator.
3. Interpreters, translators, and transliterators should also look at the person to whom they are communicating (i.e., the client and then responsively to you).
4. Use short, concise sentences to allow for careful, thorough interpretation or translation.
5. Allow sufficient time for the interpreter or transliterator to convey your message to the client in the client's language and to relay the client's message back to you in English.

Wrap-Up Session

1. Plan sufficient time at the end of your session to review with the interpreter, translator, or transliterator.
2. If the client or family has brought in written material, ask for it to be translated for you. This can be done after the session.
3. Review the session and answer any questions the interpreter, translator, or transliterator may have.
4. Thank the interpreter, translator, or transliterator and congratulate him or her on a job well done.

Cultural informant: A person with whom a professional may consult to learn more about a cultural community, a linguistic community, or both. The cultural informant should be a member of that community. To avoid bias, more than one cultural informant may be used. The goal in using information about the community is to optimize services for the client (ASHA, n.d.-a). The informant may provide information relative to topics such as child-rearing, language and dialect usage, and attitudes toward disabilities (Anderson, 2002).

Dialect: A dialect is defined as "a rule governed variation of a language used by a definable group of people characterized by their culture, ethnicity, or geographical region" (Haynes et al., 2012, p. 426).

Cultural humility: Cultural humility refers to a dynamic and lifelong process focusing on self-reflection and personal critique, acknowledging one's own biases. It encourages ongoing curiosity rather than an end point, thus recognizing that a clinician will never be fully competent about the evolving and dynamic nature of a patient's experiences (Khan, 2021).

D+I: This acronym stands for diversity and inclusion.

Ethnicity: Ethnicity is variously defined as the affiliation with a population group; having a common cultural heritage or nationality; or distinguished by customs, characteristics, languages, and common history.

Ethnographic methods or ethnography: An ethnographic method allows an individual to observe and conscientiously collect information about the life and culture of a specific group. Observations and data collection occur over time and can reveal the mores, beliefs, and interactional styles of a group. Ethnographic or qualitative study is descriptive and thus can be especially useful in understanding linguistically and culturally diverse communities (Brice, 2002).

Heritage language: A heritage language, sometimes referred to as the native or home language, is one used by a family, cultural group, or both and usually the first language to which a child is exposed. Heritage refers to the fact that the language is passed down from generation to generation.

Interpreter: An interpreter is a bilingual person specially trained to translate convey spoken or signed communications from one language to another (ASHA, n.d.-b).

Intersectionality: The complex, cumulative way in which the effects of multiple forms of discrimination (such as racism, sexism, and classism) combine and overlap, or intersect, especially in the experience of marginalized individuals or groups (https://www.merriam-webster.com). According to Crenshaw (2017), who introduced the term, intersectionality is the social components that make a person.

Language difference: As opposed to a language disorder, a language difference is characterized by variations from General American English in phonology, morphology, syntax, semantics, and pragmatics, as the result of the influence of another language or dialect.

Language disorder: A language disorder is defined as "impaired comprehension and/or use of spoken, written, signed, and/or other symbol systems. The disorder may involve: (1) the form of language (phonology, morphology, syntax), (2) the content of language (semantics), and/or (3) the function of language in communication (pragmatics) in any combination" (ASHA, 1993).

Latinx, Latino, Hispanic: These are all terms used to identify persons of Spanish and/or mixed heritage. Latinx is a relatively new term used to refer to people of Spanish and/or mixed heritage without regard for gender and thus is differentiated from Latino, a general term for all people of the group, or a male member of the group. *Hispanic* is a word that came into use during the 1970s as a means of identifying a group of persons of Spanish or mixed heritage as a conglomerate (i.e., individuals whose families emanate from Mexico, Cuba, Central America, Puerto Rico, et al.).

Linguicism: An unconscious bias toward certain dialect variations.

Linguistic broker: A linguistic broker is a person knowledgeable about the client's/patient's speech community or communication environment who can provide valuable information about language and sociolinguistic norms in the client's/patient's speech community and communication environment.

Macrolanguage: A language consisting of widely varying dialects; a group of mutually intelligible speech varieties that are sometimes considered distinct languages. Example: Mandarin, Cantonese, Taiwanese, et al.

Microaggression: A comment or action that subtly and often unconsciously or unintentionally expresses a prejudiced attitude toward a member of a marginalized group (such as a racial minority) (https://www.merriam-webster.com).

Translator: A translator, as opposed to an interpreter, is a person trained to translate written text from one language to another.

Transliterator: A transliterator is a person trained to facilitate communication for individuals from one form to another form of the same language. This person would be typically used to address the communication interactions of persons who are deaf or hard of hearing and who use oral, cued, or manual communication systems rather than a formal sign language.

REFERENCES

Agar, M. (1986). *Speaking of ethnography.* Sage.

American Community Survey. (2019). *5-Year data 2019.* www.census.gov/.../data-sets/acs-5 year/2019.html

American Speech-Language-Hearing Association. (n.d.-a). *Learning two languages.* https://www.asha.org/public/speech/development/learning-two-languages/

American Speech-Language-Hearing Association. (n.d.-b). *Collaborating with interpreters, transliterators, and translators* [Practice portal]. https://www.asha.org/Practice-Portal/Professional-Issues/Collaborating-With-Interpreters/

American Speech-Language-Hearing Association. (n.d.-c). *Phonemic inventories across languages.* http://www.asha.org/practice/multicultural/Phono/

American Speech-Language-Hearing Association. (n.d.-d). *Bilingual service delivery.* https://www.asha.org/practice-portal/professional-issues/bilingual-service-delivery/#collapse_4

American Speech-Language-Hearing Association. (1993). *Definitions of communication disorders and variations* [Relevant paper]. http://www.asha.org/policy.

American Speech-Language-Hearing Association. (2003). *American English dialects* [Technical report]. https://www.asha.org/policy.

American Speech-Language-Hearing Association. (2016). *Code of ethics.* https://www.asha.org/code-of-ethics/

American Speech-Language-Hearing Association. (2020). *Assistants code of conduct.* https://www.asha.org/policy/assistants-code-of-conduct/

American Speech-Language-Hearing Association. (2021). *Demographic profile of ASHA members providing multilingual services.* https://www.asha.org/siteassets/surveys/demographic-profile-bilingual-spanish-service-members.pdf

American Speech-Language-Hearing Association. (2022). *Speech-language pathology assistant scope of practice.* https://www.asha.org/policy/slpa-scope-of-practice/

Anderson, R. (2002). Practical assessment strategies with Hispanic students. In A. Brice (Ed.), *The Hispanic child: Speech, language, culture and education* (pp. 143–184). Allyn & Bacon.

Angelou, M. (2021). *We all should know that diversity makes for a rich tapestry, and we must understand that all the threads of* [Tweet]. Twitter.com

Bhatia, T., & Ritchie, W. (Eds.). (2006). *The handbook of bilingualism.* Blackwell.

Bogulski, C., Bice, K., & Kroll, J. (2019). Bilingualism as a desirable difficulty: Advantages in word learning depend on regulation of the dominant language. *Bilingualism: Language and Cognition, 22*(5), 1052–1067. https://doi.org/10.1017/S1366728918000858

Brice, A. (2002). Clinician as a qualitative researcher. In A. Brice (Ed.), *The Hispanic child: Speech, language, culture, and education* (pp. 85–99). Allyn & Bacon.

Colby, S. L., & Ortman, J. M. (2015). *Projections of the size and composition of the U.S. population: 2014 to 2060. Current Population Reports. Projections of the size and composition of the U.S. population: 2014 to 2060.* https://mronline.org/wp-content/uploads/2019/08/p25-1143.pdf

Crenshaw, K. W. (2017). *On intersectionality: Essential writings.* The New Press.

Gambino, C. (2017). *Inside the American Community Survey: 2016 language data overhaul.* www.census.gov.../2017/09/inside-the-american.html

Genesee, F. (2003). Rethinking bilingual acquisition. In J. Dewaele, A. Housen, & L. Wei (Eds.), *Bilingualism: Beyond basic principles* (pp. 204–229). Multilingual Matters.

Grover, V., Namasivayam, A., & Madendra, N. (2022). A viewpoint on accent services: Framing and terminology matter. *American Journal of Speech-Language Pathology, 31*(2), 639–648. https://doi.org/10.1044/2021_AJSLP-20-00376

Haynes, W., Moran, M., & Pindzola, R. (2012). *Communication disorders in educational and medical settings: An introduction for speech-language pathologists, educators, and health professionals.* Jones & Bartlett Learning.

Hoodin, R. (2011). *Intervention in child language disorders: A comprehensive handbook.* Jones & Bartlett Learning.

Khan, S. (2021). *Cultural humility vs cultural competence—and why providers need both.* https://healthycity.bmc.org/policy-and-industry/culturalhumility-vs-culturalcompetence-provider

Langdon, H. (2002). Language interpreters and translators: Bridging communication with clients and families. *ASHA Leader, 7,* 14–15. http://doi.org/10.1044/leader.FTR4.0706 2002.14

Lipson, J., & Dibble, S. (2005). *Culture and clinical care.* University of California San Francisco Nursing Press.

Madding, C. (2002). Socialization practices of Latinos. In A. Brice (Ed.), *The Hispanic child: Speech, language, culture, and education* (pp. 66–84). Allyn & Bacon.

Marian, V., Faroqi-Shah, Y., Kaushanskaya, M., Blumenfeld, H., & Sheng, L. (2009). *Bilingualism: Consequences for language, cognition, development, and the brain.* http://leader.pubs.asha.org/doi/10.1044/leader.ftr2.14132009.10

Oetting, J. (2020). *From my personal perspective/opinion: General American English as a dialect: A call for change.* http://leader.pubs.asha.org/do/10.1044/leader.FMP.25112020.12/full

Pappas, S., & McKelvie, C. (2021). *What is culture?* Live Science. www.livescience.com

That's Unheard of. (n.d.). *Care without cultural competence?* https://www.thatsunheardof.org/

Uchikoshi, Y., & Maniates, H. (2010). How does bilingual instruction enhance English achievement? A mixed-methods study of Cantonese-speaking and Spanish-speaking bilingual classrooms. *Bilingual Research Journal, 33*(3), 364–385. http://doi.org/10.1080/15235882.2010.525294

U.S. Census Bureau. (2021a). *2014 National Population Projections Tables.* https://www.census.gov/data/tables/2014/demo/popproj/2014-summary-tables.html

U.S. Census Bureau. (2021b). *Detailed languages spoken at home and ability to speak English for the population 5 years and over: 2009–2013.* American Community Survey. https://www.census.gov/data/tables/2013/demo/2009-2013-lang-tables.html

Westby, C., Burda, A., & Mehta, Z. (2003). Asking the right questions in the right ways: Strategies for ethnographic interviewing. *The ASHA Leader, 8,* 8, https://doi.org/10.1044/leader.FTR3.08082003.4

Womankind. (n.d.). *Womankind: 40 years.* https://www.iamwomankind.org/

APPENDIX 5–A
Chapter Review Self-Test

Number	Question	T/F
1.	*Interpreter* and *translator* are synonymous terms.	
2.	Clinicians should suggest that non-English-speaking families speak to their children in English in the home.	
3.	Being bilingual indicates that a person will be an appropriate interpreter or translator.	
4.	The development of cultural competence and cultural humility is an ongoing process.	
5.	Only a bilingual SLPA may work with a non-English-speaking client or student.	
6.	The interpreter, translator, or transliterator should be acquainted with the procedures of the upcoming session before it begins.	
7.	The interpreter, translator, or transliterator must be neutral, ethical, and maintain confidentiality.	
8.	A bilingual child may have a language disorder in just one of his/her languages.	
9.	A student using a dialect other than the General American English (GAE) dialect, should receive speech-language services in order to develop GAE.	
10.	Most students or clients in the United States cannot be served in their first or home language by certified bilingual speech-language pathologists.	
11.	A bilingual or multilingual student may be assessed in only his/her dominant language.	
12.	In most bilingual or multilingual individuals, one language is dominant.	

Self-Test Answers: 1. F; 2. F; 3. F; 4. T; 5. F; 6. T; 7. T; 8. F; 9. F; 10. T; 11. F; 12. T

APPENDIX 5–B
Cultural Consciousness Activities

1. Think about your own culture (specific to the geographic and familial environment in which you were raised) and list five rules or mores of your culture. (Examples: father is head of the house; church on Sunday is a must, education of children #1 goal, etc.)

2. Thinking of your responses to Question 1, can you think of some cultures where the rules or mores are different?

3. Describe an ideal family in the culture of your childhood.

4. Describe the attitude of your culture toward disabilities.

5. Check the culturally linked attitudes and behaviors that are associated with your culture:

_____ Punctuality

_____ Elders have final authority

_____ Informal child rearing (few rules)

_____ Birthright inheritance

_____ Assertiveness, directness

_____ High expectations for child

_____ Formality in family relationships

_____ Nuclear family most important

_____ Greater family (all relatives) most important; family cohesiveness

_____ Independence valued

_____ Religious family orientation

_____ Respect for elderly

_____ All older people considered as parents

_____ Matriarchal family structure

_____ Patriarchal family structure

_____ Competition between siblings valued

_____ Equality in family structure

_____ Adults defined by occupation

_____ Marriage affirmed by children

_____ Divorce acceptable

_____ Unmarried children should live with parents

_____ Privacy valued

_____ Freedom of opinion

_____ Family democracy

_____ Importance of tradition

_____ Family above personal gain

CHAPTER 6

Health and Safety

Pei-Fang Hung

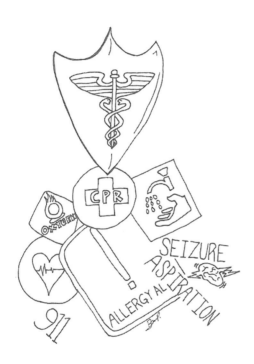

An ounce of prevention is worth a pound of cure.
—Benjamin Franklin (scientist/inventor and
Founding Father of the United States)

The aim of this chapter is to describe various health-related matters that a speech-language pathology assistant (SLPA) may encounter when working with clients in various clinical settings, such as childcare centers, schools, community clinics, long-term care facilities, private homes, and hospital settings. The purpose is to provide an overview of common medical conditions related to your work as an SLPA and practical information to ensure a safe working environment for you and the clients you serve. In the following sections, we will discuss infection control, standard precautions, first aid procedures, cardiopulmonary resuscitation (CPR), common medical conditions related to SLPA work, and additional considerations about working with clients who have special medical needs.

INFECTION CONTROL AND STANDARD PRECAUTIONS

Infectious diseases are caused by microorganisms called pathogens, which infect their hosts (Signore, 2013). The most common pathogens include various bacteria, viruses, fungi, and protozoa (Signore, 2013). For example, severe acute respiratory syndrome coronavirus 2 (SARS-CoV-2) is the name of the new virus that causes coronavirus disease 2019 (COVID-19). These microorganisms are transmitted via several routes, which

can be direct or indirect. Direct disease transmission can either be direct contact or droplet spread. Indirect disease transmission can be airborne, vehicle borne, or vector borne. Box 6–1 summarizes the modes of transmission. According to the World Health Organization (WHO, 2020a), SARS-CoV-2 can be transmitted through both direct and indirect transmission (i.e., direct contract, droplet, airborne, and fomite transmission through infected secretions).

The purpose of infection control is to ensure the protection of individuals who are at risk of acquiring an infection in various settings, such as in the general community or while receiving health care treatment (CDC, 2021a). When receiving health care treatment, clients/patients are vulnerable to health care–associated infections (HAIs). Many HAIs are caused by

---

Box 6–1. Modes of Transmission
(Centers for Disease Control and Prevention [CDC], 2012; WHO, 2020b)

Contact Transmission

Contact transmission is divided into direct and indirect contact. Two examples of contact transmissible infectious agents include methicillin-resistant *Staphylococcus aureus* (MRSA) and vancomycin-resistant enterococcus (VRE).

- Direct contact transmission refers to the transfer of infectious agents through physical contact with an infected individual. An example of direct body-to-body physical contact includes touching an infectious person. It also refers to contact with soil or vegetation harboring infectious organisms. Examples of direct contact diseases include sexually transmitted infection (STIs) and rubella (German measles).
- Indirect contact transmission (a.k.a. fomite transmission) occurs when there is no direct human-to-human contact

and involves the transfer of infections agents by making physical contact with contaminated items and surfaces. Frequently touched surfaces (fomites) include door knobs, computer keyboards, handles, washroom surfaces, phones, and so on.

Droplet Transmission

Droplets are produced when talking, coughing, or sneezing. Infectious droplets can travel through air but cannot remain suspended in the air because they are large particles (>10 micrometers). Some diseases (e.g., common cold, influenza, etc.) can be transferred by infected droplets contacting surfaces of the eye, nose, or mouth. When these droplets drop, they can contaminate the surrounding environment and cause indirect contact transmission.

Airborne Transmission

Airborne (aerosol) transmission occurs when very small particles (microorganisms <10 micrometers) containing infectious agents spread in the air and remain suspended in the air for a long period of time. The pathogens enter the respiratory tract to cause infection, such as tuberculosis (TB), measles, influenza, pertussis (whooping cough), and so on. It is important to note that airborne transmission does not require face-to-face contact with an infected individual.

Vehicle-Borne Transmission

Vehicle-borne infections result from contact with vehicles, which are contaminated, nonmoving objects. Vehicle-borne transmission is a type of indirect transmission of an infectious agent that occurs when microorganisms are transmitted by ingesting or contacting contaminated items, such as food or water sources. Examples of vehicle-borne diseases include hepatitis A and cholera.

Vector-Borne Transmission

Vector-borne transmission occurs when pathogens are transmitted through vectors, such as mosquitoes, flies, ticks, or rats. Vectors are living organisms that can transmit infectious pathogens between humans or from animals to humans (WHO, 2020b). Examples of vector-borne diseases include West Nile virus, Lyme disease, yellow fever, malaria, and so on.

the most urgent and dangerous antibiotic-resistant bacteria (e.g., methicillin-resistant *Staphylococcus aureus* [MRSA]) and may lead to sepsis or death. According to the U.S. CDC (2017), about 1 out of 25 hospitalized patients is diagnosed with at least one HAI. Fortunately, many HAIs are preventable.

All health care providers, including SLPAs, are responsible for providing safe care to clients. According to the World Health Organization, infection prevention and control is a practical, evidence-based approach that prevents spread of infection and ensures the protection of individuals who might be vulnerable to infection (WHO, 2009). The American Speech-Language-Hearing Association (ASHA) includes infection control within program operation in its policy documents: Quality Indicators for Professional Service Programs in Audiology and Speech-Language Pathology: Section III. D. Physical Facilities, Equipment, and Program Environment. It states that "the program establishes and maintains an environment that protects the health and safety of persons served and program personnel by implementing policies that address universal precautions, infection control, risk management, radiation exposure, and emergency preparedness" (ASHA, 2005, para. 1).

SLPAs may be exposed to a variety of infectious diseases when performing their duties. As such, it is critical to protect yourself and your clients from the spread of disease in all forms. If you do not take effective precautions against infection, you are at high risk of becoming infected. Similarly, without effective protection, there is a high possibility that the infectious disease can further spread to your clients, colleagues, family members, and the community at large. Therefore, infection control is essential to all health care providers, including SLPAs.

Standard precautions (previously known as universal precautions) are "the minimum infection prevention practices that apply to all patient care, regardless of suspected or confirmed infection status of the patient, in any setting where healthcare is delivered" (CDC, 2016a, Standard Precautions, para. 1). Standard precautions are designed to protect health care providers and to prevent infections from being spread. Key standard precautions important to an SLPA include hand hygiene, use of personal protective equipment, safe handling of potentially contaminated equipment or surfaces, and respiratory hygiene/cough etiquette.

Hand Hygiene

Hand hygiene is the most important and effective way to prevent infection and to reduce the risk of spreading infections (WHO, 2009). Good hand hygiene includes (a) hand washing with clean, running water and soap and (b) the use of alcohol-based hand rubs. Washing hands with soap and water is the best way to prevent health care–associated infections; using hand sanitizer cannot replace washing hands with soap and water. You should only use hand sanitizer when hands are not visibly soiled or when you cannot use or access soap and water (Wigglesworth, 2019). Table 6–1 summarizes the proper steps in hand washing and hand rubbing, as recommended by CDC (2022a) and WHO (2009). For a comprehensive review of hand hygiene, please refer to the WHO Guidelines on Hand Hygiene in Health Care (WHO, 2009). In addition, the CDC

Table 6–1. Steps for Proper Hand Washing and Hand Rubbing

Hand Washing	Hand Rubbing
1. Remove hand and arm jewelry.	1. Remove hand and arm jewelry.
2. Wet hands with warm water and apply soap.	2. Apply between one and two full pumps of alcohol-based hand sanitizer onto one palm.
3. Rub all aspects of hands for a minimum of 15 seconds, concentrating on the fingertips, between fingers, the back of hands, and the base of thumbs.	3. Spread product over all surfaces of both hands, concentrating on the fingertips, between fingers, the back of hands, and the base of thumbs.
4. Rinse and dry hands thoroughly with an air dryer or paper towel.	4. Rub hands until product is dry.
5. Turn off taps with paper towel.	

Source: CDC, 2011; Interorganizational Group for Speech Language Pathology and Audiology, 2010.

also offers an online training course for hand hygiene (the course can be accessed at https://www.cdc.gov/handhygiene/training/interactiveEducation/).

For SLPAs, hand hygiene should be performed in, but not limited to, the following conditions (CDC, 2020a; WHO, 2009):

- Before and after treating a client
- After touching objects (e.g., clinical materials, toys) or surfaces (e.g., door handles, tables) that may be frequently touched by other people (especially for mitigating SARS-CoV-2 infection)
- After touching blood, body fluids, or any contaminated items even when gloves are worn
- Immediately after removing personal protective equipment, such as gloves, masks, and so on
- Immediately if skin is contaminated or injury occurs
- After activities involving personal body functions, such as blowing one's nose

Also, SLPAs should encourage clients to perform hand hygiene at the beginning of the therapy session, prior to handling task materials, or after activities involving personal body functions.

Personal Protective Equipment

When there is a risk of coming in contact with nonintact skin, mucous membranes, or body fluids, personal protective equipment is required. According to the Occupational Safety and Health Administration (OSHA, n.d.), personal protective equipment refers to equipment designed to protect the wearer from workplace injury and to minimize exposure to hazards that cause illness. Examples of personal protective equipment include facemasks/respirators, gloves, goggles, helmets, and protective clothing.

The most commonly worn personal protective equipment is gloves. Gloves act as a barrier between the skin and potentially hazardous agents and should be worn when there is a risk of coming in contact with nonintact skin, mucous membranes, or body fluids; however, wearing gloves should not replace good hand hygiene. For SLPAs, the following common situations may require wearing gloves:

- Assisting with an oral peripheral examination or oral hygiene
- Handling dirty materials
- Working with clients who are immunocompromised or when additional precaution is needed (e.g., clients with *Clostridium difficile* infection)
- Assisting with feeding and swallowing treatment activities
- When touching someone's body fluids (such as blood, respiratory secretions, vomit, urine, or feces), certain hazardous drugs, or potentially contaminated items

Using gloves correctly is essential (CDC, 2016a). It is important to select the proper glove material. For example, vinyl gloves are designed for personal care and latex gloves are for sterile invasive procedures. Avoiding latex gloves should be considered to prevent latex allergies. Second, be sure to use the correct size of gloves and do not reuse single-use disposable gloves. Lastly, before touching a clean environment or when an activity or procedure is completed, remove gloves immediately. Some additional factors to consider before using medical gloves (U.S. Food and Drug Administration, n.d.) include:

- Wash your hands before putting on gloves.
- Make sure your gloves fit properly and you can wear them comfortably during all patient care activities.
- Be aware that sharp objects can puncture medical gloves.

- Always change your gloves if they rip or tear.
- After removing gloves, wash your hands thoroughly with soap and water or alcohol-based hand rub.
- Never reuse medical gloves.
- Never wash or disinfect medical gloves.
- Never share medical gloves with other users.
- If you or your patient is allergic to natural rubber latex, choose gloves made from other synthetic materials, such as polyvinyl chloride (PVC), nitrile, or polyurethane.

To protect your eyes, nose, and mouth from splashes and respiratory secretions of a potentially infectious material or body fluids, you can use eye protectors (e.g., goggles), face masks, and face shields (Siegel et al., 2007). Several different types of face masks are available, including cloth masks, procedure masks (a.k.a. surgical masks or medical procedure masks), and respirators. Preferred procedure masks should include multiple layers of tightly woven, breathable material and meet the requirements established by the National Institute for Occupational Safety and Health (NIOSH). NIOSH provides new performance recommendations for masks in workplace, called Workspace Performance and Workplace Performance Plus masks. Masks meeting these recommendations can help protect you from SARS-CoV-2, the virus causes COVID-19. Regarding respirators, NIOSH-approved particulate filtering respirators have different filter efficiency levels. A commonly used model is N95 respirators, which can filter at least 95% of airborne particles. P100 filtering facepiece respirators have the highest filter efficacy level; these can filter at least 99.97% of airborne particles and are strongly resistant to oil (CDC, 2021b). See Figure 6–1 for an example of NOISH-approved respirators. Appendix 6–A contains CDC's instructions for how to use N95 respirators.

It is important to wear a mask with the best fit, protection, and comfort for you. Be sure to wear a mask that completely covers your nose, mouth, and chin, along with adjusting the nosepiece, ties, bands, or ear loops to improve mask fit (no gaps between your face and mask). Box 6–2 is the summary of how to properly wear and take off a mask. A well-fitted mask can help prevent air (with respiratory droplets) from flowing freely around the edges of the mask.

Safe Handling of Potentially Contaminated Equipment or Surfaces

As an SLPA, you may be asked to participate in cleaning and disinfecting treat-ment materials and the clinical environment. Sterilization, which is defined as a process of complete elimination of all forms of microbial life, is often not required (Mohapatra, 2017). Cleaning refers to the physical removal of foreign material, such as dust, soil, or secretion, by using water and detergents (CDC, 2016b). High-traffic areas, such as furniture in the therapy room, should be cleaned frequently. Treatment materials should be placed on shelves and in bins after use. Shelves and bins should be kept clean and dust free.

Disinfection refers to the elimination of harmful microorganisms living on the surface of objects, but disinfection does not destroy all microorganisms, especially some bacterial spores (CDC, 2016c). For low-level disinfection, SLPAs can apply an Environmental Protection Agency (EPA)–registered disinfectant on equipment or surfaces and let the solution sit for at least 1 minute before wiping (CDC, 2016c). Disinfectant products from the EPA List N can

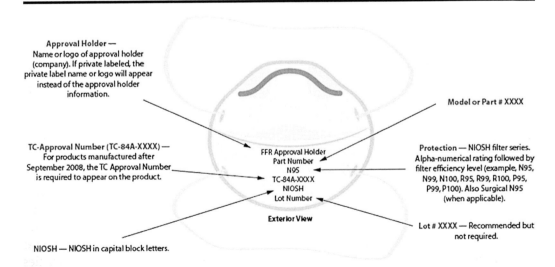

Figure 6–1. A filtering facepiece respirator with appropriate markings. Image courtesy of CDC. https://www.cdc.gov/niosh/npptl/topics/respirators/disp_part/images/FFRcorrectMarkings.jpg

---

Box 6–2. How to Properly Wear and Take Off a Mask (CDC, 2022b)

How to Properly Wear a Mask

- Wash your hands before touching the mask.
- Make sure the mask covers your nose, mouth, and chin.
- Check for gaps to prevent leaks.
- Make sure you can breathe and talk comfortably through your mask.

How to Properly Take Off a Mask

- Carefully stretch the ear loops or untie the strings.
- Grab the mask only by the ear loops or strings.
- Fold the outside corners together.
- Discard a disposable mask or wash a reusable mask when it is visibly soiled or damaged.
- Wash your hands after touching the mask.

---

kill all strains and variants of the coronavirus SARS-CoV-2 (COVID-19) when following the label directions (CDC, 2021c). While using the disinfectant, wear rubber gloves to protect hands from irritation and wash hands immediately afterward. When EPA-registered disinfectant is not available, SLPAs may use a fresh chlorine bleach solution. The formula of diluted bleach solution is 1 tablespoon of bleach to 1 quart (4 cups) of water. The CDC and the Healthcare Infection Control Practices Advisory Committee (HICPAC) provides guidelines on environmental infection control measures. A copy of the cleaning and disinfection guidelines for schools is available in Appendix 6–B. Additional information on this topic can also be found on the CDC's website (http://www.cdc.gov/hai/).

Respiratory Hygiene/Cough Etiquette

Respiratory hygiene and cough etiquette are terms used to describe infection prevention measures to decrease the transmission of respiratory illness (e.g., influenza and common cold) and should be implemented for all individuals with signs and symptoms of a respiratory infection to reduce the transmission of respiratory infections (Chavis & Ganesh, 2019). The following measures can be used to contain respiratory secretions (Healthcare Infection Control Practices Advisory Committee, 2017):

- Post signs at entrances and common areas instructing clients/patients to cover your mouth and nose when coughing or sneezing.

■ Prompt clients/patients with symptoms of respiratory infection to contain their respiratory secretions by providing tissues, masks, and hand hygiene supplies.

■ Prompt clients/patients with symptoms of respiratory infection to perform hand hygiene after contact with respiratory secretions.

■ When space permits, separate clients/patients with respiratory symptoms from others as soon as possible upon entry into the facility.

Additional information on respiratory hygiene and cough etiquette in health care settings can be found on the CDC's webpage (https://www.cdc.gov/flu/professionals/infectioncontrol/resphygiene.htm).

FIRST AID AND CARDIOPULMONARY RESUSCITATION

In case of an emergency, an SLPA should be trained in first aid and cardiopulmonary resuscitation (CPR) to respond appropriately. This section discusses the general rules for first aid and CPR use and how to get certified.

General Rules About First Aid

First aid refers to the initial care or management for an injury or illness (American Red Cross, 2016). In minor cases, the only care may be properly addressing the wound and covering it with adhesive bandages. While in serious illness or injuries, first aid may involve helping the individuals prior to professional medical help being available (e.g., paramedics arrive). The best way to prepare for these events is to get official first aid/CPR training.

Most treatment settings have a first aid kit available, which contains items for use in the event of injury. In the United States, OSHA requires all job sites and workplaces to have a first aid kit available. The kit is typically stored in a place where it is easily accessible for adults but out of reach of children. As an SLPA, you should know where this kit is and what items are in it. Key items that should be included in a first aid kit (Cronan, 2010) include a first aid manual, sterile gauze pads, adhesive tape, adhesive bandages, antiseptic wipes, alcohol wipes, antibiotic ointment, antiseptic solution, pain killers, tweezers, scissors, safety pins, disposable instant cold packs, thermometers, plastic nonlatex gloves, and a flashlight with extra batteries. The kit should be checked on a regular basis to replace low-stock items and medicines that may have expired and to check if the flashlight works properly and there are backup batteries available.

CPR/Automated External Defibrillator (AED) Certification

According to American Heart Association (AHA, 2020), CPR is an emergency procedure that manually ensures blood can continue circulating in the body after an individual experiences cardiac arrest. All the cells in our body require oxygen and nutrients to survive, which are carried in the blood. When a cardiac arrest happens, the heart stops beating, blood stops circulating, and breathing ceases after a few minutes. A cardiac arrest can be caused by a heart attack, other heart diseases (e.g., coronary artery disease, valvular heat disease), heart rhythm disturbance, drugs, blood loss, or head injury. CPR is an emergency procedure to keep the blood flowing in the body, but it cannot restart the heart. Further measures, such as defibrillation, are needed to restart the heart.

Approximately 356,000 people experience out-of-hospital cardiac arrest (OHCA) annually in the United States (Tsao et al., 2022). Signs of cardiac arrest are immediate and sudden, including sudden collapse, no pulse, no breathing, and loss of consciousness. When the heart stops, the lack of oxygen-rich blood can cause death or permanent brain damage within a few minutes (CDC, 2021d). Early CPR is an integral part of providing lifesaving aid to people having sudden cardiac arrest. In general, CPR involves chest compression and rescue breaths (AHA, 2020). Chest compressions manually pump the heart to allow blood continuing flowing throughout the body by pushing down hard and fast in the center of the chest at a rate of 100 to 120 pushes a minute and letting the chest come back up to its normal position after each push (CDC, 2021d). The AHA recommends this "hands-only" method of CPR, which does not involve breathing into the person's mouth. If you've been trained in CPR, check the person's airway and deliver rescue breaths after every 30 compressions. Rescue breaths supply air to the lungs and can be performed either by mouth-to-mouth resuscitation using a device. An automated external defibrillator (AED) is a computerized medical device that checks a person's heart rhythm. It can

recognize a rhythm that requires a shock and advises a rescuer when a shock is needed. The AED uses voice prompts, lights, and text messages to tell a rescuer what steps to take. After the AED is attached and delivers a shock, most AEDs will prompt the operator to continue CPR while the device continues to monitor the client/patient.

First aid and CPR training is easy, and it is extremely important for SLPAs to get first aid and CPR certified, so you can be prepared and know how to properly respond to emergency situations. It is also beneficial to get AED training and certification. The American Red Cross and AHA offer training and certification courses for first aid, CPR, and AED. For more information on CPR, visit the American Red Cross website (http://www.redcorss.org) and the AHA website (http://www.heart.org). Local fire departments also offer CPR training courses that are certified by the AHA.

COMMON MEDICAL CONDITIONS

When an SLPA is working with a client or patient, emergency medical situations can occur. This section covers several medical conditions that an SLPA might encounter when providing care or treatment. By understanding the causes and symptoms of these conditions, SLPAs can react to medical emergencies appropriately and seek medical attention immediately.

Stroke

According to the CDC's stroke statistics, more than 795,000 people in the United States have a stroke, and about 610,000 of these are first or new strokes (Tsao et al., 2022). A stroke, also known as cerebrovascular accident (CVA), occurs when the blood supply to part of the brain is suddenly interrupted or when a blood vessel in the brain bursts, spilling blood into the brain or the spaces surrounding the brain. There are two kinds of stroke: ischemic stroke and hemorrhagic stroke. About 87% of all strokes are ischemic strokes; an ischemic stroke is caused by obstruction of a blood vessel that supplies blood to the brain (Tsao et al., 2022). The obstruction can be caused by cerebral thrombosis or embolism. Cerebral thrombosis refers to the formation of a blood clot inside a blood vessel that blocks vascular circulation in the brain. A cerebral embolism happens when a clot breaks off from another part of body and travels to the brain, resulting in the obstruction of a blood vessel in the brain. About 13% of all strokes are hemorrhagic; a hemorrhagic stroke happens when a weakened blood vessel ruptures. Weakened blood vessels can be caused by a blood vessel malformation (e.g., arteriovenous malformation or a cerebral aneurysm). When a blood vessel that supplies the brain ruptures and bleeds, brain cells and tissues do not

get oxygen and nutrients. In addition, accumulation of blood can cause more damage to the surrounding brain tissues.

When the vascular circulation in the brain is blocked or interrupted, neurons (a.k.a. nerve cells) can no longer receive the oxygen and nutrients they need from the blood supply. This results in the death of neurons and the loss of abilities controlled by the brain area where circulation was interrupted. The effects of a stroke depend on where the stroke occurs in the brain and how much of the brain is damaged. For example, a small stroke may cause only minor weakness of an arm or leg, whereas a larger stroke can result in paralysis (total loss of muscle function) on one side of the body. A stroke can impair many important brain functions, such as speech, language, mobility, vision, and memory. Stroke is one of the main causes of several acquired speech-language disorders, such as aphasia, dysarthria, apraxia of speech, and other cognitive-communication disorders (ASHA, n.d.). Stroke is a medical emergency and prompt treatment is crucial. Box 6–3 summarizes possible signs and symptoms of stroke. If a person is experiencing those stroke-like symptoms, you should immediately call

---

Box 6–3. Common Symptoms and Signs of Stroke (CDC, 2022c)

- Sudden numbness or weakness of the face, arm, or leg, especially on one side of the body
- Sudden confusion, trouble speaking or understanding
- Sudden trouble seeing in one or both eyes
- Sudden trouble walking, dizziness, loss of balance or coordination
- Sudden severe headache with no known cause

Call 9-1-1 right away if you or someone else has any of these symptoms.

911 and get medical attention. Early treatment can minimize brain damage and other potential complications.

Heart Attack

Similar to a stroke, a heart attack, also known as a myocardial infarction, happens when the blood vessels that supply blood to the heart become blocked (National Institutes of Health [NIH], 2018). When the flow of oxygen-rich blood to a part of the heart is blocked or interrupted, the muscles of that section of the heart begin to die due to lack of oxygen and nutrients. Coronary heart disease (CHD) is the most common cause of a heart attack. CHD results from the buildup of plaque inside the coronary arteries, the major supplier of oxygen-rich blood to the heart.

If someone is experiencing symptoms of a heart attack, you should get medical attention immediately by dialing 911 or a local emergency number. This person needs to get to the hospital right away. Heart attack increases the risk for going into cardiac arrest (CDC, 2022d). Box 6–4 lists the common symptoms of a heart attack. The chest pain may move from the chest to other parts of the body, such as shoulders, arms, back, or neck. Acting quickly when a heart attack occurs can limit damage to the heart; according to the NIH (2018), treatment for a heart attack works best when given right after the symptoms occur.

Traumatic Brain Injury (TBI)

Traumatic brain injury (TBI) is caused by a bump, blow, or jolt to the head that disrupts the normal function of the brain. TBI

> ### Box 6–4. Common Signs and Symptoms of Heart Attack (NIH, 2018)
>
> - Crushing chest pain or pressure and/or discomfort or pain elsewhere in the upper body, neck, or arms
> - Shortness of breath
> - Fainting or lightheadedness
> - A cold sweat
> - Nausea

is a major cause of death and disability in the United States, and there were over 64,000 TBI-related deaths in the United States in 2020 (CDC, 2022c). Falls were the leading cause of TBI among children 0 to 14 years of age, and motor vehicle accidents were the leading cause for adolescents and adults 15 to 44 years of age (CDC, 2022e). TBI can cause impairments in attention, memory, mobility, sensation, or emotion. Common symptoms include loss of consciousness, headache, blurry vision, nausea, dizziness, sensitivity to light, and lack of energy. People with TBI may also demonstrate difficulties in thinking, concentrating, and learning new information. They may also experience mood swings, emotional disturbances, and personality change (CDC, 2022e).

When working with someone who may sustain a traumatic brain injury, SLPAs should be aware of warning signs indicating a need for immediate medical attention. The warning signs are as follows (CDC, 2022e):

- Loss of consciousness
- Headache that gets worse and does not go away

- Weakness, numbness, or decreased coordination
- Vomiting or nausea
- Slurred speech
- Very drowsy affect or inability to wake up
- Seizures
- Increased confusion, restlessness, or agitation
- Other unusual behaviors

Airway Obstruction

Airway obstruction means a blockage in either the upper or lower airway (Brady & Burns, 2021). The upper airway includes the nasal cavity, pharynx, and larynx, and the lower airway refers to the trachea, bronchial tree, and lungs. Airway obstruction can prevent air from getting into the lungs (partially or totally). This can be fatal and requires immediate medical attention. Airway obstruction may be classified as chronic airway obstruction or acute airway obstruction.

Chronic airway obstruction takes a long time to develop. Examples of chronic airway obstruction are chronic obstructive pulmonary disorders (COPD), emphysema, and abscesses in the airway. Acute airway obstruction occurs quickly. The common causes of acute airway obstruction SLPAs might encounter include inhaling, swallowing, or choking on a foreign object; allergic reactions; or a small object lodged in the nose. Children are at higher risk of foreign object obstruction than are adults (American Society for Gastrointestinal Endoscopy, 2011). Therefore, make sure to keep small items away from children when working with them and constantly monitor them for any unsafe behaviors, such as trying to put small toys into the nose or mouth or swallowing large pieces of food without chewing.

The symptoms of airway obstruction depend on the location of obstruction; Box 6–5 lists common symptoms of airway obstruction. When any of these symptoms are noticed, get medical help immediately. If trained personnel are available onsite, the Heimlich maneuver can be performed for someone choking on a foreign object and CPR can be used for someone who is not breathing.

Seizures

Seizures are caused by sudden disorganized and abnormal electrical activity in the brain, causing muscles to contract and relax repeatedly (U.S. National Library of Medicine, 2012). There are many different types of seizures, such as tonic-clonic (a.k.a. grand mal) seizures, simple focal seizures (CDC, 2020b), and so on. Seizures can occur suddenly and can result from many medical conditions, such as brain injury, stroke, brain tumor, liver or kidney

---

Box 6–5. Common Symptoms of an Airway Obstruction
(Brady & Burns, 2021)

- Difficulty breathing or no breathing
- Alterations in normal breathing pattern, whether rapid or shallow breathing
- Wheezing breathing noise
- Change of skin color (bluish-colored skin)
- Panic
- Gasping for air

failure, high fever, low blood sugar, or drug abuse. Specific symptoms of seizures depend on what part of the brain is involved. Box 6–6 lists some common symptoms. Symptoms may stop after a few seconds or minutes and usually last no longer than 10 to 15 minutes. Table 6–2 lists things that should be taken into consideration during and after a seizure.

Severe Allergic Reactions

Most of the time, people experience minor allergic symptoms when having allergic reactions. However, when a severe allergic reaction happens, it can be rapid and potentially life threatening (NIH, 2016). Allergic symptoms occur when a person's own immune system reacts to normally harmless substances. According to the NIH (2016), the most common allergy triggers include certain foods, medications, pollen, dust mites, mold, insect stings, and latex. Mild allergic symptoms include mild eye irritation, localized skin rash, and congestion. Severe allergic reactions include generalized swelling, wheezing, nausea, vomiting, fast heartbeat, and difficulty breathing.

Before working with clients/patients, an SLPA should review their medical history thoroughly to identify if they have any known allergies. Make sure to avoid

---

Box 6–6. Common Symptoms of a Seizure (Fisher et al., 2017)

- Brief blackout with confusion, drooling, eye movement, grunting, or snoring
- Sudden falling
- Uncontrollable muscle spasms with jerking limbs or shaking of the entire body
- Clenching of the teeth or jaw
- Experiencing incontinence
- During mild seizures, there may be no muscle contraction or body shaking, and the person may seem to be staring into space

---

Table 6–2. What to Do During and After a Seizure

During a Seizure	After a Seizure
• Stay calm and try to time the seizure.	• Make sure to check for any injuries or difficulty of breathing.
• If the person is pregnant or the seizure lasts longer than 3 minutes, call 911.	• Provide a safe area for the person to rest and do not give him or her anything to eat or drink until he or she is fully conscious and oriented.
• Remove objects that might hurt the person and provide postural support to prevent further injury.	
• If the person is on the ground, position him or her on his or her side to avoid saliva or vomit from entering the airway.	
• Do not attempt to open the mouth and put anything in the mouth; this could pose a choking hazard (O'Hara, 2007).	
• Do not attempt to give anything to drink or eat while the person is having a seizure (O'Hara, 2007).	

Source: Chillemi & Devinsky, 2011.

exposing clients to common allergy triggers. Severe allergic reactions require immediate medical treatment. If someone starts to have a significant allergic reaction, such as difficulty breathing or increased heart rate, call 911 immediately, or go to the nearest emergency room.

SAFETY FOR CHILDREN WITH DISABILITIES

Safe Environment

Children who have limited ability to move, see, hear, or understand pain might not realize that something is unsafe or might have trouble getting away from something unsafe (CDC, n.d.). Always ensure that every area children can reach is safe. It is also important to make sure that therapy materials are safe based on the child's age and current level of function. Additionally, only treatment-related materials should be brought into the therapy room and properly without creating safety hazards.

Safety Equipment

Children with epilepsy may experience sudden drops or falls that can cause head injury. Therefore, having the child wearing a protective helmet may be helpful to minimize consequences of unexpected seizure episodes. As an SLPA, you should talk to your speech-language pathologist (SLP) supervisor to ensure the proper use of safety equipment during therapy.

Safety Talk

Children who have difficulty understating and communicating may have limited ability to learn about danger and safety. It is beneficial to keep instructions simple, model safe behaviors, and have the child practice safety drills on a regular basis. It is also critical to educate all individuals who work with the child about how to communicate with the child if there is any danger. Some simple phrases through verbal production and augmentative and alternative communication (AAC) can also be taught, such as *"I am hurt," "I need help,"* and so forth.

ADDITIONAL CONSIDERATIONS ABOUT WORKING WITH CLIENTS WITH SPECIAL MEDICAL NEEDS

SLPAs might work with clients who have special medical needs. It is important to understand these specific needs and provide reasonable accommodation. This section discusses the precautions that SLPAs should be aware of when working with clients who have special medical needs.

Oxygen Use

SLPAs might work with clients who use oxygen. Oxygen is used for individuals who cannot keep appropriate oxygen levels in their blood. Oxygen is a prescribed drug that can improve respiration and decrease the work of heart (National Heart, Lung, and Blood Institute, 2011). Gaseous oxygen is delivered by an oxygen mask or a nasal cannula (Figure 6–2B). Common types of oxygen systems are oxygen concentrators (home and portable units), gas cylinders, and liquid oxygen systems (American Lung Association, 2018). Oxygen concentrators filter oxygen from the air and offer users an unlimited

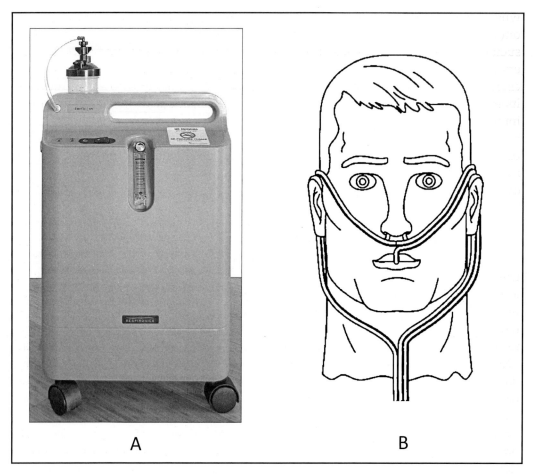

A   B

Figure 6–2. A. EverFlo oxygen concentrator (respironics). **B.** Nasal cannula. Images courtesy of Wikimedia Commons.

supply of oxygen. Larger units are made for the home (Figure 6–2A); portable oxygen concentrators are similar but smaller in size, making them better for travel. Oxygen cylinders are painted green, which is the universal color for medical oxygen cylinders. They come in many different sizes depending on the needs of the patient or client. In general, they range from 2 to 6 feet in height. Once the gas cylinder is empty, it must be refilled by trained personnel. Liquid oxygen systems are large self-contained thermos-like reservoirs that store oxygen at a very cold temperature. When clients need oxygen, they turn the unit on to warm the oxygen, which turns to a gas as it leaves the reservoir. Liquid oxygen stored in the reservoir needs to be refilled by trained personnel, usually weekly (American Lung Association, 2018).

Although oxygen is nonflammable, it makes things burn much faster than usual. Thus, smoking is prohibited in any room where oxygen is in use. "NO SMOKING" signs should be placed in treatment rooms where oxygen is used. Make sure to keep oxygen 6 feet away from any heat sources, such as heat ducts, radiators, space heaters, fireplaces, matches, and lighters. If the client uses a gas cylinder, keep the tank in its stand to avoid rolling or falling—it can injure the client or persons nearby. Also, SLPAs should pay attention to the oxygen tubing because a client may get tangled in the tubing or trip over the tubes, which can interfere with oxygen circulation.

Dysphagia and Aspiration Precautions

Dysphagia is the medical term for swallowing difficulty. Individuals with dysphagia experience difficulty transmitting food or liquid from mouth to stomach due to the tongue, throat (pharynx and larynx), or esophagus not working properly (Groher & Crary, 2020). Dysphagia can result from numerous medical conditions, such as stroke; head injury; progressive neurodegenerative diseases (e.g., Parkinson disease); oral, pharyngeal, and esophageal cancers; and other esophageal dis-

eases. Neurologic diseases can impair the nerves and muscles used for swallowing. Cancers can cause reduced movement of the tongue, pharynx, or larynx. Esophageal disorders can cause the esophagus to become narrower than usual, so food or liquid cannot travel along the esophagus smoothly. Common symptoms and signs of dysphagia are summarized in Box 6–7.

Individuals with dysphagia are at high risk of aspiration. Aspiration refers to the entry of food or liquid into the larynx or lungs. The chances of food or liquid entering the airway increase with dysphagia due to the difficulties transmitting food or liquid from the mouth to the stomach. Things that can be inhaled into the larynx or lungs include saliva, vomited stomach contents, and stomach acid, which can cause substantial damage to lungs and result in pneumonia, lung abscess (a collection of pus in the lungs), airway obstruction, and even death.

ASHA addresses dysphagia in its SLPA scope of practice document (2022), Responsibility Outside the Scope of

---

Box 6–7. Common Symptoms and Signs of Dysphagia
(Groher & Crary, 2020)

- Increasing chewing time
- Needing to swallow multiple times
- Drooling and/or liquids leaking through the nose
- Difficulty or discomfort when swallowing
- Coughing or choking when swallowing
- Difficulty breathing during feeding
- Feeling of food stuck in the throat
- Frequent clearing of the throat during and/or after meals
- Vomiting swallowed food
- Loss of appetite
- Dehydration, malnutrition, or weight loss

Practice for Speech-Language Pathology Assistants), stating that SLPAs, may <u>not</u>:

- treat medically fragile students, patients, and clients without 100% direct supervision;
- perform procedures that require specialized knowledge and training (e.g., vocal tract prosthesis shaping or fitting, vocal tract imaging);
- administer or interpret feeding and/or swallowing screenings, checklists, and assessments; and
- develop or determine the feeding and/or swallowing strategies or precautions for students, patients, and clients.

As a care provider, though, it is important you maintain a safe environment for the individuals you serve. This means when working with individuals with dysphagia, you are aware of the risk of aspiration and follow any precautions recommended by the supervising SLP. Aspiration precautions typically involve one or more of the following:

- Have the patient/client sit in an upright position when eating food or drinking liquid.
- Only allow the patient/client to consume food and liquid at the recommended consistency, such as finely chopped food and thickened liquid.
- Remind the patient/client to chew well and eat slowly.
- Eliminate distractions, such as turning off the TV or radio.
- Check the person's mouth after eating for any food residue.

- Keep the patient/client sitting upright for 30 to 45 minutes after eating.

If the client shows significant symptoms or signs of swallowing difficulty, such as coughing or difficulty breathing, ask her or him to stop eating or drinking immediately, seek medical attention, and notify your supervising SLP.

Tube Feeding

When individuals with dysphagia are at a high risk of aspiration, they can no longer consume an oral diet safely. Alternative feeding methods are implemented to meet their nutrition and hydration needs while continuing to treat their dysphagia. Feeding tubes are the most common approach of alterative feeding (Hanson et al., 2008). Different types of feeding tubes are available depending on the patient's condition and needs. Nasogastric (NG) tubes and percutaneous endoscopic gastrostomy (PEG) tubes are two frequently used types (Groher & Crary, 2020). NG tubes are plastic tubes inserted through the nose, which then pass the throat and go into the stomach. The placement of PEG tubes requires a small incision in the abdomen to insert the tube into the stomach. NG tubes are for short-term use, whereas PEG tubes can be used for a longer time or even permanently (Gomes et al., 2010).

Feeding tubes do not prevent aspiration, so it is essential for SLPAs to follow aspiration precautions when working with individuals with dysphagia and feeding tubes. Remember to keep clients with aspiration precautions in an upright position as much as possible. It's very important they do not lay flat when they are getting continuous feeding; lying flat increases the risk of food regurgitation and can further result in aspiration. If there is any leakage or blockage of the feeding tubes, contact the individuals' caregiver(s) or trained personnel for further assistance.

Ventilator Use and Tracheotomy

According to the NIH (2022), a ventilator is a machine that supports breathing for those who cannot breathe independently. They are mainly used in hospitals, though they can also be used in long-term care facilities or long term in the home. Ventilators push oxygen into the lungs and remove carbon dioxide from the body, helping the patient breathe more easily. See Figure 6–3 for a standard setup of a mechanical ventilator in hospitals. The ventilator pushes warm, moist air (or air with extra oxygen) to the patient through a breathing tube (also called an endotracheal tube) or a tightly fitting mask. Examples of diseases and conditions that can affect lung function and lead to the use of a ventilator include pneumonia, lung diseases, COPD, brain injury, stroke, or laryngeal injuries.

A tracheostomy is a surgical procedure that creates a hole through the front of the neck and into the trachea (NIH,

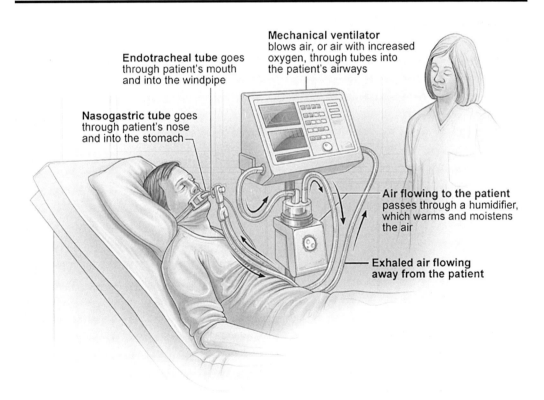

Figure 6–3. The illustration shows a standard setup of a mechanical ventilator in hospitals.

2022). The hole can be temporary or permanent. After placing a tube through the hole to provide an airway, breathing occurs through the tube rather than through the nose and mouth (Figure 6–4). One common reason for having a tracheostomy is if a ventilator needs to be used for more than a few weeks. The ventilator can connect to the tracheostomy tube to support breathing. Another possible reason for a tracheostomy tube is to help clear mucus or secretion from the lungs.

Because air no longer passes through the vocal folds, individuals who have a tracheostomy cannot easily use their voice. There are many ways to assist individuals in producing sound for speech. Certain tracheostomy tubes and many different types of valves can redirect airflow to produce speech. Trained SLPs can recommend options for communication and provide training to clients in the use of different devices to meet their communication needs.

CONCLUSION

This chapter is to provide an overview of several health-related conditions that SLPAs may encounter when working with their clients/patients. Additionally, it is critically important to create and maintain a safe working environment for you and the clients you serve. Hence, SLPAs should carefully follow infection control procedures and standard precautions when working with clients/patients. Readers who are interested in getting more information on the topics discussed in the chapter can visit the websites of Centers for Disease Control and Prevention (CDC) (https://www.cdc.gov) and World Health Organization (WHO) (https://www.who.int).

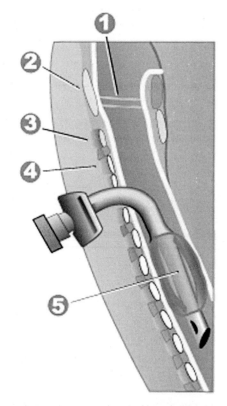

Figure 6–4. Diagram of a tracheostoma and tracheostomy tube. 1 = vocal folds; 2 = thyroid cartilage; 3 = cricoid cartilage; 4 = tracheal cartilages; 5 = balloon cuff. Image courtesy of Wikimedia Commons.

REFERENCES

American Heart Association. (2020). *2020 AHA guidelines update for cardiopulmonary resuscitation (CPR) and emergency cardiovascular care (ECC).* https://cpr.heart.org/en/resuscitation-science/cpr-and-ecc-guidelines

American Lung Association. (2018). *Oxygen therapy.* http://www.lung.org/lung-disease/copd/living-with-copd/supplemental-oxygen.html

American Red Cross. (2016). *American Red Cross first aid/CPR/AED instructor's manual.*

American Society for Gastrointestinal Endoscopy. (2011). Guideline: Management of ingested foreign bodies and food impactions. *Gastrointestinal Endoscopy, 73*(16), 1085–1091. https://doi.org/10.1016/j.gie.2010.11.010

American Speech-Language-Hearing Association (ASHA). (n.d.). *Aphasia.* https://www.asha.org/practice-portal/clinical-topics/aphasia/

American Speech-Language-Hearing Association. (2005). *Quality indicators for professional service programs in audiology and speech-language pathology* [Standards/quality indicators]. www.asha.org/policy

American Speech-Language-Hearing Association. (2022). *Speech-language pathology assistant scope of practice.* https://www.asha.org/policy/slpa-scope-of-practice/

Brady, M. F., & Burns, B. (2021). *Airway obstruction.* StatPearls Publishing.

Centers for Disease Control and Prevention (CDC). (n.d.). *Keeping children with disabilities safe.* https://www.cdc.gov/ncbddd/disabilityandsafety/child-safety.html

Centers for Disease Control and Prevention (CDC). (2012). *Respiratory hygiene/cough etiquette in healthcare settings.* https://www.cdc.gov/flu/professionals/infectioncontrol/resphygiene.htm

Centers for Disease Control and Prevention (CDC). (2016a). *Standard precautions.* https://www.cdc.gov/oralhealth/infectioncontrol/summary-infection-prevention-practices/standard-precautions.html

Centers for Disease Control and Prevention (CDC). (2016b). *Cleaning—guideline for disinfection and sterilization in healthcare facilities.* https://www.cdc.gov/infectioncontrol/guidelines/disinfection/cleaning.html

Centers for Disease Control and Prevention (CDC). (2016c). *Disinfection—guideline for disinfection and sterilization in healthcare facilities.* https://www.cdc.gov/infectioncontrol/guidelines/disinfection/disinfection-methods/index.html

Centers for Disease Control and Prevention (CDC). (2017). *Healthcare-associated infections* (HAIs). https://www.cdc.gov/winnablebattles/report/HAIs.html

Centers for Disease Control and Prevention (CDC). (2020a). *Hand hygiene guidance.* https://www.cdc.gov/handhygiene/providers/guideline.html

Centers for Disease Control and Prevention (CDC). (2020b). *Types of seizures.* https://www.cdc.gov/epilepsy/about/types-of-seizures.htm

Centers for Disease Control and Prevention (CDC). (2021a). *Current HAI progress report.* https://www.cdc.gov/hai/data/portal/progress-report.html

Centers for Disease Control and Prevention (CDC). (2021b). *NIOSH-approved particulate filtering facepiece respirators.* https://www.cdc.gov/niosh/npptl/topics/respirators/disp_part/default.html

Centers for Disease Control and Prevention (CDC). (2021c). *When to clean and when to disinfect.* https://www.cdc.gov/coronavirus/2019-ncov/community/disinfecting-building-facility.html

Centers for Disease Control and Prevention (CDC). (2021d). *Three things you may not know about CPR.* https://www.cdc.gov/heartdisease/cpr.htm

Centers for Disease Control and Prevention (CDC). (2022a). *When and how to wash your hands.* https://www.cdc.gov/handwashing/when-how-handwashing.html#:~:text=.Wet%20your%20hands%20with,at%20least%2020%20seconds

Centers for Disease Control and Prevention (CDC). (2022b). *Types of masks and respirators.* https://www.cdc.gov/coronavirus/2019-ncov/prevent-getting-sick/types-of-masks.html#masks

Centers for Disease Control and Prevention (CDC). (2022c). *Stroke signs and symptoms.* https://www.cdc.gov/stroke/signs_symptoms.htm

Centers for Disease Control and Prevention (CDC). (2022d). *Heart attack symptoms, risk, and recovery.* https://www.cdc.gov/heartdisease/heart_attack.htm

Centers for Disease Control and Prevention (CDC). (2022e). *TBI: Get the facts.* https://www.cdc.gov/traumaticbraininjury/get_the_facts.html

Chavis, S., & Ganesh, N. (2019). Respiratory hygiene and cough etiquette. *Infection Control in the Dental Office: A Global Perspective, 18,* 91–103. https://doi.org/10.1007/978-3-030-30085-2_7

Chillemi, S., & Devinsky, O. (2011). Quick tips: What to do if someone has a seizure. *Neurology Now, 7*(2), 12.

Cronan, K. (2010). *First aid kit.* http://kidshealth .org/parent/firstaid_safe/ home/firstaid_kit .html?tracking=83967_G#cat31

Fisher, R., Cross, J. H., D'Souza, C., French, J. A., Haut, S. R., Higurashi, N., . . . Zuberi, S. M. (2017). Instruction manual for the ILAE 2017 operational classification of seizure types. *Epilepsia, 58*(4), 531–542. https://doi.org/10.1111/ epi.13671

Gomes, C., Lustosa, S., Matos, D., Andriolo, R., Waisberg, D., & Waisberg, J. (2010). Percutaneous endoscopic gastrostomy versus nasogastric tube feeding for adults with swallowing disturbances. *Cochrane Database of Systematic Reviews, 10*(11), CD008096. https://doi.org/ 10.1002/14651858

Groher, M., & Crary, M. (2020). *Dysphagia: Clinical management in adults and children* (3rd ed.). Elsevier.

Hanson, L., Garrett, J., Lewis, C., Phifer, N., Jackman, A., & Carey, T. (2008). Physicians' expectations of benefit from tube feeding. *Journal of Palliative Medicine, 11*(8), 1130–1134. https:// doi.org/10.1089/jpm.2008.0033

Healthcare Infection Control Practices Advisory Committee (HICPAC). (2017, March). *Core infection prevention and control practices for safe healthcare delivery in all settings recommendations.* https://www.cdc.gov/hicpac/recom mendations/core-practices.html

Interorganizational Group for Speech Language Pathology and Audiology (2010). *Infection Prevention and Control Guidelines for Speech-Language Pathology.* https://www.caslpo.com/ sites/default/uploads/files/GU_EN_Infection_Prevention_Control_Guidelines_SLP.pdf

Mohapatra, S. (2017). Sterilization and Disinfection. *Essentials of Neuroanesthesia,* 929–944. https://doi.org/10.1016/B978-0-12-805299- 0.00059-2

National Heart, Lung, and Blood Institute. (2011). *Respiratory failure.* https://www.nhlbi.nih .gov/health-topics/respiratory-failure

National Institutes of Health. (2016). *Why food allergy is a priority for NIAID?* https://www .niaid.nih.gov/diseases-conditions/food-allergy-priority-niaid

National Institutes of Health (NIH). (2018). *What is a heart attack?* https://www.nia.nih.gov/ health/what-heart-attack

National Institutes of Health (NIH). (2022). *What is a ventilator?* https://www.nhlbi.nih.gov/ health/ventilator

Occupational Safety and Health Administration (OSHA). (n.d.). *Personal protective equipment.* https://www.osha.gov/personal-protective-equipment

O'Hara, K. A. (2007). First aid for seizures: The importance of education and appropriate response. *Journal of Child Neurology, 22,* 30S–37S.

Siegel, J., Rhinehart, E., Jackson, M., Chiarello, L., & the Healthcare Infection Control Practices Advisory Committee. (2007). *2007 Guideline for isolation precautions: Preventing transmission of infectious agents in healthcare settings.* http:// www.cdc.gov/hicpac/pdf/isolation/Isola tion2007.pdf

Signore, A. (2013). About inflammation and infection. *EJNMMI Research, 3*(1), 8. https:// doi.org/10.1186/2191-219X-3-8

Tsao, C. W., Aday, A. W., Almarzooq, Z. I., Alonso, A., Beaton, A. Z., Bittencourt, M. S., . . . Martin, S. S. (2022). Heart disease and stroke statistics—2022 update: A report from the American Heart Association. *Circulation, 145*(8), e153–e639. https://doi.org/10.1161/ CIR.0000000000001052

U.S. Food and Drug Administration. (n.d.). *Medical gloves.* https://www.fda.gov/medical-devices/personal-protective-equipment-infection-control/medical-gloves

U.S. National Library of Medicine, National Institutes of Health. (2012). *Seizures.* http:// www.nlm.nih.gov/medlineplus/ency/arti cle/003200.htm

Wigglesworth, N. (2019). Infection control 2: Hand hygiene using alcohol-based hand rub. *Nursing Times, 115*(5), 24–26.

World Health Organization (WHO). (2009). *WHO guidelines on hand hygiene in healthcare.* http:// apps.who.int/iris/bitstream/handle/10665/ 44102/9789241597906_eng.pdf?sequence=1

World Health Organization (WHO). (2020a). *Vector-borne diseases.* https://www.who.int/news-room/fact-sheets/detail/vector-borne-diseases

World Health Organization (WHO). (2020b). *Transmission of SARS-CoV-2: Implications for infection prevention precautions.* https://www .who.int/news-room/commentaries/detail/ transmission-of-sars-cov-2-implications-for-infection-prevention-precautions#:~:text= Transmission%20of%20SARS%2DCoV,%2C %20talks%20or%20sings

APPENDIX 6–A

HOW TO USE YOUR N95 RESPIRATOR | COVID-19 |

Wear your N95 properly so it is effective

N95s must form a seal to the face to work properly. This is especially important for people at increased risk for severe disease. Wearing an N95 can make it harder to breathe. If you have heart or lung problems, talk to your doctor before using an N95.

Some N95s may contain latex in the straps. If you have natural rubber latex allergies, see the manufacturers' website for information about your specific model.

Your N95 may look different than the one in these pictures. As long as your N95 has two head straps (not ear loops), these basic instructions apply.

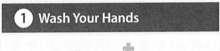

1 Wash Your Hands

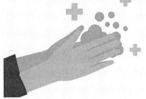

It is best to put on your N95 with clean, dry hands.

2 Check Your N95

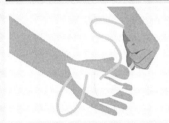

Always inspect the N95 for damage before use. If it appears damaged, dirty, or damp, do not use it.

3 Put on the N95

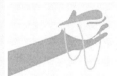

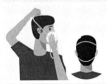

Hold the N95 in your hand with the nose piece bar (or foam) at your fingertips. If yours does not have a nose piece, use the text written on it to be sure the top end is at your fingertips.

Place the N95 under your chin with the nose piece bar at the top.

Pull the top strap over your head, placing it near the crown. Then, pull the bottom strap over and place it at the back of your neck, below your ears. Do not crisscross the straps. Make sure the straps lay flat and are not twisted.

Place your fingertips from both hands at the top of the nose piece. Press down on both sides of the nose piece to mold it to the shape of your nose.

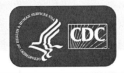

cdc.gov/coronavirus

CS329186-C | January 28, 2022 12:39 PM

Keep Your N95 Snug

Your N95 must form a seal to your face to work properly. Your breath must pass through the N95 and not around its edges. Jewelry, glasses, and facial hair can cause gaps between your face and the edge of the mask. The N95 works better if you are clean shaven. Gaps can also occur if your N95 is too big, too small, or it was not put on correctly.

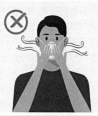

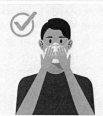

To check for gaps, gently place your hands on the N95, covering as much of it as possible, then breathe out. If you feel air leaking out from the edges of the N95, or if you are wearing glasses and they fog up, it is not snug. Adjust the N95 and try again.

If you cannot get a tight seal, try a different size or style. Even if you cannot get the N95 sealed against your face, it will provide protection that is likely better than a cloth mask. Check for gaps every time you put on your N95.

Remove the N95

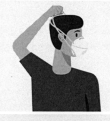

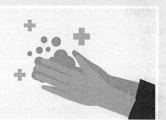

After you remove your N95, wash your hands with soap and water, or hand sanitizer containing at least 60% alcohol if soap is not available.

When to Replace Your N95

Do not wash your N95 or put it in the oven or microwave to try to sterilize it.
Replace the N95 when the straps are stretched out and it no longer fits snugly against your face or when it becomes wet, dirty, or damaged. Throw it in the trash.

You can find specific manufacturer's instructions for your N95 model at the manufacturer's website or on the CDC COVID-19 website.

This information is also available at: **https://bit.ly/3rL7tpC**

APPENDIX 6–B

How to Clean and Disinfect Schools to Help Slow the Spread of Flu

Cleaning and disinfecting are part of a broad approach to preventing infectious diseases in schools. To help slow the spread of influenza (flu), the first line of defense is getting vaccinated. Other measures include covering coughs and sneezes, washing hands, and keeping sick people away from others. Below are tips on how to slow the spread of flu specifically through cleaning and disinfecting.

1. Know the difference between cleaning, disinfecting, and sanitizing.

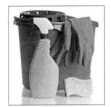

Cleaning removes germs, dirt, and impurities from surfaces or objects. Cleaning works by using soap (or detergent) and water to physically remove germs from surfaces. This process does not necessarily kill germs, but by removing them, it lowers their numbers and the risk of spreading infection.

Disinfecting kills germs on surfaces or objects. Disinfecting works by using chemicals to kill germs on surfaces or objects. This process does not necessarily clean dirty surfaces or remove germs, but by killing germs on a surface after cleaning, it can further lower the risk of spreading infection.

Sanitizing lowers the number of germs on surfaces or objects to a safe level, as judged by public health standards or requirements. This process **works by either cleaning or disinfecting** surfaces or objects to lower the risk of spreading infection.

2. Clean and disinfect surfaces and objects that are touched often.

Follow your school's standard procedures for routine cleaning and disinfecting. Typically, this means daily sanitizing surfaces and objects that are touched often, such as desks, countertops, doorknobs, computer keyboards, hands-on learning items, faucet handles, phones, and toys. Some schools may also require daily disinfecting these items. Standard procedures often call for disinfecting specific areas of the school, like bathrooms.

Immediately clean surfaces and objects that are visibly soiled. If surfaces or objects are soiled with body fluids or blood, use gloves and other standard precautions to avoid coming into contact with the fluid. Remove the spill, and then clean and disinfect the surface.

3. Simply do routine cleaning and disinfecting.

It's important to match your cleaning and disinfecting activities to the types of germs you want to remove or kill. Most studies have shown that the flu virus can live and potentially infect a person for only 2 to 8 hours after being deposited on a surface. Therefore, it is not necessary to close schools to clean or disinfect every surface in the building to slow the spread of flu. Also, if students and staff are dismissed because the school cannot function normally (e.g., high absenteeism during a flu outbreak), it is not necessary to do extra cleaning and disinfecting.

Flu viruses are relatively fragile, so standard cleaning and disinfecting practices are sufficient to remove or kill them. Special cleaning and disinfecting processes, including wiping down walls and ceilings, frequently using room air deodorizers, and fumigating, are not necessary or recommended. These processes can irritate eyes, noses, throats, and skin; aggravate asthma; and cause other serious side effects.

**U.S. Department of
Health and Human Services**
Centers for Disease
Control and Prevention
Page 1 of 2
August, 2016

4. Clean and disinfect correctly.

Always follow label directions on cleaning products and disinfectants. Wash surfaces with a general household cleaner to remove germs. Rinse with water, and follow with an EPA-registered disinfectant to kill germs. Read the label to make sure it states that EPA has approved the product for effectiveness against influenza A virus.

If an EPA-registered disinfectant is not available, use a fresh chlorine bleach solution. To make and use the solution:

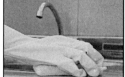

- Add 1 tablespoon of bleach to 1 quart (4 cups) of water. For a larger supply of disinfectant, add ¼ cup of bleach to 1 gallon (16 cups) of water.
- Apply the solution to the surface with a cloth.
- Let it stand for 3 to 5 minutes.
- Rinse the surface with clean water.

If a surface is not visibly dirty, you can clean it with an EPA-registered product that both cleans (removes germs) and disinfects (kills germs) instead. Be sure to read the label directions carefully, as there may be a separate procedure for using the product as a cleaner or as a disinfectant. Disinfection usually requires the product to remain on the surface for a certain period of time.

Use disinfecting wipes on electronic items that are touched often, such as phones and computers. Pay close attention to the directions for using disinfecting wipes. It may be necessary to use more than one wipe to keep the surface wet for the stated length of contact time. Make sure that the electronics can withstand the use of liquids for cleaning and disinfecting.

Routinely wash eating utensils in a dishwasher or by hand with soap and water. Wash and dry bed sheets, towels, and other linens as you normally do with household laundry soap, according to the fabric labels. Eating utensils, dishes, and linens used by sick persons do not need to be cleaned separately, but they should not be shared unless they've been washed thoroughly. Wash your hands with soap and water after handling soiled dishes and laundry items.

5. Use products safely.

Pay close attention to hazard warnings and directions on product labels. Cleaning products and disinfectants often call for the use of gloves or eye protection. For example, gloves should always be worn to protect your hands when working with bleach solutions.

Do not mix cleaners and disinfectants unless the labels indicate it is safe to do so. Combining certain products (such as chlorine bleach and ammonia cleaners) can result in serious injury or death.

Ensure that custodial staff, teachers, and others who use cleaners and disinfectants read and understand all instruction labels and understand safe and appropriate use. This might require that instructional materials and training be provided in other languages.

6. Handle waste properly.

Follow your school's standard procedures for handling waste, which may include wearing gloves. Place no-touch waste baskets where they are easy to use. Throw disposable items used to clean surfaces and items in the trash immediately after use. Avoid touching used tissues and other waste when emptying waste baskets. Wash your hands with soap and water after emptying waste baskets and touching used tissues and similar waste.

<u>www.cdc.gov/flu/school</u>

1-800-CDC-INFO

Page 2 of 2
August, 2016

PART II

Skills Development

CHAPTER 7

Deciphering Lesson Plans and Goals

Jennifer A. Ostergren and Stephanie L. Peterson

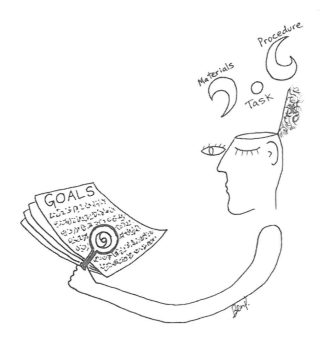

Our goals can only be reached through a vehicle of a plan, in which we must fervently believe, and upon which we must vigorously act. There is no other route to success.

—Pablo Picasso (famous artist)

As discussed in Chapter 1, one of the job responsibilities within the scope of duties of a speech-language pathology assistant (SLPA) is to follow treatment plans and protocols developed by the speech-language pathologist (SLP; American Speech-Language-Hearing Association [ASHA], 2022). Specifically, ASHA states that SLPAs may execute specific components of a treatment plan if (ASHA, 2022):

- The goals and objectives listed on the treatment plan and implemented by the SLPA are only those within the SLPA's scope of practice and are tasks the SLP has determined the SLPA has the training and skill to perform.

■ The SLP provides at least the minimum specified level of supervision to ensure quality of care to all persons served. The amount of supervision may vary and must depend on the complexity of the case and the experience of the assistant.

Before services can be implemented by an SLPA, it is the responsibility of the supervising SLP to develop an individualized treatment plan for each client. The first step in this process is an assessment (also known as an evaluation). Assessments, and screenings, can be administered by SLPAs if the SLPA meets the explicitly stated requirements in the examiner's manual and if the supervising SLP has determined that the SLPA is competent in the delivery of the assessment (ASHA, 2022). Of note is that the interpretation of assessment results and diagnosis of disorders remain solely in the scope of practice of the SLP. Further, assessment of feeding/swallowing disorders and diagnoses of this domain have been specifically defined as *outside* the scope of practice of SLPAs (ASHA, 2022). Once assessment is completed and the results have been interpreted, treatment is recommended and the SLP develops a treatment plan in which specific treatment goals are outlined. In some settings, assessment results and a treatment plan are summarized in a single document and, in other settings, in separate documents. The appendices of this chapter contain sample reports from an educational setting, including an individualized educa-

tion plan (IEP; Appendix 7–A), private practice (Appendix 7–B), and medical settings (Appendix 7–C). In some settings, these documents may be on paper, and in other settings, information is stored and accessed electronically (Krebs, 2008).

As discussed in Chapter 3, in all settings, these documents and the specifics of a client's treatment are strictly confidential and not to be shared with unauthorized individuals (ASHA, 2022). You may not bring these documents home to review, nor may you send them or discuss their content with anyone not authorized to access this information. As an SLPA, you should familiarize yourself with the form of documentation used in your setting and how to access it. If you are asked to provide services to a client, you should review the client's assessment report(s) and treatment plan in detail. Be sure to ask your supervising SLP if you have any questions about it.

LESSON PLANS

After a treatment plan is developed by your supervising SLP, the next step is to explore specific details on how to implement the plan for each individual client. How this information is conveyed to you will vary across settings and supervisors. In some settings, a lesson plan is used to outline additional information needed to implement treatment (ASHA, 2009). It may be that you are required to develop a draft of this plan for your supervisor to review, prior to implementing treatment. In other settings, this plan will be developed for you by your supervising SLP. In both instances, collaboration between you and your supervising SLP is required.

The concept of a lesson plan is borrowed from the field of education and was originally designed as a detailed description of the instruction to be provided by a teacher during a given class session (Karges-Bone, 2000). When applied to the field of speech-language pathology, lesson plans highlight important details and procedures for a single treatment session or to be provided over a short period (e.g., over 1 or 2 weeks; Hegde & Davis, 2010; Meyer, 2004). A lesson plan recommended by ASHA (2009) for use by SLPAs has several columns, including the core components of the treatment goals (Goals and Objectives), a description of the materials and equipment needed that session (Materials/Equipment), a description of the activity or task to be used (Activity/Task), and columns used to suggest modifications (Make It Easier/Make It More Difficult). Commonly, the column for modifications is also referred to as "Prompts/Modifications." Lesson plans can also include information on the client's performance (Data Collection), which may include a description of data to be collected that session and a summary of the client's actual performance during the session.

Figure 7–1 is an example of a lesson plan containing these components. Depending on the setting, some or all of these categories are used. The companion website of this textbook has additional blank copies of lesson plans applicable for SLPA use. The following sections address each component of the plan in greater detail. It is important that you clearly understand each component before you have any contact with a client. The importance of this cannot be overemphasized. To understand it in detail, as the picture and title of this chapter sug-

gests, you must decipher the information very carefully.

Goals and Objectives

The Goals and Objectives section of a lesson plan lists the goals and objectives to be targeted during the treatment session(s). Understanding goals and objectives can be very challenging for a new SLPA, as the language used is often unfamiliar and complex. Take heart, though: With time and exposure to this terminology, the process gets easier. Goals and objectives are important because they guide the selection of therapy materials, content, and procedures (Mager, 1997). They also serve as the basis for determining if a behavior has been accomplished and, importantly, provide those involved (including the client and the clinician) a full description of the desired outcome(s) of treatment (Mager, 1997). In some settings, they are also used directly for insurance reimbursement purposes (Cornett, 2010). Although SLPAs do not write or modify goals, it is still valuable to review their format to help you to decipher them.

Defining Goals

Treatment goals are statements of an outcome to be obtained. Traditionally defined, goals describe a behavior to be accomplished over the course of treatment (Roth & Worthington, 2018). Goals may or may not state a terminal behavior to be accomplished but generally are targeted over months or often, as in the case of a school setting, within an academic term. For example, a traditionally defined goal might be, "By X date, the client will decode grade-level reading material. . . . "

Client Name: Joseph Jones			Teacher/Room #: Wilson 12		
SLPA: Sarah S. Assistant			Supervising SLP: Samantha A. Supervisor		
Session Date(s): Week of 2/18/2018					
Goal/Objective	Activity/Task	Materials/Equipment	Make it Easier	Make it More Difficult	Data Collection
Joseph will produce /ʃ/ in the initial positions of words with 90% accuracy, across 10 attempts in 2 separate sessions.	Go Fish: Have Joseph ask for cards with words containing the /ʃ/ in the initial position (e.g., ship, shell, she). If he accurately produces the target, reinforce this by stating yes I have a ____, or, No I don't have a ____ (as applicable), emphasizing the /ʃ/ sound. If he inaccurately produces the target sound, model a correct version and an incorrect version and ask him to clarify by re-attempting (e.g., "did you want a ____ (/ʃ/ accurately produced) or a ____ (/ʃ/ distorted production?")	Go Fish cards containing CVC words with /ʃ/ in the initial position of words (e.g., ship, shell, she) Reminder card with picture of hand over lip to represent /ʃ/ Mirror	Point to the reminder card and/or model lip rounding before each production and after production error. Give him cards with the word written on it and the /ʃ/ underlined	Require him to have accurate production for the target word AND Go Fish When he lays down his pairs, reference it as "shelving" and have him name the pairs he obtained in the sentence, "I'll shelve 2 ____, with correct production of /ʃ/ in shelve and the target word.	+ = Accuracy (no cues/modification) +C = Accurate with cues. Note cues • M = verbal model • V = visual reminder • W = Written word CA = close approximation – = Inaccurate, Despite cues

Figure 7–1. Sample SLPA lesson plan.

By their nature, goals are broad statements of behavior. However, increasingly, the term *long-term goal* is used to identify the behavior to be accomplished, additional measurable terms (e.g., increase, decrease, maintain), and an expected ending level of performance, such as, "The student will increase the number of conversational topics that he spontaneously initiates from one to four (with no verbal or other prompts) in a student-adult conversation" (Minneapolis Public Schools, 2009). In some settings, the terms *goal* and *long-term goal* are used interchangeably, and in other settings, a general goal is followed by a set of specific long-term goals. The term *annual goal* denotes a goal that is to be accomplished that year, such as "By (annual IEP date), [the student] will listen attentively in class by using appropriate eye contact, body language, and/or proximity during oral communication in [8 out of 10] opportunities" (Porter & Steffin, 2006, p. 13).

Defining Objectives

Objectives accompany goals and are a series of steps needed to accomplish the goal's specified behavior. Objectives are also referred to as *short-term objectives* or, in some settings, are called *short-term goals* or *benchmarks*. Objectives include very precise and measurable language to state not only the behavior to be obtained but also at what level, by when, and under what conditions (Meyer, 2004; Roth & Paul, 2007; Roth & Worthington, 2018). Box 7–1 lists three key components of objectives: the performance (or do statement), the condition, and the *criterion* (singular) or *criteria* (plural; Meyer, 2004; Roth & Paul, 2007; Roth & Worthington, 2018). Appendix 7–D contains examples of goals and objectives from real-world settings.

To decipher goals and objectives, ask yourself specific questions about what is written and what additional information is needed, such as the questions listed in Box 7–2. The performance statement needs to be something that you can actually observe, meaning you can see or hear it (Meyer, 2004; Roth & Paul, 2007). If the performance is not something observable, the objective cannot be implemented. For example, verbs that describe performance, such as *understand*, *analyze*, and *process*, are not something you can see or hear, and as such, without further clarification, you would have no way of knowing if the client was performing the required task(s). Hence, in terms of the performance (or do) portion of an objective, ask yourself the following:

1. Is the performance stated?
2. What is the performance?
3. Is the performance observable (e.g., can I see it or hear it)?
4. What additional information is needed?

Similarly, a condition statement must be something that you as an SLPA can reproduce. For example, in an objective targeting pragmatics, the condition of "when speaking with grade-level peers" cannot be replicated in a one-on-one session with the clinician. Similarly, if a fluency goal included a condition of "during episodes of blocking" but you do not know what an episode of blocking is, you would not be able to replicate that condition. As such, it is important to ask yourself the following:

1. Is the condition stated?
2. What is the condition?
3. Can I replicate the condition?
4. What additional information is needed?

Box 7–1. Key Components of Behavioral Objectives

Performance: States what a client is expected to do to demonstrate mastery of the objective, including the quality and nature of performance. This is sometimes referred to as the "do" statement (e.g., the client will . . .).

Examples:

    Independently identify the names of primary colors

    Legibly write the numbers 1 to 10

    Spontaneously greet members of the social group

    Accurately produce the phoneme /t/ in the final positions of words

Condition: States what the client will be provided with (or denied) when performing the behavior, including (as applicable) terms to define the location, with whom, and given what type of assistance

Examples:

    In the community, with a same-age peer

    During a classroom group-reading activity, given a story starter

    In a one-on-one setting, given a verbal model from the clinician

    In response to a written command, without verbal cues to initiate

Criterion: States how the objective will be evaluated and in some cases a time frame in which the behavior will be accomplished, including as applicable the frequency, duration, accuracy, latency, speed, and intensity of a behavior

Examples:

    With 80% accuracy, given at least 20 attempts

    Within 2 minutes of a verbal prompt, in 8 of 10 opportunities

    For 2 minutes on two separate occasions

Lastly, the criterion of an objective must be stated in a way that you can measure it. The information you record is often referred to as data. Data is the information that is typically listed under "Data Collection" in the lesson plan. In order for you to record the client's performance on a given task, the criterion portion of an

---

> ## Box 7–2. Deciphering Goals/Objectives: Questions to Ask
>
> ### PERFORMANCE
>
> Is the performance stated?   □ YES □ NO
>
> What is the performance required? _____
>
> Can I observe the performance?   □ YES □ NO
>
> Additional information needed?   □ YES □ NO
>
> ### CONDITION
>
> Is the condition stated?   □ YES □ NO
>
> What is the condition?   _____
>
> Can I replicate the condition?   □ YES □ NO
>
> Additional information needed?   □ YES □ NO
>
> ### CRITERION
>
> Is the criterion stated?   □ YES □ NO
>
> What is the criterion?   _____
>
> Can I measure the criterion?   □ YES □ NO
>
> Additional information needed?   □ YES □ NO

objective must be something that you can effectively measure. For example, if a criterion states, "identify various types of stuttering," but you are not familiar with the types of stuttering, you will not be able to record the client's performance accurately. Similarly, if the criterion calls for "80% accuracy" in the accurate production of /r/, but you cannot accurately distinguish between correct, partially correct, and incorrect production of /r/, you will not be accurate in recording information about the client's performance. It also is impossible to record data accurately if parts of the criterion are missing. As such, in deciphering the criterion of an objective, ask yourself the following:

1. Is the criterion stated?
2. What is the criterion?
3. Can I measure the criterion (e.g., collect data)?
4. What additional information is needed?

Any time you have a question or need additional clarification, be sure to ask your supervisor before you implement any treatment activity. The companion website of this textbook contains a sample worksheet with these questions. Appendix 7–D contains sample goals and objectives from real-world settings. The sample reports in Appendices 7–A to 7–C also contain samples of goals and objectives. A good way to develop your skills in deciphering goals and objectives is to use these examples and identify the performance, condition, and criterion, asking important questions about each.

Activity/Task

This section of a lesson plan contains information relative to the type of activity or task to be used during treatment in addressing a specific goal or objective. Although objectives are detailed in their format and language, they can often be addressed utilizing a variety of activities or tasks, selected based on the client's interests, age, and specific needs. For example, consider the objective, "The client will request objects by pointing to an icon in his AAC device, in 9 of 10 opportunities." If this is implemented with a 6-year-old boy with autism who likes trains, an activity to target this goal might be to have the client build a train track by requesting different colors and types of trains, track, and other building materials, using a train theme page from his AAC notebook. In contrast, if this same objective is implemented with an adult with aphasia who enjoys cooking, the activity may be to bake a cake following a recipe and requesting needed items from the cooking page on her voice output AAC device.

Your supervising SLP will assist you in determining the type of activity or task most appropriate for each client. The following chapters on play and literacy (Chapter 16), speech sound remediation (Chapter 13), and group therapy (Chapter 12) each provide some sample tasks and activities. A review of sample activities across all ages and disorders is beyond the scope of this book; however, here are a few suggestions that will help familiarize you with an activity/task prior to implementing treatment:

1. *Self-study.* Before you engage in treatment activities with a new client, review treatment information specific to the client's disorder and unique presentation. Many resources, both online and in traditional treatment textbooks for communicative disorders, provide both a general framework of treatment techniques and a list of sample activities/tasks to use with specific treatment objectives or approaches. If you are not familiar with how to access this information, ask your supervising SLP for assistance.

2. *Observe.* Observe your supervising SLP engaging in the activity/task prior to implementing it yourself. This is valuable in helping you understand nuances that are not easily conveyed in a written description. Be sure to take notes so that you can refer back to them prior to implementing treatment.

3. *Role-play.* Role-play the activity/task with your supervising SLP. This is also an excellent way to become comfortable with implementing an activity/task. Be sure to play the role of the therapist, as this is the role you will play when implementing treatment.

4. *Ask questions.* During supervisory conferences, be sure to clarify any questions you may have about a specific activity or task. Ask, too, about the "whys" of the activity/task. This will help you understand the SLP's rationale for selecting that particular activity or task.

Materials/Equipment

This section of a lesson plan lists any materials or equipment needed to implement treatment. This could be wide ranging, including items specific to the activity or task itself, such as pictures, worksheets, toys and games, and tokens for reinforcement. It may also include items needed to record a client's performance, such as a specific score sheet or audio recorder. Materials used specifically to elicit a target response are referred to as *stimuli* (plural) or *stimulus* (singular). You should ensure you have these items ready and accessible before the treatment session begins. Be sure to review your materials and equipment well ahead of time to make sure they are in good working order. This ensures that no time is wasted locating, repairing, or troubleshooting missing items or malfunctioning equipment once the session begins. Chapter 10 provides some general principles for selecting appropriate stimuli, as do Chapters 12, 13, and 16. As discussed in Chapter 6, remember that all equipment and materials used must be properly cleaned for use in any treatment session.

Prompts and Modifications (Also Known as Make It Easier/ Make It More Difficult)

This section of an SLPA lesson plan includes any suggested modifications to the activity or task that could be used to reduce or increase task demands, including any recommended prompts or assistance appropriate to the task. Remember, treatment is a dynamic process. It may be that a given activity or task needs to be adjusted slightly to increase the client's participation and thereby address the desired objective. These modifications are not intended to alter the treatment goals or objectives but rather to enhance participation in the designated activity or task.

As with all aspects of a client's treatment, these should be discussed with the supervising SLP. Recognize as well that formats of a lesson plan vary across settings, and not all supervising SLPs will use or require this information on a lesson plan. If not, discuss any needed modifications with your supervising SLP to ensure that you understand how to modify an activity or task appropriately so that it remains consistent with the SLP's treatment plan for that particular client. Chapter 10 provides information on prompts and cues, as well as a discussion on the use of reinforcement in shaping behaviors. These are an important part of task/activity modification. Box 7–3 has additional examples of techniques to modify an activity or task, by altering the time constraints, tasks demands, or reinforcement. Not all modifications are equally applicable to all objectives, particularly if the modification changes the task sufficiently to alter a treatment objective's condition, performance, or criterion. That is not the purpose of modifications. For example, if the objective were, "The student will use the present progressive when describing pictures not visible to the clinician in 18 of 20 attempts," but you made the task easier by requiring the client to say a list of 20 verbs in present progressive tense after you say them, the activity would no longer be targeting the desired objective. As an SLPA, you must not modify elements of a treatment activity or task in any way that alters the treatment plan (ASHA, 2013).

Data Collection

Recording data about the client's performance is critical (Mowrer, 1982). Accurate data collection is particularly important in that, as an SLPA, you are the eyes and

---

Box 7–3. Potential Modifications in Activity/Task

1. Increase or decrease time constraints

   EXAMPLES

   - Give the client more time to respond (make it easier)
   - Require a quicker response (make it more difficult)
   - Give more breaks between responses (make it easier)
   - Require more responses in a shorter period (e.g., fewer breaks) (make it more difficult)

2. Increase or decrease the task demands

   EXAMPLES

   - Require a fully correct response (make it more difficult)
   - Accept a partially correct response (make it easier)
   - Require a shorter or less complex response (make it easier)
   - Require a longer or more complex response (make it more difficult)

3. Increase or decrease the reinforcement provided

   EXAMPLES

   - Provide reinforcement after every response (make it easier)
   - Provide intermittent reinforcement (make it more difficult)
   - Provide tangible reinforcement (make it easier)
   - Provide token reinforcement (make it more difficult)

---

ears for your supervising SLP when you are implementing treatment and she or he is not present to observe the client's performance. The Data Collection section of a lesson plan might include a description of any specific or important aspects of information recorded that session. In some cases, the lesson plan itself may also have space to record the data from a specific session. In that case, it doubles as a data collection sheet. Chapter 8 discusses data collection in detail and Chapter 9 addresses how to summarize this information effectively in a note about treatment.

REFERENCES

American Speech-Language-Hearing Association (ASHA). (2009). *Practical tools and forms for supervising speech-language pathology assistants.*

American Speech-Language-Hearing Association (ASHA). (2013). *Speech-language pathology assistant scope of practice.* https://www.asha.org/policy/sp2013-00337/

American Speech-Language-Hearing Association. (2022). *Scope of practice for the speech-language pathologist assistant (SLPA).* https://www.asha.org/policy/slpa-scope-of-practice/

Cornett, B. S. (2010). Health care reform and speech-language pathology practice. *ASHA*

Leader, 15, 14–17. https://doi.org/10.1044/leader.FTR2.15092010.14

Hegde, M. N., & Davis, D. (2010). *Clinical methods and practicum in speech-language pathology* (5th ed.). Cengage Learning.

Karges-Bone, L. (2000). *Lesson planning: Long-range and short-range models for Grades K–6.* Allyn & Bacon.

Krebs, J. M. (2008). Paper, paper everywhere? How to go paperless in your private practice. *ASHA Leader, 13,* 20–22. https://doi.org/10.1044/leader.FTR3.13122008.20

Mager, R. F. (1997). *Preparing instructional objectives: A critical tool in the development of effective instruction.* Center for Effective Performance Press.

Meyer, S. M. (2004). *Survival guide for beginning speech-language clinician* (2nd ed.). Pro-Ed.

Minneapolis Public Schools. (2009). *Consensus points on language goals.* https://www.asha.org/uploadedFiles/Consensus-Points-on-Language-Goals.pdf

Mowrer, D. E. (1982). *Methods of modifying speech behaviors: Learning theory in speech pathology.* Waveland.

Porter, J., & Steffin, B. (2006). *Speech-language pathology goals and objectives written to the California standards.* https://prakovic.edublogs.org/files/2015/06/SLPGoalsandObjectives update-1plo8wj.pdf

Roth, F., & Paul, R. (2007). Communication intervention. In R. Paul & P. Cascella (Eds.), *Introduction to clinical methods in communication disorders* (pp. 157–178). Paul H. Brookes.

Roth, F. P., & Worthington, C. K. (2018). *Treatment resource manual for speech-language pathologists* (5th ed.). Cengage Learning.

CHAPTER ENDNOTES

1. ASHA (n.d.-b).
2. Roth & Paul (2007); Roth & Worthington (2018).

Educational Setting—Sample Reports

XXXX School District
XXXX Elementary School

Student:	Student
DOB:	XX/XX/XXXX
Parents:	Parents
Address:	XXXXXXX
Assessment Conducted By:	Speech-Language Pathologist, M.A., CCC-SLP
Assessment Date:	January 2020
Report Date:	January 2020

Brief Background Information

Reason for Referral:
Student received a comprehensive speech-language evaluation across the three linguistic parameters of form (phonology, morphology, syntax), content (semantics), and use (pragmatics), in order to assist in the determination of the least restrictive educational environment based on his current academic and social needs.

History:
Student is a 7-year; 4-month-old boy enrolled in a first-grade, general education class. In addition to repeating kindergarten, Student receives speech-language therapy, and weekly RtI support in English Language Arts. Student resides with his parents and two siblings. English is the native, primary, and home language of the family. Student has been receiving special education services under the eligibility of Speech-Language Impairment since January 2017.

Testing Behavior:
Testing took place over multiple sessions lasting between 25 to 45 minutes each. During the assessment process, Student was given breaks as needed. In each assessment session, Student demonstrated behaviors consistent with inattention.

Assessment Procedure:

Assessment involved the use of multiple language-based instruments, record review, teacher interview, and observation. Assessment was conducted at Vessels Elementary School in the speech-language therapy room, which is well-lit and broadly free of distractions.

Language of Assessment:

As detailed above, English is Student's native, home, and primary language, which supports the use of English as the language of assessment.

Assessment Selection:

Selection of assessment instruments is based on the individual characteristics or profile of a specific child. Norm-referenced assessments maintain their validity and reliability when used with children who mirror the normative sample characteristics. The determination to use an assessment instrument in a standardized versus non-standardized manner includes consideration of the inclusionary requirements for the normative sample, as well as other factors that can preclude the use of standardized delivery.

When a child's profile does not align with the normative sample characteristics, norm-referenced assessments are useful in providing generalized guidance on specific behaviors or performance but cannot be used to provide standardized scores. The use of an assessment instrument in a non-standardized manner, in combination with the professional judgment of the specialist, criterion referenced norms, and an analysis of language use provide valid and reliable insight into a child's level of performance and can be considered accurate estimates of a child's performance.

Assessments Administered:

Standardized

Goldman-Fristoe Test of Articulation-3rd Edition (GFTA-3)

Montgomery Assessment of Vocabulary Assessment: Receptive Vocabulary (MAVA-R)

Montgomery Assessment of Vocabulary Assessment: Expressive Vocabulary (MAVA-E)

Comprehensive Assessment of Spoken Language 2nd Edition (CASL-2)

Informal Measures

Intelligibility

Voice, fluency

Oral Peripheral Exam

Pragmatic Language

Record review

Articulation

Norm-Referenced Assessment

The GFTA-3 was administered to assess Student's speech production at the word and phrase level with a standardized instrument. The GFTA-3 is a norm-referenced systematic means of assessing an individual's speech sound production of Standard American English for individuals aged 2;0 through 21;11 years. The chart below details the normative sample of the assessment used to assess Student's articulation abilities:

GFTA-3: Normative Requirements for Standardized Score Reporting	Child Characteristics	Exclusionary Cause(s)
Child is able to respond within standardized delivery as detailed in the testing manual (No modifications/adaptations required)	✓	
Child is identified as typically developing	✓	
English is the most frequently used language	✓	
Child speaks and understands English well or very well	✓	
Child is considered a simultaneous bilingual speaker		
Child acquired both languages in the United States		

Score Summary:

Subtest	Raw Score[1]	Standard Score (SS)	SS Range[2]	Percentile
Sounds-in-Words	12	75	70–82	5th

Based on a standard score range of 85 to 115, the score detailed above indicates that Student demonstrates a standard score range below what would be expected for his chronological age.

---

[1] Raw score equals the number of erred productions.
[2] Standard score range is based on a 95% confidence interval.

Consonant Inventory:

Single phonemes: As demonstrated in the following chart, which classifies phonemes by typical age of acquisition, Student's performance on the GFTA-3 revealed the following specific and consistent articulation errors:

Typical Age of Mastery*	Phonemes	Initial	Medial	Final
2 to 3 Years	/p/, /b/, /m/, /w/, /h/			
4 to 4.5 Years	/t/, /d/, /n/, /k/, /g/, /y/, /ng/			
4.5 to 5 Years	/f/			
4 to 7 Years	/ch/, /dg/	/ch/	/dg/	
6 to 6.5 Years	/l/, /v/, /sh/, /zh/			
6.5 to 7 Years	/th$_{v-}$/, /th$_{v+}$/ /s/, /z/	/th$_{v-}$/, /s/, /z/	/s/, /z/	/th$_{v-}$/, /s/, /z/
7 Years or later	/r/, vocalic /r/			

Based on data compiled from Weiss Articulation Test, Goldman-Fristoe Test of Articulation, commonly cited studies from Templin 1957; Poole 1934; Articulation Differences & Disorders Manual, San Diego)

As seen above, Student demonstrates errors on the fricatives /s,z,th$_{v-}$/ and the affricate /ch/.

Consonant Clusters:

Student demonstrated errors on a single consonant cluster, /sl/:

Typical Age of Mastery (males)	Word-Initial Consonant Cluster
3.6 Years	/tw/
5.6 Years	/kw/
6.0 Years	/pl, bl, kl, gl/
7.0 Years	/fl/
8.0 Years	/pr, br, tr, dr, kr, gr, fr/
9.0 Years	/sp, st, sl, skw, spl/
Older than 9.0 Years	/sk, sm, sn, sw, thr, spr, str, skr/

Examples of Student's productions follow:

Target	Production	Target	Production
Slide	Thlided	Chair	Shair
Thumb	Sum	Glasses	Glatheth
Cheese	Sheese	Teeth	Tees
Juice	Juith	Seven	Theven

The production of the phonemes /s,z/ require specific tongue grove formation, precise placement of the tongue tip, accurate tooth alignment, retraction of the lips, and stable jaw gradation. When one or more of these components is out of alignment, the result is a frontal lisp, which is what Student demonstrated during the assessment. Further, Student demonstrated errors on the voiceless /th/, which he altered through a change in placement by substituting the /s/ phonemes and on the affricates /ch, dg/, which he altered by substituting the corresponding fricative /sh/.

Error analysis suggests that Student is overgeneralizing the motor planning training he is receiving in intervention sessions to words with the voiceless /th/, as seen in his production of [sum] for /thumb/. Student demonstrated two voicing errors, when he produced [kituar] for /guitar/, but in the rest of the opportunities, Student produced the correct voicing, and these errors are not considered areas of concern.

Vocabulary

Montgomery Assessment of Vocabulary Acquisition (MAVA)
The MAVA was designed to measure the development of children's oral language by assessing listening (receptive) and speaking (expressive) vocabulary. Because oral language precedes reading and writing, it serves as an excellent predictor of literacy skills. The words on the MAVA were selected using the three tiers of vocabulary. Words are assigned to tier one, two, or three depending on their characteristics of meaning and use. Children acquire the three tiers as they learn and mature in both academic and real-word contexts. Results follow:

Measure	Standard Score	Standard Score Range*	Percentile
Receptive Vocabulary	86	80–82	18
Expressive Vocabulary	86	80–92	18

*Based on a 90% Confidence Interval.

A detailed analysis of Student's performance follows:

Vocabulary	Modality
Tier 1: Tier one words are the most basic words. They are the early reading words, sight words, nouns, verbs, and adjectives that students learn to identify or decode with instruction. They learn to read them—identify them in print form—because they already use them in their speaking vocabulary. Examples of tier one words are: boy, fence, happy, chicken, green, fancy, and running. There are about 8,000-word families in English in tier one.	**Receptive:** Student understood 57 of 57, or 100%, of Tier 1 words. Examples include: Winter; helmet; bounce.
	Expressive: Student identified 62 of 64, or 97%, of Tier 1 words. Examples include: firefighter; broccoli; shopping
Tier 2: Tier two words are the high frequency words that are found in many domains. They play a large role in our speaking and reading vocabulary. These words often represent multiple meanings and subtle nuances. In addition, they typically "add productivity to an individual's language ability" (Beck et al., 2002, p. 16). Tier two words are the most important ones to directly teach to students because they are assumed to be known as students progress through school. Examples of tier two words are: masterpiece, preference, fortuitous, glean, and measure. There are about 7,000-word families in English in tier two.	**Receptive:** Student understood 31 of 43, or 72%, of Tier 2 words. Examples include: court; away; anchor
	Expressive: Student identified 23 of 39, or 59%, of Tier 2 words. Examples include: trophy; vegetables; diamond
Tier 3: Tier three words are those related to specific domains and have a low frequency of use. Domains might include subject areas in school, hobbies, geographic regions, technology, weather, etc. Examples of tier three words are: ukulele, asphalt, genome, crepe, and cornice. The remaining 400,000 words in English fall in this tier.	**Receptive:** Student understood 9 of 17, or 53%, of Tier 3 words. Examples include: Cylinder; pyramid
	Expressive: Student identified 2 out of 7 or 29% Tier 3 words. Examples include tentacle, equator, and equator

The results detailed above indicate that Student's performance on the MAVA-R and MAVA-E falls within the average when compared to peers of the same chronological age and he demonstrated relatively commensurate receptive and expressive abilities. When analyzing the percentage correct of items within the tiers, Student recognized more items than he could name, and his accuracy decreased across the tiers:

Measure	Tier 1	Tier 2	Tier 3
Receptive Vocabulary	100%*	72%*	53%*
Expressive Vocabulary	97%	59%	29%

*Higher score.

These findings suggest that Student is acquiring vocabulary through exposure to the ambient language surrounding him. However, Student is not acquiring vocabulary as rapidly through exposure to the tiered language in the academic classroom. A possible contributing factor may be attentional. Over time, as children are exposed to language and vocabulary, they begin to identify new words embedded in familiar sentences. Children use the structured of the sentence to make sense of the use of these new words. This attention to individual sentences and the location of a new word within that sentence creates significant competing linguistic and cognitive demands. With the decreased focus abilities that are compromised with attention deficits, this ability to map new words decreases.

Language Functioning

Student was given a comprehensive assessment of his receptive and expressive language as detailed below:

The *Comprehensive Assessment of Spoken Language—2nd Edition* (CASL-2) is a standardized test that provides an in-depth assessment of an individual's oral language skills of: (1) oral language processing systems of auditory comprehension, oral expression, and word retrieval, (2) knowledge and use of words and grammatical structures of language, (3) ability to use language for special tasks requiring higher-level cognitive functions, and (4) knowledge and use of language in communicative contexts. Normative data is provided for English speaking students aged 3 years, 0 months to 21 years, 11 months. Average standard scores range from 85–115.

The table below details the results of each subtest used in the assessment:

Subtest	Raw Score	Standard Score (SS)	CI[3] (95%)	Percentile	Descriptor
Receptive Vocabulary	40	92	85–99	30	*Average*
Antonyms	16	91	86–98	27	*Average*
Synonyms	15	88	81–95	21	*Average*
Expressive Vocabulary	11	78	71–85	7	*Below average*
Sentence Expression	14	81	74–88	10	*Below average*
Grammatical Morphemes	19	80	72–88	9	*Below average*
Sentence Comprehension	36	100	95–105	50	*Average*
Grammaticality Judgment	12	82	80–84	12	*Below average*
Meaning from Context	2	82	74–90	12	*Below average*
Inference	23	100	97–103	50	*Average*

As seen in the scores above, Student demonstrated a range of standard scores from 78 to 100. As noted in Testing Behavior summary, Student's ability to focus on the task at hand varied significantly across the subtests. In some assessment sessions, Student was able to attend to the task, respond appropriately, and move onto the next task. In other assessment sessions, Student required frequent incentives to respond to questions, multiple movement breaks to support focus, and sat quietly in his chair in frequently. It is highly likely his performance was impacted by these issues and as such, the variability in subtest scores should be considered carefully.

Discrepant Analysis: An analysis of subtest score differences revealed a statistically significant difference between Student's receptive and expressive vocabulary scores, and his sentence comprehension and sentence expression scores. This pattern is not unexpected because receptive tasks require recognition, whereas expressive tasks require retrieval of the exact name of an item and the words required for sentence construction, which is the more difficult task.

---

[3]CI refers to Confidence Interval.

Index Scores Compared	Observed Difference	Critical Value	Significantly Different?	Percentage of Sample With this Difference
RV – EV	14	10	3	10%
SC – SE	19	11	3	10%
GM – GJ	2	7	No	N/A

Upon completion of the subtest battery, scores are compiled into indices that are seen in the table below:

Index	Sum of Standard Scores	Standard Score (SS)	CI (95%)	Percentile	Descriptive Category
General Language Ability (GLAI)	435	86	84–88	19	*Average*
Receptive Language (RLI)	280	90	85–95	25	*Average*
Expressive Language (ELI)	339	82	78–86	12	*Below Average*
Lexical/ Semantic	271	85	81–89	16	*Average*
Syntactic (SI)	343	83	79–87	13	*Below Average*
Supralinguistic (SPI)	269	88	85–91	21	*Average*

An overall analysis of Student's performance on the CASL-2 reveals a GLAI standard score range of 84 to 88, which falls just inside the range identified as *Average*, which means that his performance is within a single standard deviation from the mean of 100. This index reflects a student's general spoken language abilities. When analyzing the remaining five indices, Student's performance fell just outside the *Average* range in the ELI and the SI. The ELI reflects a student's overall skill in expressive language, with a particular emphasis on linguistic structure. This slightly below average standard score falls in line with observations by this examiner during unstructured language observations. In these observations Student consistently produced errors on irregular past tense verbs. Examples of these errors include [goed] for /went/, [putted] for /put/, [hitted] for /hit/, and [eated] for /ate/.

These errors are considered "overgeneralizations," and reflect a child's understanding of the use of morphology to mark tense, rather than the use of an irregular form that must be memorized. While this linguistic behavior is not typically observed in children Student's age, it nonetheless reflects Student's continued linguistic development.

Summary: The results above indicate that Student demonstrates a strength in his oral language skills that are largely commensurate with children in his age range. He demonstrates a relative weakness in syntactic structures, as evidenced in the Syntactic Index score and in observations by this examiner.

Informal Measures

Pragmatic Language:

Student's use of language in social contexts was analyzed through observations by this examiner in speech-language therapy session with multiple peers and during assessment sessions. Student's performance is detailed below:

Item	Skill	Always	Sometimes	Rarely
1.	Responding appropriately to questions from peers, teachers	✓		
2.	Expressing gratitude	✓		
3.	Greeting peers, teachers	✓		
4.	Polite refusal	✓		
5.	Evaluating non-verbal cues			
6.	Requesting information appropriately from peers, teachers	✓		
7.	Speaking on appropriate topics	✓		
8.	Sharing the conversational space	✓		
9.	Appropriate topic maintenance	✓		
10.	Taking turns	✓		
11.	Following directions	✓		
12.	Behaving appropriately in a variety of contexts (playground, classroom, speech-language therapy room, lunch tables)	✓		

As seen above, Student demonstrates appropriate use of language for social purposes.

Intelligibility:

Student's intelligibility was assessed on a 5-point scale: (1) completely intelligible in conversation; (2) mostly intelligible in conversation; (3) somewhat intelligible in conversation; (4) mostly unintelligible in conversation; and (5) completely unintelligible in conversation.

Per observations by this examiner and other allied professionals, Student's intelligibility is rated as a 2, *mostly intelligible in conversation*, and he successfully communicates his intent the great majority of the time across topics, contexts, and with or without context.

Voice and Fluency:

Voice quality was judged to be age and gender appropriate. No atypical disfluencies were observed.

Oral-Peripheral Examination:

The Oral-Peripheral Examination is an exam that views structures organically and functionally for speech production adequacy. Per external observation, Student's structures appear sufficiently robust for both speech production and eating.

Summary and Impressions

Student, at 7-years, 4-months of age, demonstrates overall age-appropriate language skills in content (i.e., semantics/meaning), and use (i.e., pragmatics) when compared to same-aged peers.

With respect to form (i.e., sound, word, and sentence structure), Student demonstrates speech sound errors beyond what would be expected based on his chronological age. Specifically, Student demonstrates substitution errors, /d/ for /th/, and presents with a frontal lisp. He further demonstrates errors in the production of past tense, where he is adding the ending "ed" to irregular, past tense verbs. A summary of the standardized assessments can be seen below:

Measure	Standard Score	Standard Score Range	Percentile
GFTA-3	75	70–82	5th
MAVA: Receptive Vocabulary	86	80–92	18
MAVA: Expressive Vocabulary	86	80–92	18
CASL-2: General Language Ability Index	86	84–88	19
CASL 2: Receptive Language Index	90	85–95	25
CASL 2: Expressive Language Index	82	76–86	12
CASL 2: Lexical/Semantic Index	85	81–89	16
CASL 2: Syntactic Index	83	79–87	13
CASL 2: Supralinguistic Index	88	85–91	21

An overall analysis of Student's performance on the CASL-2 reveals a General Language Ability Index standard score of 86, which falls just inside the range identified as *Average*, which means that his performance is within a single standard deviation from the mean of 100. When analyzing the remaining five indices, Student's performance fell just outside the *Average* range in the ELI and the SI. The ELI reflects a student's overall skill in expressive language, with a particular emphasis on linguistic structure.

Recommendations:
Members of the Individualized Education Program team need to review the above information along with other pertinent information to determine the Least Restrictive Environment and the most appropriate education setting and interventions to meet the student's education needs.

Respectfully submitted,

_____

Speech-Language Pathologist, M.A., CCC-SLP

EFG School District

Written Translation Requested

Language: English

Individualized Education Program

Last Name	XXXXXX
First Name	XXXXXX
Student ID	XXXXXX
IEP Date	4/14/2017
Next IEP	4/14/2018
Last Annual IEP	4/14/2018
Last Eval	4/14/2017
SPED Entry Date	4/15/2017

Purpose of Meeting: ☒ Initial ☐ Annual ☐ Triennial ☐ Transition ☐ Pre-expulsion ☐ Interim ☐ Expanded ☐ Other: _____

DOB: 11/9/2010 ☐ F ☒ M **Grade:** Kindergarten **Migrant:** ☐ Yes ☒ No

Home Language: English **EL:** ☐ Yes ☒ No ☐ Redesignated
Interpreter: ☐ Yes ☒ No

Residency: Parent or Legal Guardian
School Attending: ABC Elementary School

Parent/Guardian: XXXXXX

District of Residence: EFG School District
School of Residence: ABC Elementary School

Ethnicity: 1. <u>WHITE</u> 2. _____ 3. _____ 4. _____

Primary Disability Eligible for Special Education ☒ Yes ☐ No

☐ Autism (AUT)	☐ Hard of Hearing (HH)*	☐ Other Health Impairment (OHI)
☐ Deaf-Blindness (DB)*	☐ Mental Retardation (MR)	☒ Specific Learning Disability (SLD)
☐ Deafness (DEAF)*	☐ Multiple Disability (MD)	☐ Speech/Language Impairment (SLI)
☐ Emotional Disturbance (ED)	☐ None	☐ Traumatic Brain Injury (TBI)
☐ Established Medical Disability (EMD)	☐ Orthopedic Impairment (OI)*	☐ Visual Impairment (VI)*

Secondary Disability

☐ Autism (AUT)	☐ Hard of Hearing (HH)*	☐ Other Health Impairment (OHI)
☐ Deaf-Blindness (DB)*	☐ Mental Retardation (MR)	☒ Specific Learning Disability (SLD)
☐ Deafness (DEAF)*	☐ Multiple Disability (MD)	☐ Speech/Language Impairment (SLI)
☐ Emotional Disturbance (ED)	☐ None	☐ Traumatic Brain Injury (TBI)
☐ Established Medical Disability (EMD)	☐ Orthopedic Impairment (OI)*	☐ Visual Impairment (VI)*

*Low Incidence Disability.

Eligibility Statement:

A severe discrepancy exists between intellectual ability and academic achievement in written expression and listening comprehension. XXXXXX evidences processing disorders in attention (the ability to sustain attention and concentrate on a task or activity) and a personal weakness in auditory processing (the ability to recognize, perceive, and interpret auditory stimuli).

Describe how the student's disability affects involvement and progress in the general curriculum (or, for preschoolers, participation in appropriate activities):
He will benefit from small group and individual specialized instruction that is not available in the general class.

For Initial Placement Only

Has the student received prereferral early intervening services in the past 2 years?

☒ Yes ☐ No

Date of initial referral for special education services: 2/17/2017

Person initiating the referral for special education service:
Student study/intervention team

Date district received parental consent: 2/17/2017

Date of initial meeting to determine eligibility: 4/14/2017

PRESENT LEVELS OF ACADEMIC ACHIEVEMENT/ FUNCTIONAL PERFORMANCE

<u>Educational Strengths/Preferences/Interests</u>
He tries to work in small groups. He enjoys working on the computer and uses the DS game at home.

Concerns of parent relevant to educational progress
Mom is concerned about his reading. Mom indicated he had 2 full years of pre-school. When he doesn't want to work, he stops working completely.

State Standards

English/Language Arts	☐ Adv.	☐ Proficient	☐ Basic	☐ Below Basic	☐ Far Below Basic
Mathematics	☐ Adv.	☐ Proficient	☐ Basic	☐ Below Basic	☐ Far Below Basic
Hist./Soc. Science	☐ Adv.	☐ Proficient	☐ Basic	☐ Below Basic	☐ Far Below Basic
Science	☐ Adv.	☐ Proficient	☐ Basic	☐ Below Basic	☐ Far Below Basic

Most Recent Scores

Listening _____ Speaking _____ Reading _____ Writing _____

Fitness/PE Test (Grades 5, 7, & 9 only) _____

Other Assessment Data (e.g., curriculum assessment, other district assessment)

DRA Level 1, knows 8 of 27 kindergarten sight words, almost all capital and lower case letters

Hearing _____ ☐ Pass ☐ Fail ☐ Other: _____
Vision _____ ☐ Pass ☐ Fail ☐ Other: _____

The **Brief Written Language**-<k.0; Spelling subtest-<k.0; requires the production of single letters and words in response to oral prompts; **Writing Samples** subtest-<k.0; measures the ability to convey ideas in writing; requires the production of meaningful written sentences in responses to a variety of task criteria.

The **Listening Comprehension** cluster provides a measure of achievements including understanding directions and comprehending oral language. XXXXXX's overall listening comprehension ability is within the low average range. His performances on the Understanding Directions and Oral Comprehension subtests were within the low range.

Cognitive Functioning

The assessments results indicate that XXXXXX meets eligibility criteria for SLD. A severe discrepancy exists between intellectual ability and academic achievement in the areas of written expression and listening comprehension. XXXXXX evidences processing disorders in the area(s) of *Attention* (the ability to sustain attention and concentrate on a task or activity) as well as a personal weakness in *Auditory Processing* (the ability to recognize, perceive, and interpret auditory stimuli).

Communication Development

XXXXXX continues to exhibit decreased speech intelligibility. He exhibits difficulty producing /v/ in all word positions and he produces a frontal distortion for /s/ and /z/ in all word positions. XXXXXX is stimulable for correct production of /v/ in all word positions when given a verbal model. Additionally, XXXXXX exhibits the phonological processes of gliding, and substituting [w] for /r/ and /l/ in all word positions. Both the SLP and classroom teacher reported that his expressive and receptive language skills appear to be within normal limits. The frontal distortion of /s/ and /z/ and substitution of [w] for /r/ and /I/ is appropriate for his age.

Gross/Fine Motor Development

Gross and fine motor development appear to be within normal limits.

Social Emotional/Behavioral

XXXXXX is social, affectionate, and talkative; however, he is easily distracted. He is respectful of adults and is learning social boundaries from his peers.

Health (including medication information)

XXXXXX has general good health and parents report his hearing and vision are within normal limits.

Vocational

XXXXXX tries to be responsible and is beginning to read the calendar.

Self-Help

XXXXXX can get himself dressed and take care of his personal needs.

Area of need to be addressed in goals and objectives for student to receive educational benefit:

☐ Math Calculations ☐ Math Applications ☐ Reading Fluency ☐ Self-Help Skills

☐ Social Behavior   ☐ Attendance   ☐ Pre-vocational skills   ☒ Writing

☒ Reading Comprehension ☒ Speech and Language ☐ Other: _____

SPECIAL FACTORS TO BE CONSIDERED

Does the student require assistive technology devices and/or services?
☒ No ☐ Yes

Does the student require low incidence services, equipment, and/or materials to meet educational goals? ☒ N/A ☐ No ☐ Yes

Considerations if the student is blind or visually impaired: ☒ N/A

Considerations if the student is deaf or hard of hearing: ☒ N/A

If the child is an English learner, consider the language needs of the child as those needs relate to the IEP: ☒ N/A

Does student's behavior impede learning of self or others? ☒ No ☐ Yes

☐ Behavior Support Plan (BSP) attached

☐ Behavior Intervention Plan (BIP) attached

Statewide Testing

Participation in Math
☒ Grade Exempt (before Grade 2/after Grade 11)

Participation in Science
☒ Grade Exempt

Participation in English Language Arts
☒ Grade Exempt (before Grade 2/after Grade 11)

Participation in History (8th grade)
☒ Grade Exempt

Participation in Writing (4th and 7th grade)
☒ Grade Exempt

ANNUAL GOALS

Area of Need: Pre-Academic/ Academic Reading	Measurable Annual Goal #1
Baseline: He has trouble blending words and remembering what he reads.	By 4/14/18: In the resource room & in the general ed. class, XXXXXX will use the pictures from a story to make predictions about its content with 80% correct each opportunity as measured by work samples & observation records. ☒ Enables student to be involved/progress in general curriculum/state standard #C 0.2.2 ☒ Addresses other educational needs resulting from disability ☐ Linguistically appropriate ☒ Person(s) Responsible: *General Education Teacher & RSP*

Area of Need:	Measurable Annual Goal #2
Pre-Academic/ Academic Reading	By 4/14/18: In the resource room & in the general ed. class, XXXXXX will blend vowel-consonant sounds orally to make words or symbol with 80% correct each opportunity as measured by work samples & observation records.
Baseline: He knows sounds of words but he does not consistently blend the words in context or isolated.	☒ Enables student to be involved/progress in general curriculum/state standard #W 0.1.9 ☒ Addresses other educational needs resulting from disability ☐ Linguistically appropriate ☒ Person(s) Responsible: _General Education Teacher & RSP_ _Parents_

Area of Need:	Measurable Annual Goal #3
Pre-Academic/ Academic Writing	By 4/14/18: In the resource room & in the general ed. Class, XXXXXX will determine a reasonable spelling, using pre-phonetic knowledge, letter sounds, and knowledge of letter names with 80% correct each opportunity as measured by work samples & observation records.
Baseline: He tries to write words to form a sentence. He can write a missing word for a sentence given a review of choice of words to write.	☒ Enables student to be involved/progress in general curriculum/state standard #C 0.1.2 ☒ Addresses other educational needs resulting from disability ☐ Linguistically appropriate ☒ Person(s) Responsible: _General Education Teacher & RSP_ _Parents_

Area of Need:	Measurable Annual Goal #4
Language/ Communication	By 4/14/18, XXXXXX will independently produce /v/ in all word positions in sentences with 80% accuracy across 2 consecutive sessions.
Baseline: When on task, produces /v/ in all word positions with 30% accuracy with verbal models.	☐ Enables student to be involved/progress in general curriculum/state standard #_____ ☒ Addresses other educational needs resulting from disability ☒ Linguistically appropriate ☒ Person(s) Responsible: _Speech/Language Specialist General Education Teacher & Parents_

Area of Need:	Measurable Annual Goal #5
Language/ Communication	By 4/14/18, in the speech room, XXXXXX will produce sentences using the correct subjective pronoun to describe pictures and stories with 80% accuracy across two consecutive sessions.
Baseline: XXXXXX exhibits difficulty producing the appropriate subjective pronoun to describe stories and photographs. For example, XXXXXX frequently substitutes him for he and her for she, which detracts the reader from the message.	☒ Enables student to be involved/progress in general curriculum/state standard #S 3.1.4 ☒ Addresses other educational needs resulting from disability ☐ Linguistically appropriate ☒ Person(s) Responsible: _Speech/Language Specialist General Education Teacher & Parents_

SERVICES

Service Options considered: ☒ General Education ☒ DIS ☒ RSP ☐ SDC ☐ NPS
☐ Other _____

Services		Provider	Start/ End Date	Frequency	Duration (Total Minutes)	Location
Specialized academic instruction	I/G	a District of service	4/15/17	(4×) Weekly	30	a Special Education Room
			4/15/18			
Speech & Language	I/G	a District of service	4/15/17	(4×) Weekly	30	a Special Education Room
			4/15/18			

Special Transportation: ☐ Yes ☒ No   **Extended School Year (ESY):** ☐ Yes ☒ No

Programs and services will be provided according to when student is in attendance and consistent with the public school calendar and scheduled services, excluding holidays, vacations, conference schedules, and non-instructional days.

PLACEMENT

Physical Education: ☐ General ☐ Specially Designed (describe) _____
  ☐ APE   ☐ High School PE Requirements (2 years): ☐ Met ☐ In Progress

Service District: <u>EFG School District</u>
School of Attendance: <u>ABC Elementary School</u>
School Type   <u>Public Day School</u>
Federal Setting: <u>Regular Classroom</u>

All special education services provided at student's home school: ☒ Yes ☐ No

Other Agency Services:
  ☐ California Children's Services (CCS)   ☐ Regional Center
  ☐ Probation   ☐ Department of Rehabilitation
  ☐ Dept. of Social Services (DSS)   ☐ Other _____
  ☐ County Mental Health (CMH)

Student Eligible for Mental Health Services under Chapter 26.5 ☐ Yes ☒ No

Mental Health Services Language Included on the IEP ☐ Yes ☒ No

Transportation: ☐ None ☒ General ☐ Special Ed _____

Student Transition:
☒ N/A   ☐ PK to Elementary   ☐ Elementary to Middle School
☐ Middle to High School   ☐ High School to Adult Transition
☐ High School to Post Secondary   ☐ Other _____

GRADUATION PLAN
(Grade 8 and Higher)

Projected graduation date and/or secondary completion date _____
  ☒ Diploma
  ☐ Non-Diploma Certificate

APPENDIX 7–B
Private Practice—Sample Reports

ABC Speech Services

Speech & Language Evaluation Report

Name: XXXXXXXXXX   Date of Birth: 4/11/16

Address: XXXXXXXXXX   Chronological Age: 1.9-year-old (21 months)
        XXXXXXXXXX

Date of Report: 2/4/18

Telephone: XXXXXXXX   Assessment Date: 1/22/18

RCOC Service Coordinator: XXXXXXXXX

I. BACKGROUND INFORMATION:
The reason for the referral is to determine XXXXXX's level of functioning in the areas of speech and language. XXXXXX is a 1.9-year-old boy who lives with his mother, father, and baby sister. He was diagnosed with autism by XXXXXX at 16 months of age. At or during birth, XXXXXX may have had a brain injury, which caused left-side weaknesses of his upper and lower extremities and left eye droop (ptosis). Vietnamese is his primary language. Per parent report, there is a family history of autism (two of XXXXXX's cousins). He is currently receiving physical therapy 1 hour per week at XXXXXXX. In the past, he received feeding therapy at XXXXXXX and six sessions of speech therapy at XXXXXX. He has constipation problems and takes Miralax daily. His mom reported some sensory problems such as rubbing objects on his mouth, grabbing her hand repeatedly to rub or lick, and rubbing his face. XXXXXX passed his newborn hearing screening and there are no concerns with his hearing and vision at this time. Please refer to the Regional Center intake summary for further medical and developmental information.

II. ASSESSMENT RESULTS:
XXXXXX's speech, language, pragmatics, and informal cognitive/play skills were assessed using clinical observations, parent report, review of records, Developmental Assessment of Young Children (DAYC)–Cognitive Subtest, and The Rossetti Infant-Toddler Language Scale. The speech and language assessment was conducted in Vietnamese.

<u>DAYC–Cognitive Subtest:</u>

Age Equivalent:	23 months
Percentile:	70%ile
Standard Score:	108

<u>The Rossetti Infant-Toddler Language Scale</u>

Pragmatics:	3 months scattering to 9–12 months (86% delay)
Language Comprehension:	15 months with scattering to 33–36 mos. (29%delay)
Language Expression:	12 months with scattering to 33–36 mos. (43% delay)

A. RECEPTIVE LANGUAGE:

In the area of language comprehension, XXXXXX scored solidly at the 15-month level with scattered skills up to the 33- to 36-month level (29% delay). He is able to identify pictures, objects, action words, and body parts upon request. Also, XXXXXX follows one-step commands, recognizes family member names, understands the prepositions "in, on," and responds to simple questions. He does not identify objects by category, understand 50 words, and follow related two-step commands.

B. EXPRESSIVE LANGUAGE:

In the area of language expression, XXXXXX scored solidly at the 12-month level with scattered skills up to the 33- to 36-month level (43% delay). Although he uses up to four-word sentences to communicate wants and needs, his language is mostly scripted. As a result, his language is highly restricted. He does not spontaneously combine novel utterances. He demonstrates both immediate and delayed echolalia. XXXXXX is often off topic and will say random words out of context. If joint attention is established, then he is able to ask and answer simple questions. He is inconsistent with imitating words. Despite talking a lot, XXXXXX does not engage in a back-and-forth conversation and rarely initiates conversation with others.

C. SPEECH:

Oral structures appear adequate for speech production. XXXXXX used the age-appropriate consonants /p, b, m, w, t, d, n, h/ during the assessment. Speech intelligibility was judged to be 90% to 100%.

D. COGNITIVE/PLAY SKILLS:

According to the Rossetti, XXXXXX's pragmatics skills are at the 3-month level with scattered skills up to the 9- to 12-month level, which is considered significantly below the average range (86% delay). During play, he demonstrates limited interactions, rarely initiates play acts, and has to be prompted to maintain play. He is object oriented and his play is rigid and repetitive. He sees shapes and letters in objects and gets fixated by them. He is not able to maintain eye contact, vocalize to gain attention, consistently respond to his name, initiate turn-taking routines, or imitate other children. Results of the DAYC cognitive subtest indicated he is at the 70th percentile, which places him in the average range. He spontaneously names objects, uses pretend objects in play, counts 1 to 20, matches objects by color and shape, and stacks at least six blocks.

III. OBSERVATIONS:

XXXXXX participated in most of the test tasks and activities. His mom sat in during the testing and served as informant. He demonstrates fleeting eye contact, inconsistent joint attention, and flat affect. When excited, XXXXXX exhibits awkward arm and leg movements (e.g., when he got to play with the shape sorter). Per parent report, XXXXXX has compliance issues and tantrums at home (e.g., when there is a change in routine). When around peers, he would look at what the peers are doing but never interact with them.

IV. SUMMARY & RECOMMENDATIONS:

XXXXXX demonstrates an 86% delay in pragmatics (solid at 3 months), a 29% delay in receptive language skills (solid at 15 months), and a 43% delay in expressive language (solid at 12 months). It is recommended that XXXXXX receive 2 hours per week of speech therapy. Per parent report, there are some sensory and behavioral problems at home. It is recommended that XXXXXX receive an OT and ABA evaluation to determine if therapy is warranted.

V. GOALS:

   a. XXXXXX will follow related two-step verbal directions with 80% accuracy.
   b. XXXXXX will spontaneously produce novel utterances to communicate his wants and needs with 80% accuracy.
   c. XXXXXX will consistently imitate words upon request with 80% accuracy.
   d. XXXXXX will initiate one-step play acts during pretend play with 80% accuracy.
   e. XXXXXX will initiate one to three comments and/or questions during pretend play with 80% accuracy.
   f. XXXXXX will appropriately use words to get someone's attention with 80% accuracy.
   g. XXXXXX will initiate turn-taking games with 80% accuracy.

_____

XXXXXXXXX
Speech-Language Pathologist

PRIVATE PRACTICE
WHOLE LANGUAGE ASSESSMENT

Client:	Student
DOB:	11/10/20XX
Age:	5;6
Parents:	Parent
Assessor:	Speech-Language Pathologist, Ph.D., CCC-SLP
Assessment Date:	June 2021
Report Date:	June 2021

Brief Background Information:
Per parent report, Student is an active, engaging, and curious child. Health history is unremarkable. Her primary, native, and first language is English. She is exposed to Vietnamese via her grandparents approximately 40% of the time.

Per parent report, Student had previously been enrolled in a preschool class, but when she began to demonstrate multiple behaviors associated with anxiety, such as reduced appetite and stuttering, they decided to remove her from the program. As a result, both behaviors abated. Parent also reported that Student prefers the company of adults and has trouble interacting with peers. Examples of this interaction include Student making unsuccessful communicative bids on highly preferred topics or repeating phrases from Siri, the virtual assistant.

Student demonstrates strong literacy skills in both decoding and comprehension. She read two stories aloud to the assessor with fluency and used word attack skills when presented with an unfamiliar word (e.g., *odor*). She also demonstrated strong print literacy skills as evidenced when she commented that the presence of all capital letters indicates that the reader is supposed to speak louder.

Language of Assessment:
Per parent report, Student is exposed to both English and Vietnamese; however, the dominant home language is English. Further, in the initial session and all subsequent sessions, Student responded exclusively in English. Based on this information, it was determined that English was the appropriate language of assessment. However, given that the language of children exposed to dual languages is distributed across both languages, performance in either language alone is not expected to follow the same patterns of children of the same age who are exposed to a single language. As such, assessments are reported descriptively only.

Assessment Structure:

A. This assessment covers the following language domains:

Form	
Phonology	The speech sound system (phonemes) of a language, including the rules for combining and using phonemes
Morphology	The rules that govern how morphemes (word parts), the minimal meaning units of language, are used in language
Syntax	The rules that govern the ways words can be combined to form sentences in a language
Content	
Semantics	The meaning of words and combination of rules in a language (vocabulary)
Pragmatics	
Use	The rules associated with the use of language in conversation and broader social situations.

B. The five language domains were assessed with the following measures:

Form	
Phonology	Observation
Morphology	Narrative Procedure[1]; Language Sample Analysis (LSA)[2]
Syntax	Narrative Procedure[1]; LSA[2]
Content	
Semantics	Montgomery Assessment of Vocabulary Acquisition (MAVA)[3]: Receptive and Expressive; LSA[2]
Pragmatics	
Use	Language Use Inventory (LUI)[4]; Narrative Procedure[1]; LSA[2]

1. Narrative procedures are considered ecologically valid assessment measures across the life span (Channell et al., 2018). Narrative procedures allow clinicians to analyze multiple dimensions of language, including microstructural (e.g., grammatical word categories, mental state language) and macrostructural (e.g., story grammar, evaluations) domains. The use of wordless picture books supports expressive language production due to the structured nature of the stories (Abbeduto et al., 2012).

2. LSA has been determined to be an ecologically valid method of assessing the production of children's language when captured natural, functional language use in real-life contexts (Nippold, 2014). It has been established as an evidence-based practice by ASHA for decades (2020). For this assessment, multiple language samples were collected. For analysis, a representative sample of 50 utterances was used as seen in the table in the appendix. An additional language sample is included in the appendix.

3. The MAVA is used to assess the receptive and expressive vocabularies of children between the ages of 3;0 to 12;0. Because Student is exposed to Vietnamese 40% of the time, scores for this assessment are reported descriptively only.

4. The Language Use Inventory (LUI) is a parent-report questionnaire used to capture and analyze children's social pragmatic use of language. This measure was used for descriptive reasons only.

Results: Form

A. Phonology: Student's phonology was evaluated via observation.

Single phonemes: As demonstrated in the following chart, which classifies phonemes by typical age of acquisition, Student demonstrated phonological variation on the following phonemes:

Typical Age of Mastery	Phonemes	Initial	Medial	Final
2 to 3 Years	/p/, /b/, /m/, /w/, /h/			
4 to 4.5 Years	/t/, /d/, /n/, /k/, /g/, /y/, /ng/			
4.5 to 5 Years	/f/			
4 to 7 Years	/ch/, /dg/			
6 to 6.5 Years	/l/, /v/, /sh/, /zh/	/l/	/l/	/l/
6.5 to 7 Years	/th$_{v+}$/, /th$_{v-}$/, /s/, /z/	/th$_{v+}$/, /th$_{v-}$/		/th$_{v+}$/, /th$_{v-}$/
7 Years or later	/r/, vocalic /r/			

As indicated above, Student demonstrated variations on the phonemes /th$_{v+}$/, and /th$_{v-}$/ in the initial and final position and /l/ in all positions at the sentence level. Student substituted /d/ for the voiced phoneme ([dere] for /there/) and /f/ for the voiceless phoneme ([wif] for /with/). The substitution of /d/ for the voiced /th$_{v-}$/ is an expected interaction between Vietnamese and English. The substitution of /f/ for /th$_{v-}$/ is age-appropriate. Student substituted /ng/ for the /l/ phoneme ([yeno] for /yellow/). This is an idiosyncratic substitution and Student was able to produce the /l/ correctly with a visual and auditory model.

The production patterns described above were produced inconsistently and infrequently, which suggests she is continuing to refine her speech sound system as it moves closer to the adult model. These production patterns did not impede intelligibility, which was judged to be 100%.

Student's voice was determined to be within expected limits. A final comment is that Student demonstrated frequent use of interjections (i.e., *ummm*) and whole word repetition (i.e., *because, because . . .*), as seen in the language sample. These are considered typical dysfluencies and are not an area of concern.

B. Morphology: Student's morphology was evaluated through narrative procedure and LSA. The language sample revealed the following morphological markers:

Form	Absent	Emerging	Stable	Age of Mastery
Present progressive			P	19 to 28
Prepositions (in/on)			P	27 to 30
Regular Plural			P	27 to 33
Irregular past			P	25 to 46
Possessive 's			P	26 to 40
Uncontractible copula			P	28 to 46
Articles			P	28 to 46
Regular past –ed			P	26 to 48
Regular third person			P	28 to 50
Irregular third person (does, has)			P	28 to 50
Uncontractible auxiliary			P	29 to 48
Contractible copula			P	29 to 29
Contractible auxiliary			P	30 to 50

The above table identifies the full range of morphological markers present in the language sample. Examples of phrases with some of the markers follow:

1. He is jumping **in** the water because . . . we need to look.
2. And I have my friends at **Mommy's** school.
3. Baby **jumped** into the water.
4. No, the teacher **doesn't.**
5. **That's** a pigeon book.

However, of note was the presence of morphological errors in the sample within specific contexts. A variety of errors emerged when Student was asked questions that required accessing abstract reasoning, or inferencing. This question type was used to probe her ability to answer a question that could not necessarily be answered with information gleaned from the pictures. In these contexts, Student demonstrated morphological errors or omissions, as seen in the examples below:

1. No, **she got on his cheek**.
2. The big frog let baby **fell** down.
3. They're sitting on the turtle, and then the dog walks, and then the boy has his boots, and then **they're walk**.

Student's response to more abstract demands may reflect the complex interaction among Student's skill level, the story, and the targeted task. This competition for attention and resources, referred to as competing demands, often results in a drop in performance of one of the skills when one of the tasks is an area of weakness (Wallach & Ocampo, 2020).

Student demonstrated a mean length of utterance-morpheme (MLU-m) between 2 and 10 morphemes, with an average of 5.34 morphemes. These findings are considered appropriate for her age based on developmental milestones established by Brown (1973). This finding corresponds to her mastery of the expected morphological markers present in her language sample.

C. Syntax: Student's syntax was evaluated through a narrative procedure and LSA. Of note is that the interaction between Vietnamese and English was considered in this analysis.

The following sentence types were observed as noted in the table below:

Sentence Type	Observed	Example from Sample
Simple Infinitive	P	They have to go to the bath.
Full Propositional Complement	P	Maybe they're going on an adventure.
Simple Wh Clause	P	The dog hear who?
Simple Conjoining	P	Mommy and Daddy make a cabinet.
Multiple Embeddings	Not observed	
Embedded and Conjoined	P	They're sitting on the turtle and then the dog walks and then the boy has his boots and then they're walk.
Infinitive Clause with different subjects	P	Well, it's supposed to help you, the lowercase letters say stay quiet.
Relative clauses	Not observed	

Sentence Type	Observed	Example from Sample
Gerunds	P	Reading can be hard with one big eye.
Wh Infinitives	P	I don't know how to say it.
Unmarked Infinitive	P	But I can make a letter A for the puzzle

These examples reveal a wide range of sentences with increasing complexity. As well, the language sample revealed the following grammatical categories:

Adjectives   Nouns
Adverbs   Personal Pronouns
Auxiliary Verbs   Prepositions
Coordinators   Subordinators
Copula Forms   Verbs
Determiners   Verb Particles
Intensifiers   Words of Negation

Cross-Linguistic and Contrastive Analysis: Based on the structure of Vietnamese, the following grammatical features may be present based on Student's exposure to Vietnamese:

Feature	Description	Example	Observed
Possessives	Noun + prepositional phrase	I took the shoe of him	
Adjectives	Adjectives follows noun	The ball red is here	
Plurality	Quantifiers preceded noun	We saw three bird in tree	
Verb tense	Context and addition of words before and after verb convey meaning	I am eat/She eat/Boy read	
Question formation	Question words are used in intonation in subject-verb-object structure	Word inversion: What want eat?	
Negation	No precedes verbs	I no want play	

In the language samples collected, there were no instances of syntactic cross linguistic interaction; however, it would not be an unexpected outcome based on Student's dual language exposure.

Results: Content

D. Semantics: Student's semantics, or vocabulary, was evaluated through the MAVA-Receptive and Expressive and LSA. Because of her dual language exposure, results are presented descriptively only.

The MAVA was designed to measure the development of children's oral language by assessing listening (receptive) and speaking (expressive) vocabulary. The words on the MAVA were selected using the three tiers of vocabulary. Words are assigned to tier one, two, or three depending on their characteristics of meaning and use. Children acquire the three tiers as they learn and mature in both academic and real-word contexts.

On the two assessment measures, Student recognized 66 items out of 91 presented to her and she identified 76 out of 102 words presented to her. The table below provides a detailed analysis of Student's performance:

Vocabulary	Modality
Tier 1: Tier one words are the most basic words. They are the early reading words, sight words, nouns, verbs, and adjectives that students learn to identify or decode with instruction. They learn to read them—identify them in print form—because they already use them in their speaking vocabulary. Examples of tier one words are: boy, fence, happy, chicken, green, fancy, and running. There are about 8,000-word families in English in tier one.	**Receptive:** Student recognized 52/57 (91%) Tier 1 words administered. **Expressive:** Student identified 58/64 (91%) of Tier I words administered.
Tier 2: Tier two words are the high frequency words that are found in many domains. They play a large role in our speaking and reading vocabulary. These words often represent multiple meanings and subtle nuances. In addition, they typically "add productivity to an individual's language ability" (Beck et al., 2002, p. 16). Tier two words are the most important ones to directly teach to students because they are assumed to be known as students progress through school. Examples of tier two words are: masterpiece, preference, fortuitous, glean, and measure. There are about 7,000-word families in English in tier two.	**Receptive:** Student recognized 13/29 (45%) Tier 2 words administered. **Expressive:** Student identified 16/34 (47%) of Tier 2 words administered.

Vocabulary	Modality
Tier 3: Tier three words are those related to specific domains and have a low frequency of use. Domains might include subject areas in school, hobbies, geographic regions, technology, weather, etc. Examples of tier three words are: ukulele, asphalt, genome, crepe, and cornice. The remaining 400,000 words in English fall in this tier.	**Receptive:** Student recognized 1/5 (20%) of Tier 3 words administered. **Expressive:** Student identified 1/3 (33%) of Tier 3 words administered.

Examples of items Student recognized in this assessment process include *hippopotamus, twist, pyramid, and globe*. Examples of items Student did not recognize include *karate, fairy, mythical*, and *pounce*.

Examples of items Student identified in this assessment process include *blue, elbow, tall* and *fountain*. Examples of items Student was unable to identify include *soccer, repairing, pouring* and *cane*.

Discrepant Analysis: Of note is that Student demonstrated a stronger expressive vocabulary performance than receptive vocabulary performance. In monolingual children, this is a relatively unusual pattern as the receptive task requires only accessing semantic knowledge, whereas the expressive task requires accessing this semantic knowledge and producing the phonological representation of the concept, which is more taxing to the linguistic, cognitive, and motoric systems. Although it is not clear exactly what contributed to this difference profile, it may be related to: (a) the unique vocabulary development of children exposed to more than one language, as the rate of development of these children differs from that of children exposed to one language (Thordardottir, 2011); (b) attention, (c) task persistence, or (d) an inaccurate representation between vocabulary knowledge and performance. A final comment is that the receptive task was the final task of the session, which may implicate both attention and task persistence.

In addition to the MAVA, Student's vocabulary was analyzed through the LSA. The LSA revealed the presence of non-specific language in a small number of responses. For example, Student produced the sentence, "They're doing the present with the bow," when describing the boy opening a present, and "And then the boy did the sticks," when describing the boy rowing in the lake. This use of non-specific language may be linked dual language exposure or to the competing demands of the task. The latter is validated by her frequent use of the phrase, "I don't know," in this context. The LSA also revealed confusion among the subjective pronouns *he/she/they*.

Results: Use

E. Pragmatics: Student's pragmatics was analyzed through the LUI, narrative procedure, and LSA.

The table below summarized the information provided by parent report (LUI):

Communicative Function	Response
Use of gestures to accomplish wants and needs	Rarely
Types of words used	Broad range across grammatical categories
Requests for help	Language
Getting attention	Language
Commenting about self and others (Concrete contexts: who, what, where)	Consistent
Commenting about self and others (Inferential contexts; how, why, when)	Absent
Shares activities and information with others	Consistent
Sense of humor	Present
Uses language in a meta manner	Present
Unusual topics	Sometimes (comics)
Conversation repair	Consistent
Use of metacognitive verbs (think, know, wonder . . .)	Inconsistent
Story cohesion	Consistent

The table above suggests that Student uses language across multiple contexts and communicative partners. This table also indicates overall weakness in the use of language for inferential tasks, such as her use of metacognitive verbs (e.g., think, know). This finding is in line with what was revealed in the LSA, where Student demonstrated weakness when asked inferential questions that could not be answered with pictured support and when asked questions that required taking the perspective of another. Examples of this can be seen in her response, "The big frog let baby fell down" when asked what had happened. In this case, the frog had kicked the baby frog off the raft, but it was not obvious from the picture. Further, there were several instances where Student responded to a question with insufficient information or made a comment with no obvious links to the prior question/comment. For example, when asked how she got the office, she replied, "Mom drive. 'Cause mommy."

When considered together, these findings together suggest deficits in Theory of Mind (ToM), which is the ability to understand the mental states of others, such as emotions, feelings, beliefs, wishes, and thoughts (Fletcher-Watson et al., 2020). ToM enables us to explain and predict others' behavior and supports the communicative coherence. ToM also involves an understanding of shared assumptions, how much information to share with others, how much background needs to be supplied, and topics that support bidirectional interaction.

ToM reflects a broad range of knowledge and skills. It develops over time, building from foundational, precursor skills to a sophisticated understanding of how mental states and behavior interact. Foundational skills of ToM include joint attention, appreciation of intentionality, recognition that different people have different perspectives, use of metacognitive language, and pretend play (Miller, 2006).

Results: Receptive Language

Student's receptive language was assessed through the narrative procedure and in conversation with the assessor. Student responded to a broad range of questions and followed multi-step directions correctly via both spoken and written language. Student was observed to repeat questions or restate question that involved inferencing or abstract reasoning. An example of this can be seen in her response, "The dog hear who?" to the question, "Who did the dog hear?"

Summary and Impressions:

Student, at 5-years, 6-months old, is a charming, energetic, and humorous child: She was a pleasure to work with in this assessment. Student is exposed to both English (60%) and Vietnamese (40%). Student demonstrated strong literacy skills. Student presents with many strengths in her language. As revealed in the language sample, Student demonstrates a speech sound system that continues to move closer to the adult model. She produced variations on $/th_{v+}/$, $/th_{v-}/$, and $/l/$, all of which are developmentally appropriate and/or reflect the interaction between English and Vietnamese. There are no concerns with her voice or fluency.

Student demonstrates age-appropriate morphological skills as evidenced by her use of all 14 of Brown's morphemes. Student demonstrated use of a wide range of syntactic structures, including compound sentences with coordinating conjunctions and unmarked infinitives. She further demonstrated a wide range of grammatical categories, including adverbs, intensifiers, and words of negation. In the 50-utterance language sample, Student's utterance length ranged from two morphemes to 10, with an MLU-m of 5.34, which is considered age appropriate. Student demonstrated morphological errors when the question or context required inferencing or taking the perspective of another.

As revealed by the MAVA-Receptive and Expressive, Student recognized and used words across all three tiers of vocabulary, with the words from the third tier being the smallest word set. Student demonstrated stronger expressive vocabulary skills than receptive vocabulary skills. Potential causal factors may have included: (a) the unique vocabulary development of children exposed to more than one language, (b) attention, (c) task persistence, or (d) an inaccurate representation between vocabulary knowledge and performance. As revealed in the language sample, Student was observed to use non-specific language which may be linked to competing demands in the task. This is validated by her frequent use of the phrase, "I don't know," in this context. A final comment is that Student demonstrated confusion among the subjective pronouns *he/she/they*, although she responded to corrections when reminded of the character's gender.

As revealed by parent report via the LUI, Student uses language across multiple contexts and communicative partners. However, this also indicated overall weakness in the use of language for inferential tasks, such as her use of metacognitive verbs (e.g., think, know). This finding is in line with what was revealed in the LSA, where Student demonstrated weakness when asked inferential questions that could not be answered with pictured support and when asked questions that required taking the perspective of another. Further, there were several instances where Student responded to a question with insufficient information or made a comment with no obvious links to the prior question/comment. Together these findings together suggest deficits in Theory of Mind (ToM), which is the ability to understand the mental states of others, such as emotions, feelings, beliefs, wishes, and thoughts (Fletcher-Watson et al., 2020).

As revealed by the narrative procedure and in conversation with the assessor. Student responded to a broad range of questions and followed multi-step directions correctly via both spoken and written language. Student was observed to demonstrate repeats or restatement of questions that involved inferencing or abstract reasoning.

Recommendations:
Based on the findings of this assessment, it is recommended that Student receive intervention designed to support the continued development of vocabulary, abstract reasoning, inferencing, and the use of metacognitive language.

Respectfully submitted,

Speech-Language Pathologist
_____
Speech-Language Pathologist, M.A., CCC-SLP

Private Practice

Street

City, State, Zip

Phone

	Language Sample I: Reading a story and talking about the wordless book "One Frog Too Many"		
	Phrase	*MLU-m*	*Comment*
1.	To school	2	Elliptical response
2.	Yes, Chuckaboo likes school too.	5	
3.	Yes, Miss Gina school.	3	Missing information
4.	My name is who?	4	Restated question with alteration
5.	Oh, like at school?	4	
6.	Yes.	1	Elliptical response
7.	But she goes.	3	Unrelated response
8.	She's sad	3	
9.	I have to read the messages.	6	
10.	We start from here.	4	
11.	Because, she, I don't know.	5	Inferential question
12.	No, I think let's turn the page.	8	
13.	She's thinking.	4	
14.	Chuckaboo says that too.	5	
15.	Well, I know almost everything.	5	
16.	No, mommy's school.	4	
17.	And I have my friends at mommy's school.	10	
18.	I don't know.	3	
19.	No, she got on his cheek.	6	Missing information; Inferential question; Pronoun confusion
20.	No, the teacher doesn't.	4	
21.	They have school time.	4	
22.	No, that's not a real book.	7	
23.	That's a pigeon book.	5	

	Language Sample I: Reading a story and talking about the wordless book "One Frog Too Many"		
	Phrase	*MLU-m*	*Comment*
24.	She's scared of the baby.	6	Repetition and expansion of question
25.	Um, Jamia, at school.	3	Inferential question
26.	I don't know.	3	
27.	Yes.	1	
28.	They're painting.	4	
29.	Reading can be hard with one big eye.	8	
30.	Well, it's supposed to help you.	8	
31.	The lowercase letters say stay quiet.	7	
32.	Maybe a playground.	3	
33.	Those are called small, they're tiny.	8	
34.	Mommy and Daddy make a cabinet.	6	Missing information
35.	Oh, that is school.	4	
36.	Mom drive, 'cause mommy…	4	Missing information
37.	I want to drive school like the pigeon.	7	
38.	They're doing the present with the bow.	9	Non-specific language
39.	They're inside.	3	Referring to a single character
40.	It's a baby frog.	4	
41.	The big frog let baby fell down	7	Inferential question
42.	Ummmmm, I don't know.	3	
43.	And then what happened to little frog?	8	
44.	They're sitting on the turtle and then the dog walks and then the boy has his boots and then they're walk.	15	Missing information; Inferential question

	Language Sample I: Reading a story and talking about the wordless book "One Frog Too Many"		
	Phrase	*MLU-m*	*Comment*
45.	Ohhhh, Chuckaboo loves adventures!	6	
46.	Big frog jumped down into the boat-water and the boat.	11	Missing information; inferential question
47.	And then the boy did the sticks with the…	8	Non-specific language
48.	And then the turtle is sleeping.	7	
49.	Baby jumped into the water.	6	Inferential question; Describing the image rather than answering the question
50.	Touching the boy.	3	Inferential question
Total number of morphemes			**267**
MLU-m			**5.34**

Second Language Sample:

June 14

1. Do you remember this story? It's about who: And the boy, and the dog, um, the turtle.
2. And?: *A big frog and the small frog.*
3. Expectant wait: *I wonder what's the present inside.*
4. What's inside: *A baby frog!*
5. Expectant wait: *The baby, um, um, um, Ms. Em, mom. What did the boy do?*
6. What do you think he's doing?: *The boy's taking the baby frog to the big frog.*
7. Expectant wait: *And the boy said . . .*
8. What did the boy say?: *Um, I don't know.*
9. Does he look happy, mad, sad, silly? What does he look like?: *He look like she's . . . I don't know!*
10. Expectant wait: *What did the boy said?*
11. I don't know, what do you think?: *Um, I don't know.*
12. What happened here?: *Um, the frog is . . . I don't know.*
13. I think the boy said, "What are you doing big frog?": *And uh, the frog was mad.*
14. Yes, I think the boy was mad too, do you?: *Because the boy said, ummm, no.*
15. He probably said, "No, don't do that!": -
16. Everyone is mad at big frog: —
17. (Turning the page): *Maybe they're going on an adventure.*
18. Does Chuckaboo like adventures?: *No.*
19. Expectant wait: *Oh, no, again?*
20. Again! What did big frog do?: *She kicked baby frog.*
21. We don't kick friends, do we?: *Now she's crying.*
22. She is: *And then the boy said, umm, I don't know.*
23. I think he said, "Big frog, I told you to be nice!": *They all mad. And then the boy said, um, I don't know.*
24. We are going to go an adventure with the stick?: *That looks like a camping stick.*
25. Expectant wait: *Big frog catch baby frog.*
26. Expectant wait: *To the boat!*
27. He jumped onto the boat: (acted out jumping)
28. What's happening now?: *Um, I don't know.*
29. Well, what is the turtle doing?: *Sleeping.*
30. I think big frog is looking at little frog: *'Cause big frog is . . .*
31. Is what?: *I don't know.*
32. Expectant wait: *There's next page.*
33. Oh my gosh!: *Again?*

34. Expectant wait: *Number two is not be nice.*
35. That's right:—
36. Where did little frog go?: *No, little zero's, little zero might crying.*
37. I think so: *Um, what happened to the number three?* (giggling)
38. What is the turtle doing?: *Telling the boy.*
39. What is he telling the boy?: *For the baby frog. The boy said . . .*
40. What do you think the boy said?: *Help me.*
41. The boy said, "Where is baby frog?":—
42. Expectant wait: *And baby frog's in the water.*
43. Turn the page: *They're looking for baby frog.*
44. They are! They're all looking for baby frog: *Cause, cause, what happened to the number two?*
45. I know, what did he do?: *Um, um, what the number two feel?*
46. Hmm, what do you think he feels?: *Um, I don't know.*
47. Let's check and see if we can figure it out: *Big frog is not walking.*
48. He's not. What are these guys doing?: *They're walking on the adventure* (the characters are returning home).
49. I think they're going back home: *No, she feels sad.*
50. He does feel sad: *And then the number two, um how the number two feels?*
51. I think he wishes he had been nice to little frog: *Then the baby zero is gone.*
52. Expectant wait: *Um, what happened to number two?*
53. Where's the baby frog?: *But, uh, what happened to number two?*
54. Well, I think he feels bad. He feels mad and sad because he was not nice: —
55. But look, the dog hears something, what does he hear?: *I don't know.*
56. Let's turn the page and find out: *It's a baby frog!*
57. Oh my gosh! It is: *Um, because the number zero is here.*
58. He flew into the window: *Cause, the big frog sees baby frog.*
59. Is he happy or sad?: *Um, um, um, what does she feel?*
60. What do you think?: *Um, I don't know.*
61. I think they're all happy to see baby frog to come back because they thought baby frog was gone: *Because, because, she, she surprised baby frog.*
62. She is surprised: *Um, um, baby frog sat on big frog!*
63. I know, isn't that funny!: *Cause, cause, the number two like like. And then the number zero sat on the number two.*
64. Oh my gosh!: (giggling) *Now they're all safe.*
65. They are!: *The number two and the number zero are all safe now.*
66. And do you think they're friends now?: *Yes!*
67. And they are kind of like a family now, huh?: *Yes.*

ABC Speech Services

Speech & Language Evaluation Report

Name: XXXXXX

Address: XXXXXXXXXX

            XXXXXXXXXX

Telephone: XXXXXXXX

Date of Birth: 1/08/2005

Chronological Age: 12.1-year-old

Date of Report: 2/16/2017

I. BACKGROUND INFORMATION:

XXXXXX is a 12.1-year-old girl who is currently home-schooled through XXXXXX Charter School. She is in the sixth grade. She has been receiving speech and language therapy since she was 2¾ years old. She no longer receives occupational therapy. Her hearing and vision are within normal limits. She lives with both of her parents and an older sister. This assessment is for XXXXXX's triennial review.

II. ASSESSMENT RESULTS:

XXXXXX was assessed on 2/6/17 and 2/9/17 for a total of 2.75 hours. Based upon observations, she gave good effort on all of the test items. XXXXXX's speech and language skills were assessed using clinical observations, parent report, records review, Comprehensive Assessment of Spoken Language (CASL), and CELF-4 Pragmatics Profile.

A. LANGUAGE:

Comprehensive Assessment of Spoken Language (CASL):

	Standard Score	Percentile
Nonliteral language	120	91%ile
Meaning from context	117	87%ile
Inference	111	77%ile
Ambiguous sentences	114	82%ile
Pragmatic judgment	107	68%ile

Based upon parent report and observations, XXXXXX tends to perform well on standardized language tests but has difficulty using and generalizing what she knows with different people and across different situations and settings. XXXXXX scored within average range on all subtests. On the nonliteral language subtest, she had to explain the meaning behind the nonliteral language that was given. For example, When Mother heard about the accident, the ground started shifting beneath her feet. What does this mean? XXXXXX responded, "Mother was worried." On the meaning from context subtest, XXXXXX was asked to figure out the meaning of an unusual word from listening to a sentence. For example, Sara got tired of moving her head up and down to follow the saltations of the Russian dancers. Explain what saltations means. XXXXXX said, "Jumping." On the inference subtest, she had to listen to a story and make an inference to figure out clues in the story. For example, Darrell and Todd waited patiently in line for a chance to buy two of the remaining tickets for the rock concert. They left the ticket window without tickets. Why? XXXXXX responded, "The tickets were sold out." On the ambiguous sentences subtest, she had to explain two different meanings for an ambiguous sentence. For example, The man followed the tracks for three miles, and then exhaustion overcame him. XXXXXX answered, "Animal tracks and railroad tracks." On the pragmatic judgment subtest, the therapist described some events and XXXXXX had to explain the best thing to say or do in the given situation. For example, It is a hot summer day. MayLee's friend is wearing a heavy jacket. What does MayLee ask her friend? XXXXXX responded, "Why are you wearing a heavy jacket when it's hot outside?"

CELF-4 Pragmatics Profile:
Per parent report, she had a raw score of 99, but her criterion score for her age should be >142 (below average). Some test items that her mom rated as "never" include the following: initiates greetings, introduces others, and apologizes appropriately. Examples of test items that her mom rated as "sometimes" are as follows: asks for clarification during conversations; tells/understands jokes; agrees and disagrees using appropriate language; uses appropriate facial expressions, tone of voice, and body language; and uses nonverbal cues appropriate to the situation.

Clinical observations (social skills group):
During therapy, XXXXXX is able to engage in long reciprocal conversations about preferred topics (e.g., animals, books) with adults and peers. She tends to talk about preferred topics and does not realize that other people might not be interested. However, she is only able to maintain non-preferred topics (e.g., shopping, arts & crafts) with peers by making two to eight conversational exchanges. She offers significantly more comments than questions. She needs to work on asking more questions to show the listener that she is interested in what he or she is saying. Also, XXXXXX needs to practice selecting appropriate topics of conversation and play choices based on what she already knows about the other person's likes and dislikes. During conversations with people she knows, she is able to maintain eye contact. However, she avoids eye contact and does not initiate greetings or conversation with new people. XXXXXX reported that she only talks to people she knows and feels that she is too shy and does not know what to say to new people. When we go on field trips (e.g., shopping at the mall, Color Me Mine), XXXXXX demonstrates limited interactions and needs maximum prompting in order for her to talk to her friends.

Also, she tends to avoid talking to other people. For example, she needed to throw away trash at Color Me Mine. She asked me where the trash can was located and I told her to ask the store clerk. Instead of asking the store clerk, XXXXXX just held on to her trash.

In the area of nonverbal communication, XXXXXX is aware of other people's facial expressions, tone of voice, and hand and body gestures. During structured activities, she is able to read the nonverbal cues and figure out what to do or say when given different social situations with 80% accuracy. However, she continues to have difficulty reading nonverbal cues and responding appropriately to them in real-life situations. In role playing activities, XXXXXX correctly displays nonverbal cues appropriate to the social situation with 80% accuracy.

However, she demonstrates limited range of facial expression (mostly smiling or neutral facial expression) and tone of voice in real-life situations. She rarely uses hand gestures while she is talking. Generalization of learned skills to different people, situations, and settings continues to be difficult for XXXXXX.

Perspective taking (theory of mind concepts) is another area of difficulty. It is difficult for her to take someone else's perspective and infer what the other person might be thinking and/or feeling. As a result, it is difficult for her to alter her verbal and nonverbal language to accommodate to the person or situation. XXXXXX struggles with flexibility in her thinking and assumes that other people think the same way as she doesso it is difficult for her to see multiple interpretations. Despite being in multiple group activities (e.g., church, sailing, horseback riding), XXXXXX rarely interacts with her peers. She expresses a desire to have friends but does not know how to go about it. When asked who her friends are, she named her dog and her sister. XXXXXX also named acquaintances at church, in her neighborhood, and after-school activities. She mostly plays with boys who are younger than her (limited talking required). The play choices (e.g., tag, hide & seek) are immature for her age (limited talking required). Her mom reported that XXXXXX has the awareness of what it takes to make friends because she is very bright. She also is willing to integrate with peers but has significant difficulty applying what she knows to real-life situations. Parental concerns include: as social demands increase, XXXXXX will have a harder time making and keeping friends and XXXXXX might be depressed in the future if she does not have true friendships with her peers.

B. SPEECH:
Oral structures and functions are adequate for speech production. XXXXXX is able to correctly produce all of her sounds in all word positions at the conversational level and no longer needs articulation therapy.

III. SUMMARY & RECOMMENDATIONS:

XXXXXX demonstrates delays in the area of social skills and pragmatics. She would benefit from intervention to improve her social language skills and interactions with her peers. It is recommended that XXXXXX receive individual speech therapy for .5 hour per week and social skills group for 1 hour per week. It is also recommended that she receive 3 hours total of speech ESY.

IV. NEW GOALS:

1. XXXXXX will appropriately initiate greetings and conversation with new people during structured activities such as school events and after-school activities with 80% accuracy as measured by clinical observations, therapy notes, and parent report across three consecutive sessions.

2. XXXXXX will state appropriate topics of conversation and play choices depending on who she is talking to (e.g., 6 years old vs. 13 years old, boys vs. girls), with 80% accuracy as measured by clinical observations and therapy notes across three consecutive sessions.

3. XXXXXX will maintain the topic of conversation by making at least eight exchanges (emphasis on asking more questions than making comments) with non-preferred topics with adults and peers with 80% accuracy as measured by clinical observations and therapy notes across three consecutive sessions.

4. XXXXXX will appropriately use a total of five different body gestures, hand gestures, facial expressions, and/or tones of voice per conversation with 80% accuracy as measured by clinical observations and therapy notes across three consecutive sessions.

5. XXXXXX will take someone's perspective and make an inference about what he or she likes or is thinking with 80% accuracy as measured by clinical observations and therapy notes across three consecutive sessions.

6. XXXXXX will problem solve by stating two things that you should do or say and explain the consequences for each solution when given different social situations and/or conflicts with 80% accuracy as measured by clinical observations and therapy notes across three consecutive sessions.

XXXXXXXXXX
Speech-Language Pathologist

Medical Setting—Sample Reports

XYX Medical Facility
Patient ID: <u>XXXXXX</u>

Pt. was seen in the speech clinic for a cognitive evaluation on 01/28/17 sec. to pt. c/o memory problems. Patient is a 25 y/o Army Combat Veteran who was deployed to Afghanistan from 2009–2010 and to Iraq from 2012–2013. Pt. reported that he fell on his head and neck, with LOC for unknown period of time, and was treated in the ER. Pt endorses left-side numbness and neck spasms. Records also indicate subjective complaints of right-side weakness. Pt also reported a syncopal incident after his fingers were cut off in a noncombat accident in the military (see psychosocial hx for details). Pt did not endorse any other hx of head trauma prior to, or during the military.

Pt. endorsed problems with memory and attention. Pt. reported that he has difficulty remembering details of readings, how to complete math problems, new learning in school, dates, events, and tasks. Pt. also reported misplacing important items. Pt. stated that he is sleeping approximately 3 hours per night without medication and 4–5 hours (broken) with medication. Pt. eats 2 meals per day. Pt. reported that he drinks ETOH 1× per week (usually four beers). Pt. drinks ½ cup of coffee every other day. Pt. denied smoking or recreational drugs.

Pt. is currently compensating for memory difficulties by using his Blackberry smartphone; pt. utilizes the calendar application but not the task application. Pt. is currently enrolled in college; however, he is considering withdrawing from school sec. to panic attacks and difficulty learning. Pt. is unsure of goals at this time; pt. reported "living day-to-day." Pt's goals for therapy are to learn tips for memory.

I. Global Positioning System (GPS) Questionnaire:
"Are you having difficulty driving at this time?" and/or "Are you having any difficulty following directions while driving?"

[ ] NO = GPS not indicated. Discontinue assessment.

[x] YES

Comments: Pt. reported zoning out while driving. Pt. owns a GPS but he doesn't use it consistently. SLP encouraged pt. to use the GPS while driving to both familiar and unfamiliar destinations. GPS is not medically indicated.

II. Rivermead Behavioral Memory Test (RBMT-3):
SLP administered the Rivermead Behavioral Memory Test (RBMT-3). The RBMT provides a systematic method of assessing cognitive deficits associated with

nonprogressive brain injury and monitoring change over time. This test was standardized on 333 people (172 females, 161 males) ranging in age from 16 to 89. RBMT-3 subtests are converted to subtest scaled scores with a mean of 10 and a standard deviation of 3. In addition to providing scaled scores for the RBMT-3 subtests, a General Memory Index (GMI), representing overall memory performance, was also used. The GMI has a mean of 100 and a standard deviation of 15.

Subtest	Scaled Score
First and Second Names—Delayed Recall	2
Belongings—Delayed Recall	5
Appointments—Delayed Recall	8
Picture Recognition—Delayed Recognition	1
Story—Immediate Recall	4
Story—Delayed Recall	4
Face Recognition—Delayed Recognition	4
Route—Immediate Recall	7
Route—Delayed Recall	7
Messages—Immediate Recall	11
Messages—Delayed Recall	11
Orientation and Date	7
Novel Task—Immediate Recall	7
Novel Task—Delayed Recall	5

Sum of Scaled Scores: 83
General Memory Index: 64 (2.4 SD below mean)
Percentile Rank: 0.8

IMPRESSION: Pt. presented with moderate-to-severe memory deficits. Suspect pt.'s adjustment issues, lack of sleep, and dx. of PTSD are largely contributing to his cognitive deficits. Neuropsych assessment found similar results. Pt. has begun MH services and was encouraged to continue actively treating PTSD. Pt. would benefit from training to use his smartphone as a memory aid and organizational tool. Will defer cognitive therapy at this time until mental health issues are better controlled. Pt. might benefit from the College Connection program if he decides to withdraw from school this semester.

RECOMMENDATIONS: (1) SLP scheduled a f/u appt. to review test results and recommendations. (2) If pt. is agreeable, SLP will schedule 1–2 sessions to train pt. to use his Blackberry to improve organization and time management. (3) Pt. was encouraged to use the GPS while driving to both familiar and unfamiliar destinations. (4) SLP encouraged pt. to continue actively treating PTSD.

XYX Medical Facility
Patient ID: <u>XXXXXX</u>

Pt. was seen in the speech clinic on 04/23/18 for continued assessment to determine most appropriate treatment plan. Pt. was alert and an active participant in the evaluation. Pt. was fully cooperative with all assessment tasks with no frustration noted. Results are as follows:

SLP administered portions of the Boston Naming Test. Pt. responded accurately to 42% of stimuli presented (14/33 spontaneous responses); 7 of the 14 correct responses were self-corrections. Pt's incorrect responses were typically characterized by phonemic errors (e.g., holipotter for helicopter, mushumber for mushroom). Perseverations of paraphasias were typical; each attempt/repetition was closer to the correct word. Pt. was provided with semantic and phonemic cues; however, pt. was unable to accurately respond following cues. Pt. presented with reduced awareness of phonemic paraphasias; pt. showed potential to improve awareness. SLP verbally provided pt. with the correct response and incorrect response containing a phonemic error. Pt. was able to identify if the word was correct vs. incorrect 75% of the time. Pt. also spontaneously utilized compensatory strategies to improve verbal expression such as gestures, circumlocutions, or substituting the word.

SLP administered the ACLC, which is an assessment of auditory comprehension; normative data are not available for this test. Pt. correctly identified a pictured object/action/adjective from a field of 5 with 78% accuracy (39/50 trials). Pt. identified two-critical elements from a field of four with 50% accuracy (5/10 trials). Pt. identified three-critical elements with 70% accuracy. Suspect improvement with the more complex task is sec. to pt.'s increased use of strategy of asking for repeats.

IMPRESSIONS: Pt. would benefit from speech therapy to improve auditory comprehension, self-awareness/self-monitoring, and verbal expression. Pt. is motivated to improve communication skills and is stimulable to implement compensatory strategies. Pt. would highly benefit from intensive therapy 5 days per week; unsure if goals can be accomplished as an outpatient. Pt. might also benefit from occupational therapy to address cognitive skills given his high level of functioning prior to injury.

PLAN: SLP will schedule speech and language therapy 5 days per week for a minimum of 4 weeks with goals as follows:

Auditory Comprehension

STG 1a: Pt. will correctly identify a pictured object from a field of 4 at 90% accuracy while using compensatory strategies for improved auditory comprehension as needed (e.g., ask for repeat of message, ask for a written cue) across 30 trials and 2 consecutive sessions.

STG 1b: Pt. will correctly identify a pictured object from a field of 6 at 90% accuracy while using compensatory strategies for improved auditory comprehension as needed (e.g., ask for repeat of message, ask for a written cue) across 30 trials and 2 consecutive sessions.

STG 1c: Pt. will correctly identify a sequence of 2 pictures from a field of 6 at 90% accuracy while using compensatory strategies for improved auditory comprehension as needed (e.g., ask for repeat of message, ask for a written cue) across 30 trials and 2 consecutive sessions.

STG 1d: Pt. will correctly identify a sequence of 2 pictures from a field of 8 at 90% accuracy while using compensatory strategies for improved auditory comprehension as needed (e.g., ask for repeat of message, ask for a written cue) across 30 trials and 2 consecutive sessions.

Self–Awareness/Self–Monitoring

STG 2a: Pt. will reduce his perseverative errors to no more than 2 repetitions per word during a picture-naming task with 90% accuracy across 30 trials and 2 sessions.

STG 2b: Pt. will reduce his perseverative errors to no more than two repetitions per word during a phrase-level picture description task with 90% accuracy across 30 trials and two sessions.

STG 2c: Pt. will reduce his perseverative errors to no more than two repetitions per word during a sentence-level picture-description task with 90% accuracy across 30 trials and two sessions.

Self–Awareness/Self–Monitoring

STG 3a: Pt. will judge the SLP's verbal productions as correct vs. incorrect during a picture-naming task with 90% accuracy across 30 trials and two consecutive sessions.

STG 3b: Pt. will judge his verbal productions as correct vs. incorrect during a picture-naming task with 90% accuracy across 30 trials and two consecutive sessions.

STG 3c: Pt. will judge his verbal productions as correct vs. incorrect during a phrase-level picture-description task with 90% accuracy across 30 trials and two consecutive sessions.

STG 3d: Pt. will judge his verbal productions as correct vs. incorrect during a sentence-level picture-description task with 90% accuracy across 30 trials and two consecutive sessions.

Verbal Expression

STG 4a: To improve verbal expression, pt. will implement appropriate compensatory strategies (e.g., pause to plan, circumlocution, word substitution, use of gestures, writing word) during a picture-naming task in 90% of relevant instances across two consecutive sessions.

STG 4b: Pt. will implement appropriate compensatory strategies to improve verbal expression (e.g., pause to plan, circumlocution, word substitution, use of gestures, writing word) during a phrase-level picture-description task in 90% of relevant instances across two consecutive sessions.

STG 4c: To improve verbal expression, pt. will implement appropriate compensatory strategies (e.g., pause to plan, circumlocution, word substitution, use of gestures, writing word) during a sentence-level picture-description task in 90% of relevant instances across 2 consecutive sessions.

Long-Term Goals

LTG 1: To improve auditory comprehension, pt. will correctly identify a sequence of 3 pictures from a field of 8 at 90% accuracy, while using compensatory strategies as needed (e.g., ask for repeat of message, ask for a written cue), across 30 trials and 2 consecutive sessions.

LTG 2: Pt. will reduce his perseverative errors to no more than 2 repetitions per word during a wh-question response task with 90% accuracy across 30 trials and 2 sessions.

LTG 3: Pt. will judge his verbal productions as correct vs. incorrect during a wh-question response task with 90% accuracy across 30 trials and 2 consecutive sessions.

LTG 4: Pt. will implement appropriate compensatory strategies to improve verbal expression (e.g., pause to plan, circumlocution, word substitution, use of gestures, writing word) during a wh-question response task in 90% of relevant instances across 2 consecutive sessions.

XYZ Children's Hospital
Department of Pediatric Rehabilitation
Speech and Language Evaluation Report

RELATED DIAGNOSIS
Ependymoma (ICD-9-CM: 191.9)

BACKGROUND INFORMATION
Referral Concerns
XXXXXX was referred for a speech and language evaluation by Dr. Y due to concerns regarding mild cognitive communication deficits. His mother reported no concerns with regards to XXXXXX's speech and language, but she expressed concerns about his attention and memory.

Developmental History
XXXXXX reportedly reached all of his developmental milestones at an age-appropriate time, including gross and fine motor skills, and speech and language.

Social History
XXXXXX lives in an English-speaking home in Utah with his two siblings, parents, and grandparents. He enjoys hanging out with his friends, riding his bike, reading, and playing chess with his older brother.

Educational History
XXXXXX is currently in sixth grade at a local school district. XXXXXX has an active individualized educational program (IEP); he is in a special day class and has recently been placed into a higher reading and language arts class. XXXXXX is reportedly a good student across subjects, and receives good grades. Per parent report, prior to the ependymoma diagnosis, he performed well in school. When not at school, XXXXXX is cared for by his parents and grandparents.

Feeding History
XXXXXX's mother expressed no concerns regarding feeding and feeding history is unremarkable.

MEDICAL HISTORY
Medical history was obtained from a review of his chart. XXXXXX was initially diagnosed with an ependymoma in 2012. At that time, XXXXXX underwent surgical resection followed by radiation. He was not treated with chemotherapy at that time. He was followed continually over the next several years. In January 2015, scans revealed tumor recurrence. At that time he again underwent surgical resection followed by chemotherapy consisting of but not limited to Cisplatin, Vincristine, Cytoxan, and Etopiside. Chemotherapy was completed in June 2015.

In response to his mother reporting frequent episodes of falling, a stat MRI was ordered in July 2015, but no evidence of any abnormal enhancement to suggest tumor recurrence. Per parent report, XXXXXX has a significant visual impairment in his left eye.

EVALUATION

Information for this evaluation was obtained through parent/patient interview, elicitation of behaviors, and clinical observation of skills. The outpatient evaluation took place in a quiet therapy room located at the Pediatric Rehabilitation Department. The following people were present at various points during the evaluation: XXXXXX, his grandmother, his mother, and a speech-language pathologist. The evaluation was completed in English. Due to XXXXXX's visual impairment, when there was a visual stimulus in an assessment, a brightly colored (pink) piece of paper was placed to the left of the page to encourage XXXXXX to make a complete visual scan.

Formal Assessment

Tests Administered

Clinical Evaluation of Language Fundamentals (CELF-4)

The *CELF-4* is a flexible and multiperspective assessment that examines a child's language and communication strengths and weaknesses from ages 5 to 21 years and 11 months old. Areas assessed include vocabulary, syntax, morphology, pragmatics, memory, comprehension, and expression. XXXXXX's results are detailed below and are gauged to be an accurate reflection of his current skills.

Three subtests from the *Clinical Evaluation of Language Fundamentals, 4th Edition (CELF-4)* were administered to assess XXXXXX's language and cognitive skills as they compare to typical peers; Word Classes (Expressive), Word Classes (Receptive), and Concepts and Following Directions.

CELF-4 4/7/18

Subtest	Raw Score	Scaled Score	Percentile	Interpretation
Word Classes, Expressive:	7	7	16th	*Mild*
Word Classes, Receptive:	11	7	16th	*Mild*
Word Classes, Total:	18	9	37th	*Mild*
Concepts and Following Directions	54	13	84th	*High Average*

For these assessments, the mean scaled score for is 10 and the standard deviation is 3. Typical performance ranges between 7 and 13.

<u>Word Classes, Expressive & Receptive:</u>
This subtest examines the child's ability to hold a list of four words in working memory, identify the two words that are most closely related, and then describe their relationship. **For both expressive and receptive language, XXXXXX scored in the mild range compared to his same-age peers.**

<u>Concepts and Following Directions:</u>
This subtest requires the student to identify pictures of geometric shapes in response to orally presented directions. The student must wait for the entire set of directions and then follow the directions in the order that the items were presented. **XXXXXX scored in the high average range compared to his same-age peers.**

Ross Information Processing Assessment–Primary (RIPA-P)

The *Ross Information Processing Assessment–Primary (RIPA-P)* assesses impairments in information-processing skills in children from 5 to 12 years of age who have experienced neuropathologies that may affect these skills. Due to time constraints, only selected subtests from the *RIPA-P* were administered for this evaluation.

XXXXXX's results are detailed below and are gauged to be an accurate reflection of his current skills. On the individual subtests, XXXXXX's performance ranged between "within normal limits" and "moderate impairment." However, when the subtests were grouped by composite quotient, his performance fell within normal limits. His strongest performance was in his ability to remember the immediate past and his spatial orientation (e.g., the location of United States with respect to the Mexico). He was most challenged when asked to recall general information (e.g., the name of a famous American).

The RIPA-P was standardized on individuals with traumatic brain injury. As such, standard measurements of performance, such as standard scores, are not used to represent "average function."

RIPA-P 4/7/18

Subtest	Raw Score	Standard Score	Percentile	Interpretation
Immediate Memory	69	16	98	*Within Normal Limits*
Recent Memory	75	13	84	*Mild*
Recall of General Information	56	10	50	*Moderate*
Spatial Orientation	75	17	99	*Within Normal Limits*
Temporal Orientation	63	12	75	*Mild*
Organization	67	13	84	*Mild*
Problem Solving	69	12	75	*Mild*
Composite Quotients	Sum of Standard Score	Percentile	Quotient	Interpretation
Memory Quotient	39	90	119	*Within Normal Limits*
Orientation Quotient	29	97	127	*Within Normal Limits*

Immediate Memory:
This subtest requires the child to repeat numbers, words, and sentences of increasing length and complexity. Items are presented auditorily. XXXXXX's performance on this subtest can be interpreted to be within normal limits.

Recent Memory:
This subtest requires the child to recall specific new acquired information relative to his or her environment and daily activities. XXXXXX's performance on this subtest reflects a mild impairment.

Recall of General Information:
This subtest requires the child to recall general information in remote memory. The stimuli represent information that is acquired between the ages of 5 and 12. XXXXXX's performance on this subtest reflects a moderate impairment.

Spatial Orientation:
This subtest requires the child to answer questions related to spatial concepts and orientation. XXXXXX's performance on this subtest can be interpreted to be within normal limits.

<u>Temporal Orientation:</u>
This subtest requires the child to answer questions related to time-based information. XXXXXX's performance on this subtest reflects a mild impairment.

<u>Organization:</u>
This subtest requires the child to recall category members within a 1-minute time limit and recall a category type given three category members. XXXXXX's performance on this subtest reflects a mild impairment.

<u>Problem Solving:</u>
This subtest requires the child to respond to stimulus items containing day-to-day problems. XXXXXX's performance on this subtest reflects a mild impairment.

Test of Narrative Language (TNL)
The Test of Narrative Language (TNL) measures a child's ability to answer literal and inferential comprehension questions. It also is a good measure of how well children use language in narrative discourse. There are three narrative formats: no picture cues, sequence picture cues, and single picture cues. Narrative language abilities require the integration of semantic, syntactic, and pragmatic language for the construction of form—meaning relationships at the sentence and text level. Children who score below 90 on the Narrative Language Ability Index may demonstrate deficits in vocabulary and difficulty with recall, general language comprehension, and syntax. Scores in this range may also be indicative of challenges with social and academic language.

XXXXXX's results are detailed below and are gauged to be an accurate reflection of his current skills. On Narrative Comprehension, XXXXXX answered questions about a story that had been read to him. He performed within the average range on these tasks. On Oral Narration, XXXXXX was expected to retell two stories and create one of his own. He performed within the average range on these tasks. His strongest performance was in his ability to answer familiar, concrete questions about a story (e.g., remembering character names) and in his creativity in the creation of his own fictional story (e.g., the aliens wanted the two kids to take them to see the President of the United States).

TNL 4/7/18

	Raw Score	Standard Score	Interpretation
Narrative Comprehension	31	9	*Average*
Oral Narration	68	13	*Average*
Narrative Language Ability Index	22	65	*Average*

Informal Assessment Administered

Divided Attention Activity Worksheet

This worksheet required XXXXXX to maintain his focus on a task with competing requirements; he had to follow a pattern and trace a line from one target to the next in sequential order (i.e., moving from A–1–B–2–C–3, etc.). XXXXXX was able to complete this worksheet with 95% accuracy. During the task, XXXXXX repeatedly reviewed the written instructions provided on the worksheet to check his accuracy. During one of the reviews, he spotted an error, erased the line in error, and redrew the line correctly. This strategy of review was very effective on this task and may help him with homework assignments that present a greater than average challenge for him.

SKILLS RELATED TO COMMUNICATION

Attention/Behavior

Attention is a key component for developing language. To function appropriately at home and within the classroom, children are expected to focus and attend to a speaker, listen to what is being said, and then utilize and act upon information given (usually instructions or rules).

During the assessment, XXXXXX was able to sustain attention and focus on tasks at hand; he required no repetitions for directions. For example, during one of the narrative tasks, his grandmother entered the room. Although her entry caused a distraction, XXXXXX was able to continue with the task without requiring a review of the information. Further, when asked between assessments if he needed a break, he replied that he did not and continued for another 30 minutes.

Overall, XXXXXX demonstrated appropriate attention and was polite and interacted appropriately with his grandmother, mother, and the speech-language pathologist.

Memory

Memory involves encoding, storing, and retrieving information. These memory skills are important within the classroom and at home because they are required every day when teachers/parents ask their students/children to follow directions related to lessons, assignments, and activities as well as when taking notes and learning vocabulary.

Encoding/Storing/Retrieving for auditory and visual stimuli: On the Concepts and Following Directions subtest, XXXXXX was able to recall directions that increased in length and complexity (e.g., "point to the small orange car" and "point to the small black fish after you point to the big fish and then point to the shoe and ball"). Further, at the end of the session, XXXXXX was able to recall the spelling of the word *bueno* that the speech-language pathologist had talked about early in the session. His performance on this assessment is reflective of his current level of academic performance.

In general, XXXXXX demonstrates appropriate skills with regard to memory.

Executive Functions
Executive functions refer to the ability to initiate and stop actions, monitor and change behavior as needed, and plan future behavior when faced with new tasks and situations. Executive functions allow us to anticipate outcomes and adapt to changing situations. The ability to form concepts and think abstractly is often considered a component of executive function.

Per parent report, XXXXXX is very independent and helpful around the house; he is very involved with his siblings and participates in daily chores in addition to his schoolwork. He has demonstrated no problems with his homework. XXXXXX's performance on the Divided Attention Task is reflective of effective executive function.

Within this evaluation and as reported by his family, XXXXXX demonstrates appropriate executive function as evidenced in the results of the individual formal and informal assessments.

Play Skills
Play skills were not evaluated.

COMMUNICATION

Receptive Language
Receptive language refers to XXXXXX's ability to comprehend and process what others are saying. In general, XXXXXX is able to respond appropriately to questions and comments addressed to him. The Word Classes–Receptive subtest of the CELF-4 was administered to assess his receptive language skills in depth. XXXXXX was significantly more challenged by multiple-syllable words (e.g., catastrophe, latitude, and permanent) than by single-syllable words (e.g., joined and sun).

In general, XXXXXX presents with receptive language skills reflective of a mild impairment.

Expressive Language
Expressive Language refers to XXXXXX's ability to communicate and express his wants, needs, thoughts, and ideas to those around him. In general, XXXXXX is able to express himself appropriately during his daily activities. The Word Classes–Expressive subtest of the CELF-4 and the TNL were administered to obtain an in-depth understanding of XXXXXX's expressive language skills. XXXXXX was able to find relationships between words that were part of his daily life (e.g., pillow/blanket and window/glass) and struggled with words that were more abstract (e.g., connected/joined and achieving/accomplishing).

In general, XXXXXX presents with expressive language skills reflective of a mild impairment.

Oral Motor/Articulation
XXXXXX demonstrated appropriate articulation and motor speech skills.

Voice
Based on informal observations during conversational speech, XXXXXX exhibits appropriate vocal characteristics at this time, including pitch and loudness, which do not impact his overall ability to communicate with others.

Fluency
No abnormal dysfluencies were noted in running speech.

Social Communication/Pragmatics
Pragmatics refers to the way that language is used to communicate with others (the social use of language). Throughout this assessment, and as reported by his family, XXXXXX exhibited appropriate social communication.

In general, XXXXXX presents with appropriate social communication skills. He was polite and respectful during the evaluation. He willingly and actively engaged in conversation with the speech-language pathologist. Per parent report, he is well liked and respected by his peers and teachers.

SUMMARY
XXXXXX is a polite, well-behaved adolescent boy who was referred for a speech and language evaluation due to concerns regarding attention and memory. Results of this assessment indicate that both attention and memory are appropriate for his age and his recovery from an ependymoma.

Per parent report, he is receiving effective support through his IEP and the academic structure of the special day class. Based on these results, it is recommended that XXXXXX continue with his current support system through his school. If he exhibits a change in his academic performance or demonstrates any status changes in speech, language, attention, or memory, it is recommended that he be evaluated again.

Thank you for the opportunity to participate in the assessment of XXXXXX. Please feel free to contact me should you have any questions or concerns regarding the content of this report.

_____
Speech-Language Pathologist
Cc: family, (MD Name) ***, insurance

XYZ REHABILITATION HOSPITAL
COMMUNICATIVE DISORDERS SERVICE

Medical Diagnosis: Stroke

Date of Onset: April 2016   **Date of Report:** 6/12/2016

Speech/Language Pathologist: XXXXXXXXX

Referring Physician: XXXXXX   **Report:** Initial: XXX Final: XXX

1. **BACKGROUND INFORMATION/PROGRESS REPORT:** 37 y/o male, well known to speech clinician from previous LBMMC visit rehab center admit. Pt initially presented with altered LDC, nausea, and vomiting, having been out drinking with friends the previous night. Initially nonverbal and unable to sit up. Paramedics were called and reported CGS 1-5-1 and alcohol odor. Pt taken to LB Community Hospital, where a head CT was initially read as a bleed, then re-read as negative. Pt c/o chest pain or palpitations in ER. PMHx: headaches, anxiety, HTN, hyperlipidemia. Follow-up CT revealed occluded L internal carotid artery. Pt was d/c'd with residual mod-severe receptive aphasia and severe expressive aphasia, and R hemiplegia. SOHx: Pt lives with wife and 4-year-old daughter; with other family members involved.

2. **SPEECH/LANGUAGE/COGNITIVE DIAGNOSIS:** Pt was evaluated in clinic office with his wife present. Portions of the Boston Diagnostic Aphasia Exam (BDAE), the Boston Naming Test, and the Reading Comprehension Battery for Aphasia (RCBA) were given. The following results were obtained:

   Cognition: Difficult to fully assess all areas secondary to expressive language. However, immediate recall of short paragraph was 100% accurate for y/no responses. Problem solving during functional activities is at min assist-to-supervised.

   Speech: Verbal attempts were 100% accurate during non-structured tasks, such as picture description of "cookie theft" from BDAE. Pt was 20% accurate for verbal attempts in response to automatic phrases in structured task. Imitations of short sentences, verbally presented, were 30% accurate, with apraxic distortions. Pt was 100% accurate for automatics (i.e., counting, days, months).

   Lang.: Pt was 75% to 100% accurate for y/no responses to questions regarding complex ideational material, verbally presented. Pt was 40% accurate reading sentences and pointing to printed pictures from field of 3.

3. **PROGNOSIS:** ____ Excellent __X__ Good __X__ Fair ____ Guarded ____ Poor

   Secondary to: above results and pt.'s progress over time

4. RECOMMENDATIONS:
Speech/Language/Cognitive therapy <u>3×</u> times weekly for <u>4</u> weeks.

5. GOALS:
<u>Patient/Family:</u> To talk.   **Discharge Goals Met:** ____ Yes ____ No

<u>Treatment:</u>

↑ reading comprehension of survival words/signs to min assist (75%–80% acc.).

↑ automatic speech thru melodic intonation therapy to mod assist.

↑ naming of family members & common household items to mod assist.

Thank you for referring this patient.

NAME: XXXXX
M.D.: XXXXX
MMC NO.: XXXXX   AGE: <u>37</u>

_____
Speech-Language Pathologist

APPENDIX 7–D
Sample Goals and Objectives

Target Area: Spoken Language Expression

Objective 1: Given a visual prompt (e.g., picture) and not more than three cues (e.g., written, semantic, phonemic), the patient will say the names of familiar people, in 7 of 10 opportunities.

Objective 2: Given a visual prompt (e.g., picture) and not more than three cues (e.g., semantic, phonemic) in a clinic setting, the patient will say the names of 10 familiar places in 7 of 10 opportunities.

Objective 3: Given a visual prompt (e.g., picture) and not more than three cues (e.g., semantic, phonemic) in a clinic setting, the patient will say the names of 10 familiar objects in 7 of 10 opportunities.

Objective 4: Given a visual prompt (e.g., picture) and not more than three cues (e.g., semantic, phonemic) in a clinic setting, the patient will say the names of 10 familiar activities in 7 of 10 opportunities.

Target Area: Multimodal Communication

Goal: To improve communicative effectiveness, XXXXXX will switch communication modalities to writing, drawing, or description when word retrieval difficulties occur in conversation.

Objective 1: In response to word retrieval difficulties, XXXXXX will switch communication modalities to writing, drawing, or description during picture description in 8 of 10 opportunities.

Objective 2: In response to word retrieval difficulties, XXXXXX will switch communication modalities to writing, drawing, or description during conversation in 8 of 10 opportunities.

Target Area: Auditory Comprehension

STG 1a: Pt. will correctly identify a pictured object from a field of four at 90% accuracy while using compensatory strategies for improved auditory comprehension as needed (e.g., ask for repeat of message, ask for a written cue) across 30 trials and two consecutive sessions.

STG 1b: Pt. will correctly identify a pictured object from a field of six at 90% accuracy while using compensatory strategies for improved auditory comprehension as needed (e.g., ask for repeat of message, ask for a written cue) across 30 trials and two consecutive sessions.

STG 1c: Pt. will correctly identify a sequence of two pictures from a field of six at 90% accuracy while using compensatory strategies for improved auditory comprehension as needed (e.g., ask for repeat of message, ask for a written cue) across 30 trials and two consecutive sessions.

STG 1d: Pt. will correctly identify a sequence of two pictures from a field of eight at 90% accuracy while using compensatory strategies for improved auditory comprehension as needed (e.g., ask for repeat of message, ask for a written cue) across 30 trials and two consecutive sessions.

AUGMENTATIVE AND ALTERNATIVE COMMUNICATION

Target Area: AAC Use

Goal: Given access to an AAC system with graphic icons, the student will label and use 15 novel concepts related to daily activities and familiar routines in 4/5 opportunities.

Objective 1: Given access to an AAC system with graphic icons, the student will label 15 novel concepts related to daily activities and familiar routines in 4/5 opportunities with verbal and gestural cues.

Objective 2: Given access to an AAC system with graphic icons, the student will use 15 novel concepts related to daily activities and familiar routines in 4/5 opportunities with verbal and gestural cues.

Target Area: Functional/Expressive Communication

By May 2014, he student will incorporate aided language/graphic symbols to accomplish the communicative purposes of requesting and protesting in 4/5 opportunities across 3 trial days, as measured by observation and data collection.

Target Area: Receptive Language

By May 2014, during daily activities and routines, XXXXXX will use her AAC device to answer factual yes/no questions, given visual supports in four of five trials across 3 trial days as measured by observation and data collection.

By May 2014, during daily activities and routines, XXXXXX will use her AAC device to answer familiar "who" and "what" questions given visual supports in four of five trials across 3 trial days as measured by observation and data collection.

By May 2014, during structured speech-language activities, XXXXXX will use her AAC device to answer basic "wh" comprehension questions (i.e., who, what doing, where, when) related to a short passage/story, given visual supports as needed in four of five trials over three consecutive sessions as measured by observation and data collection.

AUTISM SPECTRUM DISORDERS

Target Area: Play

Goal: The client will perform sequences of common play scripts (e.g., restaurant, store, library), in response to a video self-model in the clinic setting.

Objective 1: The client will imitate a minimum of four actions and four verbalizations of imaginative play sequences of common play scripts (e.g., restaurant, store, library), following a video self-model, in at least two play scripts, in the clinic setting.

Target Area: Social Skills

Goal: To improve social skills, the client will demonstrate appropriate use of social conventions in conversations with familiar and unfamiliar communication partners.

> *Objective 1:* When presented with a visual stimulus (i.e., video modeling), the client will demonstrate appropriate use of social conventions (e.g., greetings, introductions, and asking questions) given moderate (3–5) verbal cues and gestures, in three of five opportunities with the clinician in the clinic setting.

> *Objective 2:* When presented with a visual stimulus (i.e., video modeling), the client will demonstrate appropriate use of social conventions (e.g., greetings, introductions, and asking questions) given minimal (1–2) verbal cues and gestures, in four of five opportunities with the clinician in the clinic setting.

Target Area: Language

By December 2018, during naturalistic activities (e.g., play, snack, library), given no more than two prompts (e.g., visual, phonemic, questioning), XXXXXX will produce two-word semantic relations (e.g., agent + action; action + object; attribute + entity), with 70% accuracy.

By December 2018, during two of three naturalistic activities (e.g., play, snack, library), with no more than two prompts

(e.g., visual, phonemic, questioning), XXXXXX will produce semantic relations within the negation + object category, using at least two-word utterances, with 70% accuracy.

CHILD LANGUAGE DISORDERS

Target Area: Auditory Comprehension

Goal: The student will follow one- to two-step instructions with verbal prompts.

> *Objective 1:* The student will follow one- to two-step instructions in 40% of opportunities with verbal and visual prompts.

> *Objective 2:* The student will follow one- to two-step instructions in 50% of opportunities with verbal and visual prompts.

> *Objective 3:* The student will follow one- to two-step instructions in 50% of opportunities with verbal prompts.

Target Area: Preliteracy / Phonology

Goal: To improve preliteracy skills, the client will demonstrate increased phonological awareness by segmenting monosyllabic words.

> *Objective 1:* To improve preliteracy skills, the client will demonstrate increased phonological awareness by categorizing words (e.g., Which one begins with a different sound: feet, five, soup, fat?) in response to print and verbal cues in 7 of 10 opportunities.

> *Objective 2:* To improve preliteracy skills, the client will demonstrate

increased phonological awareness by deletion (e.g., Say trip without the /t/) in response to print and verbal cues in 7 of 10 opportunities.

Objective 3: To improve preliteracy skills, the client will demonstrate increased phonological awareness by substitution (e.g., Replace the /m/ in man with /f/) in response to print and verbal cues in 7 of 10 opportunities.

Objective 4: To improve preliteracy skills, the client will demonstrate increased phonological awareness by manipulation (e.g., Say the word stop. Now move the /s/ to the end of the word and say it again) in response to print and verbal cues in 7 of 10 opportunities.

Target Area: Morphology

By May 2016, during pretend play activities, following therapist recasts, XXXXXX will produce the present progressive (e.g., children are singing) in at least 10 utterances across three sessions.

By May 2016, during pretend play activities, XXXXXX will complete cloze procedures with the present progressive (e.g., we are . . .) in at least 10 utterances across three sessions.

By May 2016, during pretend play activities, the client will spontaneously produce the present progressive (e.g., puppy jumping) in at least 10 utterances across three sessions.

Target Area: Pragmatics

Goal: The client will produce appropriate sentences for a variety of social functions (e.g., requesting, turn-taking, repairing conversational breakdowns).

Objective 1: The client will produce an appropriate sentence for a variety of social functions (e.g., requesting, turn-taking, repairing conversational breakdowns) when given moderate prompting (e.g., verbal and/or visual prompts), with 80% accuracy across 10 trials as measured by recorded data.

MOTOR SPEECH

Target Area: Voice

Objective 1: The patient will demonstrate controlled exhalation by sustaining phonation of the vowel /a/ for 10 seconds or longer, in 80% of trials, across two consecutive therapy sessions.

Objective 2: The patient will demonstrate controlled exhalation by sustaining phonation of the vowel /a/ for 20 seconds or longer, in 80% of trials, across two consecutive therapy sessions.

Target Area: Fluency

Goal: The client will demonstrate increased knowledge of stuttering.

Objective 1: The client correctly identifies components of the speech structures used in speaking with 80% accuracy.

Objective 2: The client will identify various types of stuttering with 80% accuracy when listening to

---

*Coleman & Yaruss, 2014.

recorded tapes of stutterers or pseudostuttering by the clinician or others in a therapy session.

Objective 3: The client will identify current feared speaking situations, define a preferred scenario, and create an action plan to attain the preferred scenario.

PHONOLOGY

Target Area: Phonological Awareness

Goal: The client will demonstrate phonological awareness skills by identifying initial and final sounds in CVC, CV, and VC words.

Objective 1: Given a visual cue and verbal prompts, the client will match the beginning sounds of words with 70% accuracy as measured by clinician observation, other informal assessments, and data collection.

Objective 2: Given a visual cue and verbal prompts, the client will identify the beginning sounds of words with 70% accuracy as measured by clinician observation, other informal assessments, and data collection.

Objective 3: Given a visual cue and verbal prompts, the client will match the ending sounds of words with 70% accuracy as measured by clinician observation, other informal assessments, and data collection.

Objective 4: Given a visual cue and verbal prompts, the client will

match the ending sounds of words with 70% accuracy as measured by clinician observation, other informal assessments, and data collection.

Target Area: Articulation

Goal: XXXXXX will produce /s/ in the initial and final position at the word level 50% of the time.

Objective 1: Given pictures, a model, and a verbal prompt, XXXXXX will produce /s/ in the initial and final position, at the word level, with 20% accuracy.

Objective 2: Given pictures, a model, and a verbal prompt, XXXXXX will produce /s/ in the initial and final position at the word level with 40% accuracy.

Target Area: Articulation

Goal: The client will produce the phonemes /r/, /l/, /s/, and /z/ in initial and final position in one-syllable words.

Objective 1: With no more than one prompt, the student will produce the phonemes /r/, /l/, /s/, and /z/ in CV and VC syllables with 80% accuracy.

Objective 2: The student will produce the phonemes /r/, /l/, /s/, and /z/ in the initial position of one-syllable words with 70% accuracy.

Objective 3: The student will produce the phonemes /r/, /l/, /s/, and /z/ in the final position of one-syllable words with 70% accuracy.

CHAPTER 8

Data Collection

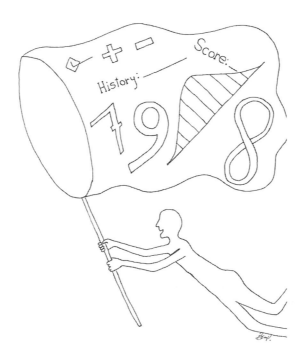

Accuracy of observation is the equivalent of accuracy of thinking.
—Wallace Stevens
(Pulitzer Prize–winning poet)

The terms *data* (plural) and *datum* (singular) refer to "factual information (as measurements or statistics) used as a basis for reasoning, discussion, or calculation" (Merriam-Webster, 2003). Hence, data collection is the process of obtaining this information. In the field of speech-language pathology, collecting, analyzing, and summarizing data is a vital part of decision-making and documentation.

As a speech-language pathology assistant (SLPA), you will learn about evidence-based practice (EBP), which is the "integration of clinical expertise, best current evidence, and client values to provide high-quality services reflecting the interests, values, needs, and choices of those we serve" (Rao, 2011, para. 4). Data collection is an integral part of EBP (Boswell, 2005; Epstein, 2008; Lemoncello & Fanning,

2011) and, as such, is a very important aspect of what speech-language pathologists (SLPs) and, in turn, SLPAs do. Box 8–1 lists some of the job responsibilities of an SLPA that may involve data collection.

Clinically, data collection begins during assessment when the SLP analyzes information about communicative or swallowing behaviors. SLPAs are qualified to conduct communicative screenings and, with the new 2022 ASHA Scope of Practice for the Speech-Language Pathology Assistant document, are now able to conduct, but not interpret, language and communicative assessments if they meet the requirements stated in the examiner's manual. However, interpreting assessment data remains outside the scope of practice of SLPAs. Further, screenings and assessments involving swallowing are outside of the SLPAs' scope of practice (ASHA, 2022). When SLPAs collaborate with SLPs in screenings and assessments, they may assist with delivery and data collection, such as tallying or recording specific behaviors, transcribing a language sample, making phonetic notations, calculating percentages, transferring data onto standardized protocols, or creating graphs or charts to display assessment or screening data.

Data collection about a client is obtained during and may continue after treatment, as the client moves toward generalization. These data are critical because they allow the SLP to monitor the client's progress from session to session and to document the efficacy of a given treatment strategy (Mowrer, 1982; Roth & Worthington, 2001). This, too, may be an area where an SLPA can assist, as it also involves tasks such as tallying or recording specific behaviors, making phonetic notations, calculating percentages, and preparing charts or graphs about treatment data. As discussed in Chapter 7, treatment objectives include information about the types of data needed to establish if a client has met a given objective. This information is present in the *criterion* portion of behavioral objectives.

As an SLPA, your role in accurately collecting data is crucial since inaccurate data will negatively influence clinical decisions. The sections that follow discuss methods for observing and recording data, including ideas for ways to record specific types of data. Chapter 9 discusses ways to summarize these data in note format. The companion website associated with this book contains samples of score sheets that can be used for charting data.

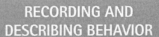

RECORDING AND DESCRIBING BEHAVIOR

There are many different methods for observing, recording, and describing communication behaviors. At the heart of each is careful observation, meaning that

---

Box 8–1. Examples of SLPA Duties Involving Data
(American Speech-Language-Hearing Association [ASHA], 2022)[1]

a. Administering and scoring screenings for clinical interpretation by the SLP.

b. Assisting the SLP during assessment of students, patients, and clients (e.g., setting up the testing environment, gathering and prepping materials, taking notes as advised by the SLP, etc.).

c. Administering and scoring assessment tools within the following parameters: (a) The SLPA meets the examiner requirements specified in the examiner's manual and (b) the supervising SLP uses to verify the SLPA's competence in administration, exclusive of clinical interpretation.

d. Administering and scoring progress monitoring tools exclusive of clinical interpretation if (a) the SLPA meets the examiner requirements specified in the examiner's manual and (b) the supervisor has verified the SLPA's competence in administration.

e. Implementing documented care plans or protocols (e.g., individualized education plan [IEP], individualized family service plan [IFSP], treatment plan) developed and directed by the supervised SLP.

f. Providing direct therapy services addressing treatment goals developed by the supervising SLP to meet the needs of the student, patient, client, and family.

g. Adjusting and documenting the amount and type of support or scaffolding provided to the student, patient, or client in treatment to facilitate progress.

h. Developing and implementing activities and materials for teaching and practice of skills to address the goals of the student, patient, client, and family per the plan of care developed by the supervising SLP.

i. Providing treatment through a variety of service delivery models (e.g., individual, group, classroom based, home based, cotreatment with other disciplines) as directed by the supervising SLP.

j. Documenting student, patient, or client performance (e.g., collecting data and calculating percentages for the SLP to use; preparing charts, records, and graphs) and reporting this information to the supervising SLP in a timely manner.

k. Sharing objective information (e.g., accuracy in speech and language skills addressed, participation in treatment, response to treatment) regarding student, patient, and client performance to students, patients, clients, caregivers, families, and other service providers without interpretation or recommendations as directed by the SLP.

you actively and directly see and listen to the client, taking care to accurately record what you observe (Kawulich, 2005; Taylor-Powell & Steele, n.d.). Careful observation requires understanding the behaviors to be observed, the type of data to be collected, and the method for summarizing the information.

Some methods for recording data in the field of speech-language pathology include frequency counts and tallies, response analysis, and transcription and narration.

Frequency Counts and Tallies

Frequency counts and tallies determine if a behavior is present (and at what rate) during a specific period (Moore & Pearson, 2003; Mowrer, 1982; Roth & Paul, 2007). These methods are also referred to as simple enumeration (Mowrer, 1982). In these techniques, the objective is to record the presence of a specific behavior, such as a client interacting with a peer, asking a question, saying a specific sound or type of word, and so forth. To record this type of data, you must know which specific behavior to observe, how long to watch for the behavior, and during which activity you need to observe the behavior. You would then record the number of times that behavior occurred in that specified period (e.g., 2 times in 1 minute, 10 times in 2 minutes, etc.) during the specified activity. Tallies, hash marks, checks, and other symbols can be used to record this information. Figure 8–1 shows an example of a chart that could be used to record this type of information.

Response Rate

Response rate is a variant of frequency counts and tallies whereby a specific behavior is counted, and the number is converted to a value that denotes responses

Client: Scott Smith (Mrs. Smith's Classroom)

Behavior/Time/Activity	Count
Behavior: Whole-word repetition Length of Time: 10 minutes Activity: Story retell Date: 12/15/17 Clinician: Sarah S. Assistant	✓ ✓ ✓ ✓ ✓ (5 in 12 min.)
Behavior: Final consonant deletion Length of Time: 10 minutes Activity: Story retell Date: 12/15/17 Clinician: Sarah S. Assistant	H̶H̶ I I (7 in 12 min.)

Figure 8–1. Sample Frequency Count/Tally Data Sheet.

per unit of time. Words per minute (WPM) is a common measurement that uses this technique (Shipley & McAfee, 2009). In this instance, the behavior is the number of words produced in a minute. To record WPM, you would count the number of words produced and divide that number by the number of minutes the person was spoke. Syllables per minute (SPM) is another measure calculated in this fashion, but the count would denote the number of syllables produced per minute (Mowrer, 1982).

Checklists

A checklist is another variant of frequency counts and tallies. This technique denotes the presence of a list of behaviors (Moore & Pearson, 2003; Roth & Paul, 2007). It could be a checklist specifically created by your supervising SLP for a specific client (or group of clients), or it may be a modi-fied version of an existing checklist. Figure 8–2 shows an example of a checklist specifically created to track behaviors in a group setting.

Of primary importance in recording behaviors using frequency counts and tallies, response rate, and checklists is that you are very clear about the behavior to be counted. For instance, in Figure 8–1, if you did not know what a whole-word repetition was or how it differs from a part-word repetition, you could not accurately record its occurrence and, in turn, would be sharing inaccurate information about the frequency of the behavior with your supervising SLP. Thus, you should always confirm that you understand the exact parameters of the behavior to be counted and ask your supervising SLP if you have any questions.

Screening. In some settings, you may be asked to assist with speech, language,

Client: John Jones

Activity: Aphasia Support Group – Thursday Session

SLPA: Sarah S. Assistant

Date: 1/3/18

Behavior	Note Y for *Yes* or N for *No*
Greets fellow group members upon entering room	Y
Finds name tag	N – located table, but needs assistance from group facilitator in locating name tag.
Finds designated seat	Y
Initiates small talk with a fellow group member	Y
Responds to a question posed by group facilitator	N
Comments during group discussion	Y – states "Like pizza" when discussing favorite foods

Figure 8–2. Sample Checklist Data Sheet.

or hearing screenings (ASHA, 2022). A screening "involves the collection of data to decide whether there is a strong likelihood that an individual does or does not have a problem that will require more in-depth assessment" (Kennedy, 2007, p. 42). Screenings are not diagnostic in nature. Rather, they are used to determine if further testing is needed. Screenings use a predetermined cutoff or expected performance level to determine if a client either passes or fails the screening. Your supervising SLP may use a setting-specific instrument or one of many commercially available screening tools.

In some cases, screenings used are similar to checklists in that specific behaviors are listed, and the screener denotes the presence or absence of each behavior in a specific context. In other cases, a screener gives the client a specific task and denotes the presence or absence of a required response. For example, in a hearing screening, the clients are instructed to raise their hand in response to a series of tones, presented at different frequencies and loudness levels. The screener presents the tones and then notes whether clients raised their hand (presence of required response) or did not raise their hand (absence of required response) for each tone. Similarly, in a kindergarten speech and language screening, a student may be asked to count from 1 to 10. The screener then notes whether the student counted from 1 to 10 (presence of required response) or did not count from 1 to 10 (absence of required response). In these instances, the screener requires a fully correct response as the criterion for the presence of a behavior. Any other response is noted as absence of the required behavior. No interpretation of the meaning behind why clients did not raise their hand or count from 1 to 10 is made.

In most cases, screeners require the use of a binary score, such as yes/no, absent/present, or correct/incorrect. In addition, some speech and language screeners require errors to be transcribed using the International Phonetic Alphabet (IPA) or written verbatim. A list of IPA symbols is available in Appendix 4–B in Chapter 4. The comments section of many screeners often requires the examiner to note any special circumstances related to the screening that may have influenced the results, such as if the client was not paying attention during a task or did not appear to understand the directions. This type of additional information can be used by the SLP to interpret the results of the screening.

Conducting screenings requires specific training on the screening tool to be used. Administration of hearing screenings also requires that you learn how to operate an audiometer.

SLPA Roles: Caution. A word of caution is in order about checklists and screenings and their use by SLPAs. Many checklists and, in some cases, commercially available screeners are used by SLPs to assess specific behaviors. These should not be confused with checklists and screenings designed for implementation by an SLPA. In cases where interpretation or diagnosis is required or implied, that is the sole domain of an SLP. For example, a common assessment tool utilized by an SLP is an oral peripheral examination, used to "identify or rule out structural or functional factors that relate to a communicative disorder or dysphagia" (Shipley & McAfee, 2009, p. 158). There are several checklists or forms available for use by SLPs for this purpose, most of which include some interpretative or diagnostic aspect. For example, Figure 8–3 contains an excerpt from the Oral-Facial Examination Form (Shipley & McAfee, 2009). In addition, some checklists contain rating scales that require the respondent to classify or rate the severity of a behavior, which is also diagnostic and interpretative in nature. Figure 8–4 is an excerpt from the Checklist for the Assessment of Clients With Clefts (Shipley & McAfee, 2009).

A diagnosis is "a concise technical description" (Merriam-Webster, 2003). The examples from Figures 8–3 and 8–4 both require interpretation and precise description. ASHA (2022) states that

SLPAs should not engage in "interpreting assessment tools for the purpose of diagnosing disability, determining eligibility or qualification of services" (Responsibilities Outside the Scope of Practice for Speech-Language Pathology Assistants, para. 1). In addition, ASHA specifically highlights the use of checklists for dysphagia (interpretative or otherwise) is outside the scope of responsibilities of an SLPA, as indicated by the statement that SLPAs are precluded from "administering or interpreting feeding and/or swallowing screenings, checklists, and

---

Evaluation of tongue

_____ Surface color: normal/abnormal (specify)_____
_____ Abnormal movements: absent/jerky/spasms/writhing/fasiculations_____
_____ Size: normal/small/large_____
_____ Frenum: normal/short _____

Tell the client to protrude the tongue.
_____ Excursion: normal/deviates to right/deviates to left _____
_____ Range of motion: normal/reduced_____
_____ Speed of motion: normal/reduced_____

(Shipley & McAfee, 2009, p. 196)

Figure 8–3. Excerpt from Oral-Facial Examination Form.

Assessment of Voice

Instructions: Evaluate the client's voice, paying particular attend to possible cleft-related problems. Check the deficits that are present and indicate severity. Record additional notes in the right-hand margin.

1 = Mild
2 = Moderate
3 = Severe

_____ Pitch variation is reduced_____
_____ Vocal intensity is reduced_____
_____ Vocal quality is hoarse/harsh/breathy (circle)_____

(Shipley & McAfee, 2009, p. 574)

Figure 8–4. Excerpt from Checklist for the Assessment of Clients With Clefts.

assessments" (Responsibilities Outside the Scope of Practice for Speech-Language Pathology Assistants, para. 1). As an SLPA, it is important that you maintain these boundaries for the benefit and safety of the clients you serve. There could be legal and ethical ramifications if you engage in practices beyond your scope of responsibilities as an SLPA.

Response Analysis

Response analysis is a type of data analysis beyond counting or denoting the presence of a behavior. Response analysis techniques look at the dimensions of correctness (response accuracy), delay (response latency), and assistance needed (response independence) to further quantify behavior. Appendix 7–D in Chapter 7 contains samples of treatment goals and objectives across a variety of response categories. After you read the sections that follow, see if you can identify what type of response analysis is used and what data collection methods you might use to record these behaviors.

Response Accuracy

To record response accuracy, you would be told about a behavior and details about what constitutes an accurate response (Mowrer, 1982). You would then count the number of correct responses and the total number of opportunities for that behavior to occur. An example of this is percent correct (Mowrer, 1982). In this method, you would divide the total number of correct responses by the total number of opportunities. This result could then be converted to a percentage of correct responses, which is helpful because it denotes if the

behavior occurred and also what portion of the time it was accurate. For example, if charting accuracy in producing /s/ in the initial position of words, you would count the number of times the client produced the /s/ correctly in the initial position of words (total correct) and divide by the total number of opportunities the client had to say words with /s/ in the initial position (total opportunities). To convert this number to a percentage, you would then multiply by 100, as follows:

$$5 \div 10 \times 100 = 50\%$$

5	÷	10	× 100 =	50%
Total Correct		Total Opportunities		Percent Correct

An example data collection sheet for this task may look similar to the sheet in Figure 8–5. Figure 8–6 contains a similar way to record these same data. You can

---

Client: Tina Thomas

SLPA: Sarah S. Assistant

Date: 1/15/18

Target: /s/ initial/single words

Key: + = correct/ – = incorrect

Word	Response
Sew	–
Say	+
Soup	+
Suit	–
Sock	–
Sub	–
Soap	+
Set	+
Sun	–
Sit	+

Score: 5/10 = 50%

Figure 8–5. Sample Percent Correct Data Sheet (targets noted).

Client: Tina Thomas   SLPA: Sarah S. Assistant

Date: 1/15/18   Objective: /s/ initial/single words

									Score
/	/	/	X	X	/	X	X	X	/	50%

Key: X = correct   / = incorrect

Figure 8–6. Sample Percent Correct Data Sheet (no targets).

see that in both examples, the client had 10 opportunities to say a word with /s/ in the initial position and did so accurately five times, resulting in a percent correct of 50%.

In Figure 8–5 the opportunities, as well as the words themselves, are recorded as a reference and the score sheet includes a key to denote that a "+" indicates times when the client produced /s/ in the initial position correctly, while a "−" indicates times when /s/ in the initial position of a word was not produced accurately. In Figure 8–6, no individual words are recorded, but an accurate production is noted with an X and an inaccurate production is noted with a /.

Another common technique that uses the concept of percent correct is a dysfluency index (Shipley & McAfee, 2009). This method counts the total number of syllables (total opportunities) and the total number of disfluencies. A percentage is then calculated, either as a measure of all types of disfluencies (e.g., % Total Disfluency) or for certain types of disfluencies (e.g., % Repetitions, % Prolongations). A similar calculation is used to determine Percent Syllables Stuttered (% SS) as follows (Jones et al., 2006):

$$\text{Syllables Stuttered/Total Syllables} \times 100 = \text{SS}\%$$

Response accuracy can also be described using an opportunity statement. In this method, correct responses and total opportunities are recorded, but the information is not displayed as a percentage. Rather, this information is summarized in a written statement, such as, "3 of 4 opportunities," "in 8 of 10 instances," or "given 20 of 25 attempts." The following objectives have criteria that use response accuracy:

- Given a verbal label of a category, the client will name three items that belong to that category in 8 of 10 opportunities.
- With a visual cue or gesture prompt, Johnny will respond to a teacher-directed question by touching an appropriate symbol on his augmentative and alternative communication

(AAC) device, in three of four opportunities, over three consecutive sessions.

■ The student will correctly use present progressive tense to describe 15 of 20 pictures not visible to the clinician.

Response accuracy can be used for almost any type of behavior, using either percent correct or an opportunity statement. In fact, response accuracy is a common measure used by SLPs in the criterion portion of treatment objectives.

The key to collecting response accuracy is understanding what constitutes a correct or an accurate response and noting how many opportunities the individual had to produce a correct response. Keep in mind that a correct response may not necessarily be synonymous with a perfect response. There are instances when a close approximation or a partly correct response may be determined by your supervising SLP as correct. This information can be noted in the client's goal. If not, you can check with your supervising SLP to confirm that you understand the parameters that constitute "correct."

Response Latency

Response latency is a method for analyzing a response, given how long it took to produce a behavior (Mowrer, 1982). This type of data collection is less common than response accuracy in the field of speech-language pathology. To calculate response latency, you would need to count the length of time between presentation of a *stimulus* and when the client responded. This is typically calculated in seconds and measured with a stopwatch. A stimulus is basically an opportunity to respond. For example, when you ask a cli-

ent to name something, like a picture of a train, a line drawing of a bed, or a real object like a cup, each of these items (the train, the line drawing, and the cup) is a stimulus. A question or command, such as, "Is grass green?" "What sound does a cow make?" or "Give me your hand," is also a stimulus as each is an opportunity for the client to respond. Figure 8–7 is an example of a data collection sheet for recording response latency. As you can see, in this instance, the task is for the client to point to a picture described by the clinician in less than 5 seconds. Data collection sheets can be very basic in this case, but the key to collecting this type of data is timing precision. In most cases, a timer is started at the end of stimulus presentation, such as at the end of a question or command, or once the picture or object stimulus is in full view. The timer is stopped at the onset of a response, although in some cases, time may be stopped once the response is completed. When collecting data on response latency, you should familiarize yourself with the timer to be used and confirm with your supervising SLP the intended start and stop times.

In some instances, a rating scale may be used to denote an immediate or delayed response. This may eliminate the need for a stopwatch, but it still requires you to monitor if the client responded right away after the stimulus was presented (immediate) or if there was a delay in responding (delayed). An example of a score sheet that uses this type of rating scale for charting response latency is shown in Figure 8–8.

Note that for both the score sheets discussed above (see Figures 8–7 and 8–8), each has a mechanism for recording response accuracy in addition to response latency. For example, in Figure 8–7, re-

Client: Tim Thomas

SLPA: Sarah S. Assistant

Target: Point to picture described by clinician in <5 seconds

Measurement: Start – End of Questions/Stop – Points to a Picture

											Average Time
Items in field: 2	5.3	4.3	2.5	3.6	6.7	3.3	11.9	3.1	4.5	3.4	
Date: 2/7/18	–	–	+	+	–	–	–	+	+	+	
Items in field: Date:											
Items in field: Date:											

Figure 8–7. Sample response Latency Data Sheet (timed).

Client: Jessica Jones

SLPA: Sarah S. Assistant

Date: 8/14/18

Target: Name familiar, real objects

Key: 1 = Immediate response
        2 = Delayed response (greater than 3 seconds
        NR = No response

Object	Response
Comb	1
Key	NR
Knife	1+
Cup	1+
Phone	1+
Fork	1
Pen	2
Shoe	NR
Sock	1
Book	2+

Figure 8–8. Sample response Latency Data Sheet (rating scale).

sponse accuracy is represented with a "+" under items that were correct and produced within the required length of time (less than 5 seconds) and a "–" for items that were either incorrect or were correct but not produced in less than 5 seconds. In Figure 8–8, response accuracy is noted with a "+" next to items named correctly. Often, potential exists to collect more than one form of data simultaneously. This can add important details to your data collection.

Response Independence

Response independence is another version of response analysis, which is fairly common in the field of speech-language pathology, particularly when clinicians use some type of assistance or prompt to achieve a desired response. Chapter 10 provides an overview of common prompts used in treatment.

In measuring response independence, you would be given details about a desired or accurate response, as well as the levels or types of assistance you can provide to help the client produce the response. You would then record if assistance was needed and, if so, what type of assistance was provided. For example, in targeting the production of prepositions, the desired or correct behavior may be for the client to produce one of four types of prepositions (e.g., in, on, over, or under) in response to a question such as, "Where is the kitten?" In this case, the desired response could be a short phrase (e.g., in the box) or a single word (e.g., in). An example of a task is using a stuffed toy kitten and a basket, eliciting different descriptions as the client moves the toy kitten to different locations (e.g., kitten in the basket, under the basket).

In terms of assistance, some options are to give the client a gestural cue, such as a hand motion representing the preposition; a phonemic cue, such as the initial sound of the appropriate preposition; or even a verbal model. Figure 8–9 shows a sample data collection sheet representing this task. As you can see, there is a code that represents three dimensions of assis-

tance: gestural assistance, represented by a *G*; a phonemic cue, represented by a *P*; and a verbal model, represented by an *M*. This example also has notation for accurate production, represented with a *3*. Inaccurate production is represented with a *0*, which indicates that despite assistance, the client was not able to produce the desired response. In the example provided, consistent cues were needed to obtain an accurate response. There are, of course, a variety of other ways to record this same task in terms of response independence, including the data collection sample depicted in Figure 8–10.

The key to recording response independence is to understand what constitutes an accurate response, the types of assistance that are appropriate, and to have a method for recording when assistance is provided. Of note as well, as with

---

Client: Florence Flower   SLPA: Sarah S. Assistant

Objective: Produce prepositions in, on, over and under

O GPM	O GPM	✓ G	✓ G	O GPM	✓	✓ GPM	✓ G	✓ GP	✓ GPM	Date/Score
										Date: 7/22/18 No Cue = 10% G = 30% GP = 10% GPM = 20%
										Date:
										Date:

Key: ✓ = correct   0 = incorrect   CUES: G = Gesture   P = Phoneme Cue   M = Model

Figure 8–9. Sample response Independence Score Sheet (key code).

Client: Florence Flower   SLPA: Sarah S. Assistant

Date: 5/18/18   Objective: Produce prepositions in, on, over and under

No Assist	Gesture	Phoneme Cue	Model	Preposition
–	–	–	–	Over
–	–	–	–	Under
–	+			In
–	+			On
–	–	–	–	Over
+				In
–	–	–	+	Under
–	+			In
–	–	+		On
–	–	–	+	Under

Figure 8–10. Sample response Independence Score Sheet (column tally).

response latency, in both the examples, you can also determine response accuracy. This combination of response accuracy and response independence within a single data collection method can be highly valuable to provide very detailed information to your supervising SLP. Furthermore, collecting data with this level of detail means that, if needed, you can categorize or summarize the client's performance based on what your supervising SLP indicates is an acceptable level of cues. For instance, in the example above, if the supervising SLP indicated that an accurate response was only a single correct response produced with no additional assistance or cues, then the client's accuracy is 10%, since in only 1 of 10 attempts was a preposition accurately produced without any assistance. However, if the supervising SLP deemed that an accurate response could include the provision of a gestural cue, then the client's response accuracy would be 40%, since she accurately produced a preposition one time without assistance and three times with only a gestural cue.

Narration/Transcription— Speech and Language Sample

The last area of data collection we will discuss is a speech and language sample. Speech and language samples are commonly used in the field of speech-language pathology (Haynes & Pindzola, 1998; Owens, 2004). Box 8–2 lists several potential uses for a speech and language sample (Shipley & McAfee, 2009). Research documents many potential advantages of speech and language samples, including ecological validity (e.g., how well it relates to real-life skills), its use in outcome and intervention measures, and sensitivity in assessment, particularly for individuals whose profiles do not align with the normative sample of the assessment tool (Costanza-Smith, 2010). A disadvantage, however, is that a speech and language

> ## Box 8–2. Potential Uses of a Speech and Language Sample
> (Shipley & McAfee, 2009)[2]
>
> ■ Identify speech sound errors.
> ■ Evaluate rate of speech, fluency, and voice.
> ■ Determine speech intelligibility.
> ■ Compare errors in structured tasks with those of connected speech.
> ■ Analyze language, including skills in the areas of semantics, phonology, morphology, syntax, and pragmatics.
> ■ Determine mean length of utterance (MLU) and type token ratio (TTR).
> ■ Identify dysarthria and apraxia.

sample is only as good as the sample collected and the skill of the person transcribing and summarizing the sample. In addition, speech and language samples can be time-consuming to record, transcribe, and analyze (Costanza-Smith, 2010). SLPAs can play an important role in collecting a speech and language sample and performing initial calculations of the sample for their supervising SLP. What follows is a discussion of ways to collect and analyze a speech and language sample.

Collecting the Sample

If your supervising SLP asks you to collect a speech and language sample, it is important that you do so in a way that is both reliable and valid. Reliable means the sample can be replicated (e.g., someone else could obtain a similar sample), and valid means the sample is a reasonable reflection of the client's actual speech and language abilities (Shipley & McAfee, 2009).

The first step in collecting a speech and language sample is asking your supervisor where, when, and what type of sample is needed. Audio recording is required for in-depth analysis and transcription. Videotaping is possible, but only if good audio quality is also available. Generally, digital audio files that can be stored and viewed on a computer-based program are preferred (Bunta et al., 2003). The advantage of this method is that specific segments of the sample (e.g., sounds, words, phrases) can be reviewed more easily than with a traditional analog recording, such as a tape recorder. Samples of the digital audio files can also be embedded within a transcription for future reference.

A word of caution is in order regarding audio or video recordings. First, it requires consent from the client or the client's guardian, typically in writing. Never audio or videotape a client without his or her knowledge and expressed consent. Second, if audio or visual information is collected, this information becomes part of the client's official records and is protected by the same confidentiality regulations discussed in Chapter 3.

In general, a sample of at least 50 utterances is needed, but 100 to 200 utterances are recommended (Constanza-

Smith, 2010; Shipley & McAfee, 2009). Samples should be collected in a variety of communication contexts (i.e., a variety of communication activities). A general rule is to collect both a conversational sample and a narrative sample (Price et al., 2010), but of course this depends on the instructions of your SLP supervisor. When collecting a sample, it is important that you help the client become comfortable interacting with you. This is particularly true with children, as the sample collected may not be a good reflection of their skills if you dominate the conversation or the client feels shy or nervous about communicating with you. Establishing a positive relationship before you collect the sample is very important (Shipley & McAfee, 2009). For young children, this may mean engaging in play before you begin collecting the sample; for older children or adults, this may mean engaging in small talk on a topic of interest. Box 8–3 contains additional recommendations for collecting a reliable and valid sample.

Conversation Sample. If you are working with adult clients or older children, you can collect a conversation sample by asking open-ended questions, such as, "Tell me about . . . " (Shipley & McAfee, 2009). Box 8–4 contains a list of additional conversation starters. For young children, incorporating pictures that depict the topic starter or pictures showing a scene with a variety of activities, such as a carnival or playground, may also be a good topic starter (Shipley & McAfee, 2009). Try to avoid, though, having the client name items in the picture, as a language sample collected during interactive conversation and a picture description task are two separate constructs. Rather, attempt to engage the client in natural conversation, with open-ended and topic-continuing statements, such as, "Tell me more about that" (Costanza-Smith, 2010; Shipley & McAfee, 2009).

Narrative Sample. A narrative is a story (Merriam-Webster, 2003). Producing a narrative requires more planning and organization than a conversation (Price et al., 2010; Shipley & McAfee, 2009). One common method for collecting a narrative sample is story retelling (Price et al., 2010;

Box 8–3. Recommendations for Collecting a Speech and Language Sample (Shipley & McAfee, 2009)[3]

- Minimize interruptions and distractions.
- Be willing to wait for the client to talk.
- Do not talk to fill silence.
- Preselect materials and topics of interest.
- Follow the client's lead.
- Vary the subject matter.
- Limit the use of yes/no questions.
- Ask open-ended questions to elicit longer responses (e.g., Tell me about X. What happened then? Why?).
- Make natural contributions to the conversation.

> ### Box 8–4. Sample Conversation Starters (Shipley & McAfee, 2009)[4]
>
> - Tell me about what you would do if you won a million dollars (you had superpowers or _____)?
> - Have you ever been to a hospital (airport, or _____)? Tell me about it.
> - Do you like video games (movies, or _____)? Tell me about your favorite one.
> - Pretend I've never had a pizza (ice cream, or _____) before. Describe it to me.
> - What is your dream vacation (home, or _____)? Describe it to me.
> - Do you have a pet (brother, sister, or children)? Tell me about him/her/them.

Shipley & McAfee, 2009). For example, you could read the client a story and then ask him or her to retell the story to you. You could also ask if the client can recall a familiar story, such as *Goldilocks and the Three Bears* or *Little Red Riding Hood*, and ask them to tell you the story. Alternatively, you could show them a wordless storybook and ask them to tell you the story depicted or give them several pictures depicting the elements of a story and ask them to place them in order and tell you the story they depict.

Sample Transcription/Analysis

To transcribe something is to make a written copy (Merriam-Webster, 2003). The first step in transcribing a speech and language sample is to listen to the audio recording and write (or type) everything said by the client and any conversation partners.

You should label who is speaking (e.g., P: _____ [Partner], C: _____ [Child], Cl: _____ [Clinician]). The initial(s) you assign to each person should be something easily recognized. Start a new line each time a new person speaks. Number the utterances and place a / at the end of each utterance. IPA symbols can be used to transcribe errors; however, for the sake of time, use IPA symbols only with errors in production rather than transcribing the entire sample using IPA symbols (Shipley & McAfee, 2009). Unintelligible utterances can be marked with a – (e.g., I like to play –). Be sure to record everything said, including repeated words and phrases (e.g., "because he [he] doesn't like me"), filler (e.g., "the girl likes [um] strawberry ice cream with [uh] sprinkles"), and revisions ("the cat has [had] a string on her tail"; Price et al., 2010). Listen carefully. Remember that our minds are specifically tuned to make sense of what we hear. As such, although a word may make sense, you need to write down what was produced. For example, in the sentence, "I go to bed," you may understand in the context of the conversation that the client meant that he "went" to bed. You should still record "I go to bed," though, because this is exactly what was said. Similarly, if a client produced a distorted production of the /r/ in the word *rabbit*, even though you may have understood the word to be rabbit despite this distortion, you would note the distorted production. In fact, that is a perfect example of an opportunity to use IPA symbols so that you can note exactly what the client said.

Once you have transcribed the sample accurately, the next step is to perform an analysis of the content. Your supervising SLP will instruct you on what type of analysis to perform. As discussed, there are many ways that a speech and language sample can be used, spanning the areas of phonology, morphology, syntax, semantics, and pragmatics. Although an extensive review of these methods is beyond the scope of this textbook, calculating MLU as a measure of morphological complexity and calculating lexical diversity using TTR are discussed in the sections that follow, as these are fairly common analyses.

Lastly, as technology advances, computer-aided language sample analysis (CLSA) is also available and may be used by your supervising SLP. With CLSA, information from a client's language sample is entered into specialized software designed to perform a wide variety of in-depth analyses. The use of CLSA requires specialized training. For readers interested in learning more about it, Price et al. (2010) provide a helpful tutorial on the topic of CLSA in clinical practice.

Mean Length of Utterance (MLU). MLU is the average number of morphemes or words produced per utterance (Shipley & McAfee, 2009). A morpheme is "a minimal meaningful unit of language" (Paul et al., 2007, p. 121). For example, in the sentence, "The cats are brown," there are five morphemes, as follows:

1. the
2. cat
3. -s (to denote the meaning of more than one)
4. are
5. brown

To calculate the MLU based on morphemes (MLUm), you first count the total number of morphemes (total morphemes) and then divide by the total number of utterances (total utterances). For example:

$$200 \text{ morphemes (total morphemes)} /$$
$$43 \text{ utterances (total utterances)}$$
$$= 4.6 \text{ MLUm}$$

SLPs use MLU as a general indicator of language development, which corresponds to a child's chronological age in young children up to approximately 6 years of age (Brown, 1973; Klee et al., 1989; Miller & Chapman, 1981). SLPAs do not interpret MLUs, but as a general reference, Appendix 8–A contains information about MLUs relative to chronological age and the age of acquisition of common morphological features. Box 8–5 contains additional recommendations for counting morphemes.

Some SLPs prefer to calculate MLU using words (MLUw). In this case, you count the total number of words (total words) and divide by the total number of utterances (total utterances), as follows:

$$115 \text{ words (total words)} / 41 \text{ utterances}$$
$$\text{(total utterances)} = 2.8 \text{ MLUw}$$

Type Token Ratio (TTR). TTR, developed by Johnson (1944), is a ratio of the different words (or types) compared with the total words produced (or tokens). SLPs use this information to assess the semantic aspects of a speech and language sample

---

Box 8–5. Recommendations for Counting Morphemes
(Lund & Duchan, 1993; Paul et al., 2007)

1. Only use intelligible utterances.
2. Count the morphemes in the first 50 consecutive utterances.
3. Do not count
   a. Imitations
   b. Rote passages, such as nursery rhymes and songs that have been memorized
   c. Noises (unless they are integrated into meaningful verbal utterances)
   d. Utterances identical to those already said by the client; in this case, the utterance is counted only on its first occurrence and not on subsequent attempts.
   e. Counting or other sequences of enumeration (e.g., "blue, green, yellow, red, purple")
   f. Fillers (e.g., um, well, oh)
4. Count each of the following as one morpheme:
   a. Compound words (e.g., birthday, somebody)
   b. Proper names (e.g., Mickey Mouse)
   c. Ritualized reduplication (e.g., choo-choo, night-night)
   d. Diminutive forms (e.g., doggie, daddy)
   e. Catenatives (e.g., gonna, wanna)
   f. Auxiliary verbs (contracted and noncontracted forms; e.g., he is and he's)
   g. Inflections (e.g., possessives, plural s, regular past –ed)

---

from children (Hess et al., 1989; Owen & Leonard, 2002). In the sentence, "Me go go go dance," there are three types (*me, go, dance*), whereas in the sentence, "I like to go dancing," there are five types (*I, like, to, go, dancing*). Both sentences have the same number of tokens (five). TTRs closer to one represent a sample with a greater number of word types. To calculate TTR, count the total number of different words (types) and divide by the total number of words (tokens). For example:

32 different words (types)/
65 total words (tokens) = .49 TTR

EFFICIENCY/ACCURACY IN DATA COLLECTION

Each of the above sections about data collection stressed the importance of accuracy in data collection and what you can do to ensure you understand and can implement data collection that meets the needs of your supervising SLP. One additional factor, which applies to all types of data collection, is efficiency—that is, your ability to quickly (and accurately) collect data under a variety of circumstances. Hopefully, as you read about these techniques, they will make sense to you and seem manageable. However, remember that you will be collecting data while you are implementing treatment and performing other tasks. In other words, you will need to multitask! You may also be collecting data in a variety of positions and locations and, in some cases, as discussed in Chapter 12, on more than one client at a time. Having an efficient data collection system is especially important when working within the group setting. Depending on the client, you may have only a small window of time between tasks to record data. In addition, your data collection may be a distraction or negatively affect your client's performance in some cases. With time, you will refine your methods for collecting data and you improve, but this is an area that will always benefit from refinement. Data collection is not easy, but as the introduction to this chapter suggests, it is critical. The following are tips for enhancing the efficiency of data collection, regardless of the situation:

1. *Plan in advance:* Review what is needed in advance. Make sure you have a data collection sheet ready in advance of data collection. Fill in any details you can in advance, including things like the client's name, date, and goals.
2. *Make notes or cheat sheets:* If you are using different symbols or notations to represent levels of cues (e.g., S = semantic cue, P = phoneme cue), record these symbols either at the top of your data collection sheet or in a location you can easily reference. Similarly, if you are addressing more than one goal or objective, or collecting different types of data, make a note or two in a convenient location to remind you of these important details.

3. *Do not wait to summarize:* As much as possible, summarize your data and make important notes right after the session ends.
4. *Be discrete:* Use symbols or coded scoring, such as *O/Xs* or *A/B* for correct/ incorrect instead of +/–; this may be needed for some clients, particularly if you are working with a client who may be distracted by your data collection or concerned about errors in performance. Chapter 10 discusses additional techniques for positioning your data collection sheets so that they are accessible to you but out of view of your clients.
5. *Get creative:* Sometimes it is necessary to get creative with where you place your score sheet and what type of data collection sheet you use. For example, while engaging in a play activity on the floor with a group of preschoolers, it is not convenient to have a full sheet of paper located on a table in the room. Instead, try making tally marks or notes on a sticky note placed in a strategic location among the clients and the toys. It can also be helpful to create data collection sheets that are formatted to be used with a specific type of goal. For example, if you know you will be targeting articulation, create a data collection sheet specifically for articulation. This data sheet may include fields such as target sound, position within a word (e.g., initial, medial, or final), and communication level (e.g., isolation, syllable, word, phrases, sentences or conversations). Figure 8–11 is an example of a customized articulation data collection sheet to make your articulation data collection more efficient. As mentioned above, you may be working with individual clients or in a group setting. If individual data

sheets become overwhelming when working with a group, explore and experiment with group data collection sheets. This can help reduce the amount of paper you need to manage during the session. Figure 8–12 is an

STUDENT:	Ryan S.		
GOAL(S):	Ryan will correctly articulate /s/ in all positions of single words with 80% accuracy given minimal prompting (1-2 prompts) during structured activities within the speech/language therapy setting as measured by clinician data.		

Date	Sound	Position	Level	Data										%	Comments
2/22/22	/s/	(I) M F	Words	-	p	+	+	-	p	-	+	p	-	60%	needed prompts for placement
		I M F													
		I M F													
		I M F													

Figure 8–11. Sample Articulation Data Collection Sheet.

Group Artic Data Collection

Ryan S.	Date	Sound	Positions	Level	Data										%
Ryan will correctly articulate /s/ in all positions of single words with 80% accuracy given minimal prompting.	1/20/22	/s/	I M (F)	syllables	-	-	+	+	p	-	-	p	+	p	60%
			I M F												
			I M F												
			I M F												
			I M F												
			I M F												
			I M F												
			I M F												
			I M F												

Jeff P.	Date	Sound	Positions	Level	Data										%
Jeff will correctly articulate /r/ in all positions of single words with 80% accuracy given minimal prompting.	1/20/22	/r/	(I) M F	words	-	p	+	+	+	p	+	-	-	+	70%
			I M F												
			I M F												
			I M F												
			I M F												
			I M F												
			I M F												
			I M F												
			I M F												

Melissa C.	Date	Sound	Positions	Level	Data										%
Melissa will correctly articulate /s/ in all positions of phrases with 80% accuracy given minimal prompting.	1/20/22	/s/	I (M) F	phrases	p	p	-	-	+	+	-	p	-	-	50%
			I M F												
			I M F												
			I M F												
			I M F												
			I M F												
			I M F												
			I M F												
			I M F												

Figure 8–12. Sample Group Articulation Data Collection Sheet.

example of a group data sheet that can be used for an articulation group. Each client will be different, but think creatively about the circumstances and ways that you can improve efficiency with alternative solutions.

6. *Employ continuous quality improvement:* Data collection is not easy. It takes time and experience to develop skills. Take every opportunity to learn from your mistakes and improve your skills. Talk to your supervising SLP about the quality of your data collection. If data collection is an area to improve, use the techniques suggested in Chapter 4 for self-assessment to evaluate your skills and find ways to improve.

REFERENCES

American Speech-Language-Hearing Association (ASHA). (2022). *Speech-language pathology assistant scope of practice* [Scope of practice]. http://www.asha.org/policy

Boswell, S. (2005, September 27). Show me the data: Finding the evidence for school-based clinical decision making. *ASHA Leader.* https://doi.org/10.1044/leader.SCM2.10132005.26

Brown, R. (1973). *A first language.* Harvard University Press.

Bunta, F., Ingram, K., & Ingram, D. (2003). Bridging the digital divide: Aspects of computerized data collection and analysis for language professionals. *Clinical Linguistics and Phonetics, 17*(3), 217–240. https://doi.org/10.1080/0269920031000094926

Costanza-Smith, A. (2010). The clinical utility of language samples. *Perspectives on Language Learning and Education, 17*(1), 9–15. https://doi.org/10.1044/lle17.1.9

Epstein, L. (2008). Clinical therapy data as learning process: The first year of clinical training and beyond. *Topic in Language Disorders, 28*(3), 274–285.

Haynes, W. O., & Pindzola, R. H. (1998). *Diagnosis and evaluation in speech pathology* (5th ed.). Allyn & Bacon.

Hess, C. W., Haug, H. T., & Landry, R. G. (1989). The reliability of type-token ratios for the oral language of school-age children. *Journal of Speech and Hearing Research, 32*(3), 536–540. https://doi.org/10.1044/jshr.3203.536

Johnson, W. (1944). A program of research: Studies in language behavior. *Psychological Monographs, 56*(2), 1–15.

Jones, M., Onslow, M., Packman, A., & Gebski, V. (2006). Guidelines for statistical analysis of percentage of syllables stuttered data. *Journal of Speech, Language, and Hearing Research, 49*(4), 867–878. https://doi.org/10.1044/1092-4388(2006/062)

Kawulich, B. B. (2005). Participant observation as a data collection method. *Forum: Qualitative Social Research, 6*(2). https://doi.org/10.17169/fqs-6.2.466

Kennedy, M. (2007).Principles of Assessment. In R. Paul & P. Cascella (Eds.), *Introduction to clinical methods in communication disorders* (pp. 39–84). Paul H. Brookes.

Klee, T., Schaffer, M., May, S., Membrino, I., & Mougey, K. (1989). A comparison of the age MLU relation in normal and specifically language-impaired preschool children. *Journal of Speech and Hearing Disorders, 54*(2), 226–233. https://doi.org/10.1044/jshd.5402.226

Lemoncello, R., & Fanning, J. L. (2011, November). *Practice-based evidence: Strategies for generating your own evidence.* Paper presented at the 2011 ASHA Convention, San Diego, CA.

Lund, N. J., & Duchan, J. F. (1993). *Assessing children's language in naturalistic contexts* (3rd ed.). Prentice-Hall.

Merriam-Webster. (2003). *Merriam-Webster's collegiate dictionary* (11th ed.).

Miller, J., & Chapman, R. (1981). The relation between age and mean length of utterance in morphemes. *Journal of Speech and Hearing Research, 24*(2), 154–161. https://doi.org/10.1044/jshr.2402.154

Moore, S. M., & Pearson, L. (2003). *Competencies and strategies for speech-language pathology assistants.* Thomson Delmar Learning.

Mowrer, D. E. (1982). *Methods of modifying speech behaviors: Learning theory in speech pathology.* Waveland.

Owen, A. J., & Leonard, L. B. (2002). Lexical diversity in the spontaneous speech of children with specific language impairment: Application of D. *Journal of Speech, Language and Hearing Research, 45*(5), 927–937. https://doi.org/10.1044/1092-4388(2002/075)

Owens, R. E., Jr. (2004). *Language disorders: A functional approach to assessment and intervention* (4th ed.). Allyn & Bacon.

Paul, R., Tentnowski, J., & Reuler, E. (2007). Communication sampling procedures. In R. Paul & P. Cascella (Eds.), *Introduction to clinical methods in communication disorders* (pp. 111–156). Paul H. Brookes.

Price, L. H., Hendricks, S., & Cook, C. (2010). Incorporating computer-aided language sample analysis into clinical practice. *Language, Speech, and Hearing Services in Schools, 41*(2), 206–222. https://doi.org/10.1044/0161-1461(2009/08-0054)

Rao, P. R. (2011, June 7). From the president: Evidence-based practice: The coin of the realm in CSD. *ASHA Leader.* https://doi.org/10.1044/leader.FTP.16072011.7

Roth, F., & Paul, R. (2007). Communication intervention. In R. Paul & P. Cascella (Eds.), *Introduction to clinical methods in communication disorders* (pp. 1–18). Paul H. Brookes.

Roth, F. R., & Worthington, C. K. (2001). *Treatment resource manual for speech-language pathology.* Delmar.

Shipley, K. G., & McAfee, J. G. (2009). *Assessment in speech-language pathology: A resource manual.* Delmar Cengage Learning.

Taylor-Powell, E., & Steele, S. (n.d.). Collecting evaluation data: Direct observation. *Program Development and Evaluation: University of Washington, Cooperative Learning.* http://learningstore.uwex.edu/assets/pdfs/G3658-5.PDF

CHAPTER ENDNOTES

1. American Speech-Language-Hearing Association. (2022). *Speech-language pathology assistant scope of practice.* Available from http://www.asha.org/policy. © Copyright 2022 American Speech-Language-Hearing Association. All rights reserved. Reprinted with permission.

2. Adapted from Shipley and McAfee (2009).

3. Adapted from Shipley and McAfee (2009, pp. 161–162).

4. Adapted from Shipley and McAfee (2009, p. 163).

APPENDIX 8–A
Mean Length of Utterance (MLU) and Age Equivalent

MLU	Age Equivalent (Within 1 Month)
1.31	18 months
1.62	21 months
1.92	24 months
2.54	30 months
2.85	33 months
3.16	36 months
3.47	39 months
3.78	42 months
4.09	45 months
4.40	48 months
4.71	51 months
5.02	54 months
5.32	57 months
5.63	60 months

Source: Miller, 1981, as cited in Williamson, 2009.

APPENDIX 8–B
Common Morphological Features and Age of Mastery

Rank	Morphological Feature	Example	Age of Mastery (months)
1	present progressive -ing	daddy sing<u>ing</u>, mummy play<u>ing</u>	19–28
2	in	key <u>in</u> cup, ball <u>in</u> box	27–30
3	on	ball <u>on</u> bed, cup <u>on</u> table	27–33
4	regular plural -s	two cat<u>s</u>, three dog<u>s</u>	27–33
5	irregular past tense	mummy <u>fell</u>, daddy <u>went</u>	25–46
6	possessive -'s	mummy<u>'s</u> hat, daddy<u>'s</u> car	26–40
7	uncontractible copula	she <u>is</u> (response to who is happy?)	28–46
8	articles	mummy got <u>a</u> dog, <u>the</u> ball	28–46
9	regular past tense -ed	daddy walk<u>ed</u>, a car crash<u>ed</u>	26–48
10	regular third person -s	mummy walk<u>s</u>, daddy play<u>s</u>	28–50
11	irregular third person	mummy <u>does</u>, daddy <u>has</u> a ball	28–50
12	uncontractible auxiliary	she <u>is</u> (response to *who is coming?*)	29–48
13	contractible copula	he<u>'s</u> happy (cf. *he is happy*)	29–49
14	contractible auxiliary	mummy<u>'s</u> playing (cf. *mummy is playing*)	30–50

Source: Brown, 1973; Miller, 1981, as cited in Williamson, 2009.

CHAPTER 9

Note Writing

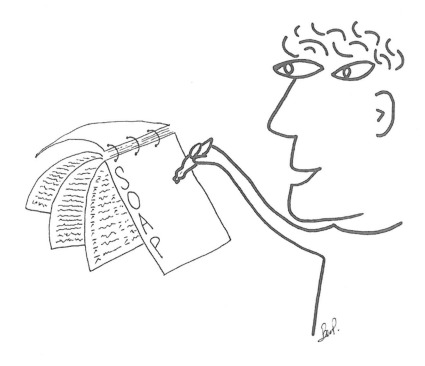

*Observe, record, tabulate, communicate. Use your five
senses. Learn to see, learn to hear, learn to feel, learn to smell,
and know that by practice alone you can become expert.*

—William Osler
(one of the fathers of modern medicine)

As mentioned in Chapter 1, speech-language pathology assistants (SLPAs) may be asked to assist their supervising speech-language pathologist (SLP) in providing treatment or screening and data collection for individuals with communication disorders (American Speech-Language-Hearing Association [ASHA],

2022). In some cases, this may be with your supervisor present. In other cases, you may provide these services when your supervising SLP is not physically present in the room but has given you specific instructions. In either case, as Chapters 7 and 8 suggest, it is critical that you perform these tasks as instructed and that you accurately record important aspects of the client's performance. It is equally important that you effectively summarize and consolidate this information, both as formal documentation of the services you provided and as a means of conveying important information to other professionals, including your supervisor. Writing a clinical note is often used for this purpose. The format of these notes can vary across settings and with the mechanism(s) for reimbursement of services (ASHA, n.d.-a, n.d.-b; Sutherland Cornett, 2006). In addition, as an SLPA, how often you write a note for a client will be directed by your supervisor. Depending on the setting, notes are written after every encounter with the client, on a weekly basis, or as needed, given the specific type of interaction.

A common format in the field of speech-language pathology for writing notes is a *SOAP note* (Moon-Meyer, 2004; Roth & Worthington, 2001; Shipley & McAfee, 2009). SOAP is an acronym for the following: subjective (S), objective (O), assessment (A), and plan (P) (Shipley & McAfee, 2009). SOAP notes are often used in medical settings (Roth & Worthington, 2001) but can be modified in form and content to fit the needs of an educational setting. Understanding the SOAP format and how to convey information effectively in a note in your setting is an important skill for an SLPA. However, as will be discussed, specific aspects of the SOAP note format are not consistently applicable to an SLPA's role or scope of services. The sections that follow discuss each aspect of a SOAP note from the perspective of an SLPA. The companion website of this textbook contains a blank version of an SLPA-applicable SOAP note for your use.

SUBJECTIVE (S)

The subjective (S) portion of a SOAP note contains "non-measurable and historical information" important for understanding the client's performance (Shipley & McAfee, 2009, p. 138). This portion of the note provides context to help the reader interpret what will follow in the remaining portions of the note. The dictionary defines subjective as "arising out of or identified by means of one's perception" (Merriam-Webster, 2003). The definition fits well, as the subjective portion of a SOAP note contains your opinions, observations, and information reported to you by others.

Key areas to include in the subjective section of a SOAP note (Moon-Meyer, 2004; Roth & Worthington, 2001; Shipley & McAfee, 2009) and corresponding examples are as follows:

Your observations about the client's mood:

- The client smiled and laughed frequently throughout the session.
- The patient was tearful today.
- Melissa greeted the clinician in the waiting area with a hug and was eager to begin the session.

Statements about clients' behavior or their current status, from the perspective of the client, family member(s), or others involved in the client's care (e.g., teachers, nurses, aides):

- Johnny's mother indicated that he has been remembering to close his mouth while breathing.
- The client indicated that he was successful with his homework

and felt it helped him recall the relaxation techniques, which he used during his classroom science fair presentation.

■ The patient's wife indicated that the patient is talking more at home and is regaining movement of his right arm.

■ Mrs. Smith reported that Susan experienced three seizures this week, with one resulting in admittance to the emergency room.

A description of the client's level of cooperation and participation:

■ Rebecca appeared reluctant to engage with her peers during the group reading activity, often averting her eyes or looking away when asked questions by her peers.

■ The client was cooperative and participated fully with all tasks.

■ The client refused to participate in the oral reading task.

■ Steven appeared distracted by the noise from the playground during screening. He frequently turned to look at the window and asked several times to be excused from the session.

A description of any factors in the environment, or other relevant conditions, that may have influenced the client's performance:

■ Due to a fire drill, screening was interrupted for 10 minutes while the SLPA and the client evacuated the building. Screening resumed after the drill.

■ The client's wife, Susan, was present during treatment.

■ Henry arrived 15 minutes late for the session, due to an assembly during the home period.

In this section of the note, you should describe what you see and not simply label the behavior. For example, if the client appeared happy to you, rather than writing, "Johnny was happy," describe the behaviors that you think lead you to that opinion, such as, "Johnny smiled and laughed frequently during the session." When you are reporting information shared with you, be sure to identify the source of this information in your statement. For example, instead of writing, "The patient was tired as he did not sleep well last night," report instead, "The nurse on duty indicated that the patient did not sleep well last night," or "The patient reported that he felt tired from not sleeping well the night before." Remember, too, that your verb choice in this section and the objective (O) section (below) should be past tense, as you are describing something that already occurred.

Lastly, note that in the examples provided, the client is sometimes referred to by first name and other times by *the client* or *the patient*. This will apply to all other sections of the note as well and will depend on the setting. In most hospital and clinical settings, the client's name is not used within the body of the medical records, in SOAP notes, or in other reports. As such, in those settings, *the client* or *the patient* is the preferred term. In most educational settings, however, the client is referred to by first name. You should check with your supervising SLP to confirm which form is appropriate for your setting.

OBJECTIVE (O)

The objective (O) section of the SOAP note contains facts and measurable findings about the session (Moon-Meyer, 2004; Roth & Worthington, 2001; Shipley & McAfee, 2009). Typically, data collected during the session (see Chapter 8) are reported in this section. As the definition of objective suggests, this section contains observable and measurable information about the client's performance during that session (in contrast to subjective opinions or reports from others).

This section typically begins with a brief summary of what occurred during the session. If screening was performed, state the name of the screener used or describe the screening methods. Describe any other forms of data collected as instructed by your supervising SLP. If this was a treatment session, state the goal(s) or objective(s) targeted during that session. Follow the summary with the actual data collected. Examples from objective (O) sections of SOAP notes are as follows:

- Johnny's augmentative and alternative communication (AAC) goals were targeted today. For Objective 3 (requesting an activity using eye gaze), Johnny requested Bingo and Candy Land using eye gaze when the SLPA presented a field of two icon choices. For Objective 5 (switch activation), Johnny answered 10 yes/no questions accurately using his yes/no voice output device.
- Objective 1a (word opposites): 15 of 20 (75%) using picture cards.

- Fluency count was performed during morning story time in David's classroom (Figure 9–1).
- Goal: The client will correctly produce the /r/ phoneme in all positions of a word with 100% accuracy. Performance: The client was 75% accurate for this task during a Go Fish activity requiring the client to request cards containing one- and two-syllable words with /r/ in the initial, medial, and final position of the word.
- Prepositions (Objective 5) (Figure 9–2).

In some of the examples provided, the information is very brief, and in others, more detail is provided. In some instances, the information is provided in text format, and in others, tables and charts are used. The level of detail needed, as well as the actual format of this section, varies from setting to setting and depends on your supervisor's needs and her or his instructions. In some settings, the content of a SOAP note is incorporated within the actual data collection sheets used to record client performance (Appendix 9–A). In that case, an additional SOAP note may not be required. The companion website of this textbook contains a blank version of the form for your use. In preparation

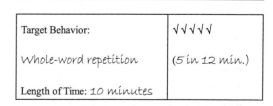

Target Behavior:	√ √ √ √ √
Whole-word repetition	(5 in 12 min.)
Length of Time: 10 minutes	

Figure 9–1. Sample frequency count table for objective (O) section of a SOAP note.

No Assistance	Gestural Cue	Sound Cue	Modeled Production	Preposition
–	–	–	–	Over
–	–	–	–	Under
–	+			In
–	+			On
–	–	–	–	Over
+				In
–	–	–	+	Under
–	+			In
–	–	+		On
–	–	–	+	Under
TOTALS: 1/10 (10%)	3/10 (30%)	1/10 (10%)	2/10 (20%)	

Figure 9–2. Sample cue record table for objective (O) section of a SOAP note.

for writing a SOAP note, you should review typical notes in your setting and discuss with your supervisor the depth, format, and type of information she or he needs in each section.

Note that in some of the examples provided, the third-person personal pronoun is used to describe the SLPA's actions (e.g., "when the SLPA presented a field of two icons to choose from" in the first example). Third-person pronoun use is common in professional writing in the field of speech-language pathology and may be the preferred form in your setting. If that is the case, instead of writing, "I gave the client paragraphs to read," which uses a first-person pronoun (I), you would reword the note and refer to yourself as the SLPA, as in "The SLPA gave the client paragraphs to read." You should model your style of writing to match acceptable standards for your setting.

ANALYZE (AZ)

This section of the SOAP note and the one that follows (P) require modification for SLPA use as they differ substantively from the forms suggested for use by SLPs. In most references about SOAP notes, the "A" portion of the note refers to "assessment" (Moon-Meyer, 2004; Roth & Worthington, 2001; Shipley & McAfee, 2009). As discussed in Chapters 1 and 2, SLPAs are not to engage in assessment for the purpose of diagnosing a disability or to write, develop, or modify a patient's (or client's) plan of care in any way (ASHA, 2022, Responsibilities Outside the Scope of Practice for Speech-Language Pathology Assistants). As such, changes in content and wording of this section are required to align with the duties and responsibilities of an SLPA. Revision of this section to reference analyze (Az) brings it in line with the scope and responsibilities of an SLPA. It is appropriate and within the scope of an SLPA to analyze the session itself given (1) an objective summary of the client's current performance compared with a previous session(s) (statement of performance) and/or (2) a description of whether the prescribed task, stimulus, or reinforcement was easy or difficult to implement during that session (description, task, stimulus, reinforcement).

In terms of a statement of performance, Table 9–1 contains a comparison of an "A" (assessment) that an SLP may write regarding the client's performance versus an "Az" (analysis), appropriate for an SLPA to write.

As you can see in the table, for the SLPA Az section, there is no interpretation of information regarding progress made toward achieving goals or in relation to the client's current status. Appropriate SLPA format in this section limits the discussion to a summary of objective information from today's session as it relates to a previous session(s).

Also, it is appropriate for the SLPA to comment in the Az section on the tasks, materials, and reinforcement that were easy or difficult to implement (description of task, stimulus, reinforcement).

Table 9–1. Assessment Versus Analyze (Statement of Performance)

Assessment (A) Appropriate for an SLP	Analyze (Az) Appropriate for an SLPA
Susan has made good progress in achieving Goal 2 (Objective 5). Her production for /s/ initial sounds has increased in accuracy from initial sessions, with some generalization noted for nontarget positions (e.g., /s/ final production). She is stimulable for /s/ final position sounds and was noted on one occasion during today's session to produce an /s/ initial word accurately in a conversational context.	Susan's performance on Goal 2 (Objective 5—/s/ in initial position of words) was 70%. During the previous session, her performance was 50% on this same objective.
The client remains with significant aphasia and significant difficulty verbally naming pictured items; however, he has improved in his use of multiple modalities, such as gestures, drawing, and writing. His performance on Objective 3 (use of gestures) indicates an increase in performance from the previous sessions.	This session, the client's scores on Objective 3 (use of gestures) increased from a score of 1 of 10 during last week's session to a score of 5 of 10 during today's session.

This may be helpful to your supervising SLP in planning future sessions or understanding the objective data in more detail. Table 9–2 shows a comparison of a description of tasks, stimuli, or reinforcement A (assessment) that an SLP may write versus an Az (analysis), appropriate for an SLPA for this type of information.

Note that for each of the examples in Table 9–2, the information under Az for an SLPA is limited to a description of some aspect of the task itself, the stimulus or materials used, or the reinforcement. It does not extend to interpreting what this information means or generalizing what was observed to a statement about the client's overall performance or status. That is limited to the scope of an SLP (ASHA, 2022).

MY PLAN (PM)

The final section of a SOAP note is indicated by the letter "P." Similar to the

"A" portion of a SOAP note, this section requires modification compared with the version that would be written by an SLP. Traditional textbooks on the topic of SOAPs, written for SLPs, state that the "P" portion of a SOAP note consists of the plan for the future course of treatment (Moon-Meyer, 2004; Paul & Cascella, 2007; Roth & Worthington, 2001; Shipley & McAfee, 2009). As was mentioned above, developing, modifying, or altering a client's plan of care from that specifically prescribed by an SLP is not within the scope of an SLPA (ASHA, 2022). As such, discussing the future course of treatment for a client in the *P* section of a note is outside the scope of practice for an SLPA. A reasonable modification, however, would be to include a plan of action specific to the needs of the SLPA, using *Pm*, to indicate *my* plan (as an SLPA).

An excellent use of the Pm section of an SLPA note is to relay any specific concerns or requests conveyed to you by the client, family members, or other team members

Table 9–2. Assessment Versus Analyze (Description of Task, Stimulus, Reinforcement)

Assessment (A) Appropriate for an SLP	Analyze (Az) Appropriate for an SLPA
The client continues to need cues to employ communication strategies during a group context and may benefit from a written reminder or one-on-one training in the scripted language needed to initiate questions or to ask for clarification/assistance in group contexts.	During the barrier communication task (Objective 5), the client needed several reminders (5) to *describe* the picture to fellow group members and to ask group members for questions if he did not understand their descriptions. (*Task*)
Jane's participation during speech sessions has increased with the use of personally relevant stimuli and given treatment activities using social structure and reinforcement. She may also benefit from treatment during small group sessions with peers.	Jane appeared to enjoy using the Sponge Bob cartoons to elicit the /s/ sound. She requested additional turns in making sentences with these cards. (*Stimulus*)
Steven benefits from the use of token reinforcement to increase on-task behaviors during speech sessions. This may be an area to discuss with his classroom teacher for increasing on-task participation during classroom activities as well.	Steven began following directions and participating more fully when tokens were provided for on-task behaviors. (*Reinforcement*)

involved in the client's case. Counseling or the provision of "providing interpretative information to the student, patient, client, family, or others regarding the student's, patient's, or client's status or service" is outside the scope of duties of an SLPA (ASHA, 2022, Responsibilities Outside the Scope of an SLPA, para. 2). For example, if a client or family member expresses a concern or request for information about services, SLPAs should first inform the client or family member that they will relay this information directly to their supervising SLP. In most cases, this information should be given verbally, and immediately, to your supervising SLP. The Pm portion of your note is a place to document this information, as in the following examples:

- The client requested additional information about options for additional days of service.
- Alice's mothers asked to speak with the supervising SLP about Alice's performance in the classroom and impending individualized educational plan (IEP) meeting.
- Stephen's teacher (Mr. Collings) requested information about the client's treatment goals and progress.
- The client indicated he is concerned that his speech is not improving with treatment. He indicated that he fears he will not improve further.
- Mrs. Smith asked about developmental milestones and if Susan's language and speech have met them.

You should also check with your supervising SLP to confirm her or his preference as to the location of this information. Some supervisors may prefer this information go in the S section of the note. As in the S section, when you are reporting information shared with you, be sure to identify the source of in your statement. Be sure to also indicate how you responded to the request or concern, such as, "The SLPA indicated she would ask her supervising SLP to contact the client's mother immediately with these details," or "The SLPA informed the client that this information was not within her scope of duties to discuss but that she would convey his concerns directly to her supervisor," or "The SLPA provided Mr. Collings with the SLP's direct phone number and indicated that she would relay this request directly to her as well."

The Pm section is also used to request additional information, assistance, or resources from your supervising SLP. In this respect, statements in the Pm section would start with, "Plan to discuss with supervisor . . . " or like the following examples:

- Plan to discuss with supervisor Johnny's distraction during treatment tasks and ways to increase his participation during group activities.
- Plan to discuss with supervisor how the client's AAC system should be used during reading activities.
- Plan to clarify what would be classified as a whole-word repetition during Stephen's conversational speech.
- Plan to request additional information about facilitating techniques referenced in Scott's treatment plan.

■ Plan to review with the supervisor current data collection methods to ensure accuracy in recording information requested.

Lastly, the Pm section of an SLPA note can be used to detail any specific preparation you need before the next session with this client, such as the following:

■ Plan to place game choices under the table before beginning a session so they are not a source of distraction during the group treatment session.
■ Plan to presort stimulus cards into three piles (sounds, words, phrases) to facilitate easy access while targeting Objective 5.
■ Plan to code data collection sheet ahead of time with required scoring parameters to make data collection more efficient and effective during the treatment session.
■ Plan to use a timer to ensure treatment activities end with enough time to review assigned homework activities.
■ Plan to start next treatment with a review of good listening rules.

These statements would most likely begin with "Plan to. . . . " They may be preparations you have already identified as applicable to a future session. If not, you can list them as an area to discuss with your supervising SLP. However, consistent with an SLPA scope of practice, any plan of action outlined by an SLPA must not be related to the client's course of treatment, such as, "Plan to modify short-term Goal 5," or "Plan to discharge Goal 3 due to achievement," or "Plan to

modify literacy objective to include sound letter correspondence training." Each of those statements is the specific domain of the supervising SLP (ASHA, 2022).

As discussed in Chapter 4, the use of a reflection journal to document your performance during a clinical session may be a good source of information to include in the Pm section of an SLPA note. The companion website of this textbook has a blank reflection journal sheet for your use and Box 9–1 shows the sample reflection journal entry provided in Chapter 4. The bolded sections are examples of items that may carry over into a Pm note for a particular session, such as the following:

■ Plan to discuss with supervisor methods for effective data collection.
■ Plan to rearrange position of table in treatment room, facing away from the window to ensure students are not distracted during treatment.
■ Plan to change instruction and procedures for group activity, including preselecting order of activities and assigning turns for who goes first in each activity.

TIPS FOR EFFECTIVE NOTE WRITING

Appendix 9–B has sample SLPA notes written following the format described above. Note that they vary in length and complexity, but all roughly follow an S, O, Az, Pm format. It is valuable to review examples of notes in your setting to ensure your notes are consistent with setting-specific expectations. Keep in mind that many of the tips on professional writing discussed in Chapter 4 also apply to writing a clinical note. Specific to clinical notes, Figure 9–3 contains a checklist of tips to make your note writing effective in any setting. This information is also available in a checklist on the companion website of this chapter.

Box 9–1. Reflection Journal Entry

Date: *2/14/2018*
Task: *10:00 a.m. Small Group Session (JL, AS, TM)*

Successes:
JL and AS participated fully and had high levels of accuracy for target sounds. The session ended on time. The students appeared to enjoy the session and were eager to begin. I felt relaxed and was able to stay focused on each student's targets during the session.

Difficulties:
TM was distracted during the session. He left the table several times to look out the window. I wasn't sure how to shape this behavior, other than reminding him that he needed to participate. I had difficulty keeping track of errors and the number and type of cues I gave for sound production. When I listened to the audio recording of the session, I provided many more models than I had noted on my data sheet. I also said "okay" twice when JL's target sound was not correct. The time spent on preparing for the session's activities took too long (10 minutes). The students argued about which activity to do first and who would start in each activity.

Areas to Improve:
1. *Increase structure of the session at the onset.* **Make sure to briefly instruct the students in the rules of the activity. Don't allow them to choose the order of the activities. Rotate who goes first per session or have them draw from a deck of cards and whoever gets the highest card goes first.**
2. *Improve data collection methods. Collect additional examples of data collection sheets used for group sessions.* **Check with supervisor about her methods for effectively and quickly noting both errors and cues in group settings.** *Possibly rearrange data collection sheet in advance with a column to place an X under each type of cue. Place a sticky note reminder on my data collection sheet for next time, reminding me not to say "okay." Listen to the audio recording from next week's session and record the number of "okays."*
3. *Close the blinds in the room or* **move the table so the students aren't distracted by the things happening outside the window.**

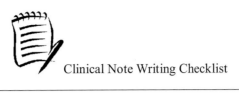 Clinical Note Writing Checklist

_____ Note is dated.

_____ Note is free of spelling errors.

_____ Note is free of grammatical errors.

_____ Note is free of any interpretation, assessment, or recommendation about a specific course of treatment.

_____ Note is free of slang and colloquialism.

_____ Note uses standard forms of medical abbreviation and phonetic notation.

_____ As applicable, third person personal pronoun is used to describe your actions (e.g., "The SLPA . . . ").

_____ Setting specific terms are used to reference the client (e.g., referring to the client by his first name, full name, or by using the terms "the client" or "the patient").

_____ Information conveyed to you by others is referenced as such (e.g., The client's family reports . . . , Susan stated . . . , etc.).

_____ Note uses language that describes a behavior observed and does not label or diagnosis the behavior.

_____ Note contains a description of what was done.

_____ Note states specific treatment goals and objective targeted.

_____ Note states specific tools or procedures used.

_____ Note contains a summary of the client's performance in objective terms (e.g., percentages, frequency counts, etc.).

_____ Note uses past tense in applicable sections (typically O and S, and sometimes Az section).

_____ Note uses future tense in the Pm section.

Figure 9–3. Clinical Note Writing Checklist.

REFERENCES

American Speech-Language-Hearing Association. (n.d.-a). *Documentation in school settings: Frequently asked questions*. http://www.asha.org/SLP/Documentation-in-Schools-FAQs

American Speech-Language-Hearing Association (ASHA). (n.d.-b). *Private health plans frequently asked questions: Speech-language pathology*. http://www.asha.org/practice/reimbursement/private-plans/php_faqs_slp.htm#7

American Speech-Language-Hearing Association (ASHA). (2022). *Speech-language pathology assistant scope of practice* [Scope of practice]. http://www.asha.org/policy

Merriam-Webster. (2003). *Merriam-Webster's collegiate dictionary* (11th ed.).

Moon-Meyer, S. (2004). *Survival guide for the beginning speech-language clinician*. Pro-Ed.

Paul, R., & Cascella, P. W. (2007). *Introduction to clinical methods in communication disorders* (2nd ed.). Paul H. Brookes.

Roth, F. R., & Worthington, C. K. (2001). *Treatment resource manual for speech-language pathology*. Delmar Cengage Learning.

Shipley, K. G., & McAfee, J. G. (2009). *Assessment in speech-language pathology: A resource manual*. Delmar Cengage Learning.

Sutherland Cornett, B. (2006). Clinical documentation in speech-language pathology: Essential information for successful practice. *ASHA Leader, 11,* 8–25. https://doi.org/10.1044/leader.FTR3.11122006.8

APPENDIX 9–A
Data Sheet Incorporating SOAP Format

Student: _____ **Teacher:** _____ **Room #:** _____

Date: _____ (Length of Session: _____)

Session goal(s)	Comments (S)	Data (O) Results (A)	Plan

Date: _____ (Length of Session: _____)

Session goal(s)	Comments (S)	Data (O) Results (A)	Plan

Date: _____ (Length of Session: _____)

Session goal(s)	Comments (S)	Data (O) Results (A)	Plan

APPENDIX 9–B
Sample SOAP Notes

SOAP NOTE EXAMPLE 1

S:/ The patient's wife indicated that the patient is talking more at home and is regaining movement of his right arm. The patient greeted group members with a smile as he entered the treatment room.

O:/ Target Goal 2a (in response to word-finding difficulties during group conversation, the patient will independently use a related gesture in three of five opportunities):

Word Retrieval Difficulty	Spontaneous Gesture	Gesture With Cue (# of Cues)
1.	+	
2.	+	
3.	–	+ (cues: 2)
4.	–	–
5.	+	

Az:/ This session, the client's scores on Objective 2a (spontaneous gestures) increased from a score of 1 of 5 during last week's session to a score of 3 of 5 (criteria) during today's session. Spontaneous gestures included swinging his arms to represent "home run," a motion to his head to represent "baseball cap," and a thumbs-up letting the group know his dinner last night was good.

Pm:/ Plan to discuss with supervisor how to change procedures for initiating the group's conversation activity, including potentially preselecting the order of activities before the session or assigning who goes first in each activity. This may decrease time spent organizing these aspects of the conversation during the session. The patient's wife asked to speak with the supervising SLP about additional community resources for physical therapy. The SLPA told the wife that she would share this request with her supervising SLP. The SLPA also gave the patient's wife her supervisor's direct phone line.

SOAP NOTE EXAMPLE 2

The client smiled and laughed frequently throughout the session. He indicated he was successful with his homework and felt it helped him recall relaxation techniques, which he indicated he used during his classroom science fair presentation. Stutter-free speech in 2-minute narratives (Goal 4) was targeted during today's session. The client completed 10 of 13 2-minute narratives, with zero (0) disfluencies (76% accuracy). Using narratives about NASCAR (describing features of favorite teams) elicited ample client narration. Plan to review with supervisor current data collection methods for noting number and type of disfluency.

SOAP NOTE EXAMPLE 3

Subjective: Jill was tearful today and reluctant to leave her mom to participate in treatment. Jill's mom attended the first 15 minutes of treatment.

Objective:

Goal 1 (phonologic awareness—syllable identification)
Jill was 100% accurate (20/20) for clapping once per syllable for words read by the SLPA.

Goal 2 (phonologic awareness—identification of initial sound)
Jill was 75% accurate (15/20) for pointing to the initial sound of words read by the SLPA, given a choice of five printed letters.

Goal 3 (phonologic awareness—sound blending)
Jill was 90% accurate (18/20) for blending and producing the correct target word from syllable segments read to her by the SLPA.

Analysis: Jill appeared to enjoy the use of Sponge Bob-related vocabulary during sound blending and initial letter identification tasks. Her scores across all goals have improved from the previous session when accuracy for Goals 1, 2, and 3 were all less than 50%.

Plan: Plan to identify additional topic areas to incorporate into future sessions. Plan to discuss with supervisor the potential use of crayons and drawing during treatment tasks. During the first portion of the session, when Jill experienced difficulty separating from her mom, her om initiated a drawing activity. Jill's mom indicated that Jill enjoys drawing at home and has started writing the letters of her name within drawn images.

CHAPTER 10

Implementing Treatment

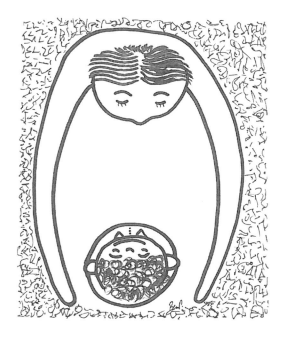

To do something, however small, to make others happier and better, is the highest ambition, the most elevating hope, which can inspire a human being.

—John Lubbock

As a speech-language pathology assistant (SLPA), you may be called upon to implement treatment services with individuals who have communicative disorders (American Speech-Language-Hearing Association [ASHA], 2022). This, of course, will be under the direct supervision and instruction of your supervising speech-language pathologist (SLP) (ASHA, 2022). Often, the thought of this is both exciting and intimidating to new SLPAs. When you see an experienced and effective SLP implementing services, it may seem effortless and easy, but in fact, it requires very careful planning, specific training, and, in many cases, years of experience.

The term *service delivery model* is used to describe "where, when, and with whom" clinical services in speech-language pathology are provided (Cascella et al., 2007, p. 259). In terms of *where* treatment is provided, this can vary greatly with the population you serve and the setting in which you are employed. Treatment may be provided within the client's environment, such as in his or her classroom, community, home, or work setting. In some settings, this is referred to as a *push-in* (Cirrin et al., 2010) or an *integrated* (Buysse & Bailey, 1993) service delivery model. This contrasts with treatment services provided outside a client's environment, such as in a clinical treatment space. This is often referred to as a *pull-out* (McGinty & Justice, 2006) or a *clinical* (Cascella et al., 2007) service delivery model.

In recent years, telepractice has emerged as a new methodology that replaces physical venues for treatment services. For SLPs, telepractice refers to "the application of telecommunications technology to the delivery of speech-language pathology and audiology professional services at a distance by linking clinician to client/patient or clinician to clinician for assessment, intervention, and/or consultation" (ASHA, n.d., Telepractice: Overview, para. 1). According to ASHA's scope-of-practice guidelines, if training, supervision, and planning are appropriate, SLPAs may provide "services via telepractice to students, patients, and clients who are selected by the supervising SLP" (ASHA, 2022, Service Delivery, para. 1). If you are asked to provide treatment services via telepractice, many of the concepts discussed in this chapter relative to treatment implementation are applicable to telepractice, but specialized training will also be required (ASHA, n.d.). As an SLPA, you may also be asked to serve as a facilitator for treatment services provided by an SLP via telepractice (ASHA, n.d., Telepractice: Key Issues, Facilitators in Telepractice for Audiology and Speech-Language Services, para. 1). In these instances, you are not the one providing treatment, but rather, you are at the client's location to assist the client while the SLP provides treatment remotely via telecommunication technology. Specialized training is also required to serve as a facilitator for telepractice. A helpful overview for school-based clinicians on this topic is available from Garcia (2013).

The *when* of the service delivery model refers to when treatment is provided and addresses the frequency and duration of services, such as the amount of time per session, the number or sessions per week or month, and the total duration of treatment. The *with whom* in service delivery refers to which professional is most appropriate to provide services. In the case of an SLPA, this may mean a decision about whether services are provided solely by an SLP or with the assistance of an SLPA.

Your supervising SLP will determine the optimum delivery model for each client, including where, when, and with whom treatment services are provided. You should familiarize yourself with each of these aspects of your client's service delivery format. How treatment is implemented is also highly variable and determined by your supervising SLP. Treatment may be provided to an individual or to a small group of individuals, using a wide array of methods and intervention models (Cascella et al., 2007). How treatment is provided can be described along a spectrum between the two extremes of clinician-directed or client-centered approaches (Roth & Paul, 2007).

Clinician-directed approaches are highly structured and directed by a clinician. The most common forms of clinician-directed approaches are either *drill* or *drill and play* (Roth & Paul, 2007, p. 164).

In drill activities, a very specific chain of events occurs. First, the clinician presents a stimulus, such a picture, a written word, a question, or some other method of eliciting a desired response from the client. This is known as the antecedent. The client then produces the required response. This is referred to as the behavior. The clinician responds to this behavior with reinforcement or corrective feedback (also known as the consequence). Generally, this same procedure of antecedent-behavior-consequence is then repeated multiple times in a very similar fashion until a required level of accuracy is obtained.

A similar procedure, called drill and play, embeds the antecedent-behavior-consequence sequence within some type of motivating activity. For children, this is typically a game or play activity. For example, a game using a small sponge and several bags labeled with a target word can elicit a response from clients (Roth & Paul, 2007). The clinician gives the client the small sponge and asks the client to throw the sponge into one of the bags to select a word to be produced (the antecedent). The client then produces the word labeled on the bag (the behavior). Then the clinician reinforces or provides feedback about the client's production (the consequence).

In client-centered approaches, clinicians give less direction. The emphasis of this approach is on eliciting a desired behavior in a natural context and then responding in a communicative way (Roth & Paul, 2007). The sequence of antecedent-behavior-consequence is modified at the levels of the antecedent and consequence. In client-centered approaches, the clinician waits for the client to initiate a behavior spontaneously instead of directly eliciting it. Generally, this is accomplished by structuring the environment to facilitate meaningful and enjoyable communication attempts in a naturally occurring context. For children, this usually means engaging in play activities that are rewarding and motivating and then encouraging communication during play. For adults, this may mean engaging in conversation about topics the client finds meaningful and interesting. In terms of consequences, rather than providing specific corrective feedback or reinforcement, such as saying *good* or *correct* (as is typical in clinician-directed approaches), the clinician responds to the client's behavior in a communicative manner. For example, if while engaging in a play activity with trains, a client spontaneously uses a targeted behavior, such as saying "my train is going under the bridge" (behavior), the clinician would respond in a manner consistent with the communicative context, such as, "I see your train is going under the bridge. My train is traveling over the bridge" (the consequence).

In real-world settings, SLPs and SLPAs engage in a blended approach, incorporating elements of both clinician-directed and client-centered approaches, as applicable to the service delivery model, goals of intervention, and the client's needs and preferences. Using either approach requires careful planning and consideration relative to the client, the environment, and your actions as the clinician. The sections that follow highlight some general concepts and factors to consider in each aspect.

FACTORS TO CONSIDER: THE CLIENT

When it comes to thinking about the client in the scope of successful treatment sessions, there are many avenues to explore, such as the client's age, goals, interests, strengths, weaknesses, and so forth. Many of these details will be discussed in the client's assessment report and treatment plans, compiled by your supervising SLP. In addition to considering the client's individual treatment plan, one of the most important questions is, "Is the client ready to participate in the treatment session?" Although a simple question, it is the most basic and minimal requirement for any successful treatment session.

Cognitive researchers describe two important principles related to client readiness: low-road processing and high-road processing (Cox, 2007; Meltzer, 2010; Ward, 2009). Low-road processing entails attention to basic biologic and physiologic need states, such as hunger, thirst, fatigue, pain, and fear. In contrast, high-road processing refers to the set of mental processes that allow people to regulate their thinking and learning. Collectively, high-road processes are referred to as executive control, which includes the ability to pay attention, plan, prioritize, organize, shift between tasks, access working memory, and monitor performance (Cox, 2007; Meltzer, 2010; Ward, 2009). Regardless of the task, these skills are all important to fully participate in treatment sessions and are key components of learning. Of course, the level of complexity demanded of each skill is tailored to the client's abilities, but it is important to understand that if the clients' resources are diverted to low-road processing, they will have limited ability to engage in high-road processing (Ward, 2009). For example, if a client is hungry, in pain, tired, angry, upset, scared, or frustrated, high-road processing becomes challenging and the client's ability to learn is dramatically reduced. As such, a key first step in a successful treatment session is ensuring the clients'

basic needs are met so that they can focus on high-road processing.

Developing a strong clinician–client relationship (as discussed below) will address some of the emotional aspects of low-road processing, such as anxiety, frustration, and fear. In terms of biologic needs such as hunger, fatigue, pain, and the need to use the restroom, if these are things you can address in the moment during a session, do so. If not, work with your supervising SLP, the client, the client's family, and related professionals to see how these needs can be met before the client attends the treatment session.

Another important factor related to a client's readiness to participate in treatment is motivation. Motivation plays a key role in successful treatment sessions. Two important elements of motivation are (1) understanding the purpose of treatment and (2) seeing a benefit from participation (Moon-Meyer, 2004; Ragan, 2011). As an SLPA, it is outside your scope of practice to discuss the outcomes of treatment overall, but this does not preclude you from explaining the tasks and intended activities of a specific session (ASHA, 2022). Taking time to explain what is planned for an individual session is valuable in helping clients understand what to expect from the session. This, in turn, may carry over to helping the client understand the purpose of treatment and, hopefully, seeing the benefit of participating. This will be particularly true if the client can see a connection between the treatment tasks in a specific session and their overall personal goals (Thomas & Storey, 2000).

Another important element in motivation is interest and engagement in the task (Grubbs & Paradise, 2010; Ragan, 2011). Often with young children, this means make it fun, and this can apply to adults as well. Beyond knowing why they are there and seeing the benefits of participation, participating in something that is interesting and engaging to them will have a positive impact on motivation. Think about the example of physical fitness. Although many of us understand the purpose of exercising on a regular basis and with some effort we may see the benefits of doing so, the motivation to continue participating in physical fitness activities increases if we enjoy them as well. Hence, your job as an SLPA is to get to know your clients and understand what aspects of treatment you can adjust to improve interest and, thereby, motivation in your session.

FACTORS TO CONSIDER: THE ENVIRONMENT

Your environment is your stage, and as such, it must be carefully arranged to support the services you provide. If arranged effectively, it will aid in the implementation of treatment. If not, it will detract from your effectiveness as a clinician.

All environments where treatment is provided should be clean and safe. Chapter 6 discusses procedures and requirements for disinfecting surfaces and materials. Your employer will have additional specific requirements. Most employers are required to establish minimal environmental safety standards, such as maximum occupancy in a given space, rules about exit accessibility, and procedures for evacuation in case of an emergency. You should familiarize yourself with all the applicable rules. In addition, when arranging the environment for treatment services, you should consider the nature of the sensory environment, the furniture

and seating arrangements, and your materials and stimulus presentation methods.

Sensory Environment

Sight and hearing are two important senses to consider when arranging your environment for treatment services. Visually, the environment should be well lit to allow for adequate visual processing of treatment materials. You should also minimize the level of visual distraction in the treatment environment. If there are toys or equipment that will not be used during a particular session, it is generally best to remove them or place them in an area of the room where they will not be a source of distraction for your client. It is also important to provide treatment services in an environment conducive to adequate hearing. This means an environment that is quiet enough for comfortable, conversational levels of speech. You should arrange the environment to eliminate sources of auditory distraction, such as excessive background noise. This may mean closing a door or window to eliminate noise from the outside or moving to a location that is less noisy overall.

In some instances, you may work with clients with specific vision and/or hearing needs. If so, consult with your supervising SLP, the client and his or her family, or related professionals, such as an audiologist (for hearing issues), to establish an optimum visual and/or hearing environment for that particular client.

Furniture Choice and Seating Arrangement

A big part of the environment is the furniture and seating arrangements. These can enhance or detract from the overall effectiveness of the clinical environment. Ensure that the furniture is suited to the size of your client (Moon-Meyer, 2004). You do not want an adult client seated in a child-sized chair, nor do you want a child client seated in an adult-sized chair. Generally, when tabletop activities are performed, you should select furniture that allows for comfort and free mobility of the arms and hands. The concept of proximal stability = distal mobility (Costigan, n.d., slide 27) can ensure that the client is in an optimal position. This means that if the client's trunk is supported and comfortable, he or she will have maximum free use of the upper extremities. An easy way to remember this is "90-90-90" when it comes to seating (Costigan, n.d., slide 40), meaning the hips, knees, and ankles should be in neutral positions at roughly 90-degree angles (Figure 10–1). In some cases, it is appropriate to use no furniture at all, as in the case of young children engaged in play activities. In any seating

position, if a client has unique motor or physical needs, you should consult with your supervising SLP, the client and his or her family, and related professionals, such as an occupational therapist, to ensure the client's seating and positioning allow for maximum participation. In terms of seating, maintaining an eye-level position with your clients will optimize communication between you and your client; you do not want to dominate your client by, for example, seating yourself in a tall chair while the client is seated on the floor (Moon-Meyer, 2004).

Where you place yourself in relation to the door is also important. It is generally best to position yourself with your back toward the exit (Figure 10–2). This gives the clinician control of the exit if needed, for example, in cases where a client such as a young child tries to exit the session abruptly (Moon-Meyer, 2004). In addition, there may be situations when the clinician needs to exit the session quickly to obtain assistance. Placing yourself closest to the

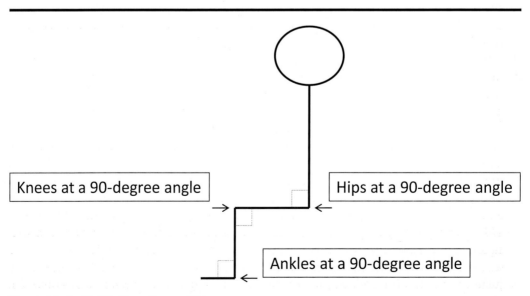

Figure 10–1. 90-90-90 seating position.

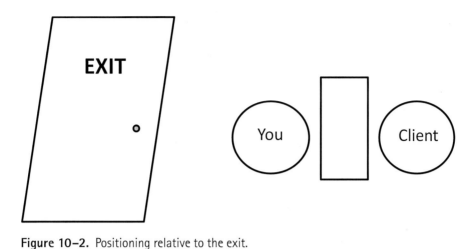

Figure 10–2. Positioning relative to the exit.

exit, with your back to the door, ensures you will have a clear path to do so (Moon-Meyer, 2004).

Your position for data collection is also something to consider when arranging furniture and seating. Data collection sheets should be placed to the side of the hand you use to write (Figure 10–3; Moon-Meyer, 2004), regardless of your seating location (e.g., at a table or seated on the floor). This allows you to easily record information and leaves your nondominant hand free for manipulating materials, as needed. In addition, the client and data collection sheet should be positioned so that what you are writing is out of view of the client (Moon-Meyer, 2004). In cases where you are seated at a table and the client is positioned directly across from you, positioning a clipboard at a slight angle may be appropriate to block the client's view of what you are writing. Figure 10–3 depicts a variety of options for positioning the client in relation to your data sheet, in both individual and group treatment settings. These positions can be adjusted for other seating arrangements, such as on the floor. The key is to arrange your data collection sheet so that it is easily accessible to you but not in view of, or a distraction to, your client.

Materials and Stimulus Presentation Methods

Treatment often involves the use of props, such as pictured items, written material, real objects, and a variety of games or toys (Hegde, 1998). These are often referred to as a stimulus (singular) or stimuli (plural). As discussed in Chapter 7, these items are carefully selected with the guidance of your supervising SLP, based on the unique aspects of your clients and their goals (Hegde, 1998).

Examples of pictured stimuli are things like a picture of a dog to elicit verbal production of the word *dog*, a line drawing of a summer scene to elicit conversation about a recent vacation or favored summer activity, or a set of cartoon images the client places in order and then uses to tell a story. Pictured stimuli can also display important concepts, such as a drawing of how to place the tongue

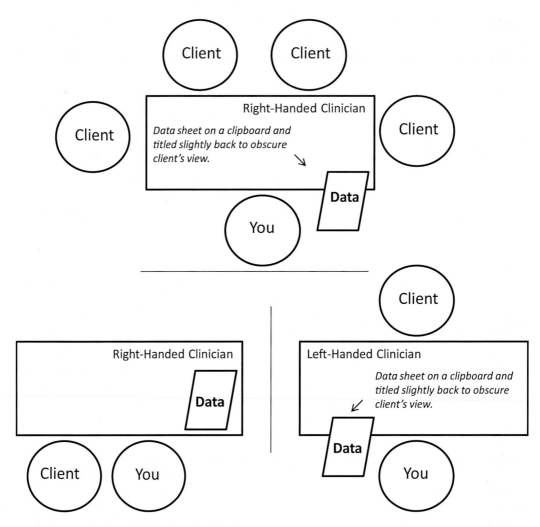

Figure 10–3. Seating and data collection sheet positions.

when producing a specific sound. Pictured stimuli can be line drawings (black and white or color), color photographs, or a combination of the two. Pictured stimuli can also be combined with written text, as applicable. The images used can be obtained from commercially available sets, magazines, or online sources such as Microsoft Clip Art, Getty Images, or Google Images.

Pictured stimuli should be "clear, simple, direct, and unambiguous" (Hegde,

1998, p. 154). This means that when clients view a stimulus, it should be obvious to them what is intended. Furthermore, pictured stimuli should be attractive and motivating for the client (Hegde, 1998). For example, if a young child is interested in a specific cartoon character, incorporating that character into pictured stimuli may be motivating for that client. Similarly, if a client has a specific interest or hobby, using pictured stimuli with these themes may be particularly rewarding.

Whenever possible, using images and pictured stimuli from the client's environment is highly effective. Pictured stimuli should also match the client's age and level of development. Avoid selecting stimuli that are childlike in nature for adults; for young children, select pictured stimuli that are appropriate to their specific developmental level.

In some cases, real-object stimuli may be preferred, such as balls, dolls, toys, or real or simulated daily items, such as kitchen utensils and food items. Chapter 16 discusses ideas for selecting toys and stimuli used for young children engaged in play during treatment activities. Remember, too, that objects used by different clients should be cleaned and disinfected between uses, as discussed in Chapter 6.

Written stimuli can also be used. Examples of written stimuli are a textbook from the client's science class to be read by the client to target reading comprehension or to elicit description and conversation; written words, sentences, or paragraphs to be read aloud; or a worksheet with written directions targeting certain grammatical elements. Like pictured stimuli, written stimuli should be direct, effective, and designed to meet their specific intended purpose. They should also match the client's reading abilities and interests. If you are not sure what level of reading material is appropriate for a specific client, speak with your supervising SLP to gain additional details about the client's skills and needs. In addition, ensure the size of any print is appropriate for use with your client. In some cases, clients have visual impairments that necessitate larger print than would be typical in traditional reading materials. Even for young children who are not literate, presenting pictured or written stimuli in a sequence consistent with their future literacy lays a good foundation for literacy development (Moon-Meyer, 2004). For English speakers, this is a left-to-right, top-to-bottom reading order. Importantly, all stimuli, regardless of form, should be "ethnoculturally appropriate" (Hegde, 1998, p. 154). Chapter 5 provides additional explanation and instruction on this topic. Furthermore, prepare your stimuli in advance of a clinical session and make sure they are presorted in the appropriate order to save time during the session and present a professional and organized impression. For some individuals, you may want to keep the work area clear and have only the stimuli needed for one activity at a time in view. In that case, have the next set of stimuli easily accessible so that you can transition between activities quickly. Lastly, if you are presenting stimuli that require the client to choose a specific target from an array of choices, as in a receptive task where the client points to a specific pictured item named by you, carefully consider the number of choices (Moon-Meyer, 2004). For example, Figure 10–4 displays a scenario in which the client was asked to point to an item described by the clinician. You can see that in the first attempt (#1), the clinician presented four cards (also known as a "field" of four) and then gave the client a command to point to one of them. When the client pointed to one of the cards (e.g., dog), the field of choices became narrowed to the three cards that the client did not select. If the clinician does not replace the card for "dog" for the second trial (#2) before giving the next command, the client would then be selecting not from a field of four, as in the first attempt, but from a field of three choices. Similarly, in the third attempt (#3), the choices narrowed even further to only two possibilities, followed by the fourth trial

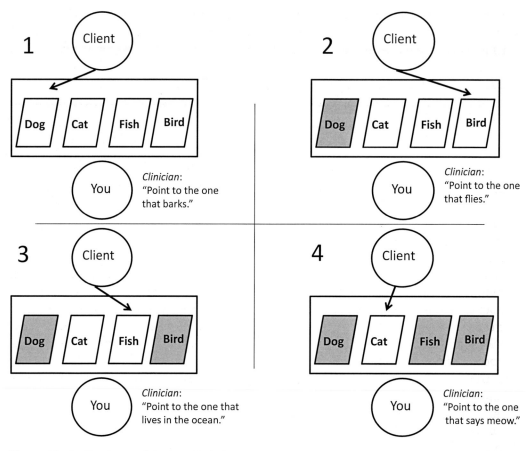

Figure 10–4. Consistency in response choices.

(#4), which was a field of one, because the client had already pointed to all but one item on the table. This decreasing field of choices makes the task easier with each successful attempt. The best method for countering this occurrence is to replace items after each attempt or present a new set of cards for each attempt.

FACTORS TO CONSIDER: THE CLINICIAN

Much of responsibility for a positive treatment session outcome rests with the clinicians and her or his behavior. When a session has not gone as anticipated or did not have a positive outcome, the best course of action is to look to your own behaviors and interactions first as the primary source of variance. Often, when you do this, you will find that there are elements of your performance that negatively affected the outcome. The good news is that if your behaviors can negatively affect the outcome, they can also positively affect. Consider developing a better clinical rapport and a refining your clinical interactions, including things like how you give instructions, model behaviors, and provide hints (also known as prompts). The use of behavioral principles is also a key factor in your interactions during therapy. This is discussed in detail in Chapter 11. Each of these areas will be discussed in the sections that follow.

Clinical Rapport

Developing a positive rapport with clients you serve can have a dramatic impact on treatment services. Rapport is not simply whether your clients *like* you (Pattison & Powell, 1990). Rather, rapport is "the establishment and maintenance of an interactive, harmonious, and communicative relationship" (p. 77). Importantly, rapport can change over time (Pattison & Powell, 1990), meaning that you must work to develop a positive clinician-client rapport initially and then work to maintain the positive relationship over time. Chapter 4 discussed tips for effective communication, which will be very helpful in establishing a strong communicative relationship with your clients.

In addition, an important element of establishing and maintaining a positive rapport is to be sensitive to the client's physical and emotional needs (Pattison & Powell, 1990). The sections above about the environment and the client discussed considerations such as clients' physical needs, such as a supportive and comfortable environment, and making sure clients' basic needs are met. In terms of emotional needs, keep in mind that clients vary in their feelings and emotions about treatment. Some individuals view it positively and are excited to attend treatment, whereas others feel anxious about treatment activities and communicative tasks (Brumfitt, 2010; Flasher & Fogle, 2004; Holland, 2007). In addition, some individuals may be depressed or have strong emotional reactions to their communicative impairment (Brumfitt, 2010; Flasher & Fogle, 2004; Holland, 2007). The provision of counseling to individuals with communicative disorders is outside the scope of an SLPA (ASHA, 2022). If you are concerned about the psychological well-being of any client you serve, immediately notify your supervising SLP. Two important ways SLPAs can support their client's emotional needs while further establishing a positive rapport are as follows:

1. *Show that you are attentive and focused on your client's needs.* This means limiting discussion about yourself and personal topics. It is appropriate on a limited basis to share personal stories and experiences with your clients, but the focus of treatment sessions should not be on you. In fact, you should limit that total amount of time you spend talking in general (Moon-Meyers, 2004; Pattison & Powell, 1990). You can encourage shy or withdrawn clients to interact with you during a clinical session by (a) allowing for a brief period of small talk at the beginning or end of each session (tailored to their age and abilities), (b) showing a genuine interest in clients' well-being, and (c) communicating slowly, asking open-ended questions, and waiting for and encouraging clients to communicate (Pattison & Powell, 1990). This is particularly true when you first get to know a client. You should also be conscious of your nonverbal behaviors to ensure that you are welcoming. You do not want to inadvertently convey the wrong messages nonverbally by displaying behaviors such as fidgeting (e.g., tapping your pencil, twirling your hair, shaking

your legs) or resting your hands on your chin, because these can make you appear nervous or bored (Moon-Meyer, 2004). In addition, always silence your cell phone and other sources of personal electronic distraction, such as e-mail and text message notifications on electronic devices. It is also professional to place these items out of view of the client since it may give the impression that you are waiting for a call or other contact not related to the client's session. Lastly, starting and ending your clinical sessions on time gives the impression that you are focused on clients' needs and are conscious that their time is valuable.

2. *Structure the session to decrease negative emotions.* Start each session with a brief description of the tasks or activities to be included in each session (Moon-Meyer, 2004). Letting clients know what is planned allows clients who are anxious to prepare for the session's activities. It also reinforces the purpose of the session and helps facilitate shared responsibility for session goals, which in turn helps build positive client-clinician rapport (Roth & Worthington, 2001). Chapter 11 offers suggestions for reinforcement and positive support that can be used to facilitate participation and reduce negative emotions and behaviors associated with treatment. In addition, consult with your supervising SLP to ensure you are pacing sessions so that activities are not too fast or too slow for each individual client (Roth & Worthington, 2001). This serves to decrease any undue frustration for tasks that are either too easy or boring or tasks that are too difficult. In addition, in general, following a pattern

of targeting easier tasks at the beginning and end of the session allows treatment to begin and end on a positive note (Moon-Meyer, 2004; Roth & Worthington, 2001). Lastly, remember to leave time at the end of the session to do the following:

a. Provide a warning shortly before the session ends, especially for clients who may feel frustrated with ending the session or anxious in transitioning to the next activity (Moon-Meyer, 2004).

b. Provide a recap of the client's performance (Roth & Worthington, 2001). This is also an opportunity to highlight any positive accomplishments made that session (Moon-Meyer, 2004).

c. Provide a summary of any home activities or additional outside assignments recommended and assigned by your supervising SLP (Roth & Worthington, 2001).

d. Offer an opportunity for the client to ask questions.

An additional avenue for improving your clinical effectiveness and establishing a positive client-clinician rapport is to give clients an opportunity to provide feedback about the services provided. In allied health fields, this is often referred to as customer-oriented care (Reisberg, 1996). One important aspect of customer-oriented care is an opportunity for customers to give both positive and negative feedback about the services provided (Frattali, 1991; Reisberg, 1996). In the case of speech-language pathology, our clients (and their families) are our customers. Feedback from clients can be obtained in a formalized fashion through written or online client satisfaction surveys (Frattali,

1991). Often these measures are developed and administered by your employer (or your supervisor). If your setting uses a client satisfaction survey, familiarize yourself with the questions on the survey.

Informal mechanisms can also be used during individual clinical sessions to obtain client feedback (Frattali, 1991). The use of a rating scale, like those in Figure 10–5, can be helpful for receiving feedback during clinical interaction (Brumfitt, 2010; Wewers & Lowe, 1990). These are examples of visual analog scales (VAS).

A visual analog scale is "a straight line, the end anchors of which are labeled as the extreme boundaries of the sensation, feeling, or response to be measured" (Wewers & Lowe, 1990, p. 13). VAS can be modified and used with any sensa-

tion or feeling. VAS have frequently been used as a way for clients to report their pain or mood in clinical settings (Wewers & Lowe, 1990). They have also been used with pictorial representations at the ends of lines to represent applicable extremes (Brumfitt, 2010). Clarifying words, numbers, and/or written descriptors can also be added (Wewers & Lowe, 1990). Some advantages of VAS, particularly those with pictorial representations, are that they are less tied to complex language skills that would be needed, for example, to describe a specific sensation or feeling or to understand a complex verbal or written question about a sensation or feeling (Brumfitt, 2010). This makes them potentially applicable for use with clients with of varying ages and abilities.

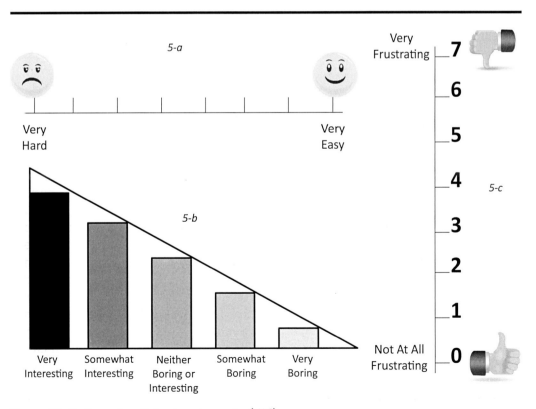

Figure 10–5. Examples of visual analog scales (VAS).

Some ways that SLPAs can incorporate VAS into their sessions could be by asking the client to give either general or specific feedback about a treatment task or session. Some senses or internal states that can be measured with VAS include the following:

- Frustration (not frustrated to frustrated)
- Pain (not painful to painful)
- Difficulty (easy to hard)
- Interest (boring to interesting)
- Comfort (comfortable to uncomfortable)

Traditionally, VAS use very specific numeric scales, but for use in speech-language pathology settings, they can simply serve as means of soliciting qualitative (e.g., nonnumeric) and subjective feedback from clients about their experiences, feelings, and attitude about anything related to the clinical session. For example, if the VAS in Figure 10–5a was used and the client pointed close to the "very easy" symbol, you could share that information with your supervising SLP, so that she or he could review the task to see if a potential modification is needed for future sessions. Similarly, if you use the scale presented in Figure 10–5c during a treatment task and the client indicated they were "very frustrated" by pointing closest to the 6, you would know that she or he is becoming frustrated with the task and a break may be needed.

As with all clinical procedures, the use of these scales should first be discussed with your supervising SLP to ensure they are appropriate for a specific client. You should obtain guidance in developing an applicable visual analog scale and in establishing how and when to request this type of feedback from the client. Generally, VAS used in this way are most effective when combined with careful instructions (Wewers & Lowe, 1990). Being given a similar visual analog scale more than once allows the client to become comfortable with offering opinions in this fashion. It also provides an opportunity to track the client's opinions over time and across tasks. A visual analog scale is not the only way to elicit client feedback about some aspect of your clinical services. You can also simply ask direct questions (e.g., Are you feeling frustrated? Is this task boring? Am I going too fast?). The key here is to offer an opportunity, appropriate to the client's abilities, for the client to express opinions about the clinical session.

Clinical Interactions

An additional and important aspect to consider when providing treatment is the nature of your clinical interaction with clients, including how you provide directions, the effectiveness of your demonstrations and modeling, and the prompts and scaffolding you deploy during treatment.

Directions

Your verbal and written directions about a treatment task can have a positive or negative impact if that task is performed accurately and as intended. Your directions to the client should be short and to the point. You should also allow sufficient time for the client to respond before repeating directions (Roth & Worthington, 2001). The form of your directions is important as well and, in general, they should be in declarative form (Roth & Worthington, 2001), such as the following:

Name this picture.

Say the word_____.

Write these words in sentences.

Let's begin.

Tell me what happened this weekend. Repeat after me.

Place the picture in the box.

Take a card from the stack of cards.

Avoid combining a command and a question, such as, "Can you name this picture?" and "Can you repeat after me?" In these instances, an appropriate response is for the client to answer yes or no, not for the individual to perform the requested task. Similarly, note that when some commands are converted to questions, such as, "Are you ready to begin?" (instead of "Let's begin."), the question form gives the client an opportunity to say no and not begin the task. In some situations, it is perfectly appropriate and acceptable to request information about a client's readiness to begin, while in others, it may be an opportunity for the client to avoid or escape an undesirable task. In those instances, it is better to avoid asking such a question and stick to a command (Roth & Worthington, 2001).

Demonstration/Modeling

Beyond clinical directions, treatment procedures typically require clinicians to demonstrate and model tasks (Hegde, 1998). The distinction between these two behaviors is that in demonstration, there is no expectation that the client immediately repeats the behavior demonstrated. In modeling, the client is expected to imitate the behavior after it is modeled.

Clinicians can provide frequent demonstrations of a desired response to help reinforce a concept or behavior (Roth & Worthington, 2001). For example, the clinician speaking at a slow rate demonstrates slow, controlled speech for an individual who stutters, or a clinician frequently using a specific grammatical form in her conversation offers repeated exposure to this form for an individual with a language impairment.

In the case of modeling, knowing when and how to model is an important skill (Hegde, 1998). Modeling is used when a client can imitate a behavior and when a question, prompt, or physical stimulus is not sufficient to elicit the desired response. Modeling occurs most frequently in the initial stages of developing a behavior (Hegde, 1998; Roth & Worthington, 2001). Box 10–1 has helpful tips for providing effective models.

We rarely use imitation in our daily conversations. As such, when using modeling to elicit a behavior, generally the client's goals will gradually transition to requiring less and less clinician support to elicit a desired response. This is known as fading (Hegde, 1998). A related technique is shaping (Hegde, 1998). Shaping occurs when a client is not able to imitate a behavior from a model or when the behavior is complex. Shaping breaks a behavior into small, progressively more complex steps, from easy to difficult, until the final level of performance is obtained (Hegde, 1998).

Prompts/Scaffolding

A *prompt* is assistance provided by a clinician to facilitate a desired response from a client (Hegde, 1998; Roth & Worthington, 2001). Prompts are generally what we

> ## Box 10–1. Providing an Effective Model
>
> 1. *Make sure the stage is set for the client to receive and imitate your model.* Model the behavior only when you have the client's attention and he or she knows that an imitation of the model is to follow. Modeling when clients are not paying attention or when they are not ready to imitate will just require a repetition of the model.
> 2. *Avoid unnatural models.* Model behaviors as you would like them imitated. For example, this means avoiding overly exaggerating or slowing certain elements to such an extent that they become distorted or inaccurate (Moon-Meyer, 2004).
> 3. *Avoid ungrammatical utterances in your models* (Moon-Meyer, 2004).
> 4. *Model language at a level appropriate to the client's abilities* (Moon-Meyer, 2004).
> 5. *As needed, emphasize target behaviors with communicative changes.* For example, when you model a behavior that is embedded in a sentence or phrase, emphasizing the model using an increased vocal pitch or loudness may be appropriate, as in the sentence, "the boy is running," when the auxiliary verb + present progressive is the target behavior (Hegde, 1998). Remember Principle 2 (above) and do not overemphasize to the extent that the model becomes unnatural.

think of as hints. Some clinicians also refer to prompts as *cues*, but generally speaking, we reserve the word *cue* to mean a behavior made by a clinician (verbal or nonverbal) to instruct clients when to respond, whereas the word *prompt* (visual, auditory, or tactile) is used to mean facilitating how to respond (Roth & Paul, 2007). For example, a clinician tapping the client's hand to signal it is the client's turn to respond would be classified as a *cue* (as it denotes *when* to respond), while a clinician using vocal emphasis to highlight a helpful feature of the required production, such as, "The boy *is running*. What is the girl doing?" would be a *prompt* (as it

offers information about how to respond). Box 10–2 lists examples of prompts.

Prompts are used when a stimulus alone is not sufficient to elicit the desired response but when more direct elicitation, such as modeling, is not preferred. The term *scaffolding* is also used to describe the use of prompts (or other assistance) from a listener (or clinician) to enable individuals to communicate a message that would not be possible otherwise (Norris & Hoffman, 1990). As the name denotes, scaffolding is thought of as a bridge of support provided to clients until they are able to receive similarly complex messages without the support of prompts. The chapters in Part III

Box 10–2. Examples of Visual, Auditory, and Tactile Prompts

Auditory prompts: Prompts *heard* by the client

- Modulating your pitch or loudness to vocally emphasize an important concept ("The girl is sad.")
- Verbal questioning to provide details about an important feature (e.g., "Where do you find these?" "The lion is hungry. What does he want to eat?")*
- Verbalizing a cloze sentence (e.g., "You bounce a ------_" or "The baby is tired. She wants to go to _____")*
- Verbalizing the first sound or syllable of a word, the first portion of a sentence, or any part of the required response*

Note. Items highlighted with an * can also be presented in written form and in that case would be considered visual prompts.

Visual prompts: Prompts *seen* by the client

- Positioning your mouth in the shape of a target phoneme (e.g., placing you lips together to demonstrate /m/)
- A picture of a concept (e.g., a drawing showing the position of the tongue)
- A written prompt, reminder, or question (e.g., "Remember to ," or "This animal lives in the jungle," or "When do we eat these?")
- Gesturing above your head with your hand to indicate a high(er) pitch
- Pantomiming an action related to a targeted response (e.g., yawning when "sleep" is the target response)

Tactile prompts: Prompts *felt* by the client

- Tapping out the syllables of a word on the client's hand
- Placing your hand on the client's throat to indicate voiced production
- Running your finger gently down the client's forearm to represent continuous sound (as in the production of /z/)
- A tactile real object that aids production or comprehension (e.g., a piece of sandpaper and silk to contrast soft versus harsh vocal production)

(Specific Populations and Disorders) provide additional information unique to certain populations, disorders, and activities. In some cases, you may need to provide more than one prompt simultaneously or present successively prompts until a desired response is obtained.

The purposeful, and importantly, documented use of prompts is a vital part of clinical interaction. New clinicians are often not aware of the level of prompting needed by a particular client and, in some cases, are not even aware that they are providing prompts to a client. This is problematic since prompts can influence how independently a client performs a task. As discussed in Chapter 8, accurate data collection about clients' performance is critical. If you assist a client in the form of prompts but do not record it in your data, it will negatively affect the accuracy of those data. These faulty data may then be used by your supervising SLP to make decisions about client care. In Chapter 7, lesson plans were outlined, including columns for "Prompts/Modifications" and "Make It Easier/Make It More Difficult," which are used to describe suggested prompts, modifications, or both that may be recommended for a specific task. Before you implement any treatment, discuss with your supervising SLP the types of appropriate prompts or modifications applicable for a specific client, as well as how these prompts should be recorded in your data. Chapter 8, particularly the section on "Response Independence," offers additional suggestions.

Presenting prompts systematically using some form of hierarchy individualized to the client is equally important. There are two general approaches to hierarchies of prompting: effortful learning and errorless learning (Abel et al., 2005; Mosall et al., 2012; Sohlberg et al., 2005). In effortful learning approaches, prompts are ordered from the least assistance to most assistance, allowing clients to respond with the greatest level of independence first. If clients are not successful, then additional prompts provide greater assistance until the desired response is obtained. For example, in a client-centered approach setting where the clinician plays with a doll and related items with a young client and is attempting to elicit the word *bottle*, the clinician might say, "Oh the baby is so hungry. What should we give her?" If the client does not respond, two potential prompts, one at each end of the spectrum, are possible. The clinician could say, "The baby needs a bottle. Say bottle." (greatest level of assistance and least level of independence). At the other end of the spectrum, the clinician could give a minimal visual prompt such as simply looking at the bottle (least assistance and greatest level of independence). In the latter example, if the client then responds by saying "a bottle," she or he has done so with minimal assistance and with greater independence than imitating the response "bottle" after it has been modeled by the clinician.

In errorless learning approaches, prompts are presented from the greatest assistance to the least assistance. For example, in a clinician-directed approach, such as teaching a client to use a memory device, the clinician might present the steps of accessing the device first by modeling each step and having the client copy the steps (e.g., opening the device, finding the applicable page, identifying information on that page). Next the clinician might provide a model for all but the final step. In that case, the greatest level of assistance (and thereby prompts) was provided first because rather than independently recalling and performing all the steps, the client only needed to perform a minimal step (the final one after all previous steps were modeled). Gradually, then, fewer and fewer prompts are provided until the client successfully performs all the steps independently. As an SLPA, you should confirm with your supervising SLP which approach is most applicable to a specific treatment target and to each client's individualized goals.

Feedback

After a client produces a desired behavior or treatment target, how the clinician responds will have an impact in helping the client to know if her or his production was correct and in increasing the likelihood of a similar response occurring again. This is referred to as clinician feedback and is based on operant conditioning and the behavioral principles discussed in Chapter 11. Several general tips in deploying effective feedback are as follows:

1. Emphasize the positive. Positive praise, particularly descriptive praise, is very powerful in shaping behaviors and in building self-esteem.
2. Use descriptive praise and avoid evaluative praise (Soclof, 2010). Descriptive praise tells clients specifically why they earned praise or reinforcement (e.g., "Great focus. That time you kept your tongue tip up," or "Good, you corrected all the spelling errors in this sentence"), whereas evaluative praise provides only a generic comment about performance, not linked to the behavior itself (e.g., "good girl," "nice work"; Soclof, 2010). Table 10–1 contains several examples of descriptive and evaluative praise.

Table 10–1. Examples of Evaluative Versus Descriptive Praise

Evaluative Praise	Descriptive Praise
"Good job."	"You worked hard on this reading comprehension sheet. You were able to determine the main point and the conclusion."
"You are so strong."	"You pushed that finger right into the playdoh, you made a pancake—that is using those fingers muscles and making them strong."
"Good girl."	"You said the /s/ sound clearly, you put your tongue right behind your teeth and that /s/ sound came right out."
"You are so smart."	"You got a match! They are the same—two horses!" or "You got two pegs into the pegboard—two more to go."
"You are a great artist."	"I like the way you used the black border around the pink. It really makes the pink color pop out."
"You are the best at coloring."	"I love to look at this picture. All the rainbow colors make me smile."
"You are so nice."	"You picked up Mark's scarf after it fell on the floor. That is a kind thing to do."
"I am so proud of you, you got all A's."	"This report card shows a lot of effort and hard work, you should be proud of yourself."

Source: Reprinted with permission from Soclof, A. (2010). *The absolute best way to motivate your clients.* Retrieved from http://www.SpeechPathology.com

3. Combine corrective feedback with descriptive praise. Corrective feedback (and in particular verbal corrective feedback) can shape the nature of production and offer suggestions for improvement (e.g., correct feedback + descriptive praise; Soclof, 2010). However, corrective feedback that is generic in nature can be perceived as criticism, which is associated with negative emotions (Soclof, 2010). Table 10–2 offers suggestions for shaping feedback from criticism to corrective feedback and combining it with descriptive praise.

4. Avoid the OK syndrome (Moon-Meyer, 2004). The "OK" syndrome is when a clinician frequently says "OK" for things such as a conversational filler (e.g., "OK, let's begin"), tagging questions (e.g., "Read this paragraph, OK?"), and in response to a client's behavior (e.g., "OK" or "OK, not quite, let's try again"; Moon-Meyer, 2004). As you can see in each of these examples, removing the "OK" actually adds clarity and specificity to the clinician's verbal statements. In particular, using "OK" in response to clients' behavior is problematic because it is a vague comment that does not assist clients in understanding whether their response was accurate or inaccurate, desired or undesired, and so on.

Table 10–2. Criticism Versus Corrective Feedback + Descriptive Praise

Criticism	Corrective Feedback + Descriptive Praise
"This is a sloppy paper!"	"This word here and this letter here are on the line. Here is a good amount of space between the words. Can you try that with the rest of the line?"
"Stop saying you can't do this, you can if you try!"	"You are halfway through the maze, only a little more to go."
"It is not enough times!"	"You said the 'r' sound five times correctly, five more to go!"
"Stop fidgeting, sit down, and finish."	"You knew baby and mommy, now show me the dog."
"Stop running and yelling."	"You walked all the way from your class to the steps using a quiet voice—only a few more steps to go using a quiet voice and steady feet."
"You won't be able to play any of the games you like if you don't hurry up and finish your work."	"You did a whole worksheet. One more to go before we play 'Operation.'"

Source: Reprinted with permission from Soclof, A. (2010). *The absolute best way to motivate your clients.* Retrieved from http://www.SpeechPathology.com

REFERENCES

Abel, S., Schultz, A., Radermacher, R., Willmes, K., & Huber, W. (2005). Decreasing and increasing cues in naming therapy for aphasia. *Aphasiology, 19*(9), 831–848.

American Speech-Language-Hearing Association. (n.d.). *Telepractice.* http://www.asha.org/Practice-Portal/Professional-Issues/Telepractice/

American Speech-Language-Hearing Association (ASHA). (2022). *Speech-language pathology assistant scope of practice* [Scope of practice]. http://www.asha.org/policy

Brumfitt, S. (2010). *Psychological well-being and acquired communication impairments.* John Wiley.

Buysse, V., & Bailey, D. B. (1993). Behavioral and developmental outcomes in young children with disabilities in integrated and segregated settings: A review of comparative studies. *Journal of Special Education, 26*, 434–461.

Cascella, R., Purdy, M. H., & Dempsey, J. J. (2007). Clinical service delivery and work settings. In R. Paul & P. Cascella (Eds.), *Introduction to clinical methods in communication disorders* (pp. 259–282). Paul H. Brookes.

Cirrin, F. M., Schooling, T. L., Nelson, N. W., Diehl, S. F., Flynn, P. F., Staskowski, M., . . . Adamczyk, D. F. (2010). Evidence-based systematic review: Effects of different service delivery models on communication outcomes for elementary school-age children. *Language, Speech, and Hearing Services in Schools, 41*(3), 233–264.

Costigan, A. (n.d.). *An introduction to seating and positioning for individuals who use assistive technology.* http://mcn.educ.psu.edu/dbm/S_P_AT_pt1/S_P_AT_HO.pdf

Cox, A. (2007). *No mind left behind: Understanding and fostering executive control—The eight essential brain skills every child needs to thrive.* Penguin.

Flasher, L. V., & Fogle, P. T. (2004). *Counseling skills for speech-language pathologists and audiologists.* Thomson Delmar Learning.

Frattali, C. (1991). Measuring client satisfaction. *ASHA Quality Improvement Digest.* http://www.asha.org/SLP/healthcare/Measuring-Client-Satisfaction/

Garcia, C. (2013). *Online manual for the school-based telepractice paraprofessional.* Unpublished manuscript. http://csd.wp.uncg.edu/wp-content/uploads/sites/6/2012/12/Online-Telepractice-Manual-for-Paraprofessionals.pdf

Grubbs, C., & Paradise, D. (2010). *Making speech therapy fun: Motivating children with autism to speak.* file:///C:/Users/000666547/Downloads/1446-GrubbsChristine.pdf

Hegde, M. N. (1998). *Treatment procedures in communicative disorders* (3rd ed.). Pro-Ed.

Holland, A. (2007). *Counseling in communication disorders: A wellness perspective.* Plural Publishing.

McGinty, A. S., & Justice, L. M. (2006). Classroom-based versus pull-out interventions: A review of the experimental evidence. *EBP Briefs, 1*(1), 1–25.

Meltzer, L. (2010). *Promoting executive function in the classroom.* Guilford.

Moon-Meyer, S. (2004). *Survival guide for the beginning speech-language clinician.* Pro-Ed.

Mosall, A., Choe, Y., Cronin, M., & Massery, M. (2012). *Effortful vs. errorless learning in computer mediated home practice* [Presentation]. file:///C:/Users/000666547/Downloads/5082%20Effortful%20vs%20Errorless%20Learning%20in%20Computer%20Mediated%20Home%20Treatment.pdf

Norris, J. A., & Hoffman, P. R. (1990). Language intervention within naturalistic environments. *Language, Speech, and Hearing Services in Schools, 21*, 72–84.

Pattison, G. A., & Powell, T. W. (1990). Establishing rapport with young children during speech and language diagnostic evaluations. *National Student Speech Language and Hearing Association Journal, 17*, 77–80.

Ragan, T. (2011). *10 ways to motivate the unmotivated student* [Web blog]. https://blog.asha.org/2011/04/05/10-waysto-motivate-the-unmotivated-student/

Reisberg, M. (1996). Customer satisfaction in health care. *Perspectives on Administration and Supervision, 6*(2), 12–15.

Roth, F., & Paul, R. (2007). Communication intervention. In R. Paul & P. Cascella (Eds.), *Introduction to clinical methods in communication disorders* (2nd ed., pp. 157–178). Paul H. Brookes.

Roth, F. R., & Worthington, C. K. (2001). *Treatment resource manual for speech-language pathology.* Delmar.

Soclof, A. (2010). *The absolute best way to motivate your clients.* http://www.SpeechPathology.com

Sohlberg, M. M., Ehlardt, L., & Kennedy, M. (2005). Instructional techniques in cognitive rehabilitation: A preliminary report. *Seminars in Speech and Language, 26,* 268–279.

Thomas, B., & Storey, E. (2000, April). Motivating the elderly client in long-term care. *Advance for Physical Therapy and Rehab Medicine.* http://physical-therapy.advanceweb.com/

Ward, S. (2009). *Executive function skills for the SLP* [Presentation]. http://www.asha.org/Events/convention/handouts/2009/1718_Ward_Sarah_2/

Wewers, M. E., & Lowe, N. K. (1990). A critical review of visual analogue scales in the measurement of clinical phenomena. *Residential Nursing Health, 13*(4), 227–236.

CHAPTER 11

Using Behavioral Principles

Jennifer A. Ostergren and Stephanie P. Davis

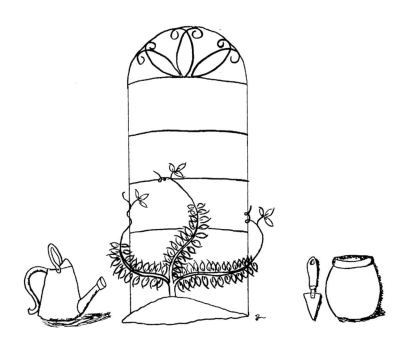

Study the past, if you would define the future.
—Confucius (Chinese philosopher)

The topic of this chapter is behavior and the application of behavior analysis in the field of speech-language pathology. Behavior analysis is broadly defined as "a natural science that seeks to understand the behavior of individuals" (Association for Behavior Analysis International, n.d., para. 1). Without further discussion, it may not be immediately obvious to the novice clinician why an entire chapter in a handbook for speech-language pathology assistants (SLPAs) is devoted to this topic. However, there are several reasons why this topic has relevance for SLPAs, including the following:

a. "There is a well-established evidence base for the efficacy of methods based on behaviorism" (Maul et al., 2016, p. 3).

b. Many preschool and school-age children with language delays are reported to demonstrate higher rates of challenging behaviors when compared to same-age peers (Curtis et al., 2018).

c. Collaboration between speech-language pathologists (SLPs) and behavior analysts can maximize outcomes for children with communication difficulties, especially autism spectrum disorder (Cardon, 2017; LaRue et al., 2009).

d. The American Speech-Language-Hearing Association (ASHA) and World Health Organization (WHO) reported interprofessional education and collaboration as part of a framework to improve quality of care provided by health organizations (ASHA, 2021; WHO, 2010).

This chapter reviews basic principles of behavior, data collection strategies, and behavioral interventions, including positive behavioral interventions and support. The information in the chapter ties back to Chapter 10 in many ways. Along with each of the recommendations discussed under the heading Things to Consider in Chapter 10, the use of behavioral principles has relevance to what SLPAs take into consideration about the clinical environment, the client, and their own behavior. This is true for any client seen by an SLPA, but data collection strategies and behavior interventions are particularly relevant in understanding and changing behaviors that interfere with successful participation in meaningful and productive activities, including behaviors that interfere with the services provided by SLPs and thereby SLPAs.

PRINCIPLES OF BEHAVIOR

How an SLPA responds to a client's communication, whether elicited or produced spontaneously, plays an important role in the treatment process. At a very basic level, the job of the SLP is to design treatment that creates, increases, and in some cases decreases specific behaviors (Hegde, 1998). Behaviors targeted by SLPs and SLPAs are typically those of communication, although in recent years, the scope of an SLP has extended to behaviors outside of communication, such as swallowing (ASHA, 2016). One foundational principle in the domain of behavior is *operant conditioning*, which is a process of increasing or decreasing a behavior based on the consequences that follow that behavior (Cooper et al., 2020). Clinician-directed treatments rely heavily on this theory and the principle of reinforcement (Roth & Paul, 2007), but these concepts are also applicable to client-centered treatment approaches. As discussed in Chapter 10, a framework of antecedent-behavior-consequence is used in both types of approaches. The principles of reinforcement and punishment explain how a consequence directly following a behavior likely impacts its occurrence and frequency in the future (Cooper et al., 2020).

Reinforcement

Reinforcement is a principle of behavior that supports an increase in the future frequency of a behavior in response to a consequence (Cooper et al., 2020). There are two types of reinforcement: positive reinforcement and negative reinforcement. Positive reinforcement consists of an item, event, or action that an individual finds rewarding when presented in direct response to a behavior, thus increasing the chance that the behavior will recur (Dozier et al., 2020). Negative reinforcement consists of the removal of an item, event, or action that an individual finds unpleasant in response to a target behavior, thereby increasing the chance that the behavior will occur in the future (Cooper et al., 2020). Although both positive and negative reinforcement increase the frequency of a desired behavior, negative reinforcement is not commonly used in clinical settings in the field of speech-language pathology (Roth & Worthington, 2001).

Positive reinforcement (and thereby positive reinforcers) is common in the field of speech-language pathology and can be classified as primary or secondary. Primary reinforcement is physiologically or biologically driven. Food and water are two examples of primary reinforcers (Cooper et al., 2020). The use of food as reinforcement, however, should be implemented with caution (Hegde, 1998) and only under the direction of your supervising SLP. Given the potential for food allergies and sensitivities, specific caregiver preferences, and religious or cultural considerations, caregiver consent is typically sought for the use of food as a reinforcement during treatment sessions.

Secondary reinforcers are items, events, or actions that a client has been conditioned to find rewarding. Secondary reinforcers are commonly used in the field of speech-language pathology and may include "sensory, tangible, activity, or social" reinforcers (Cooper et al., 2020, p. 264) (Box 11–1).

There are different schools of thought regarding the classification of reinforcers.

For example, professionals in the field of speech-language pathology frequently classify social reinforcers as any action that includes another person. Therefore, activities and sensory experiences involving social interaction are categorized as social reinforcers. Behavior analysts frequently classify reinforcers by how the client interacts with the reinforcer, thereby classifying them differently. This is an important distinction because collaboration between professionals in the field of speech-language pathology and behavior analysts frequently requires communication about vocabulary that may not be agreed upon by both disciplines. Keep in mind that agreement on assigning a reinforcer to its accurate category is much less important than knowing whether an item or activity is a reinforcer for your individual client's behavior.

Punishment

In contrast to reinforcement, punishment is a principle of behavior that describes an increase in the future frequency of a behavior in response to a consequence. Punishment is generally positive or negative. Positive punishment involves the delivery of a consequence that the individual finds aversive immediately following a target behavior, which *decreases* the future frequency of the behavior (Cooper et al., 2020). In the field of speech-language pathology, a form of positive punishment might be a variation of the word "No" in response to an incorrect answer, such as "No, try again" or "No, let me show you."

Negative punishment consists of removing a pleasant condition in response to a behavior targeted for decrease, which decreases the likelihood of the behavior

Box 11–1. Examples of Secondary Reinforcers

Sensory Reinforcers

Sensory experiences stimulate one or more of an individual's senses. Sensory experiences enjoyed by clients can be very powerful reinforcers when delivered directly following a target behavior (Cooper et al., 2020). Access to a favorite smell, tickles, squishing Play-Doh, or the sounds of nature may all function as reinforcers for behaviors.

Tangible and Activity Reinforcers

A tangible reinforcer is an item that can be held, collected, or manipulated. Examples of items that may function as tangible reinforcers are pencils, cards, small prizes, figurines, or digital items. In contrast to a tangible reinforcer, an activity reinforcer can be experienced. Examples of activity reinforcers may include an outing, game, break from demands, or opportunity to draw.

Social Reinforcers

A social reinforcer is an action such as smiling, eye contact, a high five, or verbal praise, delivered by another person. In general, clinicians utilize a variety of social reinforcers, as attention from another person functions as a potent reinforcer for many behaviors (Cooper et al., 2020). Social reinforcers of a communicative nature (such as those that would naturally occur with a successful communication exchange) are commonly used in client-centered treatment approaches.

Tokens

A token is an item given in response to a target behavior. The item itself is not particularly rewarding, but tokens can be accrued and exchanged for a variety of specific reinforcers. In behavior analysis literature, a token is termed a *generalized conditioned reinforcer* because it is reinforcing across a variety of conditions (Cooper et al., 2020). Money is an example of a generalized conditioned reinforcer, as it can be traded in for a variety of needed or desired goods and services. Examples of tokens commonly used in the field of speech-language pathology are points, check marks, stickers, and chips. The use of token systems is more common in clinician-directed than client-centered approaches to treatment and is frequently utilized to reward both communicative behaviors targeted in treatment and behaviors related to participation in treatment, such as attention and participation (Hegde, 1998).

recurring (Cooper et al., 2020). The two most common types of negative punishment used in the field of speech-language pathology were timeout and response costs (Hegde, 1998; Roth & Worthington, 2001; Box 11–2). Currently, there is a paucity of research on negative punishment in many therapeutic fields, as the benefits of using positive reinforcement to increase target behaviors frequently outweigh the risk and benefit of using positive or negative punishment (Leaf et al., 2022).

New clinicians may be reluctant to provide punishment, given the negative connotation associated with the word (Leaf et al., 2022). Keep in mind that from a behavioral analysis perspective, punishment need not involve pain or highly aversive stimuli (Leaf et al., 2022). Still, it is correct to be cautious about its use and be aware of your local and federal laws regarding its use in your occupational setting. SLPAs should follow the treatment plan provided by their supervising SLP, which most likely prioritizes increasing target or replacement behaviors. However, it makes sense for SLPAs to work closely with their supervising SLP regarding what to do when a behavior is targeted for decrease and ask questions to clarify any possible miscommunications. Generally, only very minimally aversive forms of punishment should be used with the guidance of your supervising SLP, such as saying "No" to a behavior, and only after reinforcement of a desired behavior has been ineffective (Bopp et al., 2004). Working closely with your supervising SLP to ensure you have adequate knowledge and skills in the use of reinforcement and punishment is critical.

Effective Use of Principles of Behavior

The key to using both reinforcement or punishment is to do so specifically and with an understanding of its purpose and impact. The use of these techniques first requires an understanding of what

---

Box 11–2. Timeout and Response Cost

Timeout

Timeout from positive reinforcement involves "temporary isolation or removal of a client to an environment with limited opportunity to receive positive reinforcement" (Roth & Worthington, 2001, p. 15). This is not a common practice, but a current example of this with a client might be changing from a highly preferred actively to a lesser preferred activity for a brief period (e.g., exchanging the highest preferred game for a less preferred game).

Response Cost

Response cost involves removing a previously earned positive reinforcer (Hegde, 1998; Roth & Worthington, 2001). This is commonly accomplished with the use of tokens, by removing a token earned in response to an undesired behavior.

will serve as an effective reinforcement (increase a target behavior) or punishment (decrease an undesired behavior). It is also important to understand that whether something serves as a reinforcement versus a punishment depends in part on the individual. A classic example of this concept regarding punishment is when a novice clinician inaccurately believes that a timeout from participating in treatment will be a form of punishment for an undesired behavior (e.g., a loud aggressive comment), only to find that in fact the incidence of that behavior increases. In that case, the brief and temporary removal from the treatment session was actually a reinforcer for the behavior. Similar effects can also be seen, for example, when a clinician gives attention to an undesired behavior and finds that the behavior increases. In that case, the clinicians' attention functioned as reinforcement for the behavior, resulting in an increase in the frequency of the undesired behavior in an attempt to get additional clinician attention.

Identifying what reinforcement is most applicable for a given behavior and in which context is key to using principles of behavior effectively. The underlying assumption is that behavior is produced to meet an individual's need or want (Cooper et al., 2020); therefore, discovering the function of the behavior is of the utmost importance. For example, perhaps an individual who is yelling or acting aggressively toward a classmate is attempting to say, "I want X," "I don't want X," or "I need X" (Bopp et al., 2004, p. 5). Behavior analysis addresses such challenging behavior through the lens of its function. Box 11–3 contains a description and examples of the common functions of behavior.

One way to investigate what might be maintaining the behavior is to complete an antecedent-behavior-consequence (A-B-C) chart such as the one in Figure 11–1. Behavior has a functional relationship with the environment, in that the behavior occurs to interact with the environment and cause a consequence (Johnston et al., 2020). Therefore, documenting the antecedent event, behavior that occurs in response, and the consequence that follows may provide insight regarding the function of the behavior and spark ideas for replacement behaviors or environmental changes to be addressed.

Overall, training and practical application are imperative to ensure an SLPA documents and implements behavioral techniques effectively. Specific instruction from your supervising SLP or collaborating behavior analyst, as well as having her or him evaluate your effectiveness in deploying principles of behavior, is a top priority. Several additional tips for implementing effective principles of behavior are as follows:

1. Emphasize the positive. Use positive reinforcement first and most readily (Berth et al., 2019; Hagopian et al., 2000; Leaf et al., 2022).

2. Conduct a preference assessment. The easiest, though least accurate, option is to use a caregiver/teacher interview or a self-fillable checklist in attempt to identify preferred items, which may function as reinforcers for particular behaviors (Hagopian et al., 2004). Preference assessment checklists like those in Appendices 11–A and 11–B identify several types of reinforcement (auditory, visual, tactile) that might apply to a specific behavior. If

---

Box 11–3. Common Functions of Behavior

Escape

The behavior is an attempt to get out of doing something the individual does not want to do.

> <u>Example</u>: During a pencil-and-paper task during communication group, Jorge rips his paper into small pieces and is not provided with another worksheet.

Attention

The behavior gets the attention of a caregiver, teacher, sibling, peer, or other person in the individual's environment.

> <u>Example</u>: When the SLPA is working with another student, Matilda yells. The SLPA turns her attention to Matilda.

Access to Materials

The behavior gets access to a preferred item or participation in a preferred activity.

> <u>Example</u>: While sitting with her peers at story time, Amy grabs a musical toy from the table and begins to play music on it.

Sensory Stimulation (Also Known as Automatic Reinforcement)

The behavior feels good to the individual.

> <u>Example</u>: During speech-language therapy, Bart repeatedly flips through the pages of the book because he likes the way it looks, feels, or both.

---

there is a behavior analyst on the client's team, ask if they have conducted a preference assessment and if they have permission to share the results. Conversely, with permission of his or her supervising SLP, an SLPA may consult a behavior analyst and ask to be trained in stimulus preference assessments (SPAs), as research has validated the training staff members to administer SPAs (Deliperi et al., 2015).

3. Deliver reinforcement immediately. Behaviors are more likely to increase in the future if positive reinforcement is provided within a few seconds after the behavior occurs (Cooper et al., 2020).

Sample A-B-C Data Collection

Name: Amara C.

SLPA: James W. (Assistant)

Date: 6/2/22

Target Behavior(s): projecting saliva from mouth onto objects or people, swatting open palm toward faces of staff, short bursts of high-pitch screams

Time	Activity/Setting	ANTECEDENT	BEHAVIOR	CONSEQUENCE	FUNCTION
	What was the context?	What happened first?	What was the individual's response?	What happened after the behavior?	-Access -Attention -Escape -Automatic Reinforcement
7:30am	Hospital room, patient in bed yawning	SLPA entered room and said "Good morning"	Patient projected saliva from mouth onto floor 2-3 inches from SLPA's shoe	SLPA sat in chair furthest away from hospital bed and documented	Escape?
7:35am	(same) + SLPA sitting in chair	SLP entered room and said "Good morning"	Patient projected saliva from mouth onto arm of SLP	SLP stood near SLPA away from hospital bed	Escape?
7:40am	(same) + SLP standing near SLPA	Nurse entered room smiling, walked toward curtains, slowly opened curtains	Patient smiled	Nurse looked at patient and smiled	Attention?
7:42	(same)	Nurse exited room into hallway	Patient vocalized in burst of loud high-pitched screams	Nurse entered room and asked, "Are you okay?"	Attention?

Figure 11–1. Sample A-B-C data.

DATA COLLECTION STRATEGIES

Reinforcement and punishment are principles of behavior that describe whether future behavior is likely to increase or decrease based on consequences (Cooper et al., 2020). To answer the question of whether a behavior is increasing or decreasing, a clinician must be able to see data over the course of time and compare them to earlier data of the same behavior. Visual analysis of this type requires a thorough description of the target behavior, documenting occurrences of the target behavior, and a visual display of the data over time.

Description of the Target Behavior

Description is directly applicable to an SLPA since the 2022 Scope of Practice includes "taking notes as advised by the SLP" (ASHA, 2022, p. 8). When a client is demonstrating behaviors that are interfering with speech and language services, an SLP and SLPA document the behavior by describing what is occurring. To avoid misconceptions of behavior, it is important the SLPA and SLP are both able to thoroughly define a targeted behavior, with as much detail as possible, which includes providing examples and nonexamples (i.e., a behavior that differs from the target behavior). For instance, when describing behavior that is interfering with mealtime or feeding therapy, a clinician might document, "picking up food with hands or utensils and releasing it onto any surface other than the plate or food tray." The clinician may also provide nonexamples, such as "picking up a finger food and dropping it onto the plate" or "scooping up puree with a spoon and dripping it onto the food tray."

Documentation of Occurrence of Behavior

As mentioned in Chapter 8 on data collection, there are a variety of ways to measure and record data. In the case of documenting behavior during a speech-language therapy session, an SLPA will most commonly utilize direct observation in comparison to a checklist or caregiver interview. Depending on the behavior of interest, the measure of frequency (instances over time) is often a good fit. However, behaviors of lower frequency and longer length may be measured by duration per episode. Both frequency and duration would fall into the category of continuous measurement, as the SLPA would be documenting each occurrence during the entirety of the observation (Johnston et al., 2020). Figure 11–2 is a sample data sheet for documenting frequency of behavior. When pencil and paper or digital applications are not a good fit for tallying frequency, alternative means of keeping count must be implemented.

Figure 11–3 shows an example of a bead tracker, on which one bead is pushed to the other side with each observation of the target behavior, to be documented after the session on a chart or digital graph (original design by Roger Pond).

Documenting continuous measurement of behavior may not be possible for an SLPA during a therapy session, since the SLPA may simultaneously be presenting communication, swallowing, or feeding treatment. Though not nearly as accurate as continuous measurement,

Sample Behavior Data Collection: Frequency During Routine Activities

Name: Steve S. **Target Behavior:** low growl, 2-3 seconds duration, eye contact
SLPA: Rosa M. (Assistant) **Example:** 3 second growl while facing conversation partner
Date: 5/1/22 **Non-example:** 3 short grunts while writing with a pencil

Routine Activity	Time in minutes	Target Behavior	Totals
Transition from lunch to therapy	10	llll	4
Warm-up activity	5	l	1
Shared book/story reading	8	llll	4
Categorizing vocabulary words	10	lll	3
Drawing vocabulary words	12		0
Wrap-up activity	4	ll	2
Transition from therapy to large group	6	llll	4
TOTAL:	55		18

DIRECTIONS: Place a tally in right column for each instance of target behavior during routine activity. Leave blank if no occurrences of target behavior were observed during activity.

Figure 11–2. Sample Frequency Data is a sample data sheet for documenting frequency of behavior. When pencil and paper or digital applications are not a good fit for tallying frequency, alternative means of keeping count must be implemented.

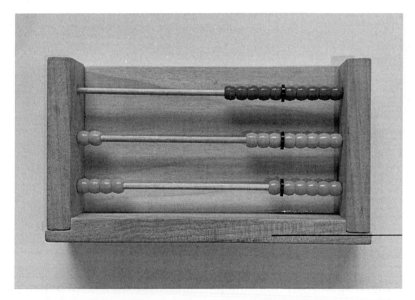

Figure 11–3. Alternative Data Strategy shows an example of a bead tracker, on which one bead is pushed to the other side with each observation of the target behavior, to be documented after the session on a chart or digital graph (original design by Roger Pond).

discontinuous measurement or interval-based recording is much less burdensome (Johnston et al., 2020). A type of discontinuous measurement called momentary time sampling (MTS) requires the least amount of attention from the recorder, thereby making it a viable option for many (Johnston et al., 2020). During MTS, the therapy session is divided into equal intervals (e.g., 30 seconds), and at the end of each interval, the recorder documents whether the behavior is occurring or absent in that moment in time (an example of this can be seen in Figure 11–4). The shorter the intervals, the more accurate the recordings since at the end of the session, MTS is reported via percentage of intervals during which behavior was recorded (Johnston et al., 2020).

Visual Display of Data Over Time

Measurement recordings from one therapy session provide only a small amount of information about behavior on a specific day. In contrast, recording data across sessions provides an opportunity to analyze whether a behavior is increasing or decreasing over time. SLPAs may consider a visual display of data taken over time to allow for faster interpretation when presenting it to their supervising SLP (see Figure 11–5 for an example of data collection across sessions).

ANTECEDENT INTERVENTIONS

Thus far, we have discussed behavior and possible consequences with little time spent discussing what happens first in the A-B-C contingency. An antecedent is any stimulus that immediately precedes

the behavior of interest and may consist of almost any environmental change such as an object, picture, smell, sound, word, phrase, movement, or combination of these (Hegde, 2018). Many antecedents function as models, prompts, or instructions (Hegde, 2018). In clinician-directed therapy sessions, the clinician is responsible for planning and presenting the antecedent event in attempt to evoke a target behavior, as well as providing the consequence once the behavior has been performed.

Antecedent interventions are employed before a behavior and independent of a planned consequence; however, it is important to know the function of the target behavior in order to implement an effective antecedent intervention (Cooper et al., 2020). A few antecedent interventions are provided in Box 11–4 for consideration. These are best implemented through collaboration with a behavior analyst after a functional behavior assessment has been conducted and must be discussed with and ultimately planned by an SLPA's supervising SLP.

POSITIVE BEHAVIORAL INTERVENTIONS AND SUPPORTS

Beyond the use of principles of behavior and antecedent interventions to impact treatment targets, professionals in the field of speech-language pathology participate in an approach known as positive behavioral interventions and supports (PBIS) (Center of PBIS, n.d.-a; Keller-Bell & Short, 2019). PBIS is designed to understand and change behaviors that interfere with successful participation in meaningful and productive activities, including the presence of a wide variety of challenging behaviors such as withdrawal,

Sample Behavior Data Collection- Momentary Time Sampling

Name: Shelby K. **Target Behavior:** sitting on the ground, under the table
SLPA: Jeff P. (Assistant) **Example:** back to therapist, sitting under the table
Start Date: 4/3/22 **Non-example:** standing near chair, leaning on table

Minutes During Session (in 1-minute increments)

Min	4/4/22 9:00am	4/6/22	4/8/22 9:30am	4/11/22 9:30am	4/13/22 11:00am	4/15/22 9:00am	4/18/22	4/20/22 9:30am					
20	11		14	16	16	18		18					
19													
18													
17	-												
16	-		-										
15	-		-			-							
14	-		-										
13	-		-	-									
12	-		-										
11	-					-							
10	-												
9													
8			-			-							
7			-	-		-							
6	-				-								
5					-								
4					-								
2					-								
2													
1		A					U						

Date and Start Time of Session

DIRECTIONS: Document date/time. Set silent timer with vibrating or light signal to quietly alert every minute for 20 minutes. When timer alerts, if behavior is present shade box, if behavior is

Figure 11–4. Sample Data MTS.

Sample Behavior Data Collection: Across Sessions

Name: Marianne P.   **Target Behavior:** one bite of food, chewed, swallowed
SLPA: Kai E.J. (Assistant)   **Example:** one spoonful of puree, swallowed, no spit up
Dates: 5/7/22- 5/13/22   **Non-example:** sip of water through straw, swallowed

Bites Swallowed Per Meal

15							
14							
13							
12							
11							
10							
9							
8							
7							
6							
5							
4							
3							
2							
1	–						
date	5/7/22	5/8/22	5/9/22	5/10/22	5/11/22	5/12/22	5/13/22
start	11:30am	11:40am	11:25am	11:20am	11:30am	11:25am	11:35am
duration	20 minutes	22 minutes	18 minutes	25 minutes	20 mins	21 minutes	19 minutes

Date and Start Time of Session

Directions: Shade one rectangle for each instance of target behavior beginning at the bottom of column. Add hyphen if no occurrences of target behavior were observed during session.

Figure 11–5. Sample data frequency across sessions.

screaming, repetitive behaviors, aggression, tantrums, and self-injury (Bopp et al., 2004; Dunlap, 2005). PBIS is a multitiered approach of evidence-based interventions most commonly implemented by schools to assist staff in proactively addressing behavior to facilitate social and academic success (Horner et al., 2010). Though not a pure behavior analytic approach, the foundations of applied behavior analysis are evidenced in staff training, data collection, early detection, functional behavior assessment, and progress monitoring (Horner et al., 2010).

PBIS has been widely studied for use with individuals with severe developmental disabilities, particularly individuals with autism spectrum disorder (ASD), but it has also been applied to children and adults with other types of

Box 11–4. Antecedent Interventions

1. Provide choices. Providing individuals with a choice regarding the order of two tasks to be completed or a choice between two reinforcers may promote positive behavior (Howell et al., 2019). See photo of an example in Figure 11–6.
2. Make the task smaller. Chunking the task by separating it into smaller assignments or pieces to be completed individually may provide small amounts of escape between smaller tasks (Cooper et al., 2020).
3. Provide the reinforcer more frequently. Delivering the reinforcer that is maintaining the behavior on a schedule that occurs more frequently than the target behavior and without the target behavior occurring is called noncontingent reinforcement (Hagopian et al., 2000). Noncontingent reinforcement has been effective in decreasing an assortment of behavior, for when the individual has access to the reinforcer, the challenging behavior is frequently no longer needed for that function (Berth et al., 2019).
4. Use the high-probability instructional sequence. Deliver two to three brief and easy tasks, prior to a "harder" task request that is generally followed by challenging behavior maintained by escape (Cooper et al., 2020). This sequence has been implemented and effective with a wide range of individuals in a large variety of environments (Cooper et al., 2020).
5. Teach functional communication. Model and reinforce alternative and multimodal forms of communication used to gain access to reinforcers (LaRue et al., 2009).

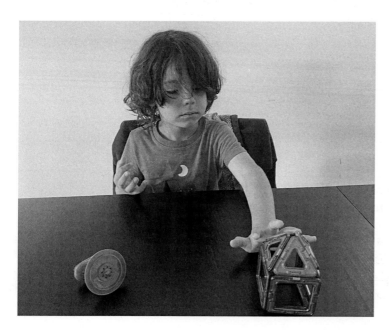

Figure 11–6. Child making choices.

disabilities and individuals without disabilities (Bopp et al., 2004; Dunlap, 2005). When used schoolwide, it is also referred to as schoolwide positive behavior supports (SWPBS) (Horner et al., 2010). PBIS is a person-centered approach (Carr et al., 2002) that focuses on:

1. Modifying specific aspects of the environment to prevent problem behaviors from occurring (antecedent)
2. Teaching new skills to replace problem behaviors (behavior)
3. Using functional consequences to encourage positive behavior (consequence)

PBIS is commonly described with three tiers (Figure 11–7). Tier 1, also known as universal or primary, targets developing a high-quality learning environment for all students. This tier focuses on schoolwide efforts, such as establishing schoolwide classroom standards, collecting data, and facilitating family involvement that encourage expected behaviors and discourage problem behaviors (Horner et al., 2010). Two common examples of supports at this level are schoolwide behavior codes (Figure 11–8) and acknowledgment reward systems (Figure 11–9; Dunlap et al., 2010).

Tier 2, also known as secondary or targeted, is focused on behaviors that interventions and supports have been unsuccessful at addressing in Tier 1. Tier 2 interventions and supports could be instruction in self-regulation and social skills, increased adult supervision, more opportunities for positive reinforcement, and increased access to academic support (Horner et al., 2010). Simple behavioral contacts might also be deployed in Tier 2 (Keller-Bell & Short, 2019) (Figures 11–10, 11–11, and 11–12).

Tier 3, also known as tertiary, is the most intensive and focuses on an individual student and behavior for which both Tier 1 and Tier 2 interventions and supports have been unsuccessful. Any successful techniques from Tier 1 and Tier 2 would continue, but Tier 3 typically includes a formal and individualized functional behavioral assessment (FBA, discussed below) for student-specific challenging behavior (Horner et al., 2010). When completed, the FBA is followed by individualized and often intensive guidance and instruction in using new skills as a replacement for the problem behavior and/or rearrangement of the antecedent environment, including staff behavior, so that problems can be prevented and desirable behaviors encouraged (Keller-Bell & Short, 2019).

Given its person-centered foundations, PBIS is established with an understanding of the "needs, goals, strengths, and preferences of the individual" (Buschbacher & Fox, 2003, p. 218). The concepts of choice, self-determination, and lifestyle enhancement are embedded within all levels of PBIS (p. 218). The essential steps of PBIS, particularly Tier 3 interventions and supports, are presented in Figure 11–13.

As the first step in PBIS illustrates, PBIS is a team effort across all levels of the approach. Studies have shown more positive outcomes for PBIS intervention when team decision-making is employed (Goh & Bambara, 2012). PBIS teams in Tier 3 are individually formed to meet the unique needs of a specific student. Members of the team include first and foremost the individual and his or her family members, as well as individuals who know the student well and who will be implementing interventions and supports (Center of PBIS, n.d.-b).

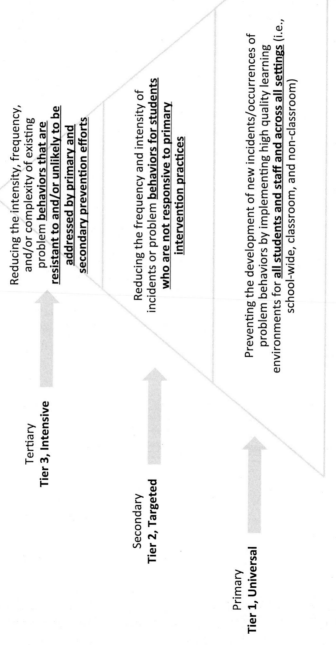

Reducing the intensity, frequency, and/or complexity of existing problem behaviors that are resistant to and/or unlikely to be addressed by primary and secondary prevention efforts

Reducing the frequency and intensity of incidents or problem behaviors for students who are not responsive to primary intervention practices

Preventing the development of new incidents/occurrences of problem behaviors by implementing high quality learning environments for all students and staff and across all settings (i.e., school-wide, classroom, and non-classroom)

Tertiary
Tier 3, Intensive

Secondary
Tier 2, Targeted

Primary
Tier 1, Universal

Figure 11–7. PBIS tiers of intervention and support. Adapted from Center of PBIS (n.d.–b, Tier 3).

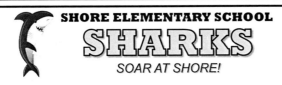

SHORE ELEMENTARY SCHOOL
SHARKS
SOAR AT SHORE!

CLASSROOM EXPECTATIONS

BE RESPECTFUL
Listen to all directions

Use quiet voices

Raise your hand and wait your turn to speak

Be friendly and polite to everyone

BE RESPONSIBLE
Be prepared by bringing all supplies

Follow directions the first time they are given

Complete all assigned tasks

Keep cubbies, desks, and classrooms clean

BE SAFE
Keep your hands, feet, and objects to yourself

Stay in assigned seat

Walk at all times

Figure 11–8. Schoolwide behavior code.

FINS UP!

_____

was being FINtastic!

Issued by: _____ Date: _____

SHORE ELEMENTARY SCHOOL

Figure 11–9. Schoolwide acknowledgment system.

POSITIVE BEHAVIOR CONTRACT

The following is an agreement between _____ and _____.

The student will _____ and the teacher will _____.

The following conditions apply:

1. _____

2. _____

3. _____

This contract is void if the student fails to achieve the goal.

The contract will be reviewed on _____.

Student Signature/Date: _____

Teacher Signature/Date: _____

Figure 11–10. Positive behavior contract (student).

★★★★★★★★★★★ MY CONTRACT ★★★★★★★★★★★★

Name: _____

Date: _____

These are my goals:

1. _____

2. _____

3. _____

These are my consequences if I don't meet my goals:

_____

_____

_____

These are my rewards/positive consequences if I meet my goals:

_____

_____

_____

My contract will be reviewed on: _____

Signatures:

_____

_____

_____

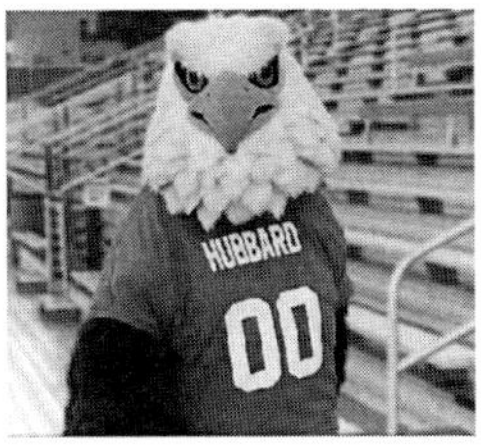

SOAR LIKE AN EAGLE
HUBBARD MIDDLE SCHOOL

Figure 11–11. Positive behavior contract (student).

HOME/SCHOOL BEHAVIOR PLAN

The school and parent(s) agree to support each other, work together, and create consistent expectations for _____ (student's name).

The reason we are developing this plan is because _____ has been having a problem with _____ (behavior in school).

Positive behaviors to be increased:

Behaviors to be decreased:

The school agrees to:

Parent(s) agree to:

When will this plan be explained to the student?

Next meeting date to review progress:

School Staff Signature: _____

Parent(s)/Guardian(s) Signatures: _____

Figure 11–12. Positive behavior contract (home/parent).

Step 1:
- **Team Building and Goal Setting.** Parent/family member involvement and person-centered goal setting

Step 2:
- **Comprehensive Functional Assessment.** Gathering information about the setting and *antecedent-behavior-consequence* chain.

Step 3:
- **Hypothesis Development.** Establishing a best guess as to the function of the behavior.

Step 4:
- **Comprehensive Support Plan.** A comprehensive plan that includes long term supports, prevention strategies, replacement skills, and consequential strategies.

Step 5:
- **Implementation, Data Collection, and Refinement.** Ongoing evaluation and refinement of support plan until objectives achieved.

Figure 11–13. Five essential steps of PBIS. Adapted from Buschbacher and Fox (2003, p. 219).

Other examples of team members include school administrators, teachers, social workers, school psychologists, applied behavioral analysis (ABA) therapists, SLPs, and support personnel such as aides and SLPAs. Though mentioned earlier in this chapter, an ABA therapist is a team member whose role may not be familiar to an SLPA. Box 11–5 contains a description of ABA therapy and the therapists who provide this service. As an SLPA, you might be called upon to collaborate with members of a PBIS team and assist with implementing interventions and supports.

Functional Behavioral Assessment

Before we review a few key PBIS treatment approaches, it is important to discuss the concept of functional behavior assessment (FBA). FBA is an individualized strategy to identify the purpose or function of a challenging behavior so that team members can develop a plan to modify the variable(s) that maintain the behavior and/or teach appropriate replacement behaviors using positive interventions (Cooper et al., 2020). Essentially, FBA is used to better understand the pattern, purpose, and function of a specific behavior by identifying events that precede (antecedents) and follow (consequences) a challenging behavior. It is an integral part of PBIS, especially Tier 3 interventions and supports. It is typically accomplished through (Cooper et al., 2020; Keller-Bell & Short, 2018):

1. Describing the behavior through observing the individual and interviewing those who know the individual to identify the events, times, and situations that give rise to the behavior(s)

and the consequences that seem to maintain the behavior(s)
2. Developing hypotheses to explain these situations and the reinforcers that maintain them
3. Collecting data through direct observation in natural settings to support or refute the hypotheses
4. Conducting a functional analysis by manipulating the variables that were hypothesized to evoke or maintain the behavior
5. Developing a behavior plan based on the findings

As noted in Box 11–5, behavior analysts have specialized training in this area, but FBA, similar to PBIS, is a team effort most commonly led by the behavior analyst or school psychologist. The outcome of FBA is commonly a behavioral intervention plan (BIP). This chapter's appendices contain samples of informal (Appendix 11–C) and more formal (Appendix 11–D) BIPs. It is important to note, however, that the scope and form of BIPs vary greatly, according to the setting and recommendations of the PBIS team. Some essential elements common to any BIP include (Robertson et al., 2020):

1. A plan for directly teaching a specific behavior(s)
2. Prevention strategies to remove or modify the antecedent triggers of the challenging behavior, which may include modifying the behavior of others
3. A planned system for reinforcement when a desired behavior occurs
4. Logical consequences if the undesired or challenging behavior occurs
5. A plan for data collection, progress monitoring, modification of the plan when needed, and generalization

Box 11–5. ABA Therapy and ABA Therapists

What is ABA?

According to ASHA, applied behavior analysis (ABA) is a "systematic application and evaluation of principles of behavior analysis for the improvement of specific behaviors" (ASHA, n.d., para 1), including the use of principles of behavior such as reinforcement, punishment, and extinction (the elimination of undesired behaviors). Common treatment techniques used in ABA therapy include prompting, modeling, chaining, shaping, differential reinforcement, and fading (Cooper et al., 2020).

What is an ABA therapist?

An *ABA therapist* is a general term used to denote an individual who provides ABA therapy. Levels of training and professional certification of those who do so vary, as noted below (Carr & Nosik, 2017):

- **Behavior Technician**
  A behavior technician is an individual who works directly with the client, implementing therapy. Professional credentials can be obtained by an individual with a minimum of a high school diploma who has met the credentialing company's requirements, which may include hours of specialized training and passing a standardized examination. Behavior technicians work under the supervision of behavior analysts to carry out therapy plans and take data on behavior.

- **Assistant Behavior Analyst**
  An assistant behavior analyst is an individual who works in a supportive role in the provision of ABA services. Professional certification can be obtained by an individual with a minimum of an undergraduate degree who meets the certification company's requirements, which may include specialized training, supervised experience, and a certification exam. An assistant behavior analyst cannot provide services alone but can work in therapeutic settings when supervised by someone who is certified at a higher level. They may also supervise behavior technicians.

- **Behavior Analyst**
  A behavior analyst is an individual with a master's-level degree or higher who completes assessments, creates

treatment plans, implements training, and supervises behavior technicians and assistant behavior analysts. Professional certification can be obtained by an individual who meets the certification company's requirements, which may include specialized coursework, supervised experience, and a certification exam. In addition to certification, some states have licensure options and requirements.

As with other aspects of PBIS, you may be asked to participate in specific aspects of a BIP. In doing so, it is critical that you work with your supervising SLP to ensure you have a good foundation in basic behavioral principles and you fully understand the tenets of PBIS in your specific setting and for the individual exhibiting challenging behaviors.

Key Approaches of PBIS

Related treatment approaches used within PBIS include functional communication training (FCT) (Keller-Bell & Short, 2019) and video modeling (Ennis et al., 2017). Given the customized nature of materials needed for these approaches, SLPAs can play a key role in the creation of materials for their supervising SLPs and PBIS team. As an SLPA, you may also be asked to assist in implementation of these techniques.

Functional Communication Training

FCT is a form of PBIS, "designed to reduce problem behaviors by replacing them with meaningful or functional communication—whether verbal or gestural" (Texas Statewide Leadership for Autism, 2009, p. 1). FCT is designed to "teach

socially acceptable communication alternatives to problem behavior" (Bopp et al., 2004, p. 6). The first step in this process is a careful assessment of the meaning or "message(s)" conveyed by a problem behavior and antecedents in the environment related to that behavior (Beukelman & Mirenda, 2013). This is achieved through a detailed and comprehensive assessment, much like FBA, described above, undertaken collaboratively with the client, his or her family, individuals in the client's environment, and related professionals such as the SLP, psychologist, and teacher (Bopp et al., 2004).

Once the message (or meaning of a behavior) is deciphered, the next step is to establish a new and more effective means of conveying that information. This new method must be equivalent in meaning and one that can be conveyed by the client effectively and efficiently in his or her environment. FCT may be used with individuals with a range of communication abilities, including individuals who are unable to use natural speech to meet their daily communicative needs, and thus, augmentative and alternative communication (AAC) is often employed to convey messages through words or short phrases, manual signs, gestures, pictured symbols, or written words (Cooper et al., 2020). Chapter 18 discusses the use of

AAC in greater detail, including elements of AAC systems that may be applicable within FCT.

Once a suitable alternative to a problem behavior is identified, an intervention plan is established. This plan addresses instruction in the use of the new behavior, as well as training and collaboration with individuals in the client's environment to ensure socially meaningful and appropriate consequences are in place to generalize the new behavior to the client's environment (Keller-Bell & Short, 2019). Typically, the intervention plan is systematic in nature and embedded within a BIP and PBIS (although it can also exist as a standalone goal and approach). Generally, it employs several principles of behavior, as well as modeling, shaping, prompting, and differential reinforcement.

Video Modeling

Video modeling is facilitated by technology that uses video recording and display equipment to provide a visual model of a targeted behavioral chain or routine (Franzone & Collet-Klingenberg, 2008). Video models can be used for a specific individual to target a specific challenging behavior or for schoolwide PBIS, such as videos that "teach and raise awareness of school-wide PBIS expectations (e.g., be safe), routines (e.g., walk in the hallway), school engagement (e.g., launch PBIS initiatives), special topics (e.g., cyberbullying), and staff responsibilities (e.g., active supervision on the playground)" (Ennis et al., 2017, p. 1).

There are several forms of video modeling, including basic video modeling, video self-modeling, point-of-view video modeling, and video prompting, and Box 11–6 describes each. Voice-overs can be included to increase comprehen-sion of the video, either as narration (e.g., "I insert 3 quarters into the machine. I select M&Ms by pressing the large button below them") or to describe the target behavior or rule (e.g., "Students in line at the cafeteria keep their hands at their sides and remain standing behind the person in front of them") (Sigafoos et al., 2007). A variety of prompts can be used before, during, or after the video is viewed, as can a series of fading techniques once the student begins to develop the target behaviors (Sigafoos et al., 2007). Each of these decisions (and the type of video to utilize) would be determined by your supervising SLP, the PBIS team, or both. In cases of Tier 3 intervention, the behavioral chain targeted within a video model is established via FBA. The BIP also includes needed details about data collection and monitoring methods for use alongside video modeling (LaCava, 2008). All these factors are critical to the success of video modeling for reducing challenging behaviors (Sigafoos et al., 2007). Figure 11–14 shows a student watching a self-modeling video recorded earlier that day.

BEHAVIOR REFERRALS

Though SLPAs may do their best to implement antecedent interventions and positive reinforcement to increase the client's overall communication skills, there will likely be many behaviors that require the specialized skills of a behavior analyst. When an individual is spending a significant amount of speech-language therapy time engaging in behaviors that interfere with their progress, an SLPA must inform their supervising SLP so the situation may be evaluated and a behavior referral made when appropriate.

Box 11–6. Types of Video Modeling
(Franzone & Collet-Klingenberg, 2008)

Basic Video Modeling

The video displays someone besides the learner engaging in the target behavior or skill.

Video Self-Modeling

The video displays the learner engaging in the target behavior or skill.

Point-of-View Video Modeling

The video displays the target behavior or skill recorded from the perspective of the learner (i.e., as if being viewed through the learner's eyes).

Video Prompting

The video displays the target behavior or skill broken down into steps, using any of the formats about, but a pause is inserted after each step for the client to attempt the step just viewed (before viewing the subsequent steps in the sequence).

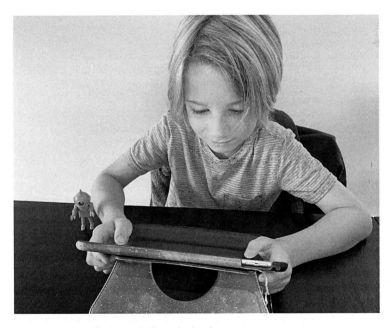

Figure 11–14. Child modeling playback.

If an SLPA believes a client or themselves to be in danger for any reason, this must be reported to the supervising SLP immediately. Safety is the highest priority for all individuals involved in speech-language therapy, especially regarding behavior. Waiting to document data across sessions regarding an unsafe behavior is not warranted at any time. An SLPA should alert their supervising SLP straightaway to begin the referral process for specialized behavior intervention per their occupational setting policies.

REFERENCES

American Speech-Language-Hearing Association. (n.d.). *Applied behavior analysis and communication services.* https://www.asha.org/NJC/Applied-Behavior-Analysis-and-Communication-Services/

American Speech-Language-Hearing Association. (2016). *Scope of practice in speech-language pathology* [Scope of practice]. https://www.asha.org/policy/slpa-scope-of-practice/

American Speech-Language-Hearing Association. (2021). *Interprofessional practice survey results: June 2021.* www.asha.org/research/memberdata/interprofessionalpractice-survey/

American Speech-Language-Hearing Association. (2022). *Speech-language pathology assistant scope of practice* [Scope of practice]. www.asha.org/policy

Association for Behavior Analysis International. (n.d.). *What is behavior analysis?* https://www.abainternational.org/about-us/behavior-analysis.aspx

Berth, D. P., Bachmeyer, M. H., Kirkwood, C. A., Mauzy IV, C. R., Retzlaff, B. J., & Gibson, A., L., (2019). Noncontingent and differential reinforcement in the treatment of pediatric feeding problems. *Journal of Applied Behavior Analysis, 52*(3), 622–641. https://doi.org/10.1002/jaba.562

Beukelman, D., & Mirenda, P. (2013). *Augmentative and alternative communication: Supporting children and adults with complex communication needs* (4th ed.). Brookes.

Bopp, K. D., Brown, K. E., & Mirenda, P. (2004). Speech-language pathologists' roles in the delivery of positive behavior supports for individuals with developmental disabilities. *American Journal of Speech-Language Pathology, 13,* 5–19. https://doi.org/10.1044/1058-0360(2004/003)

Buschbacher, P., & Fox, L. (2003). Understanding and intervening with the challenging behavior of young children with autism spectrum disorders. *Language, Speech, and Hearing Services in Schools, 34*(3), 217–227. https://doi.org/10.1044/ 0161-1461(2003/018)

Cardon, T. (2017). Speech-language pathologists and behavior analysts: Perspectives regarding theories and treatment of autism spectrum disorder. *Perspectives of the ASHA Special Interest Groups SIG 1, 2*(1), 27–46. https://doi.org/10.1044/persp2.SIG1.27

Carr, E. G., Dunlap, G., Horner, R. H., Koegel, R. L., Turnbull, A. P., Sailor, W., . . . Fox, L. (2002). Positive behavior support: Evolution of an applied science. *Journal of Positive Behavior Intervention, 4,* 4–16. https://doi.org/10.1177/109830070200400102

Carr, J. E. & Nosik, M. R. (2017). Professional credentialing of practicing behavior analysts. *Policy Insights from the Behavioral and Brain Sciences, 4*(1), 3–8. https://doi.org/10.1177/2372732216685861

Center of PBIS: Positive Behavioral Intervention and Supports. (n.d.-a). *What is PBIS?* https://www.pbis.org/pbis/what-is-pbis

Center of PBIS: Positive Behavioral Intervention and Supports. (n.d.-b). *Tier 3.* https://www.pbis.org/pbis/tier-3.

Cooper, J. O., Heron, T. E., & Heward, W. L. (2020). *Applied behavior analysis* (3rd ed.). Pearson Education.

Curtis, P. R., Frey, J. R., Watson, C. D., Hampton, L. H., & Roberts, M. Y. (2018). Language disorders and problem behaviors: A meta-analysis. *Pediatrics, 142*(2), 1–14. https://doi.org/10.1542/peds.2017-3551

Deliperi, P., Vladescu, J. C., Reeve, K. F., Reeve, S. A., & DeBar, R. M. (2015). Training staff to implement a paired-stimulus preference assessment using video modeling with voiceover instruction. *Behavioral Interventions, 30*(4), 314–332. https://doi.org/10.1002/bin.1421

Dozier, C. L., Foley, E. A., Goddard, K. S., & Jess, R. L. (2020). *The encyclopedia of child and adolescent development: Behavior in childhood—behav-*

ior principles and processes (Vol. 2). John Wiley & Sons. https://doi.org/10.1002/9781119171492.wecad062

Dunlap, G. (2005). Positive behavior supports: An overview. *Perspectives on Language Learning and Education, 12,* 3–6. https://doi.org/10.1044/lle12.1.3

Dunlap, K., Goodman, S., McEvoy Wayne, C., & Paris, F. (2010). *School-wide behavioral supports and intervention: Implementation guide.* http://www.ccresa.org/Files/Uploads/348/Positive_Behavior_Support_Impl.pdf

Ennis, R. P., Hirsch, S. E., MacSuga-Gage, A. S., & Kennedy M. J. (2017). Positive behavioral interventions and supports in pictures: Using videos to support schoolwide implementation. *Preventing School Failure: Alternative Education for Children and Youth, 62*(1), 1–12. https://doi.org/0.1080/1045988X.2017.1287048

Franzone, E., & Collet-Klingenberg, L. (2008). *Overview of video modeling.* National Professional Development Center on Autism Spectrum Disorders, Waisman Center, University of Wisconsin.

Goh, A. E., & Bambara, L. M. (2012). Individualized positive behavior support in school settings: A meta-analysis. *Remedial and Special Education, 33*(5), 271–286. https://doi.org/10.1177/0741932510383990

Hagopian, L. P., Crockett, J. L., van Stone, M., DeLeon, I. G., & Bowman, L. G. (2000). Effects of noncontingent reinforcement on problem behavior and stimulus engagement: The role of satiation, extinction, and alternative reinforcement. *Journal of Applied Behavior Analysis, 33*(4), 433–449. https://doi.org/10.1901/jaba.2000.33-433

Hagopian, L. P., Long, E. S., & Rush, K. S. (2004). Preference assessment procedures for individuals with developmental disabilities. *Behavior Modification, 28*(5), 668–677. https://doi.org/10.1177/0145445503259836

Hegde, M. N. (1998). *Treatment procedures in communicative disorders* (3rd ed.). Pro-Ed.

Hegde, M. N. (2018). *Hegde's pocketguide to treatment in speech-language pathology* (4th ed.). Plural Publishing.

Horner, R. H., Sugai, G., & Anderson, C. M. (2010). Examining the evidence base of school-wide positive behavior support. *Focus on Exceptional Children, 42*(8), 1–14. https://doi.org/10.17161/fec.v42i8.6906

Howell, M., Dounavi, K., & Storey, C. (2019). To choose or not to choose? A systematic literature review considering the effects of antecedent and consequence choice upon on-task and problem behaviour. *Review Journal of Autism and Developmental Disorders, 6,* 63–84. https://doi.org/10.1007/s40489-018-00154-7

Johnston, J. M., Pennypacker, H. S., & Green, G. (2020). *Strategies and tactics of behavioral research and practice* (4th ed.). Routledge.

Keller-Bell, Y., & Short, M. (2019). Positive behavioral interventions and supports in schools: A tutorial. *Language, Speech, and Hearing Services in Schools, 50,* 1–15. https://doi.org/10.1044/2018_LSHSS-17-0037

LaCava, P. (2008). *Video modeling: An online training module. (Kansas City: University of Kansas, Special Education Department).* Ohio Center for Autism and Low Incidence (OCALI), Autism Internet Modules. http://www.autisminternetmodules.org

LaRue, R., Weiss, M. J., & Cable, M. K. (2009). Functional communication training: The role of speech pathologists and behavior analysts in serving students with autism. *The Journal of Speech and Language Pathology–Applied Behavior Analysis, 3*(2–3), 164–172. https://doi.org/10.1037/h0100244

Leaf, J. B., Cihon, J. H., Leaf, R., McEachin, J., Liu, N., Russell, N., . . . Khosrowshahi, D. (2022). Concerns about ABA-based intervention: An evaluation and recommendations. *Journal of Autism Developmental Disorders, 52*(6), 2838–2853. https://doi.org/10.1007/s10803-021-05137-y

Maul, C. A., Findley, B. R., & Nicolson-Adams, A. (2016). *Behavioral principles in communicative disorders: Applications to assessment and treatment.* Plural Publishing.

Robertson, R. E., Kokina, A. A., & Moore, D. W. (2020). Barriers to implementing behavior intervention plans: Results of a statewide survey. *Journal of Positive Behavior Interventions, 22*(3), 145–155. https://doi.org/10.1177/1098300720908013

Roth, F., & Paul, R. (2007). Communication intervention. In R. Paul & P. Cascella (Eds.), *Introduction to clinical methods in communication disorders* (pp. 157–178). Brookes.

Roth, F. R., & Worthington, C. K. (2001). *Treatment resource manual for speech-language pathology.* Delmar.

Sigafoos, J., O'Reilly, M., & de la Cruz, B. (2007). *How to use video modeling and video prompting.* Pro-Ed.

Texas Statewide Leadership for Autism. (2009). *Texas guide for effective teaching: Functional communication training.* https://www.gvsu.edu/ cms4/asset/64CB422AED08-43F0-F795CA9D E364B6BE/functionalcommunication.pdf

World Health Organization. (2010). *Framework for action on interprofessional education and collaborative practice.* http://www.who.int/hrh/ resources/framework_action/en

APPENDIX 11–A

PREFERENCE CHECKLIST

Name of client:_____

Client identifier:_____

Date:_____

Completed by:_____

Relationship to client:_____

Directions: Circle known preferences of client. If preference is not listed, write in box labeled "Other." Add additional notes when needed.

Social Preferences

High five	Eye gaze	Smile	Other:
Knuckle bump	Head nod	Cheer	
Thumbs up	Whistle	Sing	

Tangible and Activity Preferences

Toy	Change seat	Draw	Other:
Art supply	Movement break	iPad time	
Book	Ball game	Outside	

Sensory Preferences

Bubbles	Music	Swing	Other:
Playdoh	Chewing gum	Spin	
Squishy ball	Smelly pencil	Squeeze	

Edible Preferences

Fruit	Gummy	Juice	Other:
Cracker	Cookie	Cold drink	
Pretzel	Bar	Candy	

Additional Notes:

APPENDIX 11–B

Preference Interview

Name of client:_____   **Completed by:**_____

Client identifier:_____   **Relationship to client:**_____

Date:_____   **Directions:** Fill out interview to provide team with preferences. Add additional notes when needed.

A few of my favorite

toys are: movies/shows are: characters are:

I really enjoy spending time with

these people: at these places: doing these activities:

I never want to stop

watching: listening to: doing these activities:

I do not like

When I don't like something I _____

APPENDIX 11–C

Behavior Intervention Plan

Name__Liz Schoolhouse_____   Start Date____10/5/15_____

Behavior	Liz is always blurting out in class.
Function	The function of Liz's behavior is to seek attention. She gets little attention from her classmates and has few friends.
Desired Behavior	Liz will raise her hand for permission to speak and wait for the teacher to call on her.
Proactive Plan	Liz will use a cool points chart that will allow her to self-monitor her blurting out. The chart will be checked each hour and reinforcement will be awarded contingent upon points earned. Give verbal praise each time Liz does not blurt out.
Reactive Plan	If Liz begins to blurt out, behavior will be ignored the first 2 times. After that, the teacher will correct Liz by reminding her of the appropriate behavior.
Reinforcers	A reinforcer, iPad B reinforcer, dolls C reinforcer, M&Ms
Data Collection	Cool point charts will be used as data for number of blurt outs and graphed on a frequency chart. If no progress after 2 weeks, plan will be modified.
Notes	

Behavior Intervention Plan

I. Description of targeted behavior

*Describe the behavior. What does the behavior look like?
*Identify frequency (how often it occurs), intensity (how severe is it), and/or the duration (how long the behavior lasts).

Sample

John's targeted behaviors include yelling out, screaming, making loud disruptive noises, hiding in the corner and/or running out of the classroom and around the campus.

Data taken 3/03/15 – 03/13/15
Frequency – John displayed non-compliant behaviors 7/10 days. According to frequency data collected daily for 10 days, the percentage of non-compliant behaviors displayed ranged from 40% to 100% of John's school day.

Intensity – All behaviors range from mild to moderate, with no severe incidences.

2. Functional Behavior Assessment Data

Setting:
*Where does the behavior occur? Is it a particular class, time of day, recess, bus, when child is tired?

Sample

The behaviors occur during instruction and written assignments in the self-contained classroom and during lunch.

Antecedents:
*What happens just before the behavior occurs? What triggers the behavior?

Sample

Behaviors occur when student is not allowed to change the rules or make up his own assignments, when asked to follow directions, when he does not like the lunch choices.

Function:
*What is the student trying to achieve? What are they getting or avoiding?

Sample

John exhibits these behaviors to seek control and get what he wants.

3. Replacement Behaviors (Task Analysis)

*Identify the positive behavior that will be taught to replace the negative behavior. This must be related to the function.

Sample

John will be taught to follow directions by the special education teacher through direct instruction, modeling, non-verbal cues, and practicing for at least 15 minutes, 3 times a week. He will be taught the following steps:

1. Wait patiently for the directions before beginning an activity.
2. Listen carefully to the directions given.
3. Follow the directions given, while staying calm.

4. Proactive Strategies (Individualized Positive Behavior Change Strategies)

*What positive supports will be used to encourage the replacement behavior?
*What accommodations/modifications will be made to support the student? (examples)

Sample

Use a token board reward system with John each time one of the replacement behaviors occurs.
Allow John opportunities to make up his own directions contingent upon earning his tokens.
Provide immediate positive feedback.
Provide positive teacher attention when John is following directions.
Do not focus on work completion, but reinforce following directions. Ex. Do not say,
"Good job, you finished your work." Say, "Good job, thank you for following directions" or "John, I like the way you handled that situation."

5. Positive Strategies to Modify the Environment

*What environmental supports will be used to promote the replacement behavior (seating, calm down area, room arrangement, signs)?

Sample

Display rules and expectations for following directions and review them daily.
Tape a visual reminder of the replacement behaviors on the corner of John's desk.
Provide John with a designated calm down area and a calm down kit for when he is having a difficult time following directions.

6. Reactive Strategies

*What strategies will be used when behaviors occur (prompting, loss of points, de-escalating strategies)?

Sample

Ignore minimally disruptive behaviors (planned ignoring)
Give John two choices - the first should be following directions and a reminder of the reinforcement, the second should be the inappropriate behavior and a reminder of the consequence. Give choices calmly and walk away.
Remind John of calming strategies and calm down area.
If behaviors become too disruptive to other students, TA 1 will take the students to Mrs. Wright's room while the teacher and TA 2 remain in the classroom with John.

7. Progress Monitoring

* How will progress be monitored and data collected to ensure effectiveness of the behavior plan?
*Who will collect the data?
* How often will it be collected?
* How and when will the data be reviewed (informal meeting, telephone, IEP meeting)?

Sample

The special education teacher or staff will collect data randomly throughout the week during 10 different directives, charting compliance or non-compliance.
Data will be analyzed and reviewed every two weeks by the special education teacher.
Continue with each "following directions" step in the task analysis until all steps are mastered.
The special education teacher and John's mother can make mutually agreed minor adjustments to the behavior plan via phone as needed.

8. Intervention Outcome Process

*Identify start and review dates
*Note data here

Sample

The behavior plan will begin on _____ and the special education teacher and John's parent will review the plan on _____.

CHAPTER 12

Group Therapy

Jennifer A. Ostergren and Sarah Guzzino-Herrick

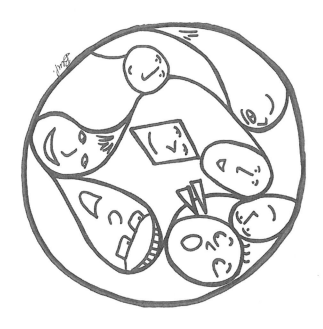

Unity is strength . . . when there is teamwork and collaboration, wonderful things can be achieved.

—Mattie Stepanek (nationally recognized poet and peace advocate. Mattie died at age 13 of complications related to dysautonomic mitochondrial myopathy, a rare form of muscular dystrophy.)

As has been mentioned, you may be asked to provide treatment services under the supervision and guidance of your supervising speech-language pathologist (SLP) (American Speech-Language-Hearing Association [ASHA], 2022). These services may be delivered to a single individual or to a small group of individuals (Cas-cella et al., 2007). Provision of treatment services to small groups of individuals is common in a variety of settings, including school settings for children (Mire, 2007) and medical and community settings for adults (Elman, 2007). Chapter 10 shares ideas for implementing treatment services that are applicable to both individual and group treatment models. The sections that follow focus on the unique aspects of group models of treatment that warrant additional consideration.

The purpose of group treatment varies (Roth & Worthington, 2001) but can include the following:

1. Teaching participants a new communication skill at an introductory level
2. Providing participants with practice in skills established in an individual session
3. Providing participants with socialization, self-help, and/or counseling

Not all groups are appropriate for a speech-language pathology assistant (SLPA) to lead. For example, groups in which counseling and adjustment is the primary (or secondary) purpose would not be appropriate for implementation by an SLPA. Group intervention can occur concurrently with individual sessions or as the sole source of intervention (Roth & Worthington, 2001). It may be provided early, late, or throughout the client's course of treatment. In some cases, group sessions will comprise individuals with similar skills, abilities, and intervention goals, whereas in other instances, group members will be individuals with diverse skills, abilities, and intervention goals (Elman, 2007; Luterman, 2008; Moon-Meyer, 2004). Groups can range in size from as small as two individuals to as large as an entire classroom, as may be the case in community-based groups or in the case of a self-contained classroom in a school setting (Cascella et al., 2007; Elman, 2007). A self-contained classroom is common for students with special needs. Self-contained classrooms place a small group of pupils with special needs with generally one instructor (often assisted

by paraprofessionals) for most of the day (Mattinson, 2011; Schubert & Baxter, 1982; Walker, 2009).

The role of the clinician during group treatment can be directive or nondirective (Roth & Worthington, 2001), based on the purpose of the group. In the case of a directive model, the clinician "sets the agenda, chooses the materials and activities, provides specific instruction, and gives corrective feedback" (Roth & Worthington, 2001, p. 25). In a nondirective role, the group members participate in these activities and the clinician serves as a facilitator in helping group members to accomplish the group's goal(s). An example of a nondirective group model is that of peer-mediated groups. According to Carter and Kennedy (2006), peer-mediated support interventions involve equipping one or more peers, without disabilities, to provide ongoing social and/or academic support to special needs peers of a similar age, under the guidance of educators, paraprofessionals, or other school staff. This intervention is thought to promote independence, due to the students involved becoming more acquainted with working together and leading their own progress. This support arrangement consists of the following: identifying students with a disability and their peers who would benefit from involvement, equipping peers to provide support, arranging opportunities for students to interact and support one another, and monitoring and offering guidance when needed (McCauley & Prelock, 2013).

In any form, clinicians working with groups maintain responsibility for ensuring that group dynamics and communication among group members support a positive learning and social environment for all members. Similar to individual sessions, group treatment activities should be driven by a specific set of goals, applicable to either individual group members or a collective group goal, shared by all members.

Table 12–1 contains a list of several advantages and disadvantages of group treatment. As with any aspect of treatment, your supervising SLP will weigh the advantages and disadvantages of group treatment in deciding when and if it is applicable to a client's needs (ASHA, 2022). She or he will also be responsible for establishing the size, composition, and purpose of group intervention, as well as recommending group activities to target treatment goals.

Moon-Meyer (2004) coined an important term: "therapy in a group" (p. 262). This warrants additional consideration, in contrast with group therapy. According to Moon-Meyer, *therapy in a group* is not the same as *group therapy*. Rather, therapy in a group employs the same tenets of an individual session but with multiple clients present. As an example, consider a small group of third graders in a school setting with the following treatment goals:

- John has a treatment goal targeting /r/ sounds in the final position of words.
- Sue has a treatment goal targeting the reduction of disfluencies in conversational speech.
- Bill has a social interaction and pragmatic treatment goal.

Using a therapy in a group model, time is split between each individual in targeting treatment goals. When John is practicing /r/ sounds in words, the clinician interacts with him, providing feedback and correction to shape accurate production of target words. While this occurs, Sue and Bill wait for their turn. Next, Sue receives the clinician's attention, practicing fluent speech in short nar-

Table 12–1. Advantages and Disadvantages of Group Therapy

Advantages of Group Therapy	Disadvantages of Group Therapy
• Group participants may motivate each other or offer insight and assistance that a clinician cannot readily provide.	• Individual participants may receive less direct attention from the clinician.
• More opportunities exist for natural speaking situations, socialization, and peer interactions. This may enhance carryover and generalization of a target behavior.	• Some participants may be reluctant to participate fully in group interactions, particularly those who are shy or self-conscious.
• Participants have an opportunity to observe group members and may recognize that others have problems similar to their own.	• Some participants may monopolize group interactions.
• Group interactions, especially when the clinician takes a nondirective role; may decrease dependence of the clinician and thereby increase client independence.	• Generally, there are fewer opportunities per participant, per increment of time, to engage in a specific behavior (compared with individual sessions). This may mean fewer opportunities to address specific weaknesses and less direct practice of a specific skill.
	• The pace of the group (or the rate of progress) may not be exactly matched with each participant.

Source: Roth and Worthington, 2007, p. 26.

ratives. Again, the clinician focuses her attention on Sue, while John and Bill now wait. Finally, it is Bill's turn, and the clinician turns her efforts to discussing sample scenarios of appropriate and inappropriate personal space diagrams, while group members John and Sue now wait. As you can see from this interaction, there is very little interaction between the group members themselves, as well as a reduction in the total amount of interaction each group member has with the clinician. This is problematic, particularly when you consider the amount of treatment received per the amount of participation. If this were, for example, a 30-minute session, each participant would have received roughly 10 minutes of treatment and 20 minutes of waiting. This is not group therapy. None of the advantages of group therapy (described above) could be realized with this model (e.g., group participants motivated by each other, group participants engaging in natural speaking situations), but all of the disadvantages are magnified (e.g., less direct attention from the clinician, fewer opportunities to practice). In this instance, a group member's time is better spent engaging in other activities and attending only an individual session with the clinician for 10 minutes.

As this example shows, the main distinguishing feature of group therapy and that of therapy in a group is interaction, both between the clients and with the clinician. In terms of client interactions, Moon-Meyer (2004) outlines two types of interaction that should be considered: non-goal-related interaction and goal-related interaction. With non-goal-related interaction, as the name suggests, the interaction between clients does not target the treatment goal, as in the case of waiting their turn or performing tasks not related to their treatment goal. In contrast, goal-directed interactions target each of the client's treatment goals. Maximizing the amount of goal-directed interaction should always be your primary goal during group sessions. This, of course, is easiest when individuals share a similar goal, but with careful planning, group therapy and maximum goal-directed interaction can also be achieved when individuals do not share similar goals.

CHARACTERISTICS OF EFFECTIVE GROUP DYNAMICS

The term *effectiveness* refers to "the extent to which a specific intervention, regimen, or service, when deployed in routine practice, does what it is intended to do" (Baum, 1998, p. 237, cited in Last, 1983). Travis (1957) outlined five characteristics that aid in effective group dynamics, including creating a positive atmosphere, facilitating observation, making tools available, providing opportunities for repeated experiences, and helping to reduce barriers. Each is a factor to consider in designing and/or modifying the dynamics of a group treatment session.

In creating a *positive atmosphere*, as an SLPA, you must demonstrate acceptance, respect, and belonging for each individual. This process may be implemented through your behaviors of speech, facial expressions, postures, and so forth, which should all communicate a positive and welcoming attitude toward group members. This will set the foundation for group interaction. In addition, you must be conscious of the fact that the world is viewed differently by others. Therefore, not projecting your own attitudes on the group will benefit the group atmosphere. Furthermore, allowing group members to participate in selecting and planning activities will influence this as well and create a sense of belonging within that group.

By exhibiting these behaviors and attitudes, you also promote the next characteristic of an effective group dynamic: facilitating observation. This means that you assume that group members will be influenced by the behavior(s) they observe, both your behavior and those of the other group members. One issue in this area is placing undue pressure on a group member to respond. You can be mindful of how you introduce group activities and what will be required of group members. You want to ensure the group dynamic is such that group members can participate with ease and pleasure. In addition, as much as possible, use naturally occurring, intrinsic rewards over artificial rewards (such as tokens or "good work"). In educational settings, it is common for students to become influenced by their group members, especially if those members seem to be doing better than them (Travis, 1957). For example, when a student struggles to produce a target utterance, this may create anxiety within the student, especially when she observes overt and artificial praise given to other students. This may decrease future participation in group activities.

The third characteristic of effective group therapy dynamics is making tools available. Use of the proper tools to complement the group and individual goal(s) is critical. You can plan in advance of group sessions by listing the materials needed to implement group treatment. This information can be listed on the lesson plan for that session (see Chapter 7). You should make sure all materials are modified to meet each group member's abilities and that there are ample materials, accessible to all members. You will want to ensure, however, that emphasis is on the interactions of group members and the goals of the group session. Chapter 10 discusses the concept of the "game mirage" (Moon-Meyer, 2004). This applies to groups as well. You can avoid the game mirage and reinforce goals of group treatment by providing an introduction to the session, stating the goals to be targeted, elaborating on them during the session, and then concluding with a summary of the group session (Vinson, 2009, p. 310).

Opportunities for repeated experience is also a characteristic of effective group dynamics. This does not mean learning will take place solely through repetition of an activity, as discussed in Chapter 10, relative to clinician-directed treatment that employs drill activities. It does mean, though, that group dynamics and learning are enhanced through opportunities to practice skills with diverse peers who may differ in gender, age, and status (e.g., authority figure vs. peer).

Reducing barriers is the final factor to consider in ensuring a positive group dynamic. This can vary greatly but would include the group leader analyzing factors that impeded the effectiveness of the group, the group dynamics, or group learning. In the field of augmentative and alternative communication (AAC), researchers describe barriers that may impede the use of AAC. These principles can also be applied to group dynamics as well and include opportunity barriers and access barriers (Beukelman & Mirenda, 2005). Opportunity barriers are factors outside the individual that may affect the individual or group dynamics. Three opportunity barriers that may be particularly relevant to your work as an SLPA in group sessions are skills, attitude, and knowledge barriers. These pertain to having the skills and knowledge needed to be effective in a group situation and your attitude toward group situations. If any of these are areas of concern, you can work with your supervising SLP to ensure you have the adequate skills, abilities, and attitudes to successfully run a group session. Access barriers relate to "the capacities, attitudes, and resources" of the individual, including "a lack of ability or difficulty with manipulation and management of objects, problems with cognitive function and decision making, literacy problems, and/or sensory-perceptual impairments (i.e., vision or hearing impairments)" (Roth & Worthington, 2001, p. 116). Here, too, you can work with your supervising SLP to identify any barriers in these areas applicable to group members and their participation in group treatment.

SAMPLE GROUP ACTIVITIES

The activities used in group sessions are a vehicle for obtaining specific goals and can vary greatly, per the group's purpose. As discussed in Chapter 7, lesson plans serve the purpose of directing specific ele-

ments of a given session, such as the goals to be targeted, materials to be used, potential prompts or assistance, and data collection methods. Carefully prepared and detailed lesson plans for group treatment sessions will serve a similar purpose.

Although an extensive review of all applicable activities used within group treatment sessions, across the multitude of settings and clients an SLPA may serve, is beyond the scope of this chapter, Table 12–2 contains a sampling of activities for children. Box 12–1 contains a list of suggested activities for adults.

In addition, Chapters 13 and 16 also contain additional examples of treatment activities that can be adapted to group dynamics. Ideas for activities can also be found in resources devoted to group approaches for specific age groups or disorders. For example, *Group Treatment of Neurogenic Communication Disorders: The Expert Clinician's Approach* (Elman, 2007) provides a comprehensive review of group treatment approaches for individuals with neurogenic disorders, such as aphasia, traumatic brain injury, and dementia. Similarly, *Group Treatment for Asperger Syndrome: A Social Skills Curriculum* (Adams, 2006) provides a valuable resource in the area of group treatment for Asperger syndrome. A sample of activities suggested by Adams (2006) for social skills is listed in Appendix 12–A.

Table 12–2. Sample Group Activities for Children

Activity	Suggested Target Area(s)
Shared book reading, card games such as Go Fish, board games, and Tic-Tac-Toe (Figure 12–1) using target sounds	Articulation
Shared reading activities, story retelling rope (Figure 12–2), and comic strips (Figure 12–3)	Language comprehension, verbal expression, writing, WH-questions
Venn diagrams (Figure 12–4) and visual aids, comparing and contrasting topics like sports, foods, presidents, holidays, and so forth	Curriculum-based information, language comprehension, language expression, vocabulary, same/different, narrative writing
Theme-based art and creative endeavors, such as coloring, crafts, and building projects	Following directions, sequencing, vocabulary, and verbal expression
Obstacle course and building activities	Prepositions
Hangman	Spelling
Treasure or scavenger hunts, conversational ladder (Figure 12–5), conversational starter cards (e.g., If you could have any superhero powers, what would they be? What would you buy if you won a million dollars? If you could invent a video game, what would it be like?), off-campus outings, and role-play (e.g., student becomes the teacher)	Verbal expression, stuttering and disfluency, and social skills

Tic-Tac-Toe

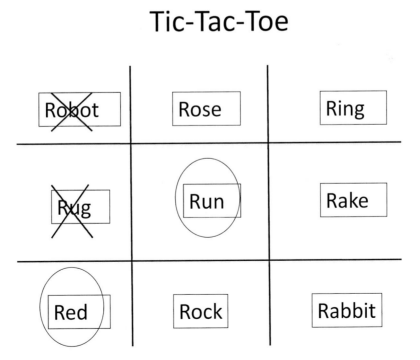

Figure 12–1. Sample group activity: Tic-Tac-Toe with target words.

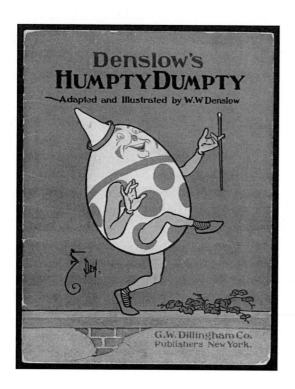

START

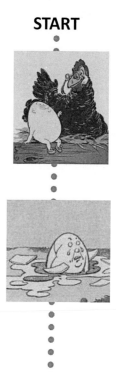

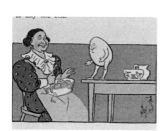

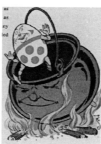

FINISH

Figure 12–2. Sample group activity: Story retelling rope, using Denslow's Humpty Dumpty. Group members engage in a shared book reading and then retell the story, placing images from the book along a rope to guide retelling. Images in the public domain. Courtesy of U.S. Library of Congress Rare Book and Special Collections Division.

Comic strip

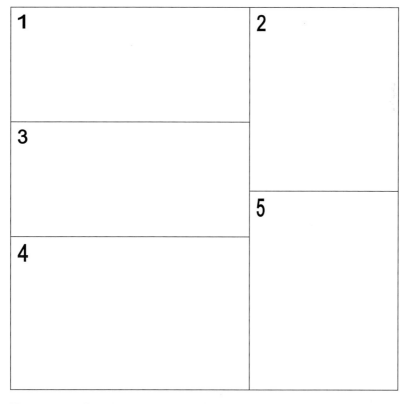

Figure 12–3. Sample group activity: Comic strip. Group members create and tell a story by drawing images in the comic strip boxes or using the provided images, arranged and placed in the boxes.

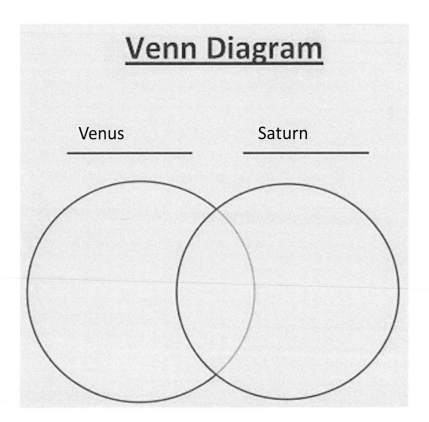

Venn Diagram

Venus
_____

Saturn
_____

1. How many moons does each planet have?
2. What is the planet made of?
3. How many rings does the planet have?

Figure 12–4. Sample group activity: Venn diagram. Group members discuss attributes of related/unrelated items.

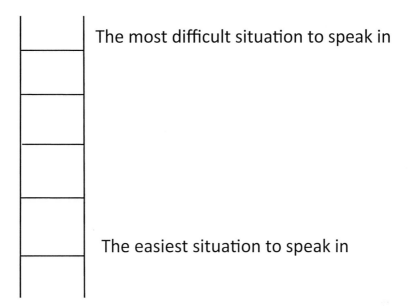

The most difficult situation to speak in

The easiest situation to speak in

Figure 12–5. Sample group activity: Conversation ladder. Group members rank and discuss contrasting concepts (e.g., easiest/most difficult speaking situations, most/least favored activity in school, etc.).

Box 12–1. Suggested Activities for Adult Groups

- Role-play real-life activities, using communication strategies, conflict resolution, self-advocacy techniques, and so forth
- Charades-based activities using gestures, drawing, writing, and description
- Facilitated discussion centered on favorite activities/hobbies, recent events, strategy use, problem solving, and so forth
- Performance, either impromptu (e.g., group script reading) or group activities centered on a specific performance (e.g., putting on a play for family, friends, community members)
- Poem reading, either impromptu or planned
- Community outings to practice daily living skills (e.g., money use, conversations with strangers, map reading, effective medical visits)
- Team activities, such as scavenger hunts, building activities, board or card games, cooking activities, and so forth
- A movie club centered on having facilitated discussion about selected movies watched by group members
- A book club centered on reading a book and facilitated discussion about its content

APPLYING CLASSROOM MANAGEMENT PRINCIPLES TO GROUP TREATMENT

In the field of education, teachers commonly work with groups of students, using techniques known as classroom management techniques. These are a set of principles that involve the actions of the teacher "to create a learning environment that encourages positive social interaction, active engagement in learning, and self-motivation" (Burden, 2006, p. 4). Many of these principles are also applicable to the services SLPs and SLPAs provide during group treatment. Research in this area suggests that several key factors underlie effective teaching and positively functioning classroom environments (Parsonson, 2012, p. 17), as follows:

1. Clear, simple rules and expectations that are consistently and fairly applied.
As an SLPA, it will be important for you to establish the rules of the group session. An example of applicable rules for children may be the following (Adams, 2006, p. 9):

- Raise your hands before you talk.
- Keep good eye contact.
- Listen when others are talking.
- Take turns talking about topics of interest.
- Use your inside voice.

These can be modified for adults as well. It is important to inform members of the rules at a level appropriate to the age, abilities, and purpose of the group. For young children, this may mean posting something in the group environment, similar to Figure 12–6, and then reviewing this information at the beginning of each session and as needed, given any potential rule violations.

2. Predictable events and routines, including cues and signals about upcoming activities.
Chapters 10 and 11 discus similar concepts in the area of visual schedules. The samples of visual schedules provided in Chapters 10 and 11 can be adapted to represent the agenda of activities planned for a group session. For adult, literate clients, this can be accomplished by providing a written agenda for group sessions, similar to those used in business meetings. You can also maintain consistency in the design of group sessions by starting each session with a consistent opening activity, such as greetings and updates, followed by a core activity (that changes on a regular basis) and then a consistent closing activity. After a few sessions, as applicable, clients can begin to actively participate (or even lead) these opening and closing activities.

3. Frequent use of specific and descriptive praise, including verbal and nonverbal praise.
Chapters 10 and 11 provide a thorough discussion of operant conditioning and positive behavioral supports, both of which are applicable to the use of reinforcement and praise. The section on the effective use of operant principles provides several helpful examples of descriptive versus evaluative praise and effective reinforcement techniques. In the area of classroom management, Bradley et al. (2006) also suggest that teachers know their students and their personalities, motives, and desires as an important factor in the use of praise and reinforcement. This is good advice for SLPAs as well.

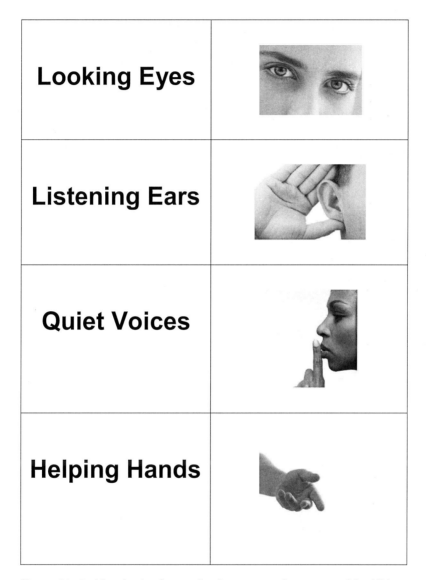

Figure 12–6. Visual rules for posting in group environments with children. Images courtesy of Microsoft Corporation © 2013.

Relative to disruptive behaviors, researchers in the area of classroom management specifically warn against the use of any of the teacher behaviors listed in Box 12–2 in response to disruptive student behavior. Instead, when student behaviors become disruptive, a Three-Step Response Plan is recommended in classroom settings (Burden, 2006; Figure 12–7). This plan employs the principles of least intervention, which states that "when dealing with routine classroom behavior, misbehavior should be corrected with the simplest, least intrusive intervention that will work" (Slavin, 2006, as cited in Burden, 2006, p. 215). Each of these suggestions can also be used by SLPAs during group sessions to restore order when disruptive behavior is present.

4. Matching tasks to the skills and abilities of the learners.

Box 12–2. Behaviors to Avoid in Response to Disruptive Behavior (Burden, 2006)

1. Harsh and humiliating reprimands
2. Threats
3. Nagging
4. Forced apologies
5. Sarcastic remarks
6. Group punishment
7. Assigning extra work
8. Reducing grades
9. Writing as punishment
10. Physical labor or exercise
11. Corporal punishment

STEP 1
SITUATIONAL ASSISTANCE
Help the student cope with the situation and keep the student on task.

Sample Teacher Actions:
• Remove distracting objects
• Reinforce desired behavior
• Boost interest
• Provide assistance
• Redirect behavior
• Modify environment

STEP 2
MILD RESPONSE
Use non-punishing actions to help the student return to the task.

Sample Teacher Actions:
• Ignore the behavior
• Use nonverbal cues (e.g., eye gaze, facial expression, etc.)
• Call on the student to respond/answer a question
• Give reminder of class rules or verbal reprimand
• Ask, "What should you be doing?"

STEP 3
MODERATE RESPONSE
Remove desired stimulus to decrease unwanted behavior.

Sample Teacher Actions:
• Withdraw privileges
• Change seating
• Place student in time-out
• Contact parents
• Have student visit the principle

Figure 12–7. Illustration of a three-step response for addressing disruptive behavior in group settings. Adapted from Burden (2006, p. 220).

In the field of education, this is known as differentiated instruction and is achieved when the teacher accommodates student differences in "readiness levels, interests, and learning profiles," thereby achieving an optimum learning environment for all learners (Subban, 2006, p. 940). Matching tasks to group members' skills and abilities also reduces frustration and/or boredom, which is often associated with disruptive behavior (Parsonson, 2012).

SLPs are generally very good at achieving differentiated instruction when given an individual treatment session. The key is to maintain this same level of differentiation during group sessions. This requires careful planning. Just as teachers plan for their classroom activities, SLPAs must also plan carefully and work with the supervising SLP to ensure an effective lesson plan is in place for each group session. In fact, as discussed in Chapter 7, the idea of lesson planning is borrowed from the field of education and the research surrounding classroom management. Remember that one element of an effective lesson plan includes ways to modify tasks, if needed. To do this in a timely fashion requires that you carefully observe group member behavior and implement modification, as needed, during group sessions. Using effective data collection is also important as this information can then be used by your supervising SLP to make additional modifications prior to the next session. Chapter 10 (particularly the sections on "Things to Consider: The Client" and "Things to Consider: The Environment") offers additional suggestions in potential modifications to ensure the environment is supportive and the client is ready and able to participate fully in treatment activities.

DATA COLLECTION DURING GROUP SESSIONS

All the techniques discussed in Chapter 8 also apply to recording the performance of group members during group sessions. The importance of doing so accurately and consistently is equally important in both group and individual sessions. Collecting data during group sessions may be even more challenging, however, given the nature of the session and the need to attend to the needs of multiple members simultaneously. Appendix 12–B and the companion website of this textbook contain a sample data collection sheet for use during a group session. Many of the sample data sheets provided in Chapter 8 can also be easily modified for group sessions. Box 12–3 contains some additional tips for collecting data during group treatment.

Box 12–3. Tips for Collecting Data in Group Sessions

■ Discuss with your supervising SLP employing different techniques, such as the following:

- ■ *Timed Data Collection:* Collecting data on one group member the first 5 minutes, the next group member the following 5 minutes, and so forth.
- ■ *Rotating Data Collection:* Collecting data on one goal, per client, per session and then rotating to a different goal, per client the next session, and so forth, until you have collected data on all goals for all clients, then start the rotating process all over again.

■ Make sure to prepare your data sheets in advance, completing as much as possible prior to the session, including prerecording group member names, goals, codes for scoring, and so forth.

■ Think creatively about where you will keep your data collection sheets within a group dynamic to ensure they are accessible to you but not readily in view of group members.

■ Be aware of the prompts you provide, both for data collection purposes (as recommended in Chapter 8) and also across group members. It may be that the prompts provided to one group member affect (either positively or negatively) the performance of another group member. For example, a student prompted using a tactile cue for the /s/ phoneme (e.g., sliding the pointer finger on the table) may influence her group mate to use the same technique for practicing her /g/ words, which would result in an error in the production of /g/. Having a way to note the relationship of all prompts is helpful if you or your supervising SLP suspect this may be the case.

REFERENCES

Adams, L. (2006). *Group treatment for Asperger syndrome: A social skills curriculum.* Plural Publishing.

American Speech-Language-Hearing Association (ASHA). (2022). *Speech-language pathology assistant scope of practice.* http://www.asha.org/policy

Beukelman, D. R., & Mirenda, P. (2005). *Augmentative and alternative communication: Supporting children and adults with complex communication needs.* Brookes.

Bradley, D. F., Pauley, J. A., & Pauley, J. F. (2006). *Effective classroom management: Six keys to success.* Rowman & Littlefield Education.

Burden, P. (2006). *Classroom management: Creating a successful K–12 learning community.* Wiley.

Carter, E. W., & Kennedy, C. H. (2006). Promoting access to the general curriculum using peer support strategies. *Research and Practice for Persons with Severe Disabilities, 31,* 284–292. https://doi.org/10.1177/154079690603100402

Cascella, R., Purdy, M. H., & Dempsey, L. (2007). Clinical service delivery and work settings. In R. Paul & P. Cascella (Eds.), *Introduction to clinical methods in communication disorders* (pp. 259–282). Brookes.

Elman, R. J. (2007). *Group treatment of neurogenic communication disorders: The expert clinician's approach* (2nd ed.). Plural Publishing.

Last, J. M. (1983). *A dictionary of epidemiology.* Oxford University Press.

Luterman, D. (2008). *Counseling persons with communication disorders and their families.* Pro-Ed.

Mattinson, R. E. (2011). Comparison of students classified ED in self-contained classrooms and a self-contained school. *Education and Treatment of Children, 34*(1), 15–33. https://www.jstor.org/stable/42900099

McCauley, R., & Prelock, P. (Eds.). (2013). *Treatment of autism spectrum disorders: Evidence-based intervention strategies for communication and social interactions.* Brookes.

Mire, S. (2007). Workload analysis: IEP and the group size factors in calculating workload. *School Based Issues, 8*(2), 18–20. https://doi.org/10.1044/sbi8.2.18

Moon-Meyer, S. (2004). *Survival guide for the beginning speech-language clinician.* Pro-Ed.

Parsonson, B. S. (2012). Evidence-based classroom behavior management strategies. *Kairanranga, 13*(1), 16–23.

Roth, F. R., & Worthington, C. K. (2001). *Treatment resource manual for speech-language pathology.* Delmar.

Schubert, N. A., & Baxter, M. B. (1982). The self-contained open classroom as a viable learning environment. *Education, 102*, 411–415.

Subban, P. (2006). Differentiated instruction: A research basis. *International Education Journal, 7*(7), 935–947.

Travis, L. E. (1957). *Handbook of speech pathology.* Appleton-Century-Crofts.

Vinson, B. P. (2009). *Workplace skills and professional issues in speech-language pathology.* Plural Publishing.

Walker, K. (2009). Self-contained classrooms: Research brief. *Education Partnerships.* https://files.eric.ed.gov/fulltext/ED538469.pdf

APPENDIX 12–A
Social Skills Group Activities (Adams, 2006)

Activity	Ages	Objective	Materials	Procedure
Dice Talk	3–5 years old	Child will use eye contact in communication.	■ A small sized box ■ Plain paper to cover box ■ Marker ■ Tape	Find a small box that can be covered with paper and used as a dice for this communication game. Use a size that is easy and fun for little hands to toss. Wrap the box in plain paper. On the faces of the dice, write questions or statements to elicit answers from the children. For example, on the six faces of the dice, you could write: ■ Name an animal that lives in the zoo. ■ Tell me a food you like to eat ■ What animal lives on a farm? ■ What is something you like to drink? ■ Tell me an animal that lives on a farm. ■ Name a toy you like to play with. Explain to the children that they each will get a turn to toss the dice, and they get to answer the question that lands on top. Tell them that they will answer to you, and they must look in your eyes as they talk to you. Explain that looking at people as they talk to them is a good thing we all need to practice.
Bowling	3–5 years old	Child will learn turn-taking in a group activity.	■ Plastic bowling pins and ball ■ Masking tape	Set up the pins, placing a piece of tape on the floor to mark where the children should stand when throwing the ball. Arrange the children in a line behind the masking tape. Explain that each child will get a turn when he or she steps up to the line.

Activity	Ages	Objective	Materials	Procedure
Bowling *continued*				Show the children how to go to the back of the line after their turn. If there are so many children that the wait in line is quite long, have two bowling sets to increase the children's turn taking and lessen the demand on their patience.
Pumpkin Decorating	6–9 years old	Child will use turn-taking in group activity.	■ One large pumpkin ■ Pretty fall leaves of various shapes and colors ■ Yarn ■ Markers ■ Construction paper ■ Scissors ■ Tape ■ Slips of numbered paper and a hat to draw them out to determine turn-taking order	Tell the group they get to decorate a pumpkin, giving it a face, hair, and ears. Instruct the children that they are free to use any of the materials, but they must take turns adding decorations to the pumpkin. Allow them a brief time to discuss possible decorating ideas; if necessary, prompt their creativity with suggestions such as, "Leaves for hair? A mouth out of yarn? Draw ears with a marker?" Draw numbers out of a hat to determine the order they go in, informing them everyone may each have as many turns as necessary to fully decorate the pumpkin.
Big Muscles!	6–9 years old	Child will participate in role-play with the group.	■ Heavy objects and light objects *Heavy/Light* cans of soup/feathers detergent jug/foam cups hammer/crayon dictionary/leaf rock/cotton balls	Talk about things that are heavy and light and ask the children for the meaning of each word. Children can pretend to be weightlifters and take turns lifting the objects. Each child can win a medal for his or her big muscles.

continues

Appendix 12–A. *continued*

Activity	Ages	Objective	Materials	Procedure
I'll Be Your Server	10–12 years old	Child will use eye contact when speaking and listening.	■ Refreshments (one item for each student to distribute to group) ■ Server's apron (optional)	Inform students that they will each have a turn being a waiter, passing out refreshments to the rest of the group. Instruct students that good communication, including eye contact, is important to being a waiter as well as being a consumer. Have students choose the refreshment items they will distribute. Let them take turns passing out the items, using eye contact as they ask each group member, "Would you like some _____?" Remind group members also to make eye contact as they are waited on.
Student Teacher	10–12 years old	Child will use eye contact, topic maintenance, and appropriate length of communication	■ None	Explain to the group that, for this activity, the teacher will be the student, and the students will give feedback to the teacher regarding topic maintenance. Instruct the students to think of topics for the teacher to present. Examples may include: what I did over the weekend, how to make a peanut butter and jelly sandwich, the reasons I became a teacher, my favorite foods, games I played when I was a child, and so on. Show the students a signal (such as raising a hand or pointing a finger at you) they may use if they hear the presentation go off topic. Be sure to wander off topic as you present and respond to students' signals to get back on topic.

APPENDIX 12–B
Group Data Collection Sheet

Group Time: _____ Location: _____ Date: _____ (Length of Session: _____)

Members Present: _____

Group Activity: _____

Member Name: _____ NOTES FOR SESSION: _____

Objective(s)	Data Tally	Data Summary	Comments

Member Name: _____ NOTES FOR SESSION: _____

Objective(s)	Data Tally	Data Summary	Comments

Member Name: _____ NOTES FOR SESSION: _____

Objective(s)	Data Tally	Data Summary	Comments

Member Name: _____ NOTES FOR SESSION: _____

Objective(s)	Data Tally	Data Summary	Comments

PART III

Treatment for Specific Populations and Disorders

CHAPTER 13

Speech Sound Remediation for Children

Lei Sun

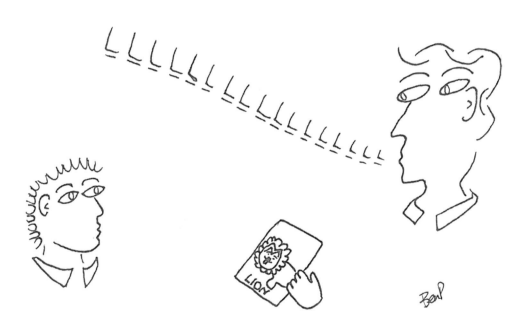

Words mean more than what is set down on paper. It takes the human voice to infuse them with deeper meaning.

—Maya Angelou (American author, poet, and recipient of the National Medal of the Arts and the President's Medal of Freedom)

The caseloads of speech-language pathologists (SLPs) commonly include individuals with speech sound disorders (SSDs), especially for SLPs working in school settings with preschoolers and young school-age children (ages 3–9 years). According to the American Speech-Language-Hearing Association's (ASHA's) 2020 schools survey, students with SSDs were among the most commonly reported individuals on the caseload of school-based SLPs (ASHA, 2020). One of the most common referral reasons from parents and teachers is a child's unintelligible speech. As such, speech-language pathology assistants (SLPAs) working in school settings must be knowledgeable about this topic. This chapter provides an overview of SSDs, including speech sound development and classification and general and specific guidelines for treating SSDs. This chapter is not meant to be a substitute for more in-depth reading and resources; rather, it can serve as a complement to your introductory coursework on the topic.

Before we discuss sound remediation, it is important to review some key concepts. A phoneme is a family of very similar sounds. For example, we produce the /t/ in *tea*, *tool*, and *take* slightly different, but we all perceive the first sound as /t/. A phoneme is the smallest linguistic unit of sound that can signal a difference in meaning. As an example, if we change the first sound of *tea* to /k/, then it will be a different word, *key*, which has a totally different meaning from *tea*. The concept of signaling a difference in meaning through a change of sound is very important for speech sound intervention. In addition to the ability to know that the combination of sounds can create different meanings, our oral motor structures must accurately execute the oral motor plan/sequence to produce the sounds accordingly. Simply put, our brain puts the phonemes together according to the intended linguistic information (e.g., /k/-/i/), and then the correct phoneme combination is produced through the accurate execution of the motor plan. Usually, we use virgules such as /t/ for the ideal description of the sound (i.e., the way the sound should be produced) and brackets [t] for the actual sound produced by an individual. The International Phonetic Alphabet (IPA) is commonly used to represent the sounds of oral language. Appendix 4–B in Chapter 4 contains a list of core IPA symbols.

Speech intelligibility is a subjective measure of how much a speech-language pathologist can understand the individual's speech. It can be targeted directly or indirectly, depending on the goals and objectives set by an SLP. The priority of treatment goals may vary across children in speech and language therapy. In some instances, speech sounds are not directly targeted if, for example, a child has limited use of natural speech or if language intervention is the priority. A lack of speech intelligibility is often addressed in younger children because of the significant negative impact it can have on social interaction and future academic performance (e.g., literacy). Usually, typically developing children can be easily understood by age 5 years with some later developing sounds still in the development (e.g., /r, z, ʃ, ð/) (Peña-Brooks & Hegde, 2007). However, children diagnosed with various speech-language related impairments (e.g., intellectual disabilities, autism spectrum disorder, developmental delay) may require more time to develop speech sounds even though these children tend to follow the same sequence of sound development (Bernthal et al., 2013). Persistent use of phonological processes beyond the expected age of expected suppression, such as liquid gliding (using /w/ to replace /r/), final consonant deletion (deleting sounds in the final position), and stopping of fricatives (using /d/ to replace /s/), must be addressed because of the negative impact on children's daily life, social interaction, and academic learning.

To consider individual differences in acquiring speech sounds, it is important to become familiar with speech acquisition norms and realize that there is no cutoff age for the development of a single sound. For example, /s/ starts to emerge around age 3 years and may not be mastered until age 8 years. It usually takes longer to develop later developing sounds compared with early developing sounds, such as /h, m, w, p/. It is also important to be mindful of the dialectical variations due to children's linguistic and cultural backgrounds, which are typically considered during SLPs' evaluation and goal-setting process. As a foundation for a discussion of speech sound remediation, the following section provides an overview about speech sound classification, speech sound acquisition, and common phonological processes.

SPEECH SOUND CLASSIFICATION

Classifications of sounds, based on place (where along the vocal tract the consonant is formed), voicing (whether the vocal folds are vibrating during the production), and manner (how the sound is formed; Peña-Brooks & Hegde, 2007), is an important foundation for understanding how to elicit target sounds. Figure 13–1 contains a place-voice-manner (PVM) chart, denoting place of articulation, whether the consonant shown is voiced or voiceless, and manner of articulation

for different sounds (Bauman-Waengler, 2020).

Familiarity with this classification system is helpful for understanding the similarity and differences across sounds. For example, if a child's target sound is /s/ and the child is able to produce /t/ consistently, clinicians can take advantage of place similarity and use /t/ to elicit /s/. Similarly, clinicians can use voice on and off to train the voiced sounds by helping the child feel the vibration of the voice box by, for example, having the child touch his or her own neck when the child produces voiced sounds. A vowel chart is also provided for review, as vowels can be used to elicit consonants in similar articulation places (Figure 13–2).

SPEECH SOUND DEVELOPMENT

Consonants

SLPs frequently use speech sound developmental norms and sequences to determine eligibility for treatment of SSDs, such as Sander (1972), Templin (1957), and Smit et al. (1990; Gordon-Brannan & Weiss, 2007). Due to different methodologies

PLACE	MANNER								
	Stop		Nasal		Fricative		Affricate		Approximate	Lateral Approximate
Bilabial	p	**b**		**m**					**w**	
Labiodental					f	**v**				
Dental					θ	**ð**				
Alveolar	t	**d**		**n**	s	**z**			**ɹ**	**l**
Postalveolar					ʃ	**ʒ**	tʃ	**dʒ**		
Palatal									**j**	
Velar	k	**g**		**ŋ**						
Glottal					h					

Figure 13–1. Consonants in bold are voiced.

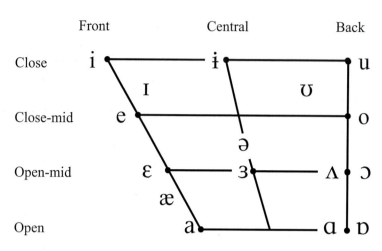

Figure 13–2. English vowels, classified based on position of the tongue. Image courtesy of Wikimedia Commons.

and criteria used when researchers developed speech norms, different sequences of speech sound acquisition have been reported. Despite these minor differences, the order of acquisition of sounds and sound classes is very similar across researchers. For example, in general, stops, nasals, and glides develop early, and liquids, fricatives, and affricates develop later. Clinicians must keep in mind, though, that the position of the sound (e.g., whether the sound appears in the initial, medial, or final position of a word) can also affect how long it takes children to acquire a sound. As an example, /t/ in initial position (*tea, toy, tale*) may be mastered around age 3 years, but /t/ in final position (*cat, feet*) may not be mastered until around age 4 years. Generally speaking, if the sound emerges in one position, sound production in other positions should be expected to follow. Medial sounds usually (but not always) take slightly longer to acquire, compared with sounds in initial and final positions.

A helpful classification of sound development was that developed by Shri-berg (1993), who divided the 24 English speech sounds into three categories: early eight, middle eight, and late eight. Lof (2017) used this classification to compare common speech acquisition norms and found that children master the early eight sounds around age 3 years; the middle eight sounds between ages 3 and 7 years, with /t, k, g, ŋ, f/ often acquired by age 4 and /v, tʃ, dʒ/ developing between ages 5 and 7; and the late eight sounds usually between 6 and 8 years of age (Table 13–1).

Consonant Clusters/Blends

Consonant clusters, or blends (e.g., combination of consonants), usually develop

Table 13–1. Shriberg's Three Categories of Speech Sound Developmental Sequence

Early eight	/m, b, j, n, w, d, p, h/
Middle eight	/t, k, g, ŋ, f, v, tʃ, dʒ/
Late eight	/ s, z, l, r, ʃ, ʒ, θ, ð/

Source: Shriberg, 1993, as cited in Lof, 2003.

after the children's oral motor control and coordination are more mature. Box 13–1 contains a list of common consonant clusters.

Consonant clusters can be in the initial position or final position (-pt, -ks, -ft, -sk, etc.) and can be a combination of two consonants or three consonants (spr-, spl-, thr-, -kst). Like single-consonant acquisition, consonant clusters follow a general acquisition sequence, which varies based on the position of the cluster. Usually, consonant clusters begin to develop between 3:6 and 4:0 years, when children have developed a good number of consonants and are ready to combine them. Therefore, it is unrealistic to work on consonant clusters when a child has only a limited number of consonants in her or his phonetic inventory (i.e., sounds that the child is able to produce consistently), has not yet developed the sounds included in the clusters, or when the child is too young. It is always good to practice single consonants (e.g., /s/) until their sound production stabilizes and then introduce associated consonant clusters (e.g., sm-, sn-, sp-, st-, etc.). However, based on complexity treatment approach, targeting clusters may facilitate the production of the production of singleton. For example, /s/ clusters may facilitate the production of /s/. Therefore, during therapy, it is important to consider different approaches and carefully monitor the client's response to intervention to select the best approach that works best for each client.

Keep in mind that consonant clusters take longer to develop, and some may be mastered after age 8 years for some children (e.g., thr-, skw-, str-, spr-, etc.; Peña-Brooks & Hegde, 2007). In addition, clinicians generally consider consonant acquisition when working on clusters. As an example, it is appropriate for a 5-year-old to say [fwog] instead of /frog/, as /r/ is still developing. In general, it is more important to help children be aware of a cluster that has two or three sounds in it, rather than the perfect production of each individual phoneme in the cluster at the beginning of the treatment. The correct production of each cluster element may be addressed later. For example, it is more critical to produce /f/ and /r/ in /frog/ even though it sounds like [fwog] than only producing one sound in the cluster as in *fog*, because *fog* is a different word and carries a very different meaning from *frog*. In contrast, *fwog* still carries the meaning of *frog* even though it does not sound the way it should.

Vowels

Most children have no difficulty acquiring vowels. Vowels usually develop early, except /ə, ɚ/, which are usually mastered before 5 years of age because tongue retraction is required to produce these two r-colored vowels. If a child shows difficulty producing vowels, more serious speech issues or structural issues may be indicated. When a child has difficulty producing vowels, sounds that carry real meanings can be used to elicit the vowels—for example, "haha," "uhoh," "ouch," and "owie." C (consonant), V (vowel), and VC (vowel-consonant) words that represent

---

> ### Box 13–1. Common Consonant Clusters
>
> - L blends: pl-, kl-, fl-
> - S blends: sp-, sm-, sn-, st-, sk-
> - R blends: gr-, br-, dr-, kr-

different daily utterances should also be included to facilitate both vowels and early developing consonants to expand the child's sound inventory—for example, *up, hi, bye, no, boo, my, nana, mama, dada.* If a child cannot differentiate between two vowels, minimal contrasts or pairs (which will be reviewed under the phonemic, linguistically based, and phonology treatment approaches) are often used in treatment to target perception and production training.

COMMON PHONOLOGICAL PROCESSES

During the time when children learn to talk like adults, they simplify adults' speech by using predictable *error* patterns called phonological processes. The use of phonological processes is related to speech sound acquisition. For example, a child uses /t/ to replace /k/ (velar fronting) when the child is still in the process of developing the /k/ sound. All children use phonological processes when developing their speech sounds. However, children with speech delays or SSDs use phonological processes beyond an appropriate age range, which makes the speech errors inappropriate. Keep in mind that some children who have impairments in other areas, such as cognition and language, may use the processes for a much longer period of time. Some phonological processes may be eliminated early, such as initial and final consonant deletion and velar fronting, but some phonological processes may take longer to be suppressed, such as liquid gliding and stopping of voiced and voiceless interdental fricative, /ð/ and /θ/. As such, sometimes goals may target specific patterns or phonological processes instead of particular sounds, such as "XX will improve speech intelligibility by reducing final consonant deletion." As an SLPA, it is important to have a basic concept of some common phonological processes (Table 13–2).

Table 13–2. Common Phonological Processes

Phonological Process	Description	Examples
Final consonant deletion	A final consonant is omitted/deleted from a word	ca for cat, cu for cup
Initial consonant deletion	An initial consonant is omitted/deleted from a word	at for fat, ake for lake
Syllable deletion	A syllable (especially a weak/unstressed syllable) is omitted/deleted from a word	puter for computer, nana for banana
Cluster reduction	One phoneme of the cluster is deleted from the cluster	fag for flag, fog for frog
Stopping of fricatives	Uses stops to replace fricatives and affricates	top for sop, poo for zoo
Velar fronting	Uses alveolar stops (/t, d/) to replace velar sounds (/k, g, ŋ/)	tea for key, do for go
Liquid gliding	Uses a glide (/w, j/) to replace a liquid (/l, r/)	wake for lake, yeg for leg
Devoicing	Uses a voiceless consonant to replace a voiced consonant	nos for nose, pik for pig
Assimilation	One sound becomes more like a neighboring sound. It could be due to place or manner.	lellow for yellow, take for cake

Source: Peña-Brooks & Hegde, 2007.

GENERAL TREATMENT PRINCIPLES

In general, treatment can be viewed as "a continuum of activities comprising three stages: establishment, facilitation of generalization, and maintenance" (Bernthal et al., 2013, p. 270). Figure 13–3 presents this continuum. Treatment starts with eliciting the target sound, gradually moves to stabilizing the speech sound production in all word positions and increasing linguistic levels (from words to conversation), and then maintains consistent speech sound production in different settings, contexts, and with different communication partners, through self-monitoring.

The first step in the treatment process is to establish appropriate treatment goals and objectives. This is the job of your supervising SLP (ASHA, 2020). As an SLPA, it is critical that for each treatment objective, you are able to accurately identify target sounds, production level (i.e., syllable, word, phrase or sentence, spontaneous speech), accuracy level (e.g., 70%, 7 of 10 trials), prompt level (e.g., minimal, maximal prompting), and setting (usually in speech-language therapy). Chapter 7 offers general suggestions in this regard.

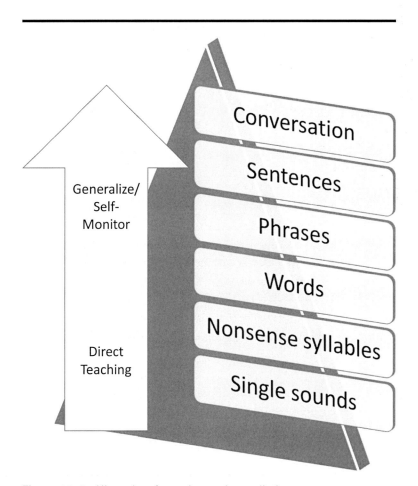

Figure 13–3. Hierarchy of speech sound remediation.

Remember that an objective may be written in various ways, but it should always contain those elements. An example of a common speech sound remediation objective is, "L.B. will produce /s/ and /s/-blends at word level in all positions with 80% accuracy with minimal prompting in three consecutive speech therapy sessions." Using this objective as an example, can you identify the elements listed above?

Intervention remediating SSDs is generally divided into two major treatment approaches: phonetic/motor-based/ articulation treatment approaches and phonemic/linguistically based/phonologic treatment approaches. Although the two treatment approaches stem from distinctive theories and clinical observations, it is impossible to separate the func-

tion (linguistic/phonemic) from the form (motor based/phonetic) as they are two sides of the same coin. As you implement treatment, it is important to keep this in mind. Phonology is only one aspect of language, and intervention to remediate SSDs should always be considered in the larger scope of language and its purpose. The ultimate goal is to improve a child's overall speech intelligibility, in order to convey meaning efficiently and effectively, and to assist the child to function better in her or his daily life. The World Health Organization's International Classification of Functioning, Disability and Health (World Health Organization, 2001) highlights this relationship, which should be the cornerstone of speech sound remediation (Figure 13–4). Effective and func-

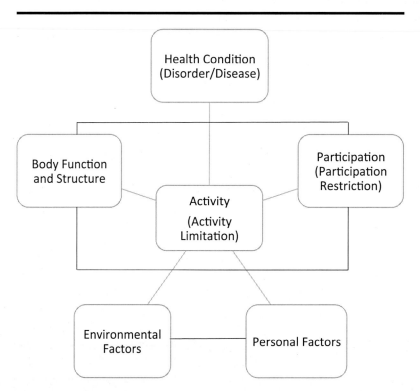

Figure 13–4. Model of the International Classification of Functioning, Disability, and Health.

tional intervention targets both language form (body structures and functions) and language function (meaningful use of speech sounds, along with language rules, to function well in daily activities).

A traditional view of remediating speech errors uses discrete skills (e.g., not viewing phonology as part of language) and a *drill-and-kill* method. Although maximizing accurate production is key to improving speech intelligibility, it may be that with this method, students overgeneralize speech sound production (e.g., use the target sound in words that do not contain the target sound). This further compromises effective communication. Students may also respond poorly to drill activities. The gold standard in speech sound remediation should always be effective, efficient, and functional treatment activities. Box 13–2 depicts an example of this approach within a treatment session.

PRIMARY TREATMENT APPROACHES

Although we divide treatment approaches into two main categories (phonetic/motor based/articulation; phonemic/linguistically based/phonologic), it is impossible to work on form and function separately. The difference across different treatment approaches is in how each approach organizes and sequences treatment targets, which is determined according to the severity of the speech-sound disorder. For example, clinicians use phonetic treatment approaches, such as using a variety of cues (e.g., visual, tactile, verbal) or external tools (e.g., tongue depressor), to elicit a target sound. Once the sound is stimulable and produced correctly, phonemic treatment approaches should be used to facilitate target discrimination and sound production. Therefore, a combination of the phonetic and phonemic

---

Box 13–2. Sample Speech Sound Remediation Session

1. Start the treatment session by having the child practice target sounds at the appropriate linguistic level (e.g., word, phrase, sentence) for a short amount of time.
2. Have the child use target words in naturalistic activities. For younger children, play-based activities are an excellent option. Language-based activities, such as shared book reading, are especially good for children with language disorders and SSDs. Literacy-based treatment activities, incorporating phonological awareness activities for preschoolers and conventional reading and writing for older children, are also highly valuable. Chapter 16 offers additional suggestions.
3. End the session by reviewing target sounds and speech homework.

approaches is recommended, depending on the child's needs and strengths. Table 13–3 briefly summarizes the general differences between the phonetic and phonemic treatment approaches.

Phonetic/Motor-Based/Articulation Treatment Approach

A traditional approach to phonetic training has been commonly used since the 1970s (Van Riper & Erickson, 1996). Using this approach, the child gradually moves along the continuum of treatment from perceptual/ear training, sound establishment, sound stabilization, transfer/carryover, and then maintenance. Some elements of the traditional approach can be separately incorporated into treatment as needed, without implementing the entire method.

Perceptual Training/Ear Training

Perceptual training is used at the beginning of a traditional approach if the child has difficulty discriminating between the desired sound (i.e., the target speech sound) and the undesired sound (i.e., the sound that the child produces instead).

If the child discriminates the sounds correctly, treatment moves forward to the sound establishment phase. Before perceptual training, training words should be selected based on the child's present level. However, it may not be an appropriate activity if the child has difficulty understanding what you expect him or her to do. Your modeling is always necessary to ensure each child's understanding of the task in order to successfully implement the activity. During perceptual training, the child's correct responses and errors should be carefully monitored. It is important to keep in mind that perceptual training does not automatically lead to correct sound production and improved speech intelligibility. However, perceptual training can increase awareness of the target phoneme and can be added before or during production training. The use of perceptual training may or may not be evident in a child's treatment objectives. An example of an objective including perceptual training may be, "XX will distinguish one sound (desired sound) from a different sound (undesired sound) with minimal prompting when presented with picture cards, with 80% accuracy in two consecutive sessions." Even though the prompting level in goals/objectives can

Table 13–3. Core Differences: Phonetic Versus Phonemic Approaches

Phonetic Approach	Phonemic Approach
Focus on teaching correct production of an individual sounds	Focus on learning correct production through contrasting sounds
Use of nonsense/made up syllables/words is allowed	Only use meaningful real words
Appropriate for limited speech errors	Appropriate for identified erred patterns
Good for nonstimulable sounds	Good for stimulable sounds
Start with phonemes or nonsense syllables	Start with words

Sources: Bernthal, Bankson, & Flipsen, 2013; Peña-Brooks & Hegde, 2007.

be written differently, maximal/moderate/minimal prompting is suggested by Paul et al. (2018) based on ASHA's National Outcomes Measurement System (ASHA, n.d.). Maximal prompting is defined as frequent cues (80%–100% of trials being prompted), moderate prompting is defined as intermittent cues (25%–75% of trials being prompted), and minimal prompting refers to occasional cues (5%–20% of trials being prompted). Besides tracking how often the client has to be prompted in one session, the type of cue should be documented. For example, direct and explicit instructions are considered maximal prompting, and using cloze, semantic, or phonological cues is classified as moderate prompting. Minimal prompting often requires subtle cues such as verbal reminders, tactile cues, or visual cues. Table 13–4 summarizes different methods for ear training.

Sound Establishment/Sound Elicitation

Sound elicitation often starts with a phoneme (e.g., fricatives), syllable (e.g., target phoneme + schwa, especially stops /pə/ and liquids /lə/), or word (e.g., meaningful and functional consonant-vowel-consonant [CVC] words). Your supervising SLP will determine which level facilitates production more easily for each child and the child's ultimate goal in communication. A common treatment objective at this level of training may be, "XX will produce_____ sound in _____position (initial or final) at word (or syllable-CV, VC

Table 13–4. Perceptual Ear Training Methods

Traditional Approach	Identification	Clinician directs the child's attention to how the speech sound feels in the mouth. Clinician uses objects to describe the characteristics of the speech sound (e.g., /t/ is a ticking sound, /f/ is an angry cat sound). A common task may be for the child to ring a bell or raise his or her hand when hearing a target sound.
	Isolation	Child is asked to identify the target sound in increasing linguistic levels (syllables, words, phrases, sentences).
	Stimulation	Similar to auditory bombardment, child is provided with maximal auditory stimuli of the target sound, through varying loudness, stress (e.g., add stress to syllable containing the target sound), and duration of the sound (prolong the target sound).
	Discrimination	Child is asked to make judgments of correct and incorrect productions made by the clinician.
Auditory Bombardment		Tasks blend the target sound into all activities and emphasize the target sound through shared book reading, language/literacy games, play, conversation, and so forth. For example, if the target sound is /s/, the clinician may read a book about superheros (Superman, Spiderman, Sandman, etc.), highlighting /s/ while reading the book. Similarly, the clinician may emphasize /s/ in conversation (it'S Super Silly, iSn't it? That'S hiS not yourS).
Minimal Pair		Clinician uses pairs of words containing undesirable sound (e.g., use [t] to replace /s/, [t] is the undesirable sound) and desirable sound (/s/ is the desirable sound) along with written words and corresponding pictures. As an example, the child is asked to hand pictures named to the clinician (sea-tea, sue-two).

Source: Bernthal, Bankson, & Flipsen, 2013.

[consonant-vowel or vowel-consonant]) level with minimal prompting with 70% accuracy in two consecutive sessions." Table 13–5 summarizes several techniques used to elicit target sounds. Keep in mind, though, that more than one technique may be needed. The combination of techniques depends on the child's needs and how the child responds to each technique. All the techniques listed are used to elicit speech sounds in isolation. Conversational speech is dynamic and variable; it considers the influence from neighboring sounds (i.e., the consonant or vowel that comes before and after the sound) and suprasegmental features (e.g., stress, intonation), rather than the combination of isolated speech sounds. Therefore, addi-

tional attention is generally given to transferring learned, isolated speech sounds to more connected running speech and then to generalization to different settings and with varied communication partners. As an additional reference, consult *Articulatory and Phonological Impairments: A Clinical Focus* by Jacqueline Bauman-Waengler (2020) and *Eliciting Sounds: Techniques and Strategies for Clinicians* by Secord et al. (2007).

Sound Stabilization

Once the target sound is successfully elicited, phonetic treatment then focuses on stabilizing sound production in all positions of words and at varied levels of complexity. Generally, objectives start with the

Table 13–5. Common Techniques for Eliciting Speech Sounds

Sound-Evoking Technique	Procedures
Imitation	Ask the child to watch, listen, and repeat the target sound. A mirror can be used (e.g., watch me, listen, and make the sound just like I do-/s/).
Phonetic Placement	Clinician describes where to place the articulators in order to produce the target sound, along with visual and tactile cues. A mouth puppet and mirror can be used with younger children. Oral structure graphs can be used with older children (first grade and up). External tools such as a tongue depressor should be used as the last resort.
Contextual Cues/ Co-Articulation	Clinician identifies key words (words in which the child can produce the target sound correctly) and word contexts (the neighboring sounds that can facilitate the correct production of the target sound, without additional training). Clinician uses this advantage to help the child feel and hear the target sound and attempt to transfer the correct target production to other words. Usually the information can be gathered from contextual testing done by the SLP. For example, /s/ may be produced easily in clusters/blends (st, sp, sn, etc) rather than singletons (sun, sit, etc) (Williams, 1991). /s/ may be produced easily after /t/ due to similar placement (bright-sun, hot-soup, etc.). Velar sounds may be easily produced after high-back vowels (/u, ʊ/).
Sound Modification/ Shaping	Clinician uses the sound that is already in the child's phonetic inventory (the child can produce the sound correctly and independently) and shapes it to the target sound. For example, if the child can produce /l/, /l/ is shaped into /r/ by asking the child to slide the tongue tip slowly back along the roof of the mouth.
Tactile-Kinesthetic	Clinician manipulates the child's articulators externally on the face and neck to guide the speech sound production.

Sources: Bauman-Waengler, 2012; Bernthal, Bankson, & Flipsen, 2013; Gordon-Brannan & Weiss, 2007.

lowest level (i.e., when the child requires great assistance from the clinician) and progresses to higher levels (i.e., when the clinician starts to fade prompting, in order to achieve correct independent speech sound production). For example, if the child successfully produces /s/ in final position (*kiss*, *face*), treatment then moves forward to initial (*sun*, *see*) and then medial position (*seesaw*, *castle*), which automatically incorporates two-syllable words. Once the child finishes the sound production in one position or one level (syllable, word), the clinician incorporates a review to ensure sound stabilization while moving forward to the next level. An example of a common treatment objective at this level would be, "XX will produce sound in position (initial, medial or final) at word level with minimal prompting with 70% accuracy in two consecutive sessions" or "XX will produce sound in all positions at sentence level with minimal prompting with 70% accuracy in two consecutive sessions." Words used in treatment should be selected from the words commonly used in the client's daily activities and school curriculum. Table 13–6 provides treatment suggestions for this type of objective.

Speech Homework

To improve speech intelligibility, clients must practice correct speech sound production. Because 30 minutes or an hour a week of treatment does not provide sufficient practice, speech homework is necessary. Creating a speech file for the child and sending home a list of practice words after each session is recommended. As an SLPA, you may be asked to assist your supervising SLP in creating these materials (ASHA, 2020). The practice words should be words that were practiced

in treatment sessions for which correct sound production has been established. Usually, 10 to 15 minutes of practice a day is sufficient to maintain and stabilize correct sound production. A note for the parent or caregiver regarding how to use the speech homework and a signature and/or initial line for the parent or caregiver to confirm the completion of the speech homework is recommended. Appendix 13–A contains a sample speech homework sheet.

Phonemic/Linguistically Based/ Phonologic Treatment Approach

The focus of phonemic/linguistically based/phonology treatment is to replace erred patterns and to establish sound contrasts (Bernthal et al., 2013). This treatment approach is more appropriate for children whose speech errors can be identified by patterns and phonological processes, such as final consonant deletion, velar fronting, liquid gliding, and cluster reduction. Because the child uses patterns, his or her speech intelligibility is usually much lower than the child who has articulation disorders with fewer speech errors. Children with phonological disorders usually have difficulty distinguishing targets sound from error sounds. For example, a child who uses liquid gliding may have difficulty distinguishing the difference between *lake* and *wake*, which results in incorrect production. In contrast, a child with an articulation disorder may be able to differentiate between /w/ and /r/ but struggle to produce /r/. Therefore, which treatment approach (phonetic or phonemic) is most effective and beneficial depends on the child's ability to contrast the sounds and produce the target with minimal assistance (i.e., the sound is

Table 13–6. Sound Stabilization Sample Activities

Level	Treatment Suggestions
Word	*Target sound can first be elicited in final or initial position and then gradually moved to medial position. The purpose of treatment is to stabilize the sound production in all word positions.* *Potential Activities:* 1. Incorporate target words into board games or any type of game. For example, use target words to play Go Fish (e.g., the child must produce the word correctly to receive the correct card). 2. Use games as reinforcement to elicit maximal correct sound production. For example, the child must produce the word correctly three times before moving the pawn. *Suggested games:* Go Fish, fishing game, memory game, bowling, safari, Hangman (good for children with a large vocabulary size), etc.
Phrase/sentence	*Incorporate phrases that contain the target sound. Carrier phrases start with the same phrase and only fill in different words that contain the target sound to complete the sentence.* *Potential Activities:* 1. Set a scene that facilitates the use of carrier phrases. e.g., I see a _____ (target sound /l/: lake, lamp, line, etc). 2. To increase the difficulty, two target words can be included in one phrase. e.g., I "like" the _____ (target sound /l/: lake, lamp, line, etc).
Sentence	*Start with simple and short sentences containing one target word and then gradually increase the complexity of the sentence and the number of target words.* *Potential Activities:* 1. If the child is able to read, use ready-made materials and ask the child to read sentences. 2. If the child has higher language abilities, ask the child to make up a sentence using the practiced target word. For example, I like to go to beach and pick up "seashells" out of the "sand."
Conversation	*The purpose of conversation level is to help the child be more aware of his or her own speech errors and develop effective self-monitoring strategies. It requires a certain level of metalinguistic skills and may be more appropriate for older children and children with good language skills.* *Potential Activities:* 1. Use audio recording: record part of the session, play it back to the child, identify and discuss the speech errors. We must be cautious about the child's emotional and psychological changes when using this method. Do not make the child feel that he or she is the center of the attention (put the child on the spot). 2. Ask the child to fill out the speech rating chart to evaluate his or her own speech for each session using letter grade (A, B, C). A speech diary can be created to use at home to continue the self-monitoring process. 3. Discuss with the child developing effective strategies tailored specifically for him or her. For example, use of the secret visual code shared between the classroom teacher, the child, and the clinician as a reminder when needed.

Source: Bernthal, Bankson, & Flipsen, 2013.

stimulable). If a child understands the difference between the sounds, the clinician can facilitate sound production using the sound-evoking techniques reviewed earlier. If the child struggles with differentiating the error sound and the target sound, training on perception of contrasts and then production of contrasts will be the focus. Your supervising SLP will determine the most appropriate approach for each client (ASHA, 2020).

Providing the treatment that meets the child's needs to improve the child's overall speech intelligibility is the ultimate goal. An indication of using phonologically based treatment activities may not always be evident in an objective. An objective using this approach may look like the examples presented in the sound stabilization section, such as "XX will produce sound in position (initial, medial, or final) at word level with minimal prompting with 80% accuracy in two consecutive sessions." The use of treatment approaches depends on the child's deficits and severity of SSDs. The sections that follow provide an overview of three evidence- and phonologically based treatment approaches.

Minimal Oppositions/Minimal Pairs

Word pairs are used in a minimal opposition/minimal pair contrast approach. A phoneme already in the child's inventory is used to contrast with the target sound/desired sound (Barlow & Gierut, 2002). For example, if the child uses /w/ to replace /r/, it shows that the child is able to produce /w/ (in the child's inventory) but may not understand the contrast between /w/ and /r/. Treatment then focuses on the use of /w/ in the child's

inventory to contrast with the target sound /r/. The goal of this treatment is to help the child understand that different sounds represent different words and meanings and that correct sound production is important for successful communication. Therefore, a change of one sound will change the word and intended meaning, which may cause communication breakdowns. As an example, if the child asks for a picture of *tea* instead of *key* when she really wants *key*, receiving the wrong picture card of *tea* will be the consequence of incorrect sound production. The procedure of minimal pair training is presented in Figure 13–5.

Maximal Oppositions Contrast

Maximal oppositions contrast uses the same procedure as minimal oppositions contrast (above). The only difference is in the selection of word pairs (Gierut, 1989). The word pair *tea-key* is different only in one feature: that of place. If "k-m" pairs are used, greater phonological change in the phonology system can be made, because /k/ and /m/ differ on place, manner, and nasality of production. Therefore, in maximal opposition training, /m/ would be used if it was already in the child's inventory, to contrast with /k/ (the target sound). The purpose of this approach is to promote better generalization to other sounds and greater overall change of the child's phonological system through maximal contrast. The same flowchart for minimal oppositions contrast (see Figure 13–5) can be used for maximal oppositions contrast, with the only change being the selection of a sound already in the child's repertoire that maximally contrasts with the target sound.

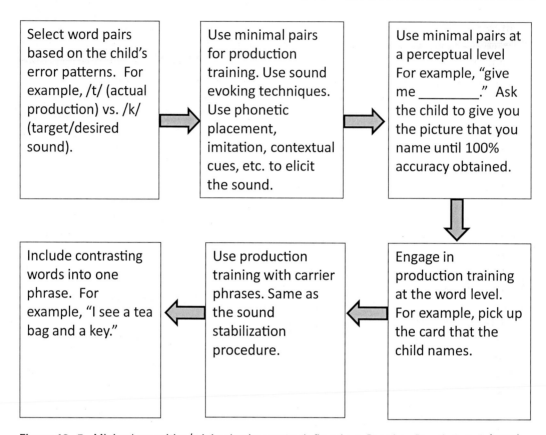

Figure 13–5. Minimal opposition/minimal pairs approach flowchart. Based on Bernthal et al. (2013).

Multiple Oppositions Therapy

The multiple oppositions approach is the expansion of minimal oppositions and maximal oppositions (as above). The aim of this approach is to achieve maximum phonological reorganization in a systematic way. Instead of targeting one contrast at a time, this approach targets several contrasts simultaneously (Williams, 1993, 2000). This approach is good for children who have multiple sound errors and tend to use one sound to replace several. For example, if the child uses /t/ to replace /s, f, k/, it is most efficient and effective to target all three substitutions at once.

In this instance, three different pairs of contrasts are used, including t-s (cheat-cheese), t-f (cheat-chief), and t-k (cheat-cheek), with 10 words in each pair. The therapy procedure is similar to minimal/maximal oppositions (see Figure 13–5). First, the clinician names words and the child sorts them into different piles for perception training (one pile for each of three target sounds: /s, f, k/). When the child is able to successfully differentiate these sound contrasts, treatment focuses on production training. Clinicians can also ask the child to sort the named words into different piles to work on perception and production simultaneously.

ADDITIONAL TREATMENT CONSIDERATIONS

Speech and Language Ability

Tying speech sound therapy to daily life and functional communication is the goal when working with children who have limited language ability. Being able to communicate needs and wants is a priority. Therefore, targeting functional words and phrases and high-frequency words is highly recommended. Treatment begins with CVC words that are highly functional and frequently used in daily life such as *hi, bye, no, help, want, go, me, mom, dad.* How intelligible the word and phrase should be depends on the child's current speech and language functioning and other related health issues. Sometimes, approximation (i.e., close production of the target word) is acceptable if the child is not able to produce clear speech sounds, but approximation of the sound or word serves the communication purpose.

Working With School-Age Children With SSDs

Children who start to develop phonics (i.e., letter sound correspondence) and phonological awareness may benefit from using phonological awareness activities to indirectly improve speech sound production. Phonological awareness is the individual's awareness of the sound structure of spoken words (Justice et al., 2013). Development of phonological awareness is important for learning to read. As phonological awareness brings the child's attention to the sound and syllable (e.g., alliteration of the sound at the beginning or at the end, syllable segmenting and blending), it is beneficial to incorporate these tasks into treatment to facilitate speech sound production and phonological awareness simultaneously. If the child uses syllable deletion, writing down the words and clapping out the syllables may increase the child's awareness of the syllable boundary and syllable structure. An example of this would be for the word *computer.* This is a three-syllable word. If the child tends to say *puter,* clinicians can show the child a picture along with the written word and clap out or highlight the syllables. Some children can quickly "fix" their speech errors through auditory and visual prompting. For alliteration, clinicians can ask the child to sort the cards into different piles based on the position of the sound and then use these target words to practice sound production. If the child enjoys spelling, spelling can also be used as a building block to facilitate awareness of speech sounds and speech errors.

Targeting Grammatical Morphemes at the Same Time

Final consonant deletion (FCD) is a one of the common phonological processes that may persist beyond the appropriate age. What makes FCD important as a treatment target is its negative impact on grammatical morphemes. Grammatical morphemes carry additional meaning, like plural-s (indicates number) and tense markers (indicate time). If a child tends to delete all final sounds, it will not only significantly affect the child's speech intelligibility but also prevent the child from delivering meaningful messages. For example, when the child is explaining what happened last night to her friend, deletion of final consonants has a negative impact, as in "I see two ca___ cha___ a mou__ " versus "I see two cats chase a mouse." Without the final consonants, the intended message is confusing. Another example is the deletion of plurals. If the child says, "my dog like to fight with each other" for "my dog*s* like to fight with each other," without producing /s/ at the end of dog*s*, the listener may be puzzled about how many dogs the child has. Thus, /t, d, ŋ, s, z/ in the final position are very important because they carry additional grammatical meaning for present progressive tense (wash<u>ing</u>), regular past tense (walk<u>ed</u>), and plurals (dog<u>s</u>). According to Tyler et al. (2002), working on morphosyntax (morphology and syntax) can lead to cross-domain change in phonology. Therefore, instead of working on FCD in general, clinicians can target those specific final sounds that carry additional grammatical meaning to also facilitate positive changes in phonology and other language components (morphosyntax and pragmatics).

The Use of Nonspeech Oral Motor Exercises and Activities (NSOMEs)

Nonspeech oral motor exercises (NSOMEs) are activities, such as blowing bubbles, sucking straws, chewing tube, tongue wagging, and kissing, used to improve speech intelligibility. NSOMEs are frequently questioned by researchers regarding the direct relationship between NSOMEs and improving speech intelligibility (Forrest, 2002; Lof, 2003). The rationales behind not using NSOMEs for children with SSDs are as follows (Forrest, 2002):

1. Speech needs more than the strength of articulators. One purpose of NSOMEs is to strengthen oral muscles to improve speech intelligibility.

2. Breaking speech production down into individual and isolated motor components is not sufficient to learn an overall skill. Speech production requires very sophisticated fine motor control and coordination in a timely fashion. Therefore, exercising each articulator separately does not improve overall skills required for speech.

3. Even though the structures used in speech and nonspeech activities may be the same, the structures are used differently in these two types of activities.

The best way to improve speech intelligibility is to actually work on speech sounds and practice the sounds in a meaningful context (e.g., words, phrases) daily, because speech movement is different from other gross motor and fine motor movements. Effective ways of treating speech errors include the following:

1. Provide ear training, if necessary.
2. Work on speech sound production intensively using meaningful words at different levels (i.e., word, phrase, sentence, conversation).
3. Incorporate curriculum-based and literacy-related activities to promote generalization of correct sound production.
4. Provide speech homework for daily practice under the parent's or caregiver's supervision.
5. Help the child develop and implement self-monitoring strategies to self-correct error sounds in daily life.

Selecting Treatment Materials

A wide selection of articulation cards is available. However, as an SLPA, you will be required to select appropriate training words for the child, either in support of your supervising SLP's session or before you implement treatment with a client (ASHA, 2020). Box 13–3 contains a list of important elements to consider in selecting these materials.

When selecting stimuli, the target word should be easily identified. Real objects or pictures of real objects and actions that contain the target sound may be more effective and functional for younger children. Line drawing pictures, word lists, or reading passages may be more suitable for older children who are reading or are beginning to read. Ready-made articulation cards are conve-

nient and can save time on preparation. However, keep in mind that selection of these materials must be done before each session to maximize learning outcomes. Appropriate training words should be selected to best facilitate target sound production. Functional target sounds used frequently in the child's daily life and words, selected from the child's curriculum, should be used to facilitate generalization and maximize treatment gains.

Individualized training materials are highly recommended, and they should always be meaningful to the child. Therefore, selection of words based on the child's language level is important in facilitating both speech and language

---

Box 13–3. Considerations When Selecting Treatment Materials

- Syllable shape: Syllable shape is the number of syllables in the word. Fewer syllables make it easier for the child to produce the target sound.
- Neighboring sounds: Neighboring sounds are the sounds that come before and after the target sound, which may influence the target sound. For example, /uk/ will be easier than /ek/ when eliciting /k/ in VC syllable production because the tongue position of /u/ is closer to the tongue position of /k/ (highback vowel /u/ vs. midfront vowel /e/).
- Stress: Stress can be used to highlight the target sound. If the target sound is stressed, it may be easier for the child to pick up the sound.
- Cluster or singleton: The use of singletons or blends depends on how easy it is to facilitate production of the target sound. For example, /s/ may be produced more easily in consonant clusters (st-, sn-) than as a singleton (Williams, 1991).
- Frequency: High-frequency words are more functional and common in daily life. However, error production from old habits may be more difficult to correct. In that case, consider staying away from the high-frequency words that are consistently produced incorrectly until the target sound can be produced consistently.

development. Using pictures with written words printed above or below may increase print awareness and sight word learning while working on the target sound. Choosing target words meaningful for the child and appropriate for the child's language level will facilitate generalization of sound production and increase the child's vocabulary repertoire. Starting with early developing words, such as concrete objects and visible action words, especially for younger children, may be helpful. If the child does not know the target word (e.g., seesaw), clinicians can talk about the word (e.g., "you can find it in the playground, one end goes up and one end goes down") and link it to the child's personal experience. Speech sound therapy should never be only drill and sound practice. When a child makes the link between the word, the letter, the sound, and the concept, the word will be stored in long-term memory more easily and become part of the child's vocabulary repertoire.

Most children who have SSDs may have comorbid language delays or disorders, which may make addressing distorted speech sound(s) through language- and literacy-based treatment activities more effective. Language- and literacy-based treatment can even facilitate and support language development and learning for children who have SSDs without other developmental or language learning issues. The focus of language- and literacy-based treatment goes beyond correct speech production. For example, through shared book reading, clinicians can highlight target sound(s) and emphasize and elaborate on related word and content knowledge. These types of activities can be blended into the treatment session to facilitate speech and language development simultaneously. Box 13–4 has suggestions for creating language- and literacy-based

---

Box 13–4. Suggestions of Language- and Literacy-Based Treatment Activities

1. *Select a book that is appropriate for the child's language and reading level.* The book can be chosen from the pool of reading materials used in the classroom or home. That way, the teacher or parent can carry over the learning to different settings to promote generalization. Collaboration with other professionals and the parent to select appropriate and motivating treatment materials is crucial.
2. *Preread the book and highlight the words containing the target sound.*
3. *While you read the book with the child, emphasize the target sound and talk about the target words* (e.g., offer definition, synonym, antonym, homonym).
4. *After reading the book, help the child retell the story using target words and pictures from the book.*
5. *Incorporate arts and crafts after the reading activities to make retelling the story fun and easy.*

treatment activities. Chapter 16 (particularly its sections on books as play) provide additional suggestions.

Making Speech Sessions Fun and Motivating

Treatment sessions should never be drill-and-kill, but maximal training opportunities and practice must be provided to stabilize the target sound production. As maximum repetition is inevitable, clinicians must keep the speech session interesting and motivational. If the child is also working on language, fun activities can be blended into the session to make the session feel less like work. As stated earlier, language- and literacy-based activities should always be part of the treatment to facilitate both speech and language production. How to divide the session and how much time to spend on speech sound production and language learning depends on the priorities for the child and how the child responds to the treatment. You can work with your supervising SLP in discussing a good balance for each child. No matter the types of activities, keeping them fun and motivational is critical. Using short games and language- and literacy-based activities creatively keeps the speech session fun and provides maximal opportunity for practice. Table 13–7 provides sample activities that can be easily modified and expanded. The purpose of these activities is to use simple and easy games and activities

Table 13–7. Sample Games and Treatment Activities

Sample Activity	Materials	General Procedure
Fishing	Fish-shape magnets Fishing poles Training words	Attach target words on the back of fish-shape magnets. Child uses fish pole to catch the fish and says the target words.
Bowling	Bowling ball and pins Training words	Attach target words on the bowling pins. Child knocks down bowling pins and says the word on the pin.
Safari	Flashlight(s) Training words	Place target words around the room. Give the child a flashlight. Turn off the light. Ask the child to find all target words using the flashlight.
Arts & Crafts	Scissors, glue, varied materials, Training words	Procedure varies depending on the art project. Use target words as part of the materials to complete the project.
Board Game	Candyland, Chutes & Ladders, Bingo, etc.	Procedure varies depending on the board game. Child has to produce the target word(s) before moving the pawn.
Card Game	Memory games, Go Fish, etc.	Procedure varies depending on the card game. Use target words as game cards to compete with each other. Minimal pairs can be used as cards for Go Fish game.
Toys/Games	Train set, Jenga, etc.	Procedure varies depending on the game. Various toys and games can be used. Child has to produce the target words before receiving or moving a game piece.

without creating additional cognitive and linguistic demands and to focus on maximizing opportunities for target sound production.

Treatment is a dynamic process. As such, clinicians need to have an open mind regarding the trial-and-error process. Keeping the speech session fun and effective is the goal; thus, finding an effective approach to facilitate target sound production through a short and quick experimental trial may be required. It is also critical to keep in mind that every child must be treated individually, even though she or he may have the same goal or work on the same sound(s) as others. It is very common to see that children respond to the same treatment approach or treatment activity differently. Therefore, creating individualized treatment activities is necessary.

In a school setting, group treatment can be used instead of individual sessions. Many of the activities discussed in Table 13–7 can be adapted for groups of children. Chapter 12 also offers suggestions for how to adapt activities. How to group children to address each child's speech and language goal(s) can be very challenging, but effective group sessions have the advantage of facilitating speech and language development through peer modeling. Using peers to model correct production and transferring practice into fun and competitive games may make training more enjoyable and motivational.

Lastly, iPads or other high-technology devices can be attractive and fun for children. Several apps designed for speech sound remediation can be used along with ready-made articulation cards. However, some children may be distracted by these devices, which may result in difficulty managing the session. Therefore, consider how to best use these devices

without creating a negative impact on speech and language learning.

Monitoring Progress and Tracking Clinical Data

To ensure the effectiveness of interventions, clinicians must consistently track the frequency of correct production of the target sound in relation to the child's progress toward speech goal(s). Creating a general clinical data sheet that can be quickly modified for each child is highly recommended. Clinical data must be collected during each session. Audio recording each session to ensure the accuracy of the data is also necessary. Appendix 13–B is a sample data sheet. All data sheets should include quantitative data (e.g., numbers, such as percentages, number of prompts) and qualitative data (e.g., clinical observations that cannot be quantified easily by numbers). Chapter 8 offers additional suggestions for data collection. The appendices of Chapter 8 contain generic data sheets that can be modified for SSD treatment. Data sheets with the following components are very helpful:

1. Target sound: the sound(s) the child was working on in the session
2. Position: initial (I), medial (M), or final (F) position
3. Accuracy of production
4. Type of prompt provided
5. Qualitative clinical observation. Clinical observation should be brief but informative. Information should include the client's level of participation (e.g., attention, behavior), the training materials used, and any noted client strengths and weaknesses evident while implementing treatment.

If language is also addressed during the session, progress regarding language learning should be documented separately. Use a separate data sheet for each goal addressed in the child's treatment plan. As stated earlier, the purpose of data collection is to ensure the effectiveness of the intervention. Therefore, if a child does not progress at a desired and reasonable pace, treatment activities need to be modified by your supervising SLP. Thus, data need to be effectively conveyed to your supervising SLP. Chapter 9 has additional suggestions on how to summarize this information in a modified subjective, objective, assessment, and plan (SOAP) note format.

REFERENCES

American Speech-Language-Hearing Association. (n.d.). *National outcomes measurement system (NOMS)*. https://www.asha.org/noms/

American Speech-Language-Hearing Association. (2020). *ASHA 2020 schools survey: SLP caseload and workload characteristics report*. https://www.asha.org/siteassets/surveys/2020-schools-survey-slp-caseload.pdf

Barlow, J., & Gierut, J. (2002). Minimal pair approaches to phonological remediation. *Seminars in Speech and Language*, 23(1), 57–67. https://doi.org/10.1055/s-2002-24969

Bauman-Waengler, J. (2020). *Articulatory and phonological impairments: A clinical focus* (6th ed.). Pearson.

Bernthal, J., Bankson, N., & Flipsen, P. (2013). *Articulation and phonological disorders: Speech sound disorders in children* (7th ed.). Pearson.

Forrest, K. (2002). Are oral-motor exercises useful in the treatment of phonological/articulatory disorders? *Seminars in Speech and Language*, 23, 15–25. https://doi.org/10.1055/s-2002-23508

Gierut, J. (1989). Maximal oppositions approach to phonological treatment. *Journal of Speech and Hearing Research*, 54, 9–19. https://doi.org/10.1044/jshd.5401.09

Gordon-Brannan, M. E., & Weiss, C. E. (2007). *Clinical management of articulation and phonologic disorders* (3rd ed.). Lippincott Williams & Wilkins.

Justice, L., Gillon, G., McNeill, B., & Schuele, C. M. (2013). Phonological awareness: Description, assessment, and intervention. In J. E. Bernthal, N. W. Bankson, & P. Flipsen (Eds.), *Articulation and phonological disorders: Speech sound disorders in children* (7th ed., pp. 355–382). Pearson.

Lof, G. (2003). Oral motor exercises and treatment outcomes. *Perspectives on Language, Learning, and Education*, 10(1), 7–12.

Lof, G. (2017, March). *What works for speech sound disorders: Using evidence to guide practice* [PowerPoint slides]. Presentation at the Mississippi Speech-Language-Hearing Association Annual Conference. https://www.z2systems.com/neon/resource/msha/files/Handouts/2017/Lof%20hand out.pdf

Paul, R., Norbury, C., & Gosse, C. (2018). *Language disorders from infancy through adolescence: Listening, speaking, reading, writing, and communicating* (5th ed.). Elsevier.

Peña-Brooks, A., & Hegde, M. N. (2007). *Assessment and treatment of articulation and phonological disorders in children: A dual-level text* (2nd ed.). Pro-Ed.

Sander, E. (1972). Do we know when speech sounds are learned? *Journal of Speech and Hearing Disorders*, 37, 55–63.

Secord, W. A., Boyce, S. E., Donohue, J. S., Fox, R. A., & Shine, R. E. (2007). *Eliciting sounds: Techniques and strategies for clinicians* (2nd ed.). Delmar Cengage Learning.

Shriberg, L. (1993). Four new speech and prosody voice measures for genetics research and other studies in developmental phonological disorders. *Journal of Speech and Hearing Research*, 36, 105–140.

Smit, A., Hand, L., Freilinger, J., Bernthal, J., & Bird, A. (1990). The Iowa articulation norms project and its Nebraska replication. *Journal of Speech and Hearing Disorders*, 55, 779–798.

Templin, M. (1957). *Certain language skills in children*. University of Minnesota Press.

Tyler, A., Lewis, K., Haskill, A., & Tolbert, L. (2002). Efficacy and cross-domain effects of a morphosyntax and a phonology intervention. *Language, Speech and Hearing Services in Schools*, 33, 52–66. https://doi.org/10.1044/0161-1461(2002/005)

Van Riper, C., & Erickson, R. (1996). *Speech correction: An introduction to speech pathology and audiology* (7th ed.). Prentice-Hall.

Williams, A. L. (1991). Generalization patterns associated with training least phonological knowledge. *Journal of Speech and Hearing Research, 34,* 722–733.

Williams, A. L. (1993). Phonological reorganization: A qualitative measure of phonological improvement. *American Journal of Speech-Language Pathology, 2,* 44–51.

Williams, A. L. (2000). Multiple oppositions: Case studies of variables in phonological intervention. *American Journal of Speech-Language Pathology, 9,* 289–299.

World Health Organization. (2001). *International Classification of Functioning, Disability and Health (ICF).*

APPENDIX 13–A
Sample SSD Homework Sheet

Please give this speech homework sheet to your parent. Say each word correctly *10 times* a day with your parent. Pay attention to the sound you make. Remember to show your parent what you have learned in your speech session. Please ask your parent to put *a check mark for each word* after you say the word correctly 10 times. After you finish saying all the words correctly, please ask your parent to *initial at the bottom for each day you practice*. Please remember to bring your speech folder with you next time when you come to speech room.

Keep up the good work!!   _____/Speech Teacher

Target words—/s/ in initial position	Day 1	Day 2	Day 3	Day 4	Day 5	Day 6	Day 7
Sun							
Sea							
Say							
Saw							
Parent's Initials							

APPENDIX 13-B
Sample SSD Treatment Data Collection Form

Target Sound	Position (I/M/F)	Speech sound production (+ correct production, – incorrect production)
		Prompt system: 1. Physical (placement) 2. Visual 3. Verbal 4. No prompt/independent
/k/	I (initial)	–/3 (explanation: incorrect with physical prompt provided), –/2, –/2+3 (incorrect with visual and verbal combined), +/3 (correct with physical prompt provided), +/3, +/3 . . . _____ *correct production /_____ total number of production in one session (correct + incorrect) =* _____*% accuracy*

Clinical Observation (qualitative)
Fully participated. Word level: one- and two-syllable words used. Responds best to physical prompt (articulation placement with tongue depressor). Starting to positively react to visual prompt. Mirror used throughout.

CHAPTER 14

Early Intervention

Margaret Vento-Wilson

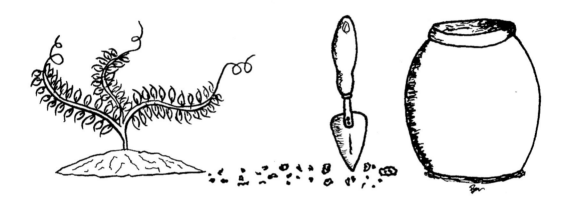

INTRODUCTION

Watch and listen to a young child talk! You may be amused, impressed, puzzled, or curious, and you are bound to learn something. You will learn that when young children talk, they interact with and influence other persons; they talk about what they are doing, or are about to do, or want someone else to do; they say sounds or words, or phrases. And having noticed these things, you will have learned something about language. (Lahey, 1988, p. 1)

So opens Margaret Lahey's textbook on language development. This quote is on the first page of the first chapter because of the primacy of the message, which serves to remind all practitioners that as much theoretical knowledge we may have about language, and as much as we have been taught by university professors about this remarkable phenomenon, children themselves are our best and truest teachers and should always inform and drive our intervention.

When I was in graduate school, I used every opportunity to interact with two of my young nieces to test out what I had recently learned. I remember one encounter with Kate, my then 3-year-old niece, who told me a complicated story about playing at the park with her best friend the day before. In the midst of the telling, she remarked with great emotion, "And then she felled me down!" Although I understood her perfectly, her sentence violated the semantic and syntactic rules of English. Upon first glance, the rule violations did not look complicated, but when I got home that evening, I analyzed what she had done in that sentence, and here is what I discovered (Goldberg & Jackendoff, 2004; Nadathur, 2017; Pinker, 1999; Smith, 1970; Wright, 2002):

1. She correctly selected a *move and change* verb to describe the event, which implies action or a change of state.
2. She further specified by using a *resultative verb*, which implies a completed action.
3. She maintained faithfulness to verb class, in that both the verbs *to fall* and *to push* involve a causative action with a resulting event.
4. She maintained faithfulness to the past-tense form of *fall* and generated the word *fell*.
5. She applied the morphological rules for marking a weak verb by adding *–ed* to a strong verb, which typically involves a vowel change—from *fall* to *fell*.
6. She incorrectly chose the verb *to fall*, rather than *to push*, and in an attempt to reconcile the morphological requirements for regular past-tense markedness, she applied the *–ed*. All of which resulted in a redundancy of markedness.
7. In selecting the verb *to fall*, she inadvertently changed the source of agency: The verb *to fall* is involuntary, which does not require an agent, and the verb *to push* is volitional and requires an agent.
8. She merged internal and external causation.
9. She altered the transitivity of the verb: The verb *to fall* is an intransitive verb, which means that the action does not transfer to an object, and the verb *to push* is transitive, which means that it requires an object to receive the action.

Unbelievably, my 3-year-old niece accomplished all this in a split second, and all before she was able to tie her own shoes!

If you had any doubts about the complexity of language before you began this chapter, I suspect that those doubts have now been erased. But I enjoin you not to let it chase you away. As complex as it is, in the end, language is simply the way we as humans use symbols to interact with others. You are a fluent speaker of your native language, and you have been manipulating linguistic symbols your whole life. And now as a speech-language pathologist assistant (SLPA), you will have the opportunity to help others use language this same way, but with a bird's-eye view of the construct of language.

Partnering in the acquisition and early development of a child's language is wonderfully fun and I cannot recommend it highly enough. I cannot think of a single day in my work with children that has not made me smile, and I can think of only a few that have not made me laugh out loud. However, I must caution you that successful outcomes never just happen. Rather, they are the result of an SLPA's strong theoretical base, well-conducted intervention, and ongoing self-reflection to support continued improvement. This chapter has been written to support your work as an SLPA in early intervention, and the information presented here addresses the first two components of successful outcomes, but only you can address the third component (Figure 14–1).

THE WORK OF CHILDREN

Upon birth, children are tasked with an immense job that seems almost impossible when described in detail. In their first few years, typically developing children make the transformation from a nonverbal state to a verbal state and learn to comprehend, manipulate, construct, and produce their native language fluently (Bates & Goodman, 1997; Brown, 1973; Pinker, 1996). This remarkable transformation involves many stages and hierarchies, several which are described below. Table 14–1 presents some of the milestones of language development as described by Bates (2003) in her extensive work on language

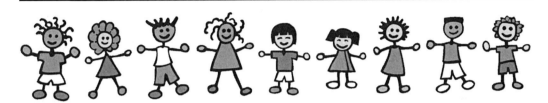

Figure 14–1. Children ready for early intervention. Courtesy of Bing Images, free to share and use commercially.

Table 14–1. Developmental Model of Language Acquisition

Age Range	Milestone	Definition
0 to 3 months	Initial state of the system	The infant prefers to listen to sounds in the native language. The infant can hear all phonetic contrasts used in the languages of the world.
3 to 6 months	Perception and production of vowels	The infant coos and imitates vowels only. Vowel perception is organized along language-specific lines.
6 to 8 months	Babbling in consonant-vowel segments (e.g., Ba, Baba)	
8 to 10 months	Word comprehension	The infant starts to lose sensitivity to consonants outside its native language.
12 to 13 months	Word production	The infant begins to name objects and people.
16 to 20 months	Word combinations	Vocabulary acceleration occurs. Relational words begin to appear (verbs and adjectives).
24 to 36 months	Grammaticization	Function words begin to appear (prepositions, articles). Inflectional morphology emerges (verb tense). Sentence complexity increases.
3 year to adulthood	Late developments	Vocabulary growth continues. The child demonstrates increases in the comprehension and use of rare and complex forms. Sentence-level grammar is reorganized for the purpose of discourse.

Source: Bates, 2003, p. 15.

acquisition. Dramatic growth occurs in receptive and expressive vocabulary in the first 30 months of life (Bates, 2003).

In this same approximate number of months (33), children begin to combine words purposefully and in the word order dictated by their native language. Additional milestones of language development in the domain of morphology follow in Table 14–2.

Throughout these early years, children move through stages that begin with a single word (often an approximation), to the use of multiple words, and then into full syntactic structures called sentences (Peters, 1995). First, children solidify the link between a concept (e.g., a small, soft, furry animal that lives in

my house) and a representation (e.g., cat). Over time, these concepts or words reach a critical mass, and they begin to put these words together into meaningful combinations (Spelke & Tsivkin, 2001; Table 14–3 provides examples of meaningful combinations). These early word combinations, or semantic relations, are defined as two- to three-word phrases with a holistic meaning that may not be obvious when looking at each individual word (Bloom et al., 1980). In other words, the sum of the utterance is greater than its parts. Soon thereafter, children add more words to these utterances, and they step into the world of syntax. Another way to think about this developmental shift follows: With a single word, children

Table 14–2. Brown's Stages of Morphological Acquisition

Age of Acquisition (Months)	Brown's Stage	Morphological Structure	Example
15–30	Stage I	One or two true words	"papa," "blankie"
28–36	Stage II	Present progressive	"singing"
		Articles "in" and "out"	
		–s Plurals	"toy<u>s</u>"
36–42	Stage III	Irregular past tense	"fell"
		's Possessive	"Riley<u>'s</u> bike"
		Uncontractible copula	"<u>is</u> it hot?"
40–46	Stage IV	Articles	"an," "the"
		Regular past tense	"talk<u>ed</u>"
		Third person regular, present tense	"he <u>rakes</u> it"
42–52+	Stage V	Third person irregular	"she <u>does</u>"
		Uncontractible auxiliary	"<u>are</u> they swimming?"
		Contractible copula	"<u>she's</u> funny"
		Contractible auxiliary	"<u>they're</u> going"

Source: Adapted from *"A first language: The early stages,"* by R. Brown, 1973 and *"Language disorders from infancy through adolescence: Listening, speaking, reading, writing, and communicating,"* by Paul, R. & Norbury, C. F., 2012.

Table 14–3. Semantic Relations

Two-Word Semantic Relations	Example
Agent + Action	Daddy go
Action + Object	Catch ball
Action + Locative	Sit chair
Entity + Locative	Cat bed
Possessor + Possession	Mommy bike
Attribute + Entity	Happy baby
Demonstrative + Entity	This book
Three-Word Semantic Relations	**Example**
Agent + Action + Object	Phoebe eat pasta
Agent + Action + Locative	Riley sleep crib
Agent + Object + Locative	Grammy key table
Action + Object + Locative	Get blanket bed

Source: Brown, 1973.

can talk about a few concepts; with two words, they can talk about a few more concepts; and with three or more words, they can talk about many concepts, but with greater specificity. A final developmental continuum demonstrating the complexity of children's work in their early years is the shift in their intentionality (Table 14–4), which is linked to their growing awareness that someone is paying attention to them, and that symbols can be used to achieve a goal (Bates et al., 1975; Bloom & Beckwith, 1989; Owens, 2004).

What these tables and figures tell us is that children are very, very busy in these early years as they work to acquire their native language by participating in the world around them. However, for a subset of children, this acquisition process is altered or delayed for various reasons that reflect their individual cognitive, motoric, sensory/perceptual, and linguistic profiles, as well as various environmental, biological, and behavioral factors, as seen in Figure 14–2.

Specific disorders that contribute to these alterations or delays can include intellectual developmental disability (IDD), language learning disorder (LLD), autism spectrum disorder (ASD), developmental language disorder (DLD), or other congenital or acquired impairments (American Speech-Language-Hearing Association [ASHA], n.d.; Rice, 2016). For these children, exposure to the language around them and participation in their worlds are not enough to support the acquisition of their native language and that is where you as an SLPA and as a member of the early intervention team become relevant. Your work will help children move to the next level in their acquisition process (Figure 14–3).

Table 14–4. Development of Intentionality

Stage	Behavior	Example
Non-Purposeful Communication		
Pre-Intentional	Behaviors are reflexive and express inner states (tired, hungry) and serve as signals for others. These behaviors are not directed to a specific person and there is no obvious expectation of an outcome.	Crying, cooing, posture changes, facial expressions
Unintentional-Intentional	Behaviors are intentional and goal orientated (reaching for a bottle), but are not conventionalized and recognized by both the speaker and listener. As above, these behaviors are not directed to a specific person and there is no obvious expectation of an outcome.	Fussing, reaching for or looking at an object
Purposeful Communication		
Non-Conventional Proto-Imperative	Non-conventional gestures, usually involving physical contact, are used with intent to affect a caregiver. The intention to communicate through behavior is confirmed when the child checks for the attention of the adult. The anticipation of an outcome is confirmed by persistence or frustration if the goal is not met. There is recognition that the caregiver provides the means to an end.	Tugging, pulling toward, pushing away
Conventional	Recognized or conventional vocalizations and gestures used to affect a caregiver's attention intentionally. There is a greater level of persistence.	Nodding, pointing, waving, alternating gaze, handing an object
Concrete	Recognizable symbols are used in a limited fashion. These symbols are used at some distance from the concept they represent. There is a range of intentions and they may be accompanied by vocalizations.	Requesting assistance/information, pointing, reaching, offering, signing
Symbolic Communication		
Abstract	Arbitrary symbols are used individually and in a limited fashion and to represent the environment and the *here and now*. There is an understanding that words have referential value. There is still some use of idiosyncratic symbols. The use of gestures and vocalizations continues.	Symbols (words)
Formal	Words are combined in a rule-bound order. These combinations are used to talk about the *there and then*, and the concept represented by the symbol does not need to be present. The use of gestures and vocalizations fades and the primary means of communication is language.	Symbol, word combinations

Source: Adapted from "The acquisition of performatives prior to speech," by E. Bates, L. Camaioni, & V. Volterra, 1975. In *Merrill-Palmer Quarterly of Behavior and Development*, *21*(3), 205–226, and "Intentionality and Language Development" by L. Bloom & R. Beckwith, 1989. In *Columbia Academic Commons* and *Language disorders: A functional approach to assessment and intervention*, by R. E. Owens, Jr., 2004, p. 89

Environmental Factors External experiences that either increase risk of disorder or that are protective in the face of biological risk	**Biological Factors** Differences in genetic risk and neurological structure and function associated with disorder
	Cognitive Factors Differences in perception and information processing associated with disorder
	Behavioral Features Overt differences in behavior that characterize the disorder

Figure 14–2. Factors affecting language development (Paul & Norbury, 2012, p. 10).

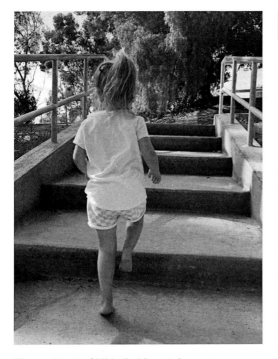

Figure 14–3. Child climbing stairs.

THE WORK OF INTERVENTION

An in-depth discussion and definition of language is well beyond the scope of this chapter; however, it is prudent to present a broad overview of what language is precisely because that is the tool with which you will be working in your role as an SLPA. Language can be viewed from many lenses: (a) Language involves multifaceted relationships between communication, linguistic forms, and world knowledge (Lahey & Bloom, 1977), (b) language is an indefinitely large system of meaning that is both created and exchanged (Halliday, 2003), and (c) language is a systematic conventionalized code of arbitrary signals agreed upon by a group (Lahey, 1988). Regardless of one's personal theory of language acquisition, a concept uniting all the theories is that language development is supported, at the very least, within human-to-human interaction (Bates et al., 1975; Eisenberg, 2004; Lightbrown & Spada, 2013). This means that there must be an interlocutor who responds to the child (Lightbrown & Spada, 2013). In intervention-based interactions, this implies a kind of mentorship where you as the SLPA provide a bridge as the child moves up the language acquisition hierarchy.

This brings us to the definition of intervention itself. According to ASHA (2008) and Ukrainetz (2015), intervention is defined as intentional actions taken to accelerate, modify, or compensate for inadequate performance. It is further defined by Lahey and Bloom (1977) as the "manipulation of the tangible non-linguistic, linguistic, and social context in ways designed to enhance the induction of regularities within and between these contexts" (p. 341). ASHA has identified four guiding principles that should serve as the foundation for early intervention:

1. Services should be family centered and culturally responsive.
2. Services should be developmentally supportive and promote children's participation in their natural environments.
3. Services should be comprehensive, coordinated, and team based.
4. Services should be based on the highest quality internal and external evidence that is available. (ASHA, 2008, para. 5)

Specific to your role as an SLPA in early intervention, and under your supervising speech-language pathologist (SLP), you are expected to provide direct treatment to children as follows (ASHA, 2022):

1. Follow and implement documented treatment plans or protocols developed by your supervising SLP.
2. Document performance of the child (e.g., tallying data, preparing charts, records, graphs, language samples) and report this information to the supervising SLP.
3. Serve as an interpreter, a translator, or a transliterator for children and their families who do not speak English or use a signed language.

In your role as an SLPA and as a language interlocutor for young children, the models described below will support your efforts and create a greater likelihood of success.

Zone of Proximal Development

The first model is called the *zone of proximal development* (ZPD), which was first identified by Vygotsky in 1978. The word *zone* refers to the space between what the child can currently do independently and what the child will be able to accomplish independently in the near future, regardless of the task, as seen in Figure 14–4. The area of overlap defines your role as a bridge between the two different states. In your work as an SLPA, you may support a child in moving from labeling items to combining words into semantic relations (i.e., early word combinations), to generating three- to four-word phrases, to producing full, syntactically correct sentences (Gentner & Boroditsky, 2003). Likewise, you may support a child's transition from an individual picture description task, to retelling a short story, to creating a personal narrative with multiple characters, similar to the one my niece told

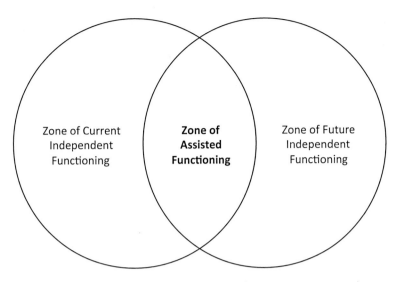

Figure 14–4. Zone of proximal development (Wass & Golding, 2014).

me. There are various intervention techniques, which are expanded on later in this chapter, that can be used when working within a ZPD. One intervention technique is called recasting, where the SLPA adds an element (or elements) to a child's utterance (Proctor-Williams & Fey, 2007), as seen below:

Child: Doggie!

SLPA: Yes, a big doggie!

In this interaction, the SLPA has incorporated a word and concept the child has acquired and added a relevant descriptor that builds complexity onto the child's original utterance.

Caregiver-Mediated Instructional Practices

A second model that can be used to frame your intervention was defined by Dunst et al. (2012) as caregiver-mediated instructional practices (CMIPs; Figure 14–5). Although Dunst et al. identified parents as the caregiver in their conceptualization, for purposes of this chapter, the role of the caregiver is being replaced by you, the SLPA. This model suggests that your intervention should reflect the interests of the child within everyday, meaningful, and familiar activities, as described in Table 14–5. These factors increase the likelihood of linguistic interactions between you and the child, which in turn increases the potential for further communicative and linguistic development (Dunst et al., 2012). In your role as an SLPA, you may interview the family to identify favorite and familiar activities of the child with whom you are working. You can also observe the child and her caregivers in a play session to gain better insight into the child's interaction style. And finally, you can use this information to engage in intervention contexts that support the child's further language development.

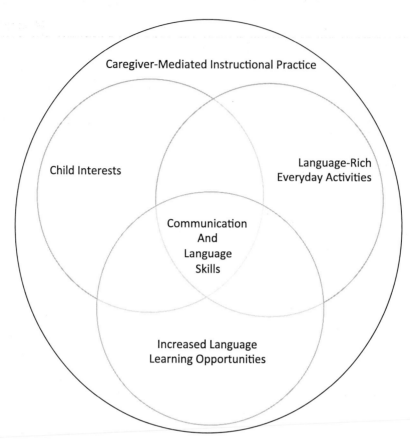

Figure 14–5. Language intervention model (Dunst et al., 2012, p. 13).

Table 14–5. Factors of Caregiver-Mediated Instructional Practices

Focus	Description
Child	Intervention targeting communicative and linguistic competence reflects the child's strengths and her personal and situational interests.
Activity	Intervention tasks increase naturalistic linguistic and communicative functioning in the child's environments.
	Intervention reflects the child's daily activities and incorporates tasks and objects that are relevant and familiar.
	Intervention allows for multiple communicative and linguistic learning opportunities within and across activities.
Methods	Intervention involves a positive affect and close attention to the child's interaction initiations to reinforce and sustain engagement.
	Intervention supports the development or refinement of reciprocal interactions between the SLPA and the child.
	Intervention follows the child's lead.

Source: Dunst et al., 2012.

Although this is good theoretical advice, it also has enormous practical value! As someone who has sat on the floor across from a 2½-year-old and attempted to entice her to engage in communication with a task that was too far removed from her daily life and much too artificial, I can attest that it does not always work. All my hard work in designing the session was met with a stony silence. However, when I stepped back and allowed this feisty toddler to guide the context and topic, our conversation took off with a bang! Going on a pretend shopping trip to Target for fruit and vegetables offered countless opportunities to use prepositions within phrases—put apple/grapes/broccoli in, take banana/strawberry/spinach out (Figure 14–6). As a result, I achieved the desired number of productions and she developed greater proficiency over prepositions. A final comment is that sometimes getting a child to engage is a bit like herding cats, but if you can bring her world into your intervention session, you are much more likely to be successful (Figure 14–7).

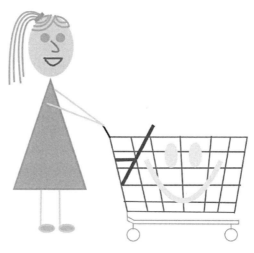

Figure 14–6. Toddler shopping for fruit.

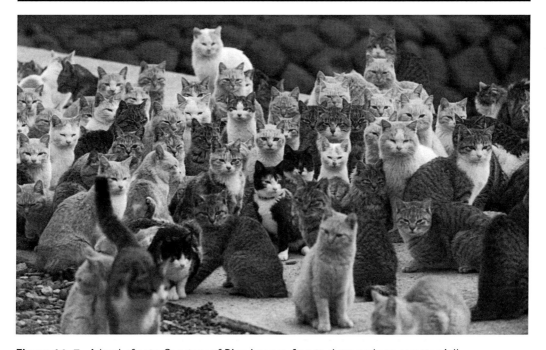

Figure 14–7. A herd of cats. Courtesy of Bing Images, free to share and use commercially.

Intervention Considerations

Competing Resources

One consideration central to language intervention, generally and specifically, is the notion of competing resources (Lahey & Bloom, 1994; Wallach, 2008; Wallach & Ocampo, 2020). When children's abilities are emerging or unstable, task demands must be carefully modulated (Wallach, 2008). When there is a mismatch between abilities and demands, the child's resources have to compete for attention, and something must give. Paul and Norbury (2012) further explained this consideration as allowing new forms to express old communicative functions or allowing new communicative functions to be expressed by an old form. Within an intervention context, this means that you must limit the task requirements. If you were working to expand a child's expressive vocabulary, it would be prudent to incorporate newly targeted words within a syntactic structure already well established in the child's repertoire. Conversely, if you were working toward an increase in utterance length, it would be best practice to incorporate familiar words into the longer, or more complex phrase (Paul & Norbury, 2012; Wallach, 2008).

Continuum of Naturalness

A final intervention consideration to be discussed is a continuum of naturalness as originally proposed by Fey (1986). This continuum describes three types of intervention that you will use in your role as an SLPA: (a) clinician directed, (b) hybrid,

and (c) child centered (Cirrin & Gillam, 2008; Paul & Norbury, 2012; Owens, 2004; Roth & Worthington, 2010). Table 14–6 contains brief descriptions and examples of each intervention type.

There is no single method or location on the continuum that is best for all children. What is needed is the best match among a specific child, a specific target, and the intervention approach (Kamhi, 1999; Paul & Norbury, 2012). For example, in the intervention context I described above, I made the wise decision to make a shift from a very clinician-directed and less natural context to a child-centered and more natural context. For that young girl, it was the right decision. However, with another child I worked with, we sat at a table across from each other and engaged in a very structured literacy routine with very predictable syntactic demands. This young boy thrived in a structured context, and this more clinician-directed structure was the best match for the child and my targets. As you become more experienced and knowledgeable, differentiating the choices become easier, but it is always best to let the child guide your intervention decisions.

A final comment regarding the continuum of naturalness is that at every point along this continuum, best practices suggest remaining mindful of the ZPD as you target specific skills to ensure a smooth transition to the next skill level. Further, this continuum parallels the intervention model proposed by Dunst et al. (2012) but acknowledges that the nature of intervention should be individualized for each child and for each task or skill being targeted.

Table 14–6. Intervention Types on the Continuum of Naturalness

Type	Definition	Intervention Method	Example
Clinician-Directed	Highly structured: The clinician selects topics, materials, acceptable forms of response, and the method of reinforcement.	Drill	Picture identification, repetitive production of similar items. Specific forms are targeted.
Hybrid	Moderately structured and naturalistic: The clinician selects a narrow set of targets and materials that tempt the child.	Milieu language therapy. Focused stimulation.	Language development is targeted by modeling and highlighting the specific forms.
Child-Centered	Naturalistic: The interests and preferences of the child dictate the topics, materials, and reinforcement method.	Indirect language stimulation.	Engagement in daily activities, facilitated play. Language development is supported by responding to the child's utterances.

INTERVENTION STRUCTURE

Language Structure

Language comprises form, content, and use, as seen in Figure 14–8. These three domains have been expanded upon in Tables 14–7, 14–8, and 14–9. In addition to clarifying the three domains of language, these tables also provide a list of targets for intervention. For example, under the domain of form, potential targets can be seen in Table 14–10. Under the domain of content, potential targets can be seen in Tables 14–11 and 14–12.

In terms of words that can be incorporated into your intervention sessions, the domains of content and form can be viewed from a perspective of semantic relations as defined above (see Table 14–3 for examples of semantic relations). Table 14–13 lists words and word combinations that can be incorporated into your intervention sessions with children in the early stages of language development.

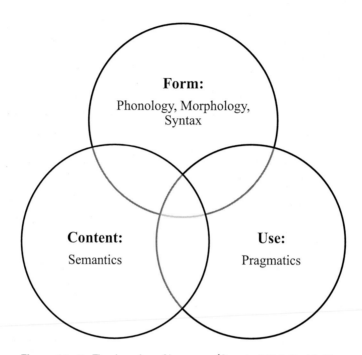

Figure 14–8. The domains of language (Owens, 2004; Paul & Norbury, 2012). Goals and intervention in the domain of phonology are addressed in Chapter 13 and thus will not be covered in this chapter.

Levels of Symbolism

Early intervention can be conceived of on a continuum of symbolic understanding and use (Owens, 2004). As detailed earlier, children move through a symbolic hierarchy that culminates with combining words in meaningful ways to express thoughts, once again moving toward greater communicative specificity. It is likely that you will work with children who demonstrate no overt communication, those who use only vocalizations or gestures, and those who are just beginning to put words together. As can be inferred, there are many states in this hierarchy, which implies many levels of intervention. Table 14–14 describes some of the intervention considerations and tasks related to a child's level of symbolic development.

Table 14–7. A Representation of Language Form (Phonology, Morphology, Syntax)

Categories of Spoken Form			
Language Domain	**Subdomain**	**Features**	**Example**
Phonology	Segmental	Phonemes	/b/, /p/, t/, /d/, ...
		Syllables	/ba/, /pa/, /ta/, /da/, ...
	Suprasegmental	Intonation	Phrase contour: rising, falling ...
		Stress	
		Pause	
Language Domain	**Word Class**	**Word Type**	**Example**
Morphology	Substantive	Content Words	Verbs, Adjectives, Adverbs, Nouns
	Relational	Function Words	Prepositions, Conjunctions, Auxiliary Verbs, Articles, Pronouns
Language Domain	**Subdomain**	**Feature**	**Example**
Syntax	Word Order	Sentence Structure	Subject-Verb-Object, Subject-Object-Verb ...
		Clauses	Coordinate, Subordinate
		Sentence Types	Active, Passive
	Inflection	Suffixes (ing, ed, ~s)	Verb: ~ing
			Noun: ~ist
			Adjective: ~able
			Adverb: ~ly

Source: Adapted from Lahey, 1988, p. 12.

Table 14–8. A Representation of Language Use (Pragmatics)

Categories of Language Use			
Language Use	**Subdomain**	**Features**	**Example**
Function	Personal/Intrapersonal	Commenting	"Book funny."
		Vocal Play	"The seat belt goes 'click, click, click.'"
		Problem Solve	"Find socks?"
	Social/Interpersonal	Request Object	"Give ball now!"
		Obtain Information	"Where is mommy?"
		Gain Attention	"I want down."
Language Use	**Subdomain**	**Features**	**Example**
Context	Nonlinguistic	Perceptual Support	Active listening, passive listening
		Adapt to Needs of Listener	Rate of speech, comprehension checks
		Social	Conversational Devices: Turn taking, initiating, terminating
			Status Relations: Politeness, direct and indirect requests
	Linguistic	Non-Contingent	N/A
		Contingent	Imitate
			Question
			Add Information

Source: Adapted from Lahey, 1988, p. 16.

Table 14–9. A Representation of Language Content (Semantics)

Categories of Language Content			
Language Domain	**Subdomain**	**Example**	
Object Knowledge	Specific Objects	Mother; father; specific siblings/friends/pets; specific familiar locations . . .	
	Object Classes	Animals, furniture, food, toys . . .	
Language Domain	**Subdomain**	**Feature**	**Example**
Object Relations	Reflexive	Existence/Disappearance	"Ball all gone."
	Interactions	Attribution Quantity	"Big pool." "Two cookies."
	Interclass	Action/State/Possession	"Drink milk." "Yummy cake." "Phoebe doll."
Language Domain	**Subdomain**	**Example**	
Event Relations	Temporal	Before, after	
	Causal	Because, since	
	Epistemic	Know, believe	

Source: Adapted from Lahey, 1988, p. 9.

Table 14–10. List of Potential Intervention Targets in the Domain of *Form*

Broad Target	Category	Example
Vocabulary	Content words	Adjectives, adverbs, nouns, verbs
	Function words	Prepositions, conjunctions, articles, pronouns, auxiliary verbs
Morphology	Plurals	Regular, irregular
	Verb tenses	Past, present, future
	Prefixes and suffixes	
Syntax	Word order	Subject-verb-object
	Clause types	Subordinate, coordinate, relative
	Sentence types	Passive, active, questions

Table 14–11. List of Potential Intervention Targets in the Domain of *Content*

Broad Target	Category	Example
Labeling	Objects, people	Family members, friends, toys
Combining words	Semantic relations	Existence, disappearance, re-occurrence, quantity, actions, possessions
	Events	Temporal (before, after), causation (because), states (knowing, being, having)

Table 14–12. List of Potential Intervention Targets in the Domain of *Use*

Broad Target	Category	Example
Language functions	Personal	Commenting, inner dialogue
	Social	Requesting, greeting, gaining attention, asking
Nonlinguistic	Implicit rules	Turn taking, initiating/ending interactions, polite behavior, tone of voice

Table 14–13. Semantic Relations That Can Be Incorporated Into Intervention

Content	Relational Words	Object–Specific Relational Words	Substantive Words
Rejection	No		
Nonexistence/disappearance	No, all gone, away		
Cessation of Action	Stop, no		
Prohibition of action	No		
Recurrence of objects and actions	More, again, another		
Noting existence or object identification	This, there, that		
Actions on objects		Give, do, make, get, throw, eat, wash, kiss	
Actions of locating objects		Put, up, down, sit, fall, go	
Attributes or descriptions of objects		Big, hot, dirty, heavy	
Persons associate with objects			Personal names

Source: Lahey & Bloom, 1977, Appendix 14-A.

Table 14–14. Considerations and Goals Related to Symbolic Developmental Levels

Developmental Levels	Considerations	Intervention Tasks
Presymbolic/Nonsymbolic	Intervention should focus on the child's family/natural settings and contexts.	Expand the number of communicative functions.
		Increase the complexity of communicative functions.
		Support the transition from nonintentional to intentional communication.
		Replace unconventional communication with conventional communication.
Symbolic	Intervention should focus on increasing the child's communicative and linguistic competence.	Expand the number of concepts expressed.
		Expand the length of utterances.
		Increase the complexity of utterances.
	Intervention should support greater communicative contexts.	Expand the child's communicative partners.
		Change the environment of the intervention.

Source: Owens, 2004.

INTERVENTION METHODS

As an SLPA, you will not be responsible for writing goals or specifying intervention targets (ASHA, 2022), but you will be implementing intervention defined and designed by your supervising SLP. Toward that end, Table 14–15 contains a list of intervention methods that can be used with children across contexts, diagnoses, and development levels. The decision to use one of these methods should be based on the child's unique characteristics and personality type, the intervention target, and your professional skill. It is important to note that these methods are not presented in an either/or fashion. There may be sessions where it is most advantageous to use more than one, or to adapt one based on a specific child's needs. Ultimately, it is your responsibility as an SLPA to engage the child, and you may have to make a change in the moment. In your work in early intervention, it is never appropriate to blame the child for lack of engagement: You are the adult and the SLPA, and it is up to you to create a successful and productive intervention session.

Language Facilitation Methods

Additional language facilitation strategies not specific to a single intervention method can be found in the following list:

1. Ask open-ended questions to offer more opportunities for interaction to continue. Asking for a child's opinion allows him to share his thoughts and ideas. You can ask the child to make a prediction about an outcome or an

Table 14–15. Intervention Methods

Drill	
Naturalness: Clinician directed	Definition: Uses discrete drill work in a highly controlled context in conjunction with relevant linguistic materials to increase the frequency of a language target with clear reinforcements

Key Factors:

Intervention targets are broken down into a series of steps.

Targets are presented in a series of a high number of trials.

Reinforcements are consistent and reflect specific performance factors, such as "You used the sign for 'more'" and "That's right, the apple is IN the basket!"

Potential Session Structure:

Engage the child in a task with many pieces (Mr. Potato Head, a train set, setting a table) and require the child to produce a target, such as the preposition "on," before they can add a piece to the task.

Focused Stimulation	
Naturalness: Hybrid	Definition: The clinician arranges the intervention context so that the child is tempted to respond with utterances.

Key Factors:

Respond to all communicative acts (gestural, vocal, symbolic).

Refer to the here and now.

Allow processing time for the child.

Describe your actions and the child's actions.

Use short sentences with words of one or two syllables.

When possible, avoid the use of telegraphic speech, or short, ungrammatical phrases ("wash hand hot").

Potential Session Structure: This method can be used in any type of task or context.

Indirect Language Stimulation	
Naturalness: Child centered	Definition: Provides a simple model within the child's ZPD that links the child's behavior with a linguistic mapping of that behavior.

Key Factors:

Describe your own and the child's actions.

Imitate the behavior, communication, or language of the child.

Expand the child's utterance with additional grammatical detail and semantics.

Extend the child's utterance by restating the utterance with additional details.

Recast the child's utterance into a different type of utterance, such as a question or a negative statement.

Potential Session Structure: This method can be used in any type of task or context.

Incidental Training	
Naturalness: Child centered	Definition: Intervention occurs within unstructured situations. The child's interests and preferences frame the focus of the intervention.

Key Factors: Input by the SLPA should match or be slightly more complex or longer than the child's current level of communication or language.

Potential Session Structure:

Hide and find objects with accompanying comments.

While putting toys away, the SLPA differentiates between singular and plural nouns (block/blocks; doll/dolls; truck/trucks).

Table 14–15. *continued*

Enhanced Milieu Teaching
Naturalness: Hybrid Definition: The use of environmental arrangement to support the development of engagement. It is used to model, prompt, and cue new language forms.
Key Factors: Choose materials of interest to the child. Arrange the environment to elicit responses. Wait expectantly for a response. Expand the child's utterances.
Potential Session Structure: Establish an interactive routine that serves as the backdrop for your session.
Behavior Chain Interruption
Naturalness: Clinician directed Definition: The intervention involves a break in an established routine.
Key Factors: The task must be familiar to the child.
Potential Session Structure: Stop playing a favorite song. Offer an empty crayon box for a drawing task. Skip the child in a turn-taking task.
Potential Session Structure: Establish an interactive routine that serves as the backdrop for your session.

Sources: Dunst et al., 2012; Hancock & Kaiser, 2006; Hart & Risley, 1975; Kaiser et al., 2000; Owens, 2004, 2009; Paul & Norbury, 2012; Peterson, 2004; Proctor-Williams & Fey, 2007; Robertson & Weismer, 1999; Schuler & Prizant, 1989.

event or to solve a problem about a story or an aspect of a play schema (Tompkins et al., 2003).

2. Incorporate the O-W-L method into your intervention scenario. **O**bserve what the child is interested in. **W**ait for his response and look at the child expectantly. **L**isten closely to the child's gestures and utterances and go from there (Rhyner et al., 2012).

3. Follow the child's lead. Join in the child's activity, imitate the child, comment on what the child is doing, and use short, grammatically correct phrases to interpret what is going on in the context. Ask questions that build on what the child has already said (Dunst et al., 2012; Fey et al., 2003).

4. Provide a running commentary of the child's actions. Do not require a response from the child and allow processing time between descriptions. Providing a language overlay onto the context offers multiple opportunities for the child to hear a new word or to hear a familiar word in a new context (Marzano, 2004).

5. Make indirect corrections in the moment during the play schema or literacy routine; however, corrections should be made with grammatically correct phrases (Fey, 2008; Owens, 2004).

6. Incorporate sensitive and positive contingent responses into the context (Kong & Carta, 2011).

Prompting

Using a least to most prompting hierarchy involves providing scaffolding with the least amount of prompting at the beginning and moving toward a greater amount of prompting over multiple trials. It is important to recognize that a child's compliance to a command, such as "Tell me what this is," is not communication; it is labeling. To determine an appropriate level of prompting, follow the following steps (Senner, n.d.):

1. Identify an appropriate time to wait before providing a prompt. This time varies greatly between children, but it can be identified through careful observation.
2. Offer the communicative bid to the child, such as "Let's play with the Play-Doh."
3. Offer a contextual cue, such as looking at a specific item, and create an expectant pause.
4. Offer an indirect verbal cue, such as remarking, "Hmm, the Play-Doh is so hard to open." This indirect cue signals to the child that something is expected from them.
5. Move the item closer to the child to bring their attention to it.
6. Ask a question, such as, "Do you need help opening the Play-Doh?"
7. Provide a model, such as, "Tell me, 'open box.'"

ADDITIONAL SOURCES

Although you work under a supervising SLP who can answer your questions and support your early intervention, Tables 14–16 and 14–17 contain links to resources within ASHA that may be helpful in guiding your intervention. You will find that ASHA is a rich source of information for early intervention through its Practice Portal (see Table 14–16) and Evidence Maps (see Table 14–17).

CONCLUSION

In my work with children, I often think of a quote that beautifully represents what we do: "If you want to build a ship, don't assign men tasks and work, but rather, teach them to yearn for the vast and endless immensity of the sea" (Bray, 2001) (Figure 14–9).

In the same vein, I work to convince children that language is their key to power and control, constructs that are often in short supply in the lives of children, more so in the lives of children with language impairments. With the uniquely human tool of language, they can share their worlds and shape their futures, and in your role as an SLPA, you play a part in their journey. I urge you to take the theoretical and practical knowledge you

Table 14–16. Topics in ASHA's Practice Portal

Topic	Link
Late Language Emergence	https://www.asha.org/practice-portal/clinical-topics/late-language-emergence/
Intellectual Disability	https://www.asha.org/practice-portal/clinical-topics/intellectual-disability/
Spoken Language Disorders	https://www.asha.org/practice-portal/clinical-topics/spoken-language-disorders/

Table 14–17. Topics in ASHA's Evidence Maps

Topic	Link
Apraxia of Speech	https://apps.asha.org/EvidenceMaps/Maps/LandingPage/b537a59d-b97c-4148-b3c5-1a69357138fe
Central Auditory Processing Disorder	https://apps.asha.org/EvidenceMaps/Maps/LandingPage/9b624ef4-5819-40eb-ae0e-172075be930a
Intellectual Disability	https://apps.asha.org/EvidenceMaps/Maps/LandingPage/d001c8ce-9d87-48d1-b2b3-1c9059f9450b
Late Language Emergence	https://apps.asha.org/EvidenceMaps/Maps/LandingPage/278c5022-32a7-4f3d-85ad-3ce292970cf5
Spoken Language Disorders	https://apps.asha.org/EvidenceMaps/Maps/LandingPage/82816e2d-0cc2-4dfa-948b-369175088a12

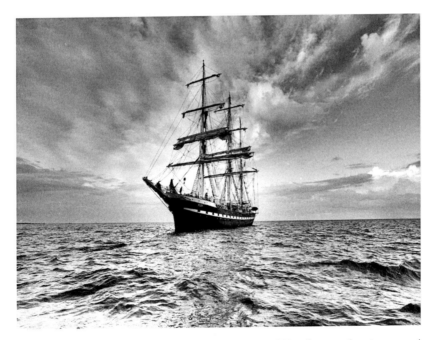

Figure 14–9. A ship in an immense sea. Courtesy of Bing Images, free to use and share commercially.

gain through this chapter and the others in this book, and use it as you sit alongside children, talk to children, play with children, read with children, tell stories with children, learn from children, and have plain old fun with children. Whether you are using clinician-directed methods or incidental teaching, whether you are targeting labeling to increase vocabulary or more complex sentences to support the development of syntax, or whether the child is presymbolic or symbolic, be present in the moment, work in concert with the child and his or her world, and support the child's transition to the next level. As I wrote in the introduction, working with children in early intervention is wonderfully fun, and I hope you will someday share those sentiments.

REFERENCES

American Speech-Language-Hearing Association (ASHA). (n.d.). *Spoken language disorders.* https://www.asha.org/practice-portal/clinical-topics/spoken-language-disorders/

American Speech-Language-Hearing Association. (2008). *Roles and responsibilities of speech-language pathologists in early intervention: Technical report* [Technical report]. http://www.asha.org/policy

American Speech-Language-Hearing Association (ASHA). (2022). *Speech-language pathology assistant scope of practice* [Scope of practice]. http://www.asha.org/policy

Bates, E. (2003). On the nature and nurture of language. In R. Levi-Montalcini, D. Baltimore, R. Dulbecco, F. Jacob, E. Bizzi, P. Calissano, & V. Volterra (Eds.), *Frontiers of biology: The brain of Homo sapiens* (pp. 241–265). Instituto della Enciclopedia Italiana Fondata de Giovanni Trecanni.

Bates, E., Camaioni, L., & Volterra, V. (1975). The acquisition of performatives prior to speech. *Merrill-Palmer Quarterly, 21*(3), 205–226.

Bates, E., & Goodman, J. C. (1997). On the inseparability of grammar and the lexicon: Evidence from acquisition, aphasia, and real-time processing. *Language and Cognitive Processes, 12*(5/6), 507–584. https://doi.org/10.1080/016909697386628

Bloom, L., & Beckwith, R. (1989). *Intentionality and language development.* Unpublished manuscript, Columbia University. https://doi.org/10.79 16/D8KH0Z8N

Bloom, L., Lahey, M., Hood, L., Lifter, K., & Fiess, K. (1980). Complex sentences: Acquisition of syntactic connectives and the relations they encode. *Journal of Child Language, 7*(2), 235–261. https://doi.org/10.1017/S030500090002610

Bray, D. (2001). *A willful volunteer: Examining conscience in an unconscious world.* iUniverse.

Brown, R. (1973). *A first language: The early stages.* George Allen & Unwin.

Cirrin, F. M., & Gillam, R. B. (2008). Language intervention practices for school-age children with spoken language disorders: A systematic review. *Language, Speech, and Hearing in the Schools, 37,* S110–S137. https://doi.org/10.1044/0161-1461 (2008/012)

Dunst, C. J., Raab, M., & Trivette, C. M. (2012). Characteristics of naturalistic language intervention strategies. *Journal of Speech-Language Pathology and Applied Behavior Analysis, 5*(3–4), 8–16. https://doi.org/10.1037/h0100047

Eisenberg, S. (2004). Structured communicative play therapy for targeting language intervention in young children. *Communicative Disorders Quarterly, 26*(1), 29–35. https://doi.org/10.1177/15257401040260010201

Fey, M. E. (1986). *Language intervention with young children.* Allyn & Bacon.

Fey, M. E. (2008). The (mis-)use of telegraphic input in child language intervention. *Revista de Logopedia, Foniatria y Audiologia, 28*(4), 218–230. https://doi.org/10.1016/S0214-4603(08) 70129-3

Fey, M. E., Long, S. H., & Finestack, L. H. (2003). Ten principles of grammar facilitation for children with specific language impairments. *American Journal of Speech-Language Pathology, 12,* 3–15. https://doi.org/10.1044/1058-0360 (2003/048)

Gentner, D., & Boroditsky, L. (2003). Individuation, relativity, and early word learning. In M. Bowerman & S. C. Levinson (Eds.), *Language acquisition and conceptual development* (pp. 215–256). Cambridge University Press.

Goldberg, A. E., & Jackendoff, R. (2004). The English resultative as a family of constructions. *Language, 80*(3), 532–568. http://www.jstor.org/stable/4489722

Halliday, M. A. K. (2003). *On language and linguistics.* In J. Webster (Ed.), *Collected works of M. A. K. Halliday* (Vol. 3). Continuum.

Hancock, T., & Kaiser, A. (2006). Enhanced milieu teaching. In R. McCauley & M. Fey (Eds.), *Treatment of language disorders in children* (pp. 203–236). Brookes.

Hart, B., & Risley, T. R. (1975). Incidental teaching of language in the preschool. *Journal of Applied Behavior Analysis, 8,* 411–420. https://doi.org/10.1901/ jaba.1975.8-411

Kaiser, A. P., Hancock, T. B., & Nietfeld, J. P. (2000). The effects of parent-implemented milieu teaching on the social communication of children who have autism. *Early Education and Development, 11*(4), 423–446. https://doi.org/10.1207/s15566935eed1104 4

Kamhi, A. G. (1999). To use or not to use: Factors that influence the selection of new treatment approaches. *Language, Speech, and Hearing Services in the Schools, 30*, 92–98. https://doi.org/10.1044/ 0161-1461.3001.92

Kong, N. Y., & Carta, J. J. (2011). Responsiveness interaction interventions for children with or at risk for developmental delays. *Topics in Early Childhood Special Education, 33*(1), 4–17. https://doi.org/10.1177/027112141142 6486

Lahey, M. (1988). *Language disorders and language development*. Simon and Schuster.

Lahey, M., & Bloom, L. (1977). Planning a first lexicon: Which words to teach first. *Journal of Speech and Hearing, 42*, 340–350. https://doi.org/10.1044/ jshd.4203.340

Lahey, M., & Bloom, L. (1994). Variability in language learning disabilities. In G. P. Wallach & K. G. Butler (Eds.), *Language learning disabilities in school-age children and adolescents: Some principles and applications* (pp. 354–372). Allyn & Bacon.

Lightbrown, P. M., & Spada, N. (2013). *Oxford handbooks for language teachers: How languages are learned*. Oxford University Press.

Marzano, R. J. (2004). *Building academic background knowledge: Facilitator's guide*. Association for Supervision and Curriculum Development. http://www.ascd.org/ASCD/pdf/siteASCD/ video/buildingacademic.pdf

Nadathur, P. (2017). *Causative verbs: Introduction to lexical semantics*. https://web.stanford. edu/~pnadath/handouts/ling130bfall17/ Nadathur-analytic-causatives.pdf

Owens, R. E. (2004). *Language disorders: A functional approach to assessment and intervention* (4th ed.). Pearson Education.

Owens, R. E. (2009). *Language disorders: A functional approach to assessment and intervention* (5th ed.). Pearson Education.

Paul, R., & Norbury, C. (2012). *Language disorders from infancy through adolescence: Listening, speaking, reading, writing, and communicating* (4th ed.). Elsevier.

Peters, A. M. (1995). Strategies in the acquisition of syntax. In P. Fletcher & B. MacWhinney (Eds.), *The handbook of child language* (pp. 475–482). Blackwell.

Peterson, P. (2004). Naturalistic language teaching procedures for children at risk for language delays. *The Behavior Analyst Today, 5*, 404–424. https://doi.org/10.1037/h0100047

Pinker, S. (1996). *Language learnability and language development*. Harvard University Press.

Pinker, S. (1999). *Words and rules*. Perseus Book Group.

Proctor-Williams, K., & Fey, M. (2007). Recast density and acquisition of novel irregular past tense verbs. *Journal of Speech, Language, and Hearing Research, 40*(4), 1029–1047. https://doi.org/10.1044/1092-4388(2007/072)

Rhyner, P. M., Guenther, K. L., Pizur-Barnekow, K., Cashin, S. E., & Chavie, A. L. (2012). Child caregivers' contingent responsiveness behaviors during interactions with toddlers within three day care contexts. *Communication Disorders Quarterly, 34*(4), 232–241. https://doi.org/10.1177/1525740112465174

Rice, M. L. (2016). Specific language impairment, nonverbal IQ, attention-deficit/hyperactivity disorder, autism spectrum disorder, cochlear implants, bilingualism, and dialectal variants: Defining the boundaries, clarifying the clinical conditions and sorting out cases. *Journal of Speech, Language, and Hearing Research, 59*, 122–132. https://doi.org/10.1044/2015_JSL HR-L-15-0255

Robertson, S., & Weismer, E. (1999). Effects of treatment on linguistic and social skills in toddlers with delayed language development. *Journal of Speech, Language, and Hearing Research, 42*, 1234–1248. https://doi.org/10.1044/ jslhr.4205.1234

Roth, F., & Worthington, C. (2010). *Treatment resource manual for speech language pathology* (5th ed.). Cengage Learning.

Schuler, A. L., & Prizant, B. M. (1989). Facilitating language: Prelanguage approaches. In D. J. Cohen & A. M. Donnellan (Eds.), *Handbook of autism and pervasive developmental disorders* (pp. 301–315). John Wiley.

Senner, J. E. (n.d.). *Least to most prompting*. http://www.talcaac.com/prompting.pdf

Smith, C. S. (1970). Jespersen's "move and change" class and causative verbs in English. In M. A. Jazayery, E. C. Polome, & W. Winter (Eds.), *Linguistic and literary studies in honor of Archibald A. Hill: Volume 2. Descriptive linguistics* (pp. 101–109). Mouton.

Spelke, E. S., & Tsivkin, S. (2001). Initial knowledge and conceptual change: Space and number. In M. Bowerman & S. C. Levinson (Eds.), *Language acquisition and conceptual development* (pp. 71–97). Cambridge University Press.

Tompkins, V., Zucker, T. A., Justice, L. M., & Binici, S. (2003). Inferential talk during teacher-child interactions in small-group play. *Early Childhood Research Quarterly, 28*(2), 424–436. https://doi.org/10.1016/j.ecresq.2012.11.001

Ukrainetz, T. A. (2015). *School-age language intervention: Evidence-based practices.* ProEd.

Vygotsky, L. S. (1978). Interaction between learning and development. In M. Cole, V. John-Steiner, S. Scribner, & E. Souberman (Eds.), *Mind and Society: The Development of Higher Psychological Processes* (pp. 79–91). Harvard University Press.

Wallach, G. P. (2008). *Language intervention for school-age students: Setting goals for academic success.* Mosby/Elsevier.

Wallach, G. P., & Ocampo, A. (2020). *Language and literacy connections: Intervention for school-age children and adolescents.* Plural Publishing.

Wass, R., & Golding, C. (2014). Sharpening a tool for teaching: The zone of proximal development. *Teaching in Higher Education, 19*(6), 671–684.

Wright, S. K. (2002). Transitivity and change of state verbs. *Berkeley Linguistics Society, 28,* 339–350. https://doi.org/10.3765/bls.v28i1.3849

CHAPTER 15

Language Intervention for Children

Margaret Vento-Wilson

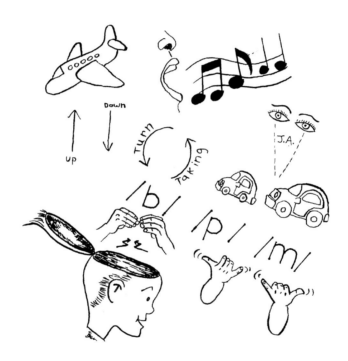

Words are not vocal labels which have come to be attached to things and qualities already given in advance by Nature, or to ideas already grasped independently by the human mind. On the contrary, languages themselves, collective products of social interaction, supply the essential conceptual frameworks for . . . analysis of reality and, simultaneously, the verbal equipment for their descriptions of it. The concepts we use are creations of the language we speak.

—Saussure (1983, p. IX)

INTRODUCTION

Why did I work in the public school system with children with language disorders for many years? It was a question I often asked myself after long days of back-to-back sessions, seemingly endless and complex Individual Education Program (IEP) meetings, and hours of report writing that began well after the students had gone home. However, the answer to that question often emerged precisely in that daily work—one time in the day's first session, in the form of a picture drawn by one of the students on my caseload, who believed—wholeheartedly—that he was as strong as a superhero and could save the world (and me!) if needed (Figure 15–1).

I worked in this setting and with this population because the work was extraordinarily rewarding and because it mattered deeply to the students on my caseload. I also worked in this setting because I remain ever fascinated by the human capacity for language and how we shape and are shaped by our language. Whether you are new to this population or very experienced in this work, I hope that in your role as a speech-language pathologist assistant (SLPA), you have the opportunity to work with a young superhero, who is not going to let a language learning disorder get in his way of saving the world—one speech-language pathologist (SLP) at a time!

LANGUAGE INTERVENTION WITH CHILDREN

Language intervention with children is complex, is far reaching, and encompasses a wide range of ages, from about 6 to 18

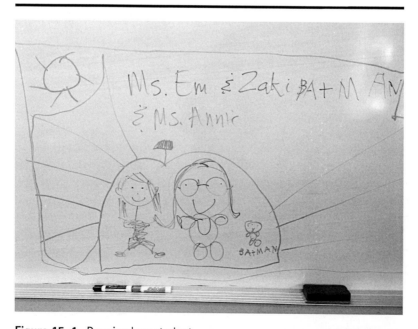

Figure 15–1. Drawing by a student.

years of age, or from 1st to 12th grade (American Speech-Language-Hearing Association [ASHA], 2001). In early intervention, one of the primary focuses is language acquisition, which supports the transition from the nonlinguistic state to the linguistic state (Pinker, 1996). Once children reside solidly in the linguistic world, the break between early intervention and language intervention emerges. As such, this chapter can be viewed as a continuation of the previous chapter on early intervention, but it is important to note that while the age of the children may change, the foundational principles of language intervention remain the same. As I often remind the undergraduate and graduate students I teach, *language is language is language.*

Whether children are in the early stages of language acquisition or developing and refining their language, it all comes down to supporting children's ability to use and produce the building blocks of language: semantics, syntax, and pragmatics (Roth et al., 2006) (Figure 15–2).

As stated above, in our early intervention with children, the focus is on establishing an early lexicon, supporting the development of syntax, and expanding their ability to use language in social contexts (Bloom & Lahey, 1978) and much of this intervention revolves around Brown's morphemes (Brown, 1973). However, as children continue to develop and move beyond the early years, intervention moves well beyond Brown's morphemes and can include any of the following (Nippold et al., 2009):

- More advanced morphological markers
- Complex syntax
- Higher-level vocabulary

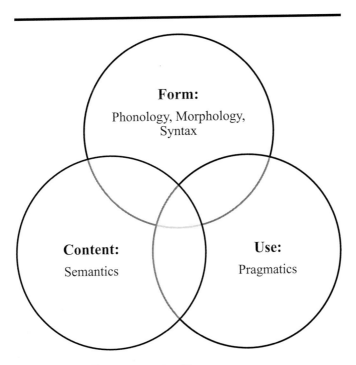

Figure 15–2. The components of language.

- Adjectival and adverbial markers
- Conjunctive and cohesive markers
- Noun phrase elaboration

Furthermore, in addition to the basic components of language described above, the following domains are well within the scope of practice for SLPAs because of the foundational nature of language (Pennington & Bishop, 2009; Sun & Wallach, 2014): spelling (Apel & Masterson, 2001), reading (Catts et al., 2002), and writing (Nelson et al., 2001). A final comment with respect to the intervention for children with language learning disorders is the multifaceted relationships between all of the domains listed above. For example, intervention in vocabulary supports complex syntax (DeKemel, 2003), and syntax has been shown to be one of the underpinnings of reading comprehension (Brimo et al., 2017). In your work as an SLPA with children with language learning disorders, be confident that the skills you target build on each other in a cohesive manner that provides a bridge to the next step.

In this chapter, the term *language learning disorder* (LLD) will be used to describe the children you will work with as an SLPA (Wallach, 2008). This specific term is used to disambiguate the broad concept of a language impairment from the terms *specific language impairment* (SLI) or *developmental language disorder* (DLD), which are used for a very specific type of language impairment. The term *language learning disorder* also differentiates this population from the special eligibility category of *speech-language impairment*.

This chapter explores and defines the following concepts: (a) foundational principles of language intervention, (b) legislative action and federal guidelines as they relate to the school-age popula-

tion, (c) broad intervention concepts, and (d) specific intervention practices that can be used across all domains of language. As a trained SLPA, you are qualified to work with these students (ASHA, 2020), and after reading this chapter, I hope you feel more confident in this work and that the intervention feels less daunting than it may have initially.

LANGUAGE INTERVENTION FRAMEWORK

Language is defined as "a dynamic system that involves the ability to integrate knowledge of phonology, morphology, syntax, semantics, and pragmatics to create sentences within conversational, narrative, and expository discourse contexts" (Gillam & Ukrainetz, 2006, p. 62). Language development can be viewed as existing on several shifting paradigms: the oral-to-literate continuum, the narrative-to-expository continuum, and the change over time in the way language disorders are defined (Fey et al., 2004; Sun & Nippold, 2012). In children, LLDs are often first revealed in their conversational contexts during the early stages of language development but continue to manifest themselves in the comprehension and production of narratives and expository texts as they grow up (Gillam et al., 1995; Wallach & Ocampo, 2020; Wallach et al., 2014).

One concept deeply central to intervention with children with LLD is the need to maintain a view toward the horizon (Sun & Wallach, 2014). Over time, young children become students, who move through the K to 12 curriculum, who may or may not attend higher education, and who eventually shift into adulthood and gainful employment (Bashir, 1989). Also over time, speakers become readers and writers, with a parallel increase in linguistic and cognitive demands (Wallach et al., 2014). Children move from the concrete world of the *here and now* to the more abstract world of the *there and then* (Gillam & Ukrainetz, 2006). And finally, children move from the familiar world of stories and narratives to the demands of expository text, where the majority of learning occurs in the school years, with very different vocabularies and morphosyntactic structures (DeKemel, 2003; Gillam & Ukrainetz, 2006; Puranik et al., 2008). On a macro level, intervention must reflect the demands of each stage, while simultaneously supporting the transition to the next stage. However, on the micro level, the time spent with an individual child may be only at a single point, which underscores that need to always ask the question, "What's next for this child?"

FOUNDATIONAL PRINCIPLES OF LANGUAGE INTERVENTION

The definition of language intervention is defined as follows: intentional actions taken to accelerate, modify, or compensate for inadequate performance (Ukrainetz, 2006). In contrast to this concise and narrow definition, children with LLDs are a heterogeneous population whose unifying characteristics include challenges in understanding, acquiring, or using oral or written language (Cirrin & Gillam, 2008; Kamhi, 2014). These challenges are seen across phonology, morphology, semantics, syntax, and pragmatics, as well as across disability category (e.g., autism spectrum disorder [ASD], developmental language disorder [DLD], intellectual

developmental disability [IDD]). While the presentation of these disorders varies considerably, the impact of reduced language abilities on the individual does not. LLDs are associated with decreases in educational outcomes, social interaction, and individual agency (Cohen, 2010; Lyons & Roulstone, 2018). As such, it is appropriate to discuss larger constructs that may be useful in framing intervention for children with LLDs.

Systems Constructs

One foundational construct that can be applied to intervention with children is Bronfenbrenner's bioecological model (Bronfenbrenner & Morris, 2006), which demonstrates the interaction between children and their environment, as seen in Figure 15–3.

This model provides a discrete separation between children and their linguistic micro-, meso-, exo-, and macrosystems; however, in reality, the boundaries between each are very permeable, and children often move seamlessly among them. The model also suggests a list of systems and people that should be considered when intervening with children (e.g., family, community, friends). Finally, this model involves several propositions describing the process of human development, with a tacit description of the process of language development that parallels human development:

Development takes place through processes of progressively more complex reciprocal interaction between an active . . . human . . . and the persons, objects, and symbols in its immediate . . . environment. To be effective, the interaction must occur on a fairly

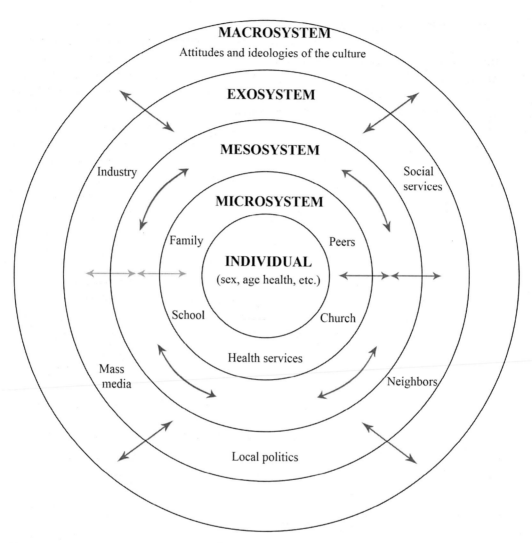

Figure 15–3. Bronfenbrenner's bioecological model. Courtesy of Bing Images, free to share and use commercially.

regular basis over extended periods of time . . . [as in] performing complex tasks, and acquiring new knowledge. (Bronfenbrenner & Morris, 2006, p. 797)

Of significance in this model is the relevance of approaching language intervention with a holistic perspective, involving multidirectional interactions among the child and his or her family, peers,

the classroom, as well as the child's cultural and linguistic background (ASHA, n.d.-b.). For example, research has demonstrated that expressive language outcomes are very similar for clinician- and parent-delivered intervention (Law et al., 2004). Based on the underlying precepts of this model, language intervention with children is best implemented within naturalistic settings and contexts and must be deeply connected to the demands and rigors of children's daily lives, regardless of the intervention setting (Dunst et al., 2012). Although this chapter is intended as a practice-based resource for language intervention with children, discussions of theoretical constructs have value in that

> theory underlies . . . interventions, whether or not we acknowledge this openly, and the theory one adopts reflects what is believed to be important. One should be aware that approaches to intervention entail certain underlying theoretical assumptions, and theory and action should be consistent with each other. (Sutton, 2008, p. 60)

Considerations for At-Risk Children

Deeply related to Bronfenbrenner's bio-ecological model are the multiple societal, biological, and psychosocial factors related to children's resilience and risk (Lyons & Roulstone, 2018; World Health Organization, 2007). The term *resilience* is defined as the process of adapting positively when faced with adversity or significant sources of stress (American Psychological Association, n.d.). Children defined as *at risk* are those who are more likely than their peers to experience poor outcomes (Harrison & McLeod, 2010; Lyons & Roulstone, 2018). When looked at within an ecological model, resilience and the at-risk status can be impacted by children's internal capacity and by the capacity of their personal ecologies (Ungar, 2015). This suggests that protective factors, such as the ability to problem solve and the presence of hope, agency, and positive relationships, can mitigate negative effects (Harrison & McLeod, 2010; Lyons & Roulstone, 2018). However, there are also ecological factors that may contribute to poorer outcomes (Figure 15–4).

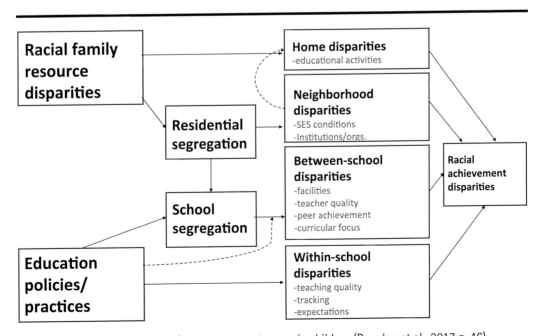

Figure 15–4. Factors contributing to poorer outcomes in children (Reardon et al., 2017 p. 46).

Statistics compiled by the National Center for Education Statistics (n.d.) and the U.S. Department of Education (n.d.-a) indicate that academic performance, retention and dropout rates, statewide assessment scores, and an eligibility of LLDs or emotional disturbance (ED) as special education categories are related to poverty. Specific to language disorders, there are multiple factors that have been linked to greater likelihoods of LLDs, as described in Table 15–1 (Stanton-Chapman et al., 2002).

In your role as an SLPA, you become part of the ecological system of the children with whom you work, and as such, you have an opportunity to support and mentor them, and provide a positive relationship as they make their way in the world.

Intervention Constructs

This next section discusses a valuable guideline in your intervention with children with LLDs: the distinction between *performance* and *learning*. As discussed by Kamhi (2014) and defined by Bjork (2004), performance should be viewed as the context-specific, short-term manifestation of a behavior, and learning can be viewed as an independent, long-term occurrence of

Table 15–1. List of Risk Factors Linked to LLDs

Individual Level Risk Factors	Environmental Risks
Male	Parental substance abuse
Low birth weight	
5-minute Apgar score	Poverty
Maternal age	Maternal educational level
Maternal educational level	
	Child abuse/neglect
Gestational age	Birth order

a specified behavior. These two constructs parallel the distinct difference between what children can do in a speech-language therapy session with a highly contrived context and what they can do in naturalistic settings and in conversations involving spontaneous novel utterances. These constructs also parallel the difference between a set of narrow rules with predictable boundaries and a broad-based set of rules that can be applied across unpredictable events (Kamhi, 2014). With respect to intervention with children with LLDs, this difference supports intervention in naturalistic settings with real-time demands. It also suggests that children benefit from repeated and varied opportunities and multiple contexts to acquire a new skill set (Yoder et al., 2012).

SCHOOL-BASED ISSUES

There are multiple settings in which SLPs and SLPAs work: schools, private practice, and hospitals (ASHA, n.d.-e, 2022; see Chapter 1 for a detailed description of the settings). Although SLPAs will encounter children with LLDs in each setting, the great majority of SLPs (53%) and SLPAs work in the K through 12 school setting (ASHA, n.d.-c), which mandates a brief overview of the major legislative acts that influence services in the schools for children with disabilities.

Legislation

Of primary importance to the work of SLPAs in the schools is the Individuals With Disabilities Education Act (IDEA) (P.L. 94–142), initially authorized in 1997 and reauthorized in 2004, which made a free and appropriate public education (FAPE) available to all children with disabilities determined to be eligible and guaranteed protections for all students in (see Table 15–2 for a list of terms and their acronyms related to special education). Within the framework of FAPE is the explicit requirement that children with disabilities receive an education designed to meet their unique needs (IDEA, n.d.). This legislation drives many of the service models observed in schools. A second legislative act, the No Child Left Behind (NCLB) (PL 107–110) (NCLB, n.d.), was designed to support children with disabilities and those considered at risk in their academic success. More recently, the Every Student Succeeds Act (ESSA) (P.L. 114–95) (U.S. Department of Education, n.d.-b.) was enacted to further support critical protections and procedural safeguards for high-need and disadvantaged students. A final legislative act that relates to services in the schools is the Americans With Disabilities Act (ADA; 1990), prohibiting discrimination against individuals with disabilities and guaranteeing similar opportunities for these individuals to those of individuals without disabilities in mainstream American life (ADA, n.d.).

While these legislative acts and terms can appear intimidating and confusing, in essence, they confirm that

> disability is a natural part of the human experience and in no way diminishes the right of individuals to participate in or contribute to society. Improving educational results for children with disabilities is an essential element of our national policy of ensuring equality of opportunity, full participation, independent living, and economic self-sufficiency for individuals with disabilities. (IDEA, n.d., para. 6)

Response to Intervention

As an SLPA in a school setting, it is likely you will be involved with the response to intervention (RtI) framework, also known as multitiered systems of support (MTSS). This framework supports instructional intensity across a continuum to support student learning (ASHA, n.d.-d.; Ehren et al., 2014; Ehern & Nelson, 2005; Scott et al., 2005; Wixson et al., 2014). Rather than being based on a *wait to fail* paradigm, RtI and MTSS are grounded in the concept of prevention that is intended to address culturally and linguistically diverse inequities that have persisted in special education in the United States (Wixson et al., 2014). According to ASHA (n.d.-d., para. 1), RtI and MTSS include the following (Figure 15–5):

- Universal screening
- High-quality instruction
- Intervention matched to student need
- Frequent progress monitoring
- Use of child response data to make educational decisions

Table 15–2. List of Terms Related to Special Education Legislation

Abbreviation	Expanded Term
ADA	American with Disabilities Act
ESSA	Every Student Succeeds Act
FAPE	Free and Appropriate Public Education
IDEA	Individuals with Disabilities Education Act
IEP	Individual Educational Plan
NCLB	No Child Left Behind Act

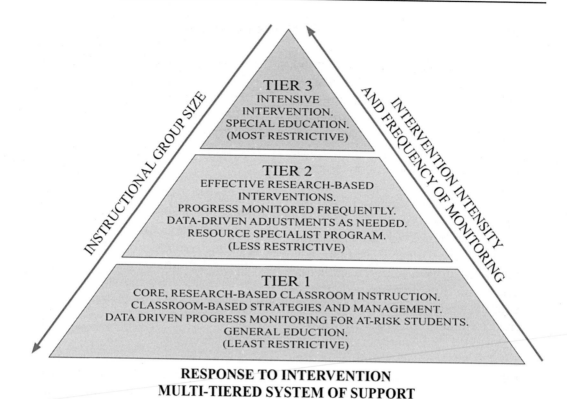

**RESPONSE TO INTERVENTION
MULTI-TIERED SYSTEM OF SUPPORT**

Figure 15–5. Model of response to intervention or multitiered system of support.

Specific to your role as an SLPA, you may be involved in the following tasks:

- Collaborating with general education teachers to support students identified as at risk
- Consulting with general education teachers to meet the needs of students identified as at risk
- Conducting small group instruction in the general education classroom for students (with and without an IEP) with similar needs (Ehren et al., 2014; Wixson et al., 2014)
- Tracking relevant data as evidence for progress

Individualized Educational and 504 Plans

The information detailed in the preceding paragraphs leads to a discussion of Individual Education Plans (IEPs) and 504 Plans, which drive the services delivered in the schools. An IEP is a plan or program developed specifically for a child with a disability that ensures specialized instruction and services (Disabilities, Opportunities, Internetworking, and Technology [DO IT], n.d.). These plans were designed to ensure appropriate accommodations supporting academic success and access to the learning environment for children with disabilities (DO IT, n.d.). A 504 Plan is based on Section 504 of the Rehabilitation Act of 1973, a federal civil rights law written to end discrimination against individuals with disabilities (Disability Rights Education & Defense Fund, n.d.). Children qualify for IEPs or 504s based on federal special education disability categories that are identified and specified through a comprehensive assessment, as detailed in Table 15–3. *See your state guidelines for the specific language used to describe these disabilities.*

As an SLPA working with children with LLD, at least some of your work will involve the goals and services detailed in IEPs, examples of which can be found in Appendices 7–A and 7–D from Chapter 7. Although your supervising SLP is responsible for the development and implementation of the goals and services addressed in each child's IEP, it would be wise to familiarize yourself with the structure and language of IEP forms to ensure appropriate delivery of intervention. Even if you do not work in a school setting, it is likely that many of the children on your caseload will have an IEP that can be shared with your supervising SLP by the parents and can be used to inform and guide your intervention decisions with those children. A final recommendation is to review the national database on Common Core State Standards (CCSS) (http://www.core standards.org), or your state-specific site, which may provide a rich source to guide your intervention.

SETTING-SPECIFIC INTERVENTION

As was discussed in Chapter 1, in your role as an SLPA, you will be conducting your intervention in multiple settings, such as private clinic, schools, rehabilitation settings, and hospitals, and in each of these settings, there are multiple service delivery models, such as those listed below (ASHA, n.d.-c.; Cirrin et al., 2010):

Direct Services:

- Individual or group therapy session
  - Pull-out
  - Push-in

Indirect Services:

- Consult or collaborative
  - Push-in

In more recent years, interprofessional collaborative practice (IPP) has been validated as an evidence-based practice (ASHA, n.d.-f.; Cirrin et al., 2010) and its use has increased. This approach gives SLPAs opportunities to learn with, from, and about their colleagues to improve outcomes for the children with whom you work (ASHA, n.d.-c). As an SLPA in a school, this may involve coteaching in the different settings (Table 15–4) and shared responsibilities among educational professionals for all students.

All professionals can experience the benefits of collaboration. In the schools, you may collaborate with general education teachers, special education teachers, audiologists, physical therapists, occupational therapists, and nurses. For example, teachers (e.g., general, special, and resource) may become more competent in providing appropriate language supports, while SLPAs may become more competent in linking their intervention to relevant classroom content (Cirrin & Gillam, 2008; Davies et al., 2004). In clinical, hospital, or private practice settings, you may collaborate with audiologists, physical therapists, occupational therapists, nurses, and social workers (Johnson, 2016).

Table 15–3. Federal Special Education Disability Categories by Incidence Level

Low-Incidence Disability	
Disability	**Definition**
Deaf-blindness	Concomitant hearing and visual impairments that cause complex communication needs that cannot be accommodated in special programs designed solely for children with deafness of children with blindness.
Deafness	A severe hearing impairment that impairs a child's ability to process spoken linguistic information with or without amplification and that adversely affects educational performance.
Hearing Impairment	A permanent or fluctuating hearing impairment that negatively impacts educational performance but that is not included under the definition of deaf.
Multiple Disabilities	A combination of concomitant impairments causing severe educational needs that cannot be accommodated in special education programs designed solely for one of the impairments.
Orthopedic Impairment	Severe orthopedic impairment that adversely affects a child's educational performance.
Visual Impairments	Visual impairments that, even with correction, adversely affect a child's educational performance.
Traumatic Brain Injury	An acquired injury to the brain caused by an external physical force, which results in partial functional impairment or psychosocial disability impacting educational performance.
Medium-Incidence Disability	
Disability	**Definition**
Autism	A disability that significantly affects verbal and nonverbal communication and social interactions.
Developmental Delay	A delay in children between 3 through 9 years of age in the development of physical abilities, cognition, communication, social or emotion abilities, or in adaptive abilities.
Emotional Disturbance	A condition exhibited over a long period of time that adversely affects educational performance. Examples of conditions include pervasive depression, anxiety, schizophrenia, or an inability to maintain relationships with peers or adults.
Intellectual Disability	Subaverage general cognitive abilities manifested in the developmental period that coexist with significant deficits in adaptive behavior affecting a child's educational performance.
High-Incidence Disability	
Disability	**Definition**
Other Health Impairment	Having limited strength, alertness, or vitality due to an acute or chronic health problem(s) that significantly affect a child's educational performance.
Specific Learning Disability	A disorder in one or more of the basic psychological processes related to understanding or using oral or written language that manifests in reduced abilities in listening, thinking, speaking, reading, writing, spelling, or performing math calculations.
Speech or Language Impairment	Communication or language disorders that adversely affect a child's educational performance, such as stuttering or disorders of the speech-sound system, articulation, voice, or language.

Source: Adapted from *California department of education (CDE): CALPADS primary disability category codes,* by CDE, n.d. retrieved from https://www.cde.ca.gov/ta/tg/ca/disablecodes.asp and *Congressional Research Service: The Individuals With Disabilities Education Act: A comparison of state eligibility criteria* retrieved from https://crsreports.congress.gov/product/pdf/R/R46566#:~:text=The%20majority%20of%20IDEA%20appropriations,multiple%20disabilities%2C%20(8)%20orthopedic

Table 15–4. A Description of the Continuum of Settings in the Schools

Setting	Definition
General Education Classroom	The majority of the classrooms in a school. The majority of children in these classrooms received generalized instruction across all curricular topics.
Resource Specialist Program Classroom	A classroom supporting children who have been identified in an IEP and whose academic needs cannot be met solely in the general education classroom. Children receive sheltered learning on various subjects to support greater access to the curriculum, but spend the majority of their day in a general education classroom.
Special Day Class	A self contained classroom providing specialized and intensive services to children identified in an IEP, and whose needs academic needs cannot be met in either the RSP setting or the general education classroom.

Source: Understanding Special Education, n.d.

This service delivery of IPP includes (a) parallel, supplemental, primary, and coteaching; (b) consulting with team members; (c) modeling targeted skills; and (d) greater inclusion of the child's peers to the benefit of all. When collaborating, SLPAs can model interactive teaching styles and support their colleague(s) by introducing listening, speaking, reading, and writing activities into instructional tasks, while ensuring that the tasks are structured to support children with LLDs (ASHA, 2020; Farber & Klein, 1999). In light of this recommendation, two concepts must remain in the forefront of all decisions: (1) Children are all individuals with unique needs and (2) targeting different skills requires unique contexts (Cirrin et al., 2010).

LANGUAGE INTERVENTION

Language intervention with children mandates broad considerations because of the wide age range and the heterogeneity of language disorders. As far as the field of speech-language pathology has come in the past 50 years, there are still no published guidelines or hard-and-fast rules governing intervention for children with language disorders (Cirrin & Gillam, 2008). Fortunately, there are evidence-based practices that have been shown to be effective at the micro and macro levels (Cirrin et al., 2010). However, just as important as identifying what language intervention with children is, it is important to identify what it is not. This chapter does not detail disorder-specific language intervention (e.g., ASD, TBI, IDD) but provides broad guidelines for intervention with children. Regardless, it would not be unexpected that many of the intervention concepts presented here would be appropriate for children with LLDs and various comorbidities.

Broad Intervention Concepts

This section of the chapter describes and discusses evidence-based intervention practices you can implement in your work with children, presented in a hierarchy that moves from broad to specific.

Language intervention with children encompasses form, content, and use, because language disorders exert influence over characteristics of phonology, morphology, syntax, semantics, and pragmatics (Paul & Norbury, 2012). This influence can result in deficits observed in (a) phonological memory, awareness, and production at the word and sentence levels (Pennington & Bishop, 2009); (b) use of morphological markers (Eisenberg, 2007; Moyle et al., 2011); (c) comprehension of complex and compound sentences, embedded and relative clauses, passive voice, and negation (Eisenberg, 2007; Paul, 2000); and (d) production of varied and complex vocabulary (Catts et al., 1999). From a broad perspective, effective language intervention can be framed through the inclusion of critical elements that can be implemented regardless of age, disorder (e.g., SLI/DLD, TBI, ASD) or language domain (i.e., form, content, use) (Ukrainetz, 2006).

Just as a rudder serves to guide a sailboat through the unfamiliar waters, familiarity with guiding intervention principles supports more effective intervention with the children on your caseload (Figure 15–6).

Although there are many guiding principles out there, the following broad principles provide a solid framework, as described by Paul and Norbury (2012):

1. Use of curricular-based instruction. Although you may not be in a school setting, considering the academic demands placed on children supports their success across all other contexts of their daily lives (Nelson, 2010; Wallach, 2010; Wallach & Ocampo, 2020). This requires familiarity with the demands of academic language and the CCSSs (Appendix 15–A). Whether the overarching goal is vocabulary acquisition or use of cohesive language, the CCSSs allow you to gain a better understanding of the demands (the CCSSs can be found at http://www.corestandards.org).

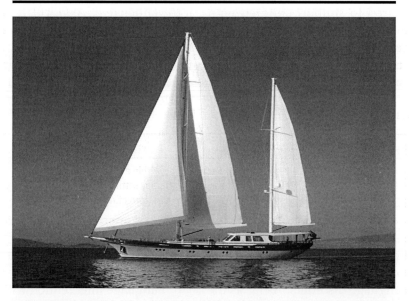

Figure 15–6. Sailboat in the ocean. Courtesy of Bing Images, free to use and share commercially.

2. Integration of oral and written language.

   Because oral and written language exist on a continuum, they cannot be truly separated in intervention (Wallach, 2008, 2014; Wallach & Ocampo, 2020). Just as children look different across the age span, so too does intervention integrating oral and written language. Integration of the two language modalities can be accomplished by providing varied activities that cross from oral language tasks (talking about the meaning of a word) to incorporating target words in a short story or poem that you and the children write together.

3. Focus on metacognitive, metalinguistic, and metapragmatic activities.

   Talking and thinking about language are metaskills (Wallach et al., 2009; Wallach & Ocampo, 2020). In the world of language, *meta* means going beyond the use of language as a function of communication and to focus on underlying structures (Wallach et al., 2009; Wallach & Ocampo, 2020). By modeling and practicing specific language structures and then taking those structures outside of the production, the focus can shift to the explicit rules of language (Wallach, 2010). Defining a sentence form and how it differs from another is an example of a metatask. Stating the unspoken rules about what one cannot say is another.

4. For SLPAs in schools, collaborative participation in response to intervention (RtI), which involves tiered instruction to support children with learning needs (Ardoin et al., 2005). For example, you can coteach with the resource specialist program teacher (RSP) or general education teacher in their setting to support expanded access for children at-risk for LLDs.

With these four principles in mind, intervention can be further guided by the following list of skill formats (Table 15–5; Ukrainetz, 2006).

Scaffolding is an instructional strategy that supports children's independent use of language-processing skills and strategies (Nelson, 2005). It is related to the socially mediated learning process identified by Vygotsky and the zone of proximal development (ZPD), which is "the distance between the level of performance

Table 15–5. Intervention Skill Formats

Skill	Task Structure
Hierarchical Skill Intervention	Skills are targeted one at a time within a hierarchy moving from simple, contrived tasks in the therapy setting to naturalistic activities with minimal to no prompting and correcting.
Skill Stimulation	Skills are practiced in simple tasks with minimal to no prompting and correcting.
Enrichment and Task Assistance	Skills are targeted in naturalistic life activities with prompts and corrections as needed.
Contextualized Skill Intervention	Several skills are targeted at a time within a mix of naturalistic and contrived contexts with prompting and correction as needed.

a child can achieve independently and the higher level that same child can achieve with effective social mediation" (Nelson, 2005, p. 328). Scaffolding techniques are as follows (Scott & Balthazar, 2015):

- Manipulating the length of the stimuli (clauses, sentences)
- Ensuring familiarity with the content (grade level, curriculum, vocabulary)
- Modulating the difficulty of the stimuli (abstractness, information density)
- Including visual supports (written modality, key words)
- Paying close attention to the amount and quality of linguistic facilitations (modeling, expansions, extensions)

The process of intervention can be further framed through these three approaches (Paul & Norbury, 2012):

1. Clinician Directed:
   The clinician identifies a skill to be targeted, selects the materials or manipulatives to use, and determines the success or failure of an outcome. The use of drills is common in this context.
2. Child Centered:
   The clinician provides appropriate scaffolding to support the child's ZPD in a particular skill. In this model, the child has a voice in the selection of targets, in selecting manipulatives and materials, and in the determination of outcome. The use of play or conversational interaction is common in this context.
3. Hybrid:
   The clinician shifts between the two previous structures according to the

situation, the child's performance, and the task demands.

A final set of principles relates to grammatical intervention for children with LLDs. However, these principles are evidence based and sufficiently broad so as to support increases in the overall behavioral, communicative, academic, and social performance of children across contexts, age, and population (Fey et al., 2003):

1. The primary focus of grammatical intervention should be to support children's increased proficiency over comprehension and use of morphology and syntax, in the naturalistic context of the oral and written modalities of conversation, narratives, exposition, and additional text-based genres. However, research has demonstrated that discrete, explicit instruction can be an appropriate method in specific situations.
2. Based on our understanding that grammatical deficits rarely exist independent of deficits in the other domains of language, grammatical intervention should never be addressed in isolation.
3. Intermediate-level goals that support language acquisition and development, rather than specific language forms, are more effective because of the possibilities of triggering shifts in a grammatical system (Bates et al., 1991). This approach parallels the use of the complexity theory used in addressing motor speech disorders.
4. Children must exhibit a readiness for a specific targeted form, as demonstrated by an emergence of this form in specific contexts, regardless of whether the emerging form is produced with errors.

5. Manipulating intervention contexts (e.g., social, physical, linguistic) increases the number of opportunities to address specific grammatical targets. An example is when a clinician becomes less cooperative in a conversation, which creates an expectation for children to "fill in the spaces."

6. Appropriate contexts for intervention can be developed by capitalizing on different genres of text and incorporating a written modality. For example, narratives often use more past tense, informational discourse uses more present tense, and higher-level grammatical forms (e.g., passives, adverbial clauses) are seen more often in written texts.

7. Manipulating the target within discourse to draw attention to specific forms. For example, change loudness, pitch, and word length for increased salience.

8. Sentence recasts are an effective method of systematically contrasting the less mature form produced by children with the more mature forms produced by adults.

9. Modeling well-formed sentences to support comprehension of both function and content words.

10. Eliciting imitation of targeted forms allows children to practice with forms that are difficult to produce. It also encourages children to use words in the natural contexts of phrases or sentences and develops a better understanding of the relationships between forms.

Specific Language Intervention Models

The R.I.S.E.+ Model

The first specific intervention framework discussed is based on repeated opportunities for practice and learning with a focus on appropriate levels of Repeated opportunities, Intensive schedule, Systematic support, and Explicit skill focus (Ukrainetz, 2015). This model, called R.I.S.E+, is described in Table 15–6.

Repeated opportunities are necessary to gain proficiency over a concept, although the actual number of opportunities

Table 15–6. Continuum of R.I.S.E.+ for Intervention and Instruction

Feature	Intervention Contexts
Repeated Opportunities	Few—some—many
Intensity of Scheduling	Clinic/Classroom—Group/Individual
	Occasional—Regular—Frequent
	Short—Medium—Long
Systematic Support	Little—Some—Significant
Explicit Skill	Implicit—Explicit—Metalinguistic/Metacognitive
+ The Learner Factor	Passive attention/minimal engagement—motivated attentive engagement—Motivated, self-directed, and sustained engagement

Source: Ukrainetz, 2015, p. 58.

is highly individualized. Intensity refers to the number of interactions between the child and the intervention, or the more holistic concept of session length and frequency. Systematic support refers to efforts of the SLPA to support success of the child in the session and includes (a) modifying the environment, (b) being aware of pause time when waiting for a response, and (c) providing scaffolding within an appropriate hierarchy. Explicit skill focus refers to the instruction provided by the SLPA and can involve (a) drill-based work, (b) strategic highlighting, and (c) a clear focus on a specified skill (Ukraintez, 2015).

In addition to the concepts described above, effective intervention should include prompting, modeling, guidance, and explanation (Ukrainetz, 2015). The modeling can be presented in the form of developmentally appropriate recasts and expansions, where the clinician either simply restates what the child says or expands on it, as seen in the exchanges below:

Recast

Child: We go*ed* to the store after school and find*ed* the kind of cake she likes.

SLPA: Oh, you went to the store and found that cake? Your mother must have been happy.

Expansion

Child: Got the special cake.

SLPA: Oh, you finally got the cake your mother likes?

Recent research by Venker et al. (2015) found that the use of telegraphic speech, which omits function words and grammatical morphemes, might have a nega-

tive impact on the development and refinement of syntax. As such, restating utterances with the correct morphosyntactic form reflects best practices (Kamhi, 2014), as seen in the exchange below:

Child: Basketball school friend.

SLPA: Oh, you played basketball with a friend? That must have been fun!

The final but important factor in the R.I.S.E.+ model is the learner factor. One of the greatest challenges in intervention is developing and maintaining the engagement, motivation, and buy-in of the child. This engagement is supported by evidence (ASHA, n.d.-a) and can be mediated by the following: (a) using relevant activities, (b) creating authentic interactions between the SLPA and the child, (c) allowing the child to make choices throughout the session, and (d) providing clear task expectations (Ukrainetz, 2015).

Literature–Based Units

Literature-based units is a contextualized language intervention based on books, reading, and discussion (Gillam & Ukrainetz, 2006). A description of the intervention follows.

Intervention Components:

1. Functional activities:
   The individual needs of children are addressed through an oral context.
2. Thematic unity:
   Activities are linked thematically, progressing from an initial reading of a story to a final parallel story generation. Thematic intervention provides structure, builds coherence, supports extended learning, and varies activities.

3. Whole-part-whole:
   The intervention begins with a piece of literature and ends with generating a parallel story. Activities are selected to target specific goals and objectives.

Many methods can facilitate language when working with literature-based units. Table 15–7 lists a series of facilitation devices that can be embedded in your intervention with storybooks.

Some final recommendations for your intervention with children who have LLDs follow (Ukrainetz, 2015):

- Relate the known to the unknown.
- Modify the complexity of the task and content.
- Make connections between ideas, content, and task.
- Call attention to specific aspects of the text.
- Incorporate graphic organizers in the tasks.
- Model the process.

Instructional Discourse

Instructional discourse is an intervention process based on strategic conversations between children and clinicians (Culatta et al., 2010). Instructional discourse is highly valuable because it can be used with both written and oral texts and across levels. The primary goals of this intervention are to support access and strengthen comprehension of a specific text by modifying the demands. Strategies that can be used include (a) engaging in exploratory discussion; (b) establishing an emotional link between children and the text; (c) acknowledging and elaborating on comments, questions, and contributions of the children; (d) encouraging all participants to engage; and (e) providing scaffolding and multiple response options.

Additional supports to consider are graphic organizers, also called thinking maps and concept diagrams. These are visual displays demonstrating relationships among concepts, terms, and facts that help children make sense of information (Kim et al., 2004). Figure 15–7 shows examples of thinking maps.

In information discourse intervention, graphic organizers can help identify cohesive structures and intertopic relationships, as well as support overall organization. Informational discourse requires an emphasis on vocabulary. Supporting children in the development of a mental schema about words increases comprehension and allows them to apply their new word knowledge in future contexts (DeKemel, 2003; Wallach & Ocampo, 2020). Linking words to synonyms and antonyms, giving examples, and creating semantic maps (Beck et al., 2002) are some methods used to target vocabulary (Figure 15–8).

Instructional strategies to support connections between ideas and content might relate (a) the familiar to the unfamiliar, (b) past experiences to the current text, (c) previously read text to the current text, (d) the concrete to the abstract, (e) the remote to the immediate, and (f) the implicit to the explicit (Culatta et al., 2010).

CONCLUSION

This chapter ends with recommendations for how best to implement the many theoretical constructs, principles, and intervention practices it described. The first is to remain informed and current on evidence-based practices; this is the best

Table 15–7. Facilitation Methods

Linguistic Facilitation	
Syntactic Expansion: The production of a syntactically correct form that parallels the student's production.	Child: Her lived in the Netherlands. Clinician: Yes, she lived in the Netherlands.
Semantic Expansion: The production of a parallel form of the student's production with additional information.	Child: Her lived in the Netherlands. Clinician: Yes, she lived in the Netherlands during World War II.
Recast: The production of a parallel form with an altered syntactic structure.	Child: Her lived in the Netherlands. Clinician: Right, Anne Frank lived in the Netherlands.
Prompt: A question or comment that elicits a correction in a previous syntactically incorrect sentence.	Child: Her lived in the Netherlands. Clinician: Who did she live with? Child: She lived in the Netherlands with her family.
Elaboration: A question that elicits an expansion of a previous response.	Child: Her lived in the Netherlands. Clinician: Whom did she have in her family? Child: She lived in the Netherlands with her parents and her sister.
Vertical Structure: A question that elicits additional information. The clinician incorporates the new response with the question to form a more complex structure.	Child: Her lived in the Netherlands. Clinician: Why did she stay in the Netherlands? Child: Because they couldn't leave. Clinician: She stayed in the Netherlands because she couldn't leave? How terrible!
Response Facilitations	
Model: A model of a targeted form or word.	Clinician: Anne Frank was hidden by Miep Gies and her family.
Question: A question used to elicit a targeted structure.	Clinician: What happened to Anne Frank when the Nazi's came to the Netherlands?
Prompt: The use of pause, repetition of the child's utterance, or a statement to elicit the targeted structure.	Clinician: Anne Frank was . . .
Regulatory Facilitations	
State the Goal/Target: Explicit statement of what the child will be working on.	Clinician: We are going to work on pronouns and passive verbs and we are going to use those to talk about "The Diary of Anne Frank."
Compare or Contrast: Highlighting differences or similarities between words or forms.	Clinician: Anne Frank lived with her family and Miep Gies lived with her family too.
Informative Feedback: Explicit feedback on accuracy.	Child: Anne Frank hid Miep Gies and her family. Clinician: No, Anne Frank was hidden by Miep Gies and her family. Those two sentences have two very different meanings.

Source: Gillam & Ukrainetz, 2006.

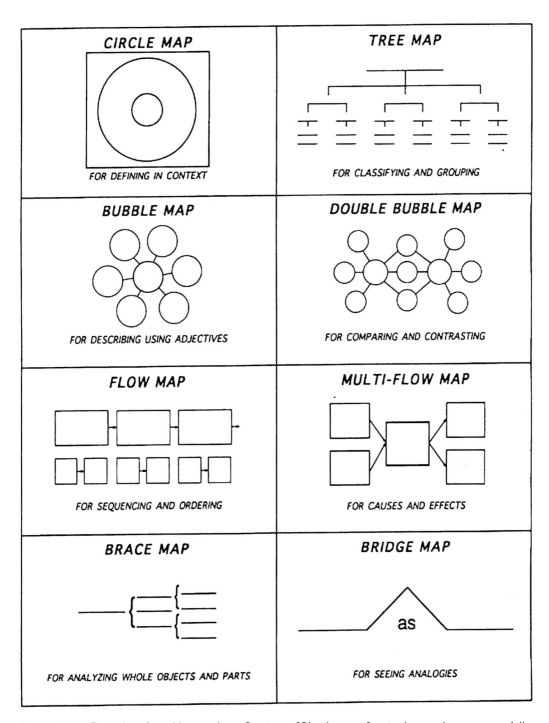

Figure 15–7. Examples of graphic organizers. Courtesy of Bing Images, free to share and use commercially.

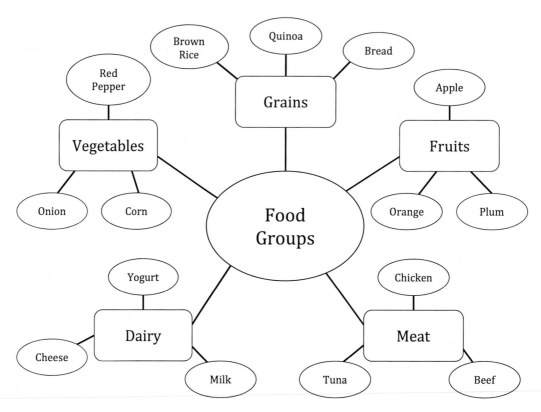

Figure 15–8. Example of graphic organizer or semantic map.

way to instill confidence in the children and families. The second is to be mindful of the worlds the children come from, the challenges they face daily because of their LLDs, and the importance of holistic approaches to intervention. A third recommendation is to build and maintain authentic, caring relationships with these children and their families—it is truly worth the effort. A final recommendation is to recognize that as much theoretical knowledge and practical experience you may have or may gain in your role as an SLPA, it is likely that you have not had the lived experience of LLDs. This lived experience gives the children and their families a level of expertise and valid-

ity that should solidify their relevance in the intervention process. And finally, I charge you to go forth and do good work, because what we do matters deeply to all the children we work with, not just those who are superheroes.

REFERENCES

American Psychological Association. (n.d.). *The road to resilience.* http://www.apa.org/help center/road-resilience.aspx

American Speech-Language-Hearing Association (ASHA). (n.d.-a). *Evidence-based practice.* https://www.asha.org/Research/EBP/Evi dence-Based-Practice/

American Speech-Language-Hearing Association (ASHA). (n.d.-b). *Cultural competence* [Practice portal]. https://www.asha.org/Practice-Portal/Professional-Issues/Cultural-Competence/

American Speech-Language-Hearing Association (ASHA). (n.d.-c). *Collaboration and teaming.* https://www.asha.org/Practice-Portal/Clinical-Topics/IntellectualDisability/Collaboration-and-Teaming/

American Speech-Language-Hearing Association (ASHA). (n.d.-d). *Response to intervention.* https://www.asha.org/slp/schools/profconsult/RtoI/

American Speech-Language-Hearing Association (ASHA). (n.d.-e). *Employment settings for SLPs.* https://www.asha.org/Students/Employment-Settings-for-SLPs/

American Speech-Language-Hearing Association (ASHA). (n.d.-f). *Interprofessional education/interprofessional practice* (IPE/IPP). https://www.asha.org/practice/interprofessional-education-practice/

American Speech-Language-Hearing Association (ASHA). (2001). *Roles and responsibilities of speech-language pathologists with respect to reading and writing in children and adolescents* [Position statement]. http://www.asha.org/policy

American Speech-Language-Hearing Association (ASHA). (2020). *Schools survey report: SLP caseload and workload characteristics.* https://www.asha.org/siteassets/surveys/2020-schools-survey-slp-caseload.pdf

American Speech-Language-Hearing Association (ASHA). (2022). *Speech-language pathology assistant scope of practice* [Scope of practice]. http://www.asha.org/policy

Americans With Disabilities Act (ADA). (n.d.). *Information and technical assistance on the American with disabilities act.* https://www.ada.gov/ada_intro.htm

Apel, K., & Masterson, J. J. (2001). Theory guided spelling assessment and intervention: A case study. *Language, Speech, and Hearing Services in Schools, 32,* 182–195. https://doi.org/10.1177/0734282905023004051 0.1044/0161-1461(2001/017)

Ardoin, S. P., Witt, J. C., & Connell, J. E., & Koenig, J. L. (2005). Application of a three-tiered response to intervention model for instructional planning, decision making, and the identification of children in need. *Journal of Psy-*

choeducational Assessment, 4, 362–380. https://doi.org/10.1177/073428290502300405

Bashir, A. S. (1989). Language intervention and the curriculum. *Seminars in Speech and Language, 10*(3), 181–191.

Bates, E., Thal, D., & MacWhinney, B. (1991). A functionalist approach to language and its implications for assessment and intervention. In T. M. Gallagher (Ed.), *Pragmatics of language: Clinical practice issues* (pp. 133–161). Singular Publishing. https://doi.org/10.1007/978-1-48997156-2_5

Beck, I. L., McKeown, M. G., & Kucan, L. (2002). *Bringing words to life: Robust vocabulary instruction.* Guilford Press.

Bjork, E. (2004). *Research on learning as a foundation for curricular reform and pedagogy.* http://reinventioncenter.miami.edu/Conference/2004Conference/2004ConferenceDetails.html#ElizabethBjork

Bloom, L., & Lahey, M. (1978). *Language development and language disorders.* Wiley. https://doi.org/10.7916/D8QZ2GQ5

Brimo, D., Apel, K., & Fountain, T. (2017). Examining the contributions of syntactic awareness and syntactic knowledge to reading comprehension. *Journal of Research in Reading, 1,*57–74. https://doi.org/10.1111/1467-9817.12050

Bronfenbrenner, U., & Morris, P. A. (2006). The biological model of human development. In R. M. Lerner (Ed.), *Handbook of child psychology* (6th ed., Vol. 1, pp. 792–828). Wiley.

Brown, R. (1973). *A first language: The early stages.* George Allen & Unwin.

California Department of Education. (n.d.). *CALPADS primary disability category codes.* https://www.cde.ca.gov/ta/tg/ca/disablecodes.asp

Catts, H. W., Fey, M. E., Tomblin, J. B., & Zhang, X. (2002). A longitudinal investigation of reading outcomes in children with language impairments. *Journal of Speech, Language, and Hearing Research, 45*(6), 1142–1157.

Catts, H. W., Fey, M. E., Zhang, X., & Tomblin, J. B. (1999). Language basis of reading and reading disabilities: Evidence from a longitudinal investigation. *Scientific studies of reading, 3*(4), 331-361. https://doi.org/10.1207/s1532799xssr0304_2

Cirrin, F. M., & Gillam, R. B. (2008). Language intervention practices for school-age children with spoken language disorders: A systematic review. *Language, Speech, and Hearing in the Schools, 37*, S110–S137.

Cirrin, F. M., Schooling, T. L., Nelson, N. W., Diehl, S. F., Flynn, P. F., Staskowski, M., . . . Adamczyk, D. F. (2010). Evidence-based systematic review: Effects of different service models on communication outcomes for elementary school-age children. *Language, Speech, and Hearing in Schools, 41*, 233–264. https://doi.org/10.1044/0161-1461(2009/08-0128)

Cohen, N. J. (2010). The impact of language development on the psychosocial and emotional development of young children. *Language Development and Literacy* [PDF document]. http://www.child-encyclope dia.com/sites/default/files/textes-experts/en/622/the-impact-of-language-development-on-the-psychosocial-and-emotionaldevelopment-of-young-children.pdf

Common Core State Standards. (n.d.). *Common core state standards initiative: Preparing America's students for college and career.* http://www.corestandards.org

Congressional Research Service. (2020). *The Individuals With Disabilities Education Act: A comparison of state eligibility criteria.* https://crsreports.congress.gov/product/pdf/R/R46566#:~:text=The%20majority%20of%20IDEA%20appropriations,multiple%20disabilities%2C%20(8)%20orthopedic

Culatta, B., Blank, M., & Black, S. (2010). Talking things through: Roles of instructional processing of expository texts. *Topics in Language Disorders, 30*(4), 308–322.

Davies, P., Shanks, B., & Davies, K. (2004). Improving narrative skills in young children with delayed language development. *Educational Review, 53*(3), 271–286. https://doi.org/10.1080/0013191042000201181

DeKemel, K. (2003). *Intervention in language arts: A practical guide for speech-language pathologists.* Mosby/Elsevier.

Disabilities, Opportunities, Internetworking, and Technology (DO IT). (n.d.). *What is the difference between and IEP and a 504 Plan?* https://www.washington.edu/doit/what-difference-between-iep-and-504-plan

Disability Rights Education & Defense Fund (DREDF). (n.d.). *Doing disability justice: Section 405 of the Rehabilitation Act of 1973.* https://dredf.org/legal-advocacy/laws/section-504-of-the-rehabilitation-actof-1973/

Dunst, C. J., Raab, M., & Trivette, C. M. (2012). Characteristics of naturalistic language intervention strategies. *Journal of Speech-Language Pathology and Applied Behavior Analysis, 53*(4), 8–16.

Ehren, B. J., Lenz, B. K. B. H., & Deshler, D. (2014). Adolescents who struggle with 21st Century literacy. In C. A. Stone, E. R. Silliman, B. J. Ehren, & G. W. Wallach (Eds.), *Handbook of language and literacy: Development and disorders* (pp. 619–636). Guilford Press.

Ehren, B. J., & Nelson, N. W. (2005). The responsiveness to intervention approach and language impairment. *Topics in Language Disorders, 25*(2), 120–131.

Eisenberg, S. (2007). How can I say that better? In T. Ukrainetz (Ed.), *Contextualized language Intervention: Scaffolding PreK-12 literacy achievement* (pp. 7–58). Pro-Ed.

Farber, J. G., & Klein, E. R. (1999). Classroom based assessment of a collaborative intervention with kindergarten and first-grade students. *Language, Speech, and Hearing Services in the Schools, 30*, 83–91. https://doi.org/10.1044/0161-1461.3001.83

Fey, M. E., Catts, H. W., Proctor-Williams, K., Tomblin, J. B., & Zhang, X. (2004). Oral and written story composition skills of children with language impairment. *Journal of Speech, Language, and Hearing Research, 47*, 1301–1318. https://doi.org/10.1044/1092-4388(2004/098)

Fey, M. E., Long, S. H., & Finestack, L. H. (2003). Ten principles of grammar facilitation for children with specific language impairments. *American Journal of Speech-Language Pathology, 12*, 3–15. https://doi.org/10.1044/1058-0360(2003/048)

Gillam, R., McFadden, T. U., & van Kleeck, A. (1995). Improving narrative abilities: Whole language and language skills approaches. In M. E. Fey, J. Windsor, & S. F. Warren (Eds.), *Language intervention: Preschool through the elementary years* (pp. 145–182). Paul H. Brookes.

Gillam, R. B., & Ukrainetz, T. A. (2006). Language intervention through literature-based units. In T. Ukrainetz (Ed.), *Contextualized language intervention* (pp. 7–58). Thinking Publications.

Harrison, L. J., & McLeod, S. (2010). Risk and protective factors associated with speech and language impairment in a nationally representative sample of 4- to 5-year-old children. *Journal of Speech, Language, and Hearing Research,*

53, 508–529. https://doi.org/10.1044/1092-4388(2009/08-0086)

Individuals With Disability Education Act (IDEA). (n.d.). *About IDEA.* https://sites.ed.gov/idea/about-idea/

Johnson, A. (2016). *Interprofessional education and interprofessional practice in communication sciences and disorders* [PDF document]. http://www.asha.org/uploadedFiles/IPE-IPP-Reader-eBook.pdf

Kamhi, A. G. (2014). Improving clinical practices for children with language and learning disorders. *Language, Speech, and Hearing Services in the Schools, 45*, 92–103. https://doi.org/10.1044/2014_LSHSS-13-0063

Kim, A. H., Vaughn, S., Wanzek, J., & Wei, S. (2004). Graphic organizers and their effects on the reading comprehension of students with LD: A synthesis of research. *Journal of Learning Disabilities, 37*, 105–118. https://doi.org/10.1177/00222194040370020201

Law, J., Garrett, X., & Nye, C. (2004). The efficacy of treatment with developmental speech and language delay/disorder: A meta-analysis. *Journal of Speech, Language, and Hearing Research, 44*(4), 924–943.

Lyons, R., & Roulstone, S. (2018). Well-being and resilience in children with speech and language disorders. *Journal of Speech, Language, and Hearing Research, 61*, 324–344. https://doi.org/10.1044/2017_JSLHR-L-16-0391

Moyle, M. J., Karasinksi, C., Weismer, S. E., & Gorman, B. K. (2011). Grammatical morphology in school-age children with and without language impairment: A discriminant function analysis. *Language, Speech, and Hearing in Schools, 42*, 550–560. https://doi.org/10.1044/0161-1461 (2011/10-0029)

National Center for Education Statistics. (n.d.). *Trends in high school dropout and completion rates in the United States.* https://nces.ed.gov/programs/dropout/

Nelson, N. W. (2005). The context of discourse difficulty in classroom and clinic: An update. *Topics in Language Disorders, 25*(4), 322–331.

Nelson, N. W. (2010). *Language and literacy disorders: Infancy through adolescence.* Pearson Education.

Nelson, N. W., Van Meter, A. M., Chamberlain, D., & Bahr, C. M. (2001). The speech-language pathologist's role in a writing lab approach. *Seminars in Speech and Language, 22*, 209–219. https://doi.org/10.1055/s-2001-16148

Nippold, M. A., Mansfield, T. C., Billow, J. L., & Tomblin, J. B. (2009). Syntactic development in adolescents with a history of language impairments: A follow-up investigation. *American Journal of Speech-Language Pathology, 18*, 241–251. https://doi.org/10.1044/1058-0360 (2008/08-0022)

No Child Left Behind Act. (n.d.). *NCLB.* https://www2.ed.gov/policy/elsec/leg/esea02/index.html

Paul, R. (2000). Understanding the "whole" of it: Comprehension assessment. *Seminars in Speech and Language, 21*(3), 10–17.

Paul, R., & Norbury, C. F. (2012). *Language disorders from infancy through adolescence: Listening, speaking, reading, writing, and communicating.* Elsevier Mosby.

Pennington, B., & Bishop, D. (2009). Relations among speech, language, and reading disorders. *Annual Review of Psychology, 60*, 283–306. https://doi.org/10.1146/annurev.psych.60.110707.163548.

Pinker, S. (1996). *Language learnability and language development.* Harvard University Press.

Puranik, C. S., Lombardino, L. J., & Altmann, J. P. (2008). Assessing the microstructure of written language using a retelling paradigm. *American Journal of Speech-Language Pathology, 17*, 107–120. https://doi.org/10.1044/1058-0360(2008/012)

Reardon, S. F., Kalogrides, D., & Shores, K. (2017). *The Geography of Racial/Ethnic Test Score Gaps* (CEPA Working Paper No.16–10). Stanford Center for Education Policy Analysis. http://cepa.stanford.edu/wp16-10

Roth, F. P., Paul, D. R., & Pierotti, A. (2006). *Let's talk: For people with special communication needs.* https://www.asha.org/public/speech/emergent-literacy.htm

Saussure, F. D. (1983). *Course in general linguistics.* Open Court Classics.

Scott, C., & Balthazar, C. M. (2015). The role of complex sentence knowledge in children with reading and writing difficulties. *Perspectives on Language and Literacy, 39*(3), 18–30.

Scott, P. A., Witt, J. C., Connell, J. E., & Koenig, J. L. (2005). Application of a three-tiered response to intervention model for instructional planning, decision making, and the identification of children in need. *Journal of Psychoeducational Assessment, 23*(4), 362–380. https://doi.org/10.1177/073428290502300405

Stanton-Chapman, T. L., Chapman, D. A., Bainbridge, N. L., & Scott, K. G. (2002). Identification of early risk factors for language impairment. *Research in Developmental Disabilities, 23*, 390–405.

Sun, L., & Nippold, M. A. (2012). Narrative writing in children and adolescents: Examining the literate lexicon. *Language, Speech, and Hearing in Schools, 43*, 2–13. https://doi.org/10.1044/01611461(2011/10-0099)

Sun, L., & Wallach, G. P. (2014). Language disorders are learning disabilities: Challenges on the divergent and diverse paths to language learning disability. *Topics in Language Disorders, 34*(1), 25–38. https://doi.org/10.1097/TLD.0000000000000005

Sutton, A. (2008). Language acquisition theory and AAC intervention. *Perspectives on Augmentative and Alternative Communication, 17*(2), 56–61. https://doi.org/10.1044/aac17.2.56

Ukrainetz, T. A. (2006). *Contextualized language intervention.* Thinking Publications.

Ukraintez, T. A. (2015). Assessment and intervention within a contextualized skill framework. In T. Ukrainetz (Ed.), *School-age language intervention: Evidence-based practices* (p. 689). Pro-Ed.

Understanding Special Education. (n.d.). *Special education terms and definitions.* http://www.understandingspecialeducation.com/special-education-terms.html

Ungar, M. (2015). Practitioner review: Diagnosing childhood resilience—A systemic approach to the diagnosis of adaptation in adverse social and physical ecologies. *The Journal of Child Psychology and Psychiatry, 56*(1), 4–17. https://doi.org/10.11 11/jcpp.12306

U.S. Department of Education. (n.d-a). *Education for homeless children and youths (EHCY) program.* https://nche.ed.gov/downloads/ehcy_profile.pdf

U.S. Department of Education (n.d.-b.). *Every student succeeds act.* https://www.ed.gov/essa?src=rn

Venker, C. E., Bolt, D. M., Meyer, A., Sindberg, H., Weismer, S. E., & Tager-Flusberg, H. (2015). Parent telegraphic speech use and spoken in preschoolers with ASD. *Journal of Speech, Language, and Hearing Research, 58*(6), 1733–1746. https://doi.org/10.1044/2015_JSLHR-L-14-0291

Wallach, G. P. (2008). *Language intervention for school-age students: Setting goals for academic success.* Mosby/Elsevier.

Wallach, G. P. (2010). It was a dark and stormy night: Pulling language-based learning disabilities out of the drifting snow. *Topics in Language Disorders, 30*, 6–14.

Wallach, G. P. (2014). Improving clinical practice: A school-age and school-based perspective. *Language, Speech, and Hearing Services in the Schools, 45*, 127–136. https://doi.org/10.1044/2014_ LSHSS-14-0016.

Wallach, G. P., Charlton, S., & Christie, J. (2009). Making a broader case for the narrow: Where to begin. *Language, Speech, and Hearing Services in Schools, 40*, 201–211. https://doi.org/10.1044/0161-1461(2009/08-0043)

Wallach, G. P., Charlton, S., & Christie, J. (2014). The spoken-written comprehension connection. In C. A. Stone, E, R. Silliman, B. J. Ehren, & G. P. Wallach (Eds.), *Handbook of language & literacy: Development and disorders* (pp. 485–501). Guilford Press.

Wallach, G. P., & Ocampo, A. (2020). *Language and literacy connections: Intervention for school-age children and adolescents.* Plural Publishing.

Wixson, K. K., Lipson, M. Y., & Valencia, S. W. (2014). Response to intervention for teaching and learning in language and literacy. In C. A. Stone, E. R. Silliman, B. J. Ehren, & G. P. Wallach (Eds.), *Handbook of language & literacy: Development and disorders* (pp. 637–653). Guilford Press.

World Health Organization. (2007). *International classification of functioning, disability, and health—Version for children and youth: ICF-CY.*

Yoder, P., Fey, M., & Warren, S. (2012). Studying the impact of intensity is important but complicated. *International Journal of Speech-Language Pathology, 14*, 410–413. https://doi.org/10.3109/17549507.2012.68589

APPENDIX 15–A
Examples of Common Core State Standards

Strand	Grade	Standard	Description
Speaking and Listening	3	Comprehension and Collaboration English Language Arts: SL.3.1	Engage effectively in a range of collaborative discussions (one-on-one, in groups, and teacher-led) with diverse partners on *grade 3 topics and texts*, building on others' ideas and expressing their own clearly.
	6	Presentation of Knowledge and Ideas English Language Arts: SL.6.4.1	Present claims and findings, sequencing ideas logically and using pertinent descriptions, facts, and details to accentuate main ideas or themes; use appropriate eye contact, adequate volume, and clear pronunciation.
	9–10	Comprehension and Collaboration English Language Arts: SL.9-10.1	Initiate and participate effectively in a range of collaborative discussions (one-on-one, in groups, and teacher-led) with diverse partners on grades 9–10 topics, texts, and issues, building on others' ideas and expressing their own clearly and persuasively.
Language	4	Conventions of Standard English Literacy: L.4.1	Demonstrate command of the conventions of standard English grammar and usage when writing or speaking.
	8	Vocabulary Acquisition and Use Literacy: L.8.4A	Determine or clarify the meaning of unknown and multiple-meaning words or phrases based on *grade 8 reading and content*, choosing flexibly from a range of strategies.

continues

Strand	Grade	Standard	Description
Language *continued*	11–12	Knowledge of Language Literacy: L.11-12.3.	Apply knowledge of language to understand how language functions in different contexts, to make effective choices for meaning or style, and to comprehend more fully when reading or listening.
History/ Social Studies	6–8	Craft and Structure Literacy: RH.6-8.4	Determine the meaning of words and phrases as they are used in a text, including vocabulary specific to domains related to history/social studies.
	9–10	Integration of Knowledge and Ideas RH.9-10.7	Integrate quantitative or technical analysis (e.g., charts, research data) with qualitative analysis in print or digital text.
Writing	6–8	Writing WHST: 6-8.2A	Write informative/explanatory texts, including the narration of historical events, scientific procedures/experiments, or technical processes.
	11–12	Writing Literacy: WHST 11.12.1.A	Introduce precise, knowledgeable claim(s), establish the significance of the claim(s), distinguish the claim(s) from alternate or opposing claims, and create an organization that logically sequences the claim(s), counterclaims, reasons, and evidence.

CHAPTER 16

Incorporating Play and Literacy in Treatment

Sara M. Aguilar

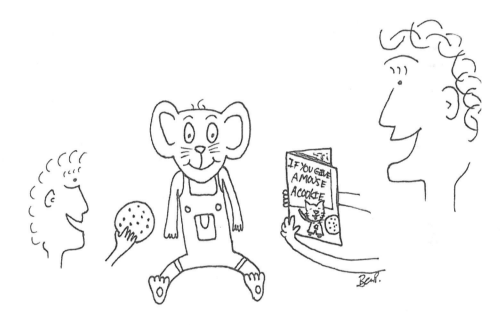

Play is a child's work.

> —Jean Piaget (prominent developmental psychologist)

Children learn about the world they live in through play. It provides them with a way to learn, experiment with, and use new information. Beginning in infancy with basic games, such as peek-a-boo, play goes on to assume a critical role in a child's physical, emotional, social, and cognitive-linguistic development. It is commonly believed that most of a child's linguistic knowledge develops in the context of play. The American Speech-Language-Hearing Association (ASHA) identifies play as a consistent activity that can be used to support the understanding and use of language by children across the early years (ASHA, n.d.). As such, the ability to incorporate play into treatment sessions is an important skill for a speech-language pathology assistant (SLPA).

DEVELOPMENT OF PLAY

As you consider how to incorporate play into treatment, it is important to understand how play develops. A child's play begins with reflexive behaviors that initially lack inherent intentionality, such as crying, cooing, and smiling (Schwartz, 2004). When these behaviors are met with meaningful reactions from caregivers, they are treated as communicative acts. With time, these behaviors mature into more complex cognitive processes, including representational thought, imagination, exploration, analysis, and problem solving. As such, the stages in a child's

cognitive development will be reflected in that child's play. Based on Piaget's work, we know that children engage in four stages of cognitive development: *sensorimotor, preoperational, concrete operational,* and *formal operational* (Table 16–1).

The ability to engage in representational thought is a cognitive skill that typically emerges by 18 months, during the sensorimotor period of cognitive development. This period is often associated with practice play, Piaget's earliest classification of play (Casby, 2003). During practice play, children explore objects in an egocentric manner as they learn about the world through their physical senses (e.g., mouthing objects, banging and throwing objects). Later in this stage, children begin to engage in simple cause-and-effect actions, such as physically moving toward a desired object, finding a toy obscured by an object, and pulling a string to get a toy located at the end of the string (Westby, 1980).

Table 16–1. Piaget's Stages of Cognitive Development

Age	Stage	Characteristics	Language Behaviors
Birth to 2 years	Sensorimotor	Begins with reflexive behaviors and motor learning. Progresses rapidly, learning object permanence, means-end behaviors, and so on.	Begins with reflexive vocal behaviors (e.g., crying/cooing) and later develops into use of true words when referents are not present (e.g., Child says "Daddy" even when he is not present).
2 to 7 years	Preoperational	Most rapid stage of language learning. Child develops representational thought and learns to solve physical problems.	Begins to engage in make believe and starts to comprehend and express temporal concepts (e.g., past, future).
7 to 11 years	Concrete Operations	Child learns to categorize and organize information; begins to be a logical thinker.	Begins to develop conversational skills; use logic to complete tasks.
11 to 15 years	Formal Operations	Learns to be an abstract thinker, tests mental hypotheses	Uses verbal reasoning to produce "if . . . then" statements.

Source: Adapted from Casby, 2003.

Representational thought serves as a foundation for children to later develop *symbolic play*. Symbolic play is associated with the preoperational period of cognitive development and includes the symbolism involved with the acquisition of true language behaviors (Westby, 1980). The presence of symbolic play indicates that a child understands that an object or entity can be used to represent something distinct from itself. For example, a child demonstrates this knowledge when using a shoebox to represent a doll's bed. This basic symbolism, used first in play, later serves as a foundation for children's understanding of the more abstract symbols involved with language, such as the words used to represent objects and ideas. For instance, a pattern of sounds such as "b-e-d" represents a piece of furniture used for sleeping. Overall, symbolic play and language share the underlying ability to engage in symbolism. In fact, observation of a child's symbolic play behaviors helps determine that child's level of functioning relative to the skills required for the development of language.

The remaining stages of cognitive development identified by Piaget are concrete operations and formal operations. These stages are associated with more advanced types of play. During the concrete operations stage, children learn to categorize and organize information. Later, in the formal operations stage, children engage in abstract thought and begin to test mental hypotheses during play (Wadsworth, 2004).

One way to better understand a child's level of play and representational abilities is through careful observations using a research-based tool, such as Westby's Symbolic Play Scale (Westby, 1980). Westby's play scale was developed out of observational research conducted on children who

were typically developing and those with intellectual impairments. Interestingly, Westby found that both groups of children progressed through the same sequence of play stages. Westby's Symbolic Play Scale was originally published as an appendix in her landmark 1980 article, "Assessment of Cognitive and Language Abilities Through Play," and the scale is now easily located using an online Web search. A description of the 10 stages of symbolic play, as depicted by Westby (1980), is summarized in Appendix 16–A. This summary can be used as an observational tool to determine a child's representational abilities, which in turn can guide the creation of developmentally appropriate treatment environments and materials. In addition, knowledge of the sequence of symbolic play allows you to engage in appropriate data collection to document children's progression through the stages of play.

PLAY IN SPEECH–LANGUAGE TREATMENT

Play can be incorporated in treatment as a platform for intervention approaches that focus on language form (i.e., phonology, morphology, syntax, semantics) and use (i.e., pragmatics). Play is a natural context for all children, since it gives them an opportunity to interact and experiment with their surroundings. Children develop language during social interactions. Hence, play in treatment provides opportunities for meaningful social scenarios that encourage language. During play scenarios, a child's communication acts elicit appropriate social responses from you, the child's communication partner. Clinicians can then expand on, and enhance, a child's communication acts to support her or him in becoming a competent language user.

Intervention in the context of play requires the provision of appropriate language input and skillful selection of materials and activities, including imaginative play scenarios, toys, and books. At its core, play in treatment should be a fun, child-directed experience and involve adult guidance and scaffolding to encourage children to experiment with new language forms to understand, describe, and manipulate the world around them.

Because play involves spontaneous and fluid interaction with a child's surroundings, clinicians must ensure that treatment is organized and systematic as intervention becomes more naturalistic and less structured (Norris & Hoffman, 1990). Without an organized and systematic approach, play in treatment merely becomes play. The balance between the spontaneity of play and the organization and methodology of intervention is a delicate one to achieve and maintain. To achieve this balance, it is critical that you work with your supervising speech-language pathologist (SLP) to (a) carefully determine a child's level of play, (b) create opportunities for meaningful communication, (c) provide effective scaffolding, and (d) select appropriate materials for use during play.

Determining the Level of Play

The first step in using play in treatment is to identify a child's current level of play and developmental abilities. You can identify where a child is functioning on the continuum of play by observing that child's behaviors, consulting with your supervising SLP, and using a play scale such as the one discussed above (Westby, 1980; Appendix 16–A). During observations, be aware that children typically engage in activities and interact with toys to the extent of their developmental level. In other words, an activity will be abandoned as soon as play reaches the capacity of that child's knowledge of the actions and relationships that can be performed or established with a particular toy. Consider this excellent example provided by Norris and Hoffman (1990):

> The child rocks a baby doll and then abandons the activity, failing to recognize that the doll's hair can be brushed, her hat can be worn, she can be placed in a stroller and taken for a walk, etc. (p. 74)

Once a child has reached her or his level of knowledge about a given situation (i.e., the relationship between objects or the actions that can be performed on objects, etc.), it is your job as the clinician to extend that child's current knowledge to new learning opportunities. Norris and Hoffman (1990) suggest the following in relation to the scenario above:

> If the child rocks the doll and begins to abandon it, the SLP might extend the child's understanding at that moment by making the child aware of some other object in relationship to the doll. The SLP can point to the doll's hair, refer to its state of messiness, and guide the child to brush the doll's hair while referring to all of the relationships between the doll and the brush ("The doll's hair is messy—it has to be brushed—you're brushing her hair— now it's looking prettier—don't brush it too hard"). (p. 74)

The actions and the accompanying language help the child to organize information about the doll in relationship to the brush that was not previously understood.

Creating Communication Opportunities

Once you have extended opportunities for play, you can create opportunities for a child to become a communicator in that environment by helping the child to (a) understand how to control and/or manipulate activities and (b) formulate the language involved in the completion of such tasks. Norris and Hoffman (1990) point out that "the goal is not to teach language, but rather to provide for active experiences with the use of language so that language may emerge" (p. 78). One way to accomplish this is to develop a set of *communication temptations* (Wetherby & Prutting, 1984). Although originally intended to be used in the assessment of children on the autism spectrum, communication temptations can be helpful in developing play scenarios for any young child.

Communication temptations are situations devised specifically to entice a child into initiating communicative acts (Wetherby & Prutting, 1984). For instance, you can present the child with a jar of bubbles, open it and blow a few bubbles, capture one and encourage the child to pop it, and then tightly close the lid on the bubble jar and hand it to the child. Next, without prompting or cueing, simply wait for the child to produce a communicative signal for help. Once the child initiates communication through vocalization, gesture, or some other means, you can respond naturally by opening the bottle and repeating the blowing and popping action with the child. After repeating

this scenario a few times, you can add an additional communication temptation by bringing the bubble wand up to your lips, waiting to blow the bubble with an expectant look on your face. Once the child produces a communicative signal, you should respond naturally by blowing the bubbles. This communication temptation scenario may be adapted to a number of activities, including balloons, wind-up toys, and peek-a-boo.

The key to creating this type of communication opportunity is to consistently view a child's behaviors as communicative (i.e., request, comment, command, question, protest, etc.) and follow through on that child's communicative act by responding in an appropriate and meaningful way. As such, play interactions should be led by the child, meaning that your goal is to focus on responding to the child's behaviors (e.g., "Oh, you want to roll the ball!") rather than requesting behaviors from the child (e.g., "What's that?" or "Say ball."). When you treat a child's behavior as a communicative act, it creates the opportunity to expose that child to more complex communication acts. For instance, a child's utterance of "ball" may have been merely produced as a label, but when you interpret it as a request (e.g., "You want the ball?") and provide that child with an appropriate consequence (e.g., giving the ball to the child), the child is immediately exposed to this new and more complex communication act.

Scaffolding Communication

After extending play and creating communication opportunities, you can also clarify any additional information needed by the child's communication partner (whether that is another child, you as the clinician, an adult, a doll, etc.). This can be done by modeling the language required to express the missing information and providing support as the child attempts to engage in this more complex communication act. In this way, you are partnering with the child to assist in the communication of more complex information. This is referred to as *scaffolding* (Pentimonti & Justice, 2010). Much like the scaffolding used in the construction of a building, therapeutic scaffolding temporarily provides adult support to a child who is learning how to perform increasingly complex communication acts. Adult support ensures the opportunity to practice using language at a higher level than a child would produce independently. The amount of adult support is adjusted as the child becomes more proficient with the targeted language forms independently. Table 16–2 outlines various approaches to supporting the development of complex communication acts. The techniques listed in Box 16–1 may also be helpful during play activities.

Box 16–1

- **Self-talk:** The clinician watches the child's play and then engages in the same behavior, but while describing her or his own actions. For example, the child is playing with a tea set and the clinician begins playing with the set, stating things like, "I'm making tea. I am going to pour some tea for everyone. The tea is so yummy, but hot."
- **Parallel talk:** The clinician describes the child's behaviors during play. For example, during the above play activity with a tea set, the clinician says, "You are making tea and pouring it into each glass. Oh, the tea must be yummy, but hot."
- **Expansion:** The clinician rephrases the child's utterance but uses a grammatically correct version. For example, if the child in the above example says, "Tea hot," the clinician can expand by saying, "Yes, the tea is hot."
- **Extension or expatiation:** Similar to expansion (above), but the clinician rephrases the child's utterance, adding additional semantic information. For example, if the child said, "Tea hot," the clinician could say, "Yes, we should be careful to sip the tea slowly."
- **Recast:** The clinician reformulates the child's utterance into a different form, such as a question. For example, if the child says, "Drink tea," the clinician can say, "Are you drinking the tea?" or "Should I drink the tea?"

Source: Adapted from Roth and Paul (2007, pp. 165–166).

Table 16–2. Scaffolding Approaches

Scaffolding Approach	Description	Example
Cloze procedures	Child and adult collaborate in creating a message. Adult omits words from phrases/sentences to allow child to provide missing information.	Adult: "Baby is tired, so she will go to _____." Child: "Bed"
Gestures and pantomime	Nonlinguistic physical cues that encourage child to produce language.	Adult: "She's tired. What should she do?" (tilting head and placing it on hands) Child: "Sleep"
Relational terms	Cues child to provide more information.	Child: "She need blanket" Adult: "So she can . . . " Child: "Go bed"
Preparatory sets	Highlights important information for child, including appropriate communication acts for particular contexts.	"You can't just take the blanket, you have to *ask* baby for it."
Constituent questioning	Encourages child to produce important details about and relationships between agents, actions, objects, and locations.	Adult: "What does baby need?" Child: "Blanket" Adult: "What does she need the blanket for?" Child: "Baby go sleep"
Comprehension questions	Monitors child's level of understanding during play.	"Why did she cry?" "Why isn't she sleeping?" "What happens next?"
Summarization or evaluation	Encourages child to summarize or evaluate information about play activity and provides additional opportunity to practice communicating the message.	"Tell mommy what the baby did."
Binary choices	Provides child with choices for communicating a message.	"You can ask nicely—'I want blanket, please' or you can be mean—'Give me the blanket!'"
Turn-taking cues	Indirectly requests more information from child.	Child: "I want blanket." Adult: "I want the blanket . . . " (with expectant pause and look) Child: "I want blanket." Adult: "Yeah?" (with rising intonation)
Phonemic cues	Provides child with beginning sound or syllable to support child's production.	Adult: "I need the bl___." Child: "-anket"

Source: Adapted from Norris & Hoffman, 1990.

Selecting Toys and Materials for Play

Another important consideration in incorporating play in treatment relates to the actual toys and materials that you use during intervention sessions. Selection of toys should be driven by the anticipated outcome(s) targeted in your treatment session and informed by the child's interests and preferences. Before selecting toys, you must first ask yourself, "What do I want the child to do or say?" Table 16–3 lists examples of language opportunities that can be targeted using particular toys. However, be sure to cautiously manage the treatment environment. It is a good idea to provide options, but be careful not to overwhelm the child with too many choices. It is also helpful to keep some toys visible but out of reach of the child to encourage the child to initiate comments and requests.

In addition, toys used in treatment must be safe for a child at a particular age (Schwartz, 2004). Clinicians should consult a toy's packaging for age recommendations; however, if packaging is not available, a good resource is the U.S. Consumer Product Safety Commission (2013). Be sure to take appropriate precautions when working with children who have developmental delays and may continue to mouth toys past the typical age of development. Chapter 6 discusses additional procedures in ensuring toys and materials are properly cleaned for use in treatment.

Lastly, Lahey and Bloom's (1977) article is an excellent resource for determining what language input to provide to a child during play. These authors suggest that clinicians focus on using words that frequently occur in the child's environment rather than more specific and less frequently used vocabulary. For example,

it is better to say *car* rather than *Toyota* and *money* instead of *quarter*. Using more general terms is valuable because they may be used in a wider variety of situations. In addition, some words express multiple meanings, allowing a child to use a single utterance in multiple ways. A good example of one such word is *no*, which can be used to reject, deny, or express disappearance.

SHARED READING AS PLAY

Young children with language disorders are more likely to experience academic difficulties later in life, particularly in the area of literacy, as spoken and written language have a close and interdependent relationship (Catts & Kamhi, 2005). It is common for children with a language impairment to experience difficulties learning to read and write, just as children who face difficulty with reading and writing often have problems with spoken language. Furthermore, the relationship between spoken and written language is established early in a child's development and continues to grow throughout childhood and into adulthood. ASHA (2001) points out that individuals engaging in early speech-language intervention can play a significant role in the prevention of future literacy problems. Table 16–4 lists various approaches to early literacy intervention that have been shown to effectively prevent future literacy problems. As an SLPA, you may be asked to engage in tasks to support literacy development. To do so effectively, you need to work with your supervising SLP to (a) incorporate print referencing into treatment sessions and (b) select appropriate books for use during shared reading activities.

Table 16–3. Activities, Toys, and Language Opportunities

Activity/Toy	Language Opportunities
Peek-a-boo	• Joint attention (fundamental skill required for language development) • Turn-taking • Cause/effect—child learns to anticipate your reappearance • Model/encourage language routines: *"Where is (child's name)? Is he under the table? There you are!"*
Blocks	• Cause/effect relationships: stack blocks, then knock them down • Model/encourage language routines: *"Uh, oh! Fall down! Oh no!"* • Color/size concepts: label and request blocks of different colors, shapes, and sizes • Prepositions: support child' in understanding and/or using prepositions (e.g., *"Let's put it on top"*)
Cars	• Cause/effect: Expand understanding of cause and effect by first stacking blocks, then using a car to knock down blocks • Model/encourage language routines: *ready, set, go!*; *crash!*; *stop/go*; *go fast/go slow* • Expand utterance: *yellow car; big car; fast car* • Sabotage: present a car with a broken wheel and see how child reacts to it. • Encourage/model language: *"Oh, no!" "What happened?" "It's broken!" "Let's fix it!"*

Bubbles	• Expand utterances:
	  ○ Actions: *open/close bubble,; blow bubble, pop bubble*
	  ○ Adjectives: *big bubble, small bubble, red bubble (with colored bubbles)*
	• Request recurrence: *more bubbles*

Puzzles	• Child identifies puzzle pieces when you request them: *"Give me the _____."* • Encourage child-initiated requests • Teach vocabulary for the puzzle pieces (e.g., farm animals, shapes) • Turn-taking

Puppets	• Feeding puppet
	  ○ Teach food vocabulary
	  ○ Identify/request foods: *"Feed him the banana" "What do you want to feed him?"*
	  ○ Use puppet to model language: *"I want more grapes! Yum, yum, yum! I like grapes!"*

Balls (various sizes, textures, weights, etc.)	• Expanding utterances:
	  ○ Actions: *roll ball, bounce ball, throw ball*
	  ○ Prepositions: *ball in, ball out, ball on, ball off*
	  ○ Adjectives: *small ball, red ball, bumpy ball*

Table 16–4. Approaches to Early Literacy Intervention

Type of Approach	Description of Approach	Examples
Joint Book Reading	Shared reading between adult and child in which adult and child jointly explore content, language, and illustrations. Adult produces models by commenting on what is being read or pictured and asks questions about the book.	• Asking questions that can be answered by either looking at pictures or using information read in book (e.g., "Who is hiding under the table?" [pointing to picture of a bear under the table]) • Asking questions that require child to go beyond what is shown in pictures or given in text (e.g., "What will happen next?")
Environmental Print Awareness	Understanding the meaning of common symbols/knowledge and that print communicates meaning.	• Community signs (STOP, EXIT, etc.) • Logos (restaurants, brands, etc.)
Conventions of Print	Teaching children about book handling and other common features of print and reading.	• Front-to-back direction of book reading • Left-to-right reading orientation • Meaning of punctuation (exclamations, etc.)
Phonemic Awareness/ Phonological Processing Skills	Drawing attention to sounds and encouraging sound play and sound recognition during reading.	• Alliteration in books • Nursery rhymes and other books with rhyming
Alphabetic Principle/Letter Knowledge	Recognition of letters and their corresponding sounds.	• Labeling letters • Drawing attention to words

Source: Adapted from ASHA, 2001.

Print Referencing

Print knowledge is an area of preliteracy development that involves a child's exposure to and basic understanding of written language (Storch & Whitehurst, 2002). It has received attention as a form of early literacy intervention that is associated with later success in word recognition and spelling (National Early Literacy Panel, 2004). *Print referencing* is an evidence-based approach for increasing print knowledge during the emergent literacy period (typically 3–5 years old) (Justice & Ezell, 2000, 2002; Justice et al., 2009;

Lovelace & Stewart, 2007). Print knowledge includes understanding the organization and functions of print in text (i.e., book title, author's name, speech bubbles, etc.), alphabet knowledge (i.e., names and features of letters), and emergent writing (i.e., expressing meaning through writing). The theory behind print referencing is that fostering a child's learning about print and literacy increases that child's awareness of, and interest in, print during shared reading activities.

Print referencing involves adult-generated cues that guide a child to notice salient features and functions of written language during shared storybook reading (Justice & Ezell, 2004). The cues may be either verbal or nonverbal. Verbal cues include commenting about print, asking questions about print, and making requests of the child regarding print. Nonverbal cues include drawing attention to print by pointing to text and tracking text with a finger. Table 16–5 has examples of how to use print referencing cues in the context of shared storybook reading.

Selecting Appropriate Books for Shared Reading

Books with *print salience* lend themselves to a print referencing approach (Zucker et al., 2009). Print salience refers to books that contain exciting print features that draw a child's attention to print in books. Examples of print-salient features include (a) bright colors, (b) interesting font changes, (c) visible speech (e.g., speech bubbles that connect illustrations and characters to text), (d) visible sounds (e.g., "meow" near a picture of a cat), and (e) environmental labels on illustrations (e.g., the word *candy* on a box). These qualities invite readers to explore, discuss, and interact with print in a meaningful way, thereby making the act of reading a rich and exciting experience rather than a passive and possibly tedious routine.

Print referencing and the use of books with print-salient material should be implemented strategically to encourage children's understanding of the forms and functions of print while introducing new vocabulary and concepts. Be mindful, though, to create a positive and fun atmosphere that encourages children's exploration of books and fosters enjoyment of reading.

Table 16–5. Print Referencing Cues

Type of Cue	Examples
Questions about print	• "Do you know what this letter is called?" • "There are words in the bear's speech bubble! What do you think he is saying?" • "Which word says *bear*?" • "What do you think this says?"
Requests of child	• "Show me where I start reading on this page." • "Look at the letters in this word. Show me one that is in your name." • "Help me read this word." • "Find the letter *C.*"
Comments about print	• "This is the title of the book. It tells us what this book is called." • "This word in the title says *bear.*" (points to word) • "That says *Eric Carle* (points to author's name). He's the author of this book." • "Uppercase *C* is the same shape as lower case *c.*"
Nonverbal cues	• Point to words and letters • Point to the first word on page (to show where you begin reading) • Track print left to right

Source: Adapted from Zucker et al., 2009.

REFERENCES

American Speech-Language-Hearing Association. (n.d.). *Activities to encourage speech and language development*. https://www.asha.org/public/speech/development/activities-to-encourage-speech-and-language-development/

American Speech-Language-Hearing Association. (2001). *Roles and responsibilities of speech-language pathologists with respect to reading and writing in children and adolescents*. http://www.asha.org/policy

Casby, M. W. (2003). The development of play in infants, toddlers, and young children. *Communication Disorders Quarterly, 24*(4), 163–174.

Catts, H., & Kamhi, A. (2005). *Language and reading disabilities*. Pearson Education.

Cazden, C. B. (1988). *Classroom discourse: The language of teaching and learning*. Heinemann.

Justice, L. M., & Ezell, H. K. (2000). Enhancing children's print and word awareness through home-based parent intervention. *American Journal of Speech-Language Pathology, 9*(3), 257–269.

Justice, L. M., & Ezell, H. K. (2002). Use of storybook reading to increase print awareness in at-risk children. *American Journal of Speech-Language Pathology, 11*(1), 17–29.

Justice, L. M., & Ezell, H. K. (2004). Print referencing: An emergent literacy enhancement strategy and its clinical applications. *Language, Speech, and Hearing Services in Schools, 35*, 185–193.

Justice, L. M., Kaderavek, J. N., Xitao, F., Sofka, A., & Hunt, A. (2009). Accelerating preschoolers' early literacy development through classroom-based teacher-child storybook reading and explicit print referencing. *Language, Speech, and Hearing Services in Schools, 40*(1), 67–85.

Lahey, M., & Bloom, L. (1977). Planning a first lexicon: Which words to teach first. *Journal of Speech & Hearing Disorders, 42*(3), 340–350.

Lovelace, S., & Stewart, S. R. (2007). Increasing print awareness in preschoolers with language impairment using non-evocative print referencing. *Language, Speech, and Hearing Services in Schools, 38*(1), 16–30.

National Early Literacy Panel. (2004, November). *The National Early Literacy Panel: A research synthesis on early literacy development.*

Norris, J. A., & Hoffman, P. R. (1990). Language intervention within naturalistic environments. *Language, Speech, and Hearing Services in Schools, 21*, 72–84.

Pentimonti, J. M., & Justice, L.M. (2010). Teachers' use of scaffolding strategies during read alouds in the preschool classroom. *Early Childhood Education Journal, 37*(4), 241–248. https://doi.org/10.1007/s10643-009-0348-6

Roth, F., & Paul, R. (2007). Communication intervention. In R. Paul & P. Cascella (Eds.), *Introduction to clinical methods in communication disorders* (pp. 157–178). Paul H. Brookes.

Schwartz, S. (2004). *The new language of toys: Teaching communication skills to children with special needs* (3rd ed.). Woodbine House.

Storch, S. A., & Whitehurst, G. J. (2002). Oral language and code-related precursors to reading: Evidence from a longitudinal structural model. *Developmental Psychology, 38*, 934–947.

U.S. Consumer Product Safety Commission. (2013, June 15). *Safety education*. http://www.cpsc.gov/

Wadsworth, B. J. (2004). *Piaget's theory of cognitive and affective development* (5th ed.). Pearson Education.

Westby, C. (1980). Assessment of cognitive and language abilities through play. *Language, Speech, and Hearing Services in Schools, 11*, 154–168.

Wetherby, A. M., & Prutting, C. A. (1984). Profiles of communicative and cognitive social abilities in autistic children. *Journal of Speech and Hearing Research, 27*, 364–377.

Zucker, T. A., Ward, A. E., & Justice, L. M. (2009). Print referencing during read-alouds: A technique for increasing emergent readers' print knowledge. *Reading Teacher, 63*(1), 62–72.

APPENDIX 16–A
Summary of Play Stages

Stage	Typical Age of Acquisition	Description	Examples
I	9–12 months	■ Development of object permanence ■ Means-ends behaviors ■ Uses some toys appropriately/ceases to mouth/bang all toys ■ Vocalizations begin to function as requests or commands	■ Child finds toy covered by scarf ■ Moves to desired object/pulls string to attain toy at end of string ■ Rolls car on table (rather than putting it in his or her mouth)
II	13–17 months	■ Explores toys ■ Understands that adults are entities who can act upon objects ■ Single words emerge but are context dependent ■ Communication becomes increasingly intentional (gestures/vocalizes to request, command, gain attention, initiate interactions with others, protest, label)	■ Identifies part of toy responsible for operation and attempts to physically activate it (push, pull, turn, pound, shake) ■ Seeks help from adult when child is unable to operate it independently
III	17–19 months	■ Representational abilities begin to emerge (pretend play) ■ Autosymbolic play emerges ■ Begins to exhibit tool use ■ True verbal language emerges ■ Marked growth in vocabulary; a variety of words used for various functions and semantic roles	■ Child pretends to sleep, eat, etc. ■ Finds toy hidden out of view ■ Obtains toy with use of a stick
IV	19–22 months	■ Symbolic play extends beyond himself or herself ■ Word combinations used to express semantic relations (possessive relation is most common) ■ Child has combined sensorimotor concepts and has acquired internalized action schemas and is now able to refer to objects and individuals who are not physically present in play scenario	■ Child pretends doll is sleeping or pretends to feed communication/play partner ■ Child says, "my baby," "my car," etc.

continues

Stage	Typical Age of Acquisition	Description	Examples
V	24 months	<ul><li>Child engages in pretend play scenarios about other individuals</li><li>Simple sequences emerge (not yet able to perform more complex realistic sequences)</li><li>Emergence of present progressive *-ing*, plural and possessive *-s*</li><li>Begins to use short sentences to describe what is presently occurring</li><li>Communicative acts begin to include simple interrogatives, often lacking proper syntactic form</li></ul>	<ul><li>Child plays house and pretends to be mommy</li><li>Child puts food in bowl, then uses a spoon to feed doll/stacks blocks, then knocks them down</li><li>With rising intonation, child says, "The doggy sleepy" in order to ask, "Is the doggy sleepy?"</li></ul>
VI	2½ years	<ul><li>Child begins to depict less-common events</li><li>Child's role in play changes quickly</li><li>Associative play begins to emerge (though parallel play remains most common)</li><li>Uses language to analyze experiences</li><li>Begins to provide syntactically and semantically appropriate answers to "who," "whose," "what," "where," and "what . . . do" questions</li><li>Begins to ask "why" questions, especially in response to negative statements, but may not yet understand adult's answer to "why" questions</li></ul>	<ul><li>Child engages in pretend play involving doctor/sick child, or teacher/student</li><li>Child switches from being teacher to child often with little indication/warning</li><li>Child asks, "Where the doggy is?"</li><li>Child participates in the same activity as another individual but plays independently (without working together cooperatively)</li></ul>
VII	3 years	<ul><li>Begins to link several play schemas in a sequence</li><li>With the use of sequences, the child begins to talk about past and future events using past and future verb tenses</li><li>Play becomes increasingly associative</li></ul>	<ul><li>Child pretends to make a pizza, bake it, cut it, serve it, and wash the dishes</li><li>Child says, "He ate pizza." and "He will eat pizza."</li></ul>

Stage	Typical Age of Acquisition	Description	Examples
VIII	3–3½ years	■ Plays with less realistic toys, which involves abstraction in order to identify similarities and differences between real and pretend objects ■ Descriptive vocabulary increases ■ Begins to take another's perspective and develops the metalinguistic ability to think about and talk about language ■ Dolls are given personalities and begin to participate in play scenarios	■ Child plays with doll house, barn ■ Child uses blocks to construct enclosures (house, fence, etc.) ■ Child pretends a row of chairs is a bus ■ Child provides dialogue during play
IX	4 years	■ Child begins to consider future events and solve problems for novel events ■ Child begins to use modal verbs*: *can, may, might, could, would, will* (*these will not be mastered until 10–12 years) ■ Child begins to use conjunctions, including *and, but, if, so, because*	■ Child begins to consider and verbalize, "What would happen if . . . ?" or "If I do this, then . . ." ■ Child builds increasingly elaborate structures with blocks and other 3D objects ■ Uses dolls to test out hypotheses ("What would happen if . . .")
X	5 years	■ Child begins to plan out sequences and play scenarios in advance ■ Identifies what will be required to carry out planned play scenarios ■ Play becomes more imaginative and the child is able to manage more than one event at a time ■ Child begins to use relative and subordinate clauses in order to link two or more prepositions ■ Child begins to use relational terms,* including *then, when, first, while, next, before, after* (*these will not be mastered until 12 years)	■ Child states that she will be the mother and while she is feeding the baby, her other children clean their room and daddy works in the yard ■ Child produces phrases such as, "I'm the princess who lives in the castle."

Source: Based on Westby, 1980.

CHAPTER 17

Autism Spectrum Disorder (ASD)

Jodi Robledo

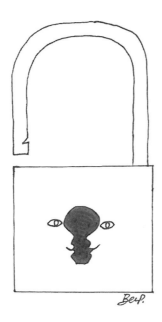

Autism isn't something a person has, or a "shell" that a person is trapped inside. There's no normal child hidden behind autism. Autism is a way of being. It is pervasive: It colors every experience, every sensation, perception, thought, emotion, and encounter, every aspect of existence. It is not possible to separate the autism from the person—and if it were possible, the person you'd have left would not be the same person you started with.

—Sinclair (1993, p. 1, as cited in Kluth, 2010, p. 3)

As a speech-language pathology assistant (SLPA), you will have the opportunity to work with individuals with autism spectrum disorder (ASD). According to the Centers for Disease Control and Pre-vention's (CDC's) Autism and Developmental Disabilities Monitoring (ADDM) Network, 1 in 44 school-aged children have been identified with ASD (CDC, 2021). ASD is more than four times more common among boys than among girls and can be found in all racial, ethnic, and socioeconomic groups. Researchers believe that the cause or causes of ASD involve both genetic and environmental factors. Current research continues to search for both its cause and a cure for ASD, as well as evidence-based practices to support individuals with ASD across the life span.

This chapter gives you a general overview of the definitions and common characteristics of ASD and foundational supports to benefit individuals with ASD. The goal is not to simply present a list of deficits that distinguish individuals with ASD from those without ASD. Rather, the goal is to present you with information to guide your learning regarding the individuals with ASD whom you will support. Remember this famous saying about ASD: "If you know one individual with autism, then you know one individual with autism" (Stephen Shore, as cited in Kolarik, 2016, p. 479). As professionals, we must continue to learn and grow in relationship with and understanding of the individuals we support. As the disability rights movement reminds us, it is imperative that we work with individuals, rather than work on them.

DEFINITIONS OF AUTISM SPECTRUM DISORDER

Clinical Definitions

Within a medical (or clinical) model, autism is described as a spectrum disorder, meaning that individuals will range in intensity of characteristics. According to the fifth edition of the *Diagnostic and Statistical Manual of Mental Disorders*

(*DSM-5*; American Psychiatric Association [APA], 2013), individuals with ASD display persistent deficits in social communication and social interaction across multiple contexts, as well as restricted, repetitive patterns of behavior, interests, and activities. Severity is described in three levels: Level 1 requiring support, Level 2 requiring substantial support, and Level 3 requiring very substantial support. In addition, the *DSM-5* specifies that symptoms must be present in the early developmental period; cause clinically significant impairment in social, occupational, or other important areas of current functioning; and are not better explained by intellectual disability or global developmental delay.

Challenges within the category of social communication and social interaction may include challenges with reciprocity (e.g., abnormal social approach and failure of normal back-and-forth conversations); reduced sharing of interests, emotions, or affect; challenges with initiation or response to social interactions; challenges with nonverbal communication used for social interaction (e.g., poorly integrated verbal and nonverbal communication; abnormalities in eye contact and body language, understanding and using gesture and facial expressions, possible lack of facial expressions and nonverbal communication); and deficits in developing, maintaining, and understanding relationships (e.g., difficulties adjusting behavior to suit various social contexts, difficulties in sharing imaginative play or in making friends, absence of interest in peers) (APA, 2013).

Challenges within the category of restrictive, repetitive patterns of behavior, interests, and activities may include stereotyped or repetitive motor movements, object use, or speech; insistence on sameness (e.g., inflexible adherence to routines, ritualized patterns of verbal or nonverbal behavior); highly restricted, fixated interests that are abnormal in intensity or focus; and *hyper*reactivity or *hypo*reactivity to sensory input or unusual interests in sensory aspects of the environment (APA, 2013).

Educational Definition

The category of autism was added to the Individuals With Disabilities Education Act (IDEA) in 1990 under P.L. 101-476 (Hall, 2009; Knoblauch & Sorenson, 1998). To receive supports and services from special education, individuals must meet the following three criteria: They must be eligible in a disability category as defined in IDEA, there must be an adverse impact on educational performance, and there must be an actual need for special education and related services to achieve a free and appropriate public education. Autism is specifically defined in IDEA as a developmental disability significantly affecting verbal and nonverbal communication and social interaction, repetitive activities, stereotyped movements, resistance to environmental change or change in daily routines, and unusual responses to sensory experiences. Generally, autism is evident before age 3 years and adversely affects an individual's educational performance (Hall, 2009).

An Insider's Perspective

I think that much of the characteristics of autism is a result of not being able to cope with the neurological impairment which autistic people seem to have. I expect that withdrawal of an autistic person into his own world is a result of the impairment. I also believe that an autistic person's inability to cope makes them less able to concentrate and therefore to learn. I hope this evaluation by an autistic individual will help other people to understand that we are intelligent even though we may not always appear to be. (Hale & Hale, 1999, p. 60)

I believe that autism results when some sort of mechanism that controls emotion does not function properly, leaving an otherwise relatively normal body and mind unable to express themselves with the depth that they would otherwise be capable of. (Williams, 1992, p. 203)

I believe Autism [sic] is a marvelous occurrence of nature, not a tragic example of the human mind gone wrong. In many cases, Autism [sic] can also be kind of genius undiscovered. (O'Neil, 1999, p. 14)

Although clinical and educational definitions are most commonly associated with the definition of ASD, they leave out one of the most important aspects of truly understanding what ASD is—the perspective and experiences of individuals with ASD—the true experts. One important aspect of including an insider's perspective is that we can better understand how ASD affects individuals in different ways—that no two people with ASD experience it the same way. As we move on to explore the common characteristics of ASD, we must remember that individuals will vary greatly in the intensity or type of characteristic and that if we are truly hoping to understand the individuals we support, we must understand their strengths and challenges.

COMMON CHARACTERISTICS

Although no two individuals experience ASD in the same way, there are nonetheless common characteristics that many individuals with ASD share. These include social differences, communication differences, sensory differences, movement differences, and learning differences, as well as unique passions, interests, and rituals. Common characteristics presented in this chapter include both the clinical description and insiders' perspectives.

Social Differences

I can't speak for other kids, but I'd like to be very clear about my own feelings. I did not ever want to be alone. And all of those child psychologists who said, "John prefers to play by himself" were dead wrong. I played by myself because I was a failure at playing with others. (Robinson, 2007, p. 211)

Some people have said that autistic people don't care about friendships. That wasn't true at all for me. I tried to make as many friends as possible . . . I just want to say that people mean more than anything to me. I always try to be as friendly as I can to people I meet. However, I still need to work more on my social skills. They are not as good as a lot of people's. (McDonnell, 1993, p. 363)

Challenges with social relationships and interactions have been paramount to the definition of ASD since it was first described. In 1943, Leo Kanner suggested that social impairment was the defining component of autism (Heflin & Alaimo, 2007; Kanner, 1943; Waterhouse et al., 1996). Social challenges associated with ASD are well documented within the literature (Bellini, 2008; Brown & Whiten, 2000; Miller et al., 2008; Rogers, 2000; Travis et al., 2001).

The major social challenges of ASD are joint attention, nonverbal communication, social initiating, social reciprocity, social cognition, behavior associated with perspective taking and self-awareness, and social anxiety and withdrawal (Bellini, 2006, 2008).

Joint Attention

Young children with ASD have shown challenges with intentional communication and joint attention (Brien & Prelock, 2021). Difficulty orienting to people in social environments, limited frequency of sharing attention, and impaired monitoring of emotional states have been noted in young children with ASD (Bellini, 2006, 2008). This early challenge with joint attention may impact the individual's ability to interact, connect with, and learn from others in their environment.

Nonverbal Communication

Individuals with ASD often have difficulty reading the body language and nonverbal cues of others. Many individuals with ASD also report that they can attend better to the speaker when they are looking away from the person's face (Robledo et al., 2012). However, in avoiding direct eye contact, individuals may miss nonverbal communication. Individuals with ASD may struggle to read and understand subtle social signals or to decode what they experience as social secrets (Kluth, 2009, 2010). Other individuals with ASD report that they also have trouble using nonverbal communication such as gestures, body language, and facial expressions (Kluth, 2009, 2010).

Social Initiation

Individuals with ASD experience two common categories of social initiation challenges: There are those who rarely initiate interactions with others and those who initiate frequently but inappropriately (Bellini, 2006, 2008). Individuals in the first category often demonstrate fear, anxiety, or apathy regarding social interactions. Within the second category, individuals may initiate often but might do so by interrupting, repeating phrases or questions, or violating other social rules or norms when initiating. In addition, some individuals with ASD may attempt to initiate, but others might not recognize their attempts to be social or interact.

Social Reciprocity

Challenges associated with social reciprocity involve the give-and-take, turn-taking, mutuality, and back-and-forth exchanges of social interactions. Many individuals with ASD engage in one-sided conversations, forgetting to ask the perspective of their social partner (Bellini, 2008). Individuals with ASD may fail to jointly attend, meaning they are not always able to shift their attention in unison to an object, event, or person when their social partner does. Many individuals with ASD report that they have difficulty keeping up with the rhythm or pace of conversation and struggle to know when it is appropriate to jump into a conversation. Others report challenges with knowing when to terminate an interaction, often reporting difficulty determining the social cues that signal the end of a conversation. Knowing how to appropriately terminate an interaction can also be challenging. An individual with ASD may walk away, change topics, or hang up the phone before the social partner believes the conversation is finished.

Social Cognition

Researchers have suggested that many social challenges displayed by individuals with ASD stem from difficulties with social cognition (Baron-Cohen, 1989; Bellini, 2006, 2008). Social cognition refers to understanding the thoughts, intentions, motives, and behaviors of ourselves and others (Flavell et al., 1993), as well as the social norms, customs, and values of the surrounding culture (Resnick et al., 1991). Challenges related to difficulty with social cognition can include difficulty analyzing social situations, understanding the jokes or humor of others, or incorrectly interpreting the intentions of others (Bellini, 2008).

Perspective Taking and Self-Awareness

Individuals with ASD often make socially inappropriate comments, have challenges expressing sympathy for others, have difficulty maintaining personal hygiene or personal space, or may fail to talk about or acknowledge the interests of others (Bellini, 2008). Difficulty with taking the perspective of another has been described as lacking a theory of mind (Baron-Cohen, 1989). However, we must consider that some of these problems might reflect an inability to show concern and care, rather than a lack of perspective taking or self-awareness. Some individuals with ASD report being so attuned to the feelings of others that they themselves can feel emotional distress just by being around others who are in distress (Kluth, 2009).

Social Anxiety and Performance Fears

Individuals with ASD may experience social anxiety, or intense fears of social situations (Bellini, 2008). Due to intense fears, they might avoid interacting with peers and might engage in solitary activities instead. It is important to remember that many of these individuals do want to engage in social interactions, but a lack of social skills or intense fears might be holding them back.

Communication Challenges

My speech really just bulges out of my mouth like a balloon, and the real thoughts in my head just keep on a direct line. The direct line and the balloon are related, but they do not correspond, and the more the balloon bulges, the less sense it makes, until it bursts, leaving nearly all my thoughts scattered, and me wild with anger and shame. (Blackman, 1999, p. 135)

There are, on occasion, still times when I want to talk, but I can't. I can try and try and try, but I can't talk. There is a fear holding me back. I do not know what it is I am afraid of, I only know that it is a feeling of fear unlike any other feeling of fear I have ever known. It is not that I do not want to talk, it is that I am unable to at that moment. (McKean, 1994, p. 39)

I am very fortunate that my friends and family are people who know me very intimately. Many times I feel as if oral communication is overrated. Much of how I express myself is through my eyes. Those close to me

are easily able to tell if I am sick, tired, or happy, by just looking at my face. My expressions are not always appropriate, yet my eyes are the windows to my soul. (Rubin, in Biklen, 2005, p. 89)

For most individuals with ASD, there are no problems with the physical form or function of the mouth, vocal cords, or other parts of the anatomy involved in speech and communication. Nonetheless, challenges with both nonverbal and verbal communication are a defining characteristic of ASD. Approximately 33% to 50% of individuals with ASD do not develop functional speech (Noens & van Berckelaer-Onnes, 2005). If an individual with ASD does use speech, there may be impairments in the ability to initiate or sustain conversations (Paul & Sutherland, 2005). According to Wegner (2021), the use of augmentative and alternative communication (AAC) has shown positive results for individuals with ASD in the areas of behavior (Bopp et al., 2004; Walker & Snell, 2013), social interaction (Therrien et al., 2016), receptive language and comprehension (Brady, 2000), and speech and expressive language (Millar, 2009; Mirenda, 2003).

The quality or tone of voice of an individual with ASD may be monotone, singsong, flat, husky, or unusual sounding. Gebauer et al. (2014) described that the prosody, pitch, or volume in speech may be unusual. Intonation may be mechanical, wooden, or arrhythmic. This can be problematic because others may believe that the individual is cold, aloof, or odd.

Individuals with ASD may also use immediate or delayed echolalia (Prizant & Rydell, 1993). Immediate echolalia refers to repeating sounds or speech that the individual has just heard. Delayed echolalia refers to repeating sounds or speech that the individual has heard in the past. There is great debate as to the purpose of echolalia, and some researchers believe it serves different functions for individuals (Prizant & Rydell, 1993). Some individuals with ASD have described it as attempts to communicate with those around them or as self-stimulatory or calming, whereas others have called echolalia "words of annoyance" that are not volitional and have little meaning. Recent research has begun to identify possible communicative functions of echolalia such as turn-taking, labeling, requesting, affirming, and protesting, and has suggested its role in gestalt language acquisition (Blanc, 2012; Stiegler, 2015).

Individuals with ASD have also reported difficulty processing speech, spanning all aspects of speech (Kluth, 2009, 2010). Many report that they hear bits and pieces of a conversation and have trouble processing and understanding the general message of the speaker. In addition, individuals with ASD often have trouble with figurative language idioms, metaphors, jokes, slang, and sarcasm (Kluth, 2009).

A review by Hall (2009) summarized common communication challenges associated with ASD. Challenges with pronoun use have been reported, in terms of using the third person when individuals are talking about themselves (Scheuermann & Webber, 2002). Gender is commonly confused in the speech of individuals with ASD, with words such as *he, she,* or *it* used incorrectly. Difficulty with word boundaries and a tendency to comprehend phrases as single chunks of speech are also common. Using bound morphemes and answering Wh-questions can present challenges for individuals with

ASD (Koegel & Koegel, 1995), and they may have a greater capacity for learning nouns over verbs.

Sensory Differences

The unmodulated sensory input often overwhelmed me, causing me mental torture, and I would begin feeling mentally confused and sluggish. My head would feel fogged so that I could not think. My vision would blur, and the speech of those around me would become gibberish. My whole body buzzed. The slight tremor that always plagued me would worsen. My hands would feel detached from my body, as if they were foreign objects. I would be paralyzed, unable to comprehend my own movements unless I could see them. I could not tell where my hand started and the table ended, or what shape the table was, or even if it was rough or smooth. I felt like I was in a cartoon world. (Hawthorne, as cited in Gillingham, 2000, pp. 21–22)

Individuals with ASD report a variety of sensory differences, compared to typically developing individuals. Some are hypersensitive and others are hyposensitive to sensory stimulation, and reports indicate that any of their senses can be affected (i.e., smell, touch, vision, taste, temperature, hearing, vestibular system, and proprioception) (Gillingham, 2000). The impact of sensory differences in the everyday life of an individual with ASD should not be underestimated and is an area in need of support. A description of each area of sensory differences will focus heavily on the experience of individuals with ASD to give you a rich understanding of how these differences affect them.

Tactile Sensitivity

Individuals with ASD can experience the sensation of touch in different ways (Robledo et al., 2012). Some may crave and seek out touch, whereas others may avoid any kind of touch. Some individuals seek out deep-pressure touch, like a firm hug or handshake, but pull away from light or soft touch. Unexpected touch can startle many individuals with ASD and should be avoided. Many individuals report avoiding activities or situations where touch may become unbearable. Sean Barron and Temple Grandin described their experiences with tactile sensitivity:

> I felt acutely uncomfortable sitting upright in the bathtub, so I didn't enjoy taking a bath in the least. I absolutely hated the way my bottom felt against the tub, and I couldn't make myself think about something else so I wouldn't feel it. When I tried to sit normally it felt "squishy" and I was extremely sensitive to this feeling. I couldn't shake it off. It was the same feeling I used to have when I couldn't stand to touch our rug with my bare feet. To make it more bearable, I shifted most of my weight onto one side so that only a part of me came into contact with the bathtub. When they insisted I "sit right," it only compounded the problem. (Barron & Barron, 1992, p. 96)

> "I'll miss you, Temple." She walked quickly to my side and kissed my cheek. I ached to be enfolded in her arms, but how could she know? I stood

rigid as a pole trapped by the approach avoidance syndrome of autism. I drew back from her kiss, not able to endure tactile stimulation—not even loving, tactile stimulation. (Grandin & Scariano, 1986, p. 65)

Individuals with tactile sensitivities also describe challenges with personal hygiene such as brushing teeth and hair. Some report avoiding certain fabrics or preferring to wear similar clothing again and again, or both. Tactile sensitivities have also been reported for eating, and many individuals with ASD seek or avoid particular food textures, which limit their diet.

Auditory Sensitivities

Auditory input typically causes anxiety for individuals with ASD. Donna Williams (1992, 1994) and Temple Grandin (1995) explained that hearing certain sounds created painful experiences. For Williams (1992), the tone of people's voice disturbed her. Grandin (1992) said her hearing felt "like having a hearing aid with the volume control stuck on super loud" (p. 107) and expressed that "sudden loud noises hurt my ears like a dentist's drill hitting a nerve" (p. 107). She described her dislike for environments that had many different noises, "such as shopping centers and sports arenas. High pitched continuous noise, such as bathroom vent fans or hair dryers, are annoying" (p. 2).

Lucy Blackman (1999) described her auditory differences:

> Because other people's sound processing was alien to me, I had no idea that sound should not be like a pressure

cooker lid. I put my hands to my ears for loud sudden noises, but the continuous clamor of everyday life was only relieved by movement. Even in the classroom there was visual stimulation and noise, which combined with my own breathing and a buzzing effect that I think was my own inner ear. (p. 51)

Matt Ward explained that sudden loud noises were very stressful:

Especially things like gunshots, loud motors, and brass bands. My mom took me through a drive-thru car wash once when I was in grade school and I was terrified. The brushes sounded to me like the sound of intense machine gunfire, but I could not communicate well enough to explain why I got so upset. (Robledo et al., 2012, p. 4)

Other individuals with ASD noted that, at times, they had an inconsistent ability to process auditory input. Darren White explained, a "trick which my ears played was to change the volume of sounds around me. Sometimes when other kids spoke to me I could scarcely hear them and sometimes they sounded like bullets" (White & White, 1987, p. 225). Donna Williams (1992) said that she sometimes needed people to repeat a particular sentence several times because she heard the message in bits. She stated that her mind segments sentences into words, leaving her with a strange and sometimes unintelligible message. She described it as, a "bit like when someone plays around with the volume switch on a TV" (p. 69). In fact, she described that she would sometimes turn the sound up and down on the television, breaking up

people's voices while keeping the picture intact. This seemed to imitate the difficulty she sometimes had hearing people consistently.

Visual Sensitivities

Individuals with ASD have described several different types of visual differences, including unique interactions with colors, lighting, stimulation, or pain caused by visual stimuli, and challenges with eye contact.

Sean Barron described his intrigue with colors and the positive emotions he felt when comparing colors for hours at a time (Barron & Barron, 1992). Donna Williams (1992) said her early memories included spending hours looking at bright spots of color that made her laugh. Years later, she learned that the spots of color were air particles of reflected light, which her hypersensitivity to color and light allowed her to see.

Other individuals with ASD experienced colors quite differently. Darren White described a situation where he received a bike as a Christmas present. He explained that he could not look at the yellow color on his bike because it was too painful. Extra red was added to make the color look orange and that color "blurred upwards making it look like it was on fire" (White & White, 1987, p. 226). He also could not see blue clearly because it "looked too light and it looked like ice" (p. 227).

Many individuals report sensitivity to lights, particularly fluorescent light. A participant in Robledo et al. (2012) pointed out,

There are certain types of light I cannot tolerate—they make me nervous.

. . . If I am in a hall and it is too bright, I can't handle it, I have to put a sun hat on. Fluorescent light absolutely turns my stomach into knots. It does a trip on my nervous system. (p. 5)

Other colors and patterns have also been reported as problematic.

A common visual characteristic in ASD is a lack of eye contact (Kluth, 2009; Robledo et al., 2012). Individuals with ASD shared their perspective on lack of eye contact related to visual sensitivity:

When I concentrated on the sound, I felt my eyes and nose shutting off. I could never do everything together at the same time. That is, I could not see you and at the same time hear you. My sense of hearing was always sharper than my sight. This is the reason I never used my eyes to interact with anybody. Psychologists call it "lack of eye contact." The result was the knowledge of a fragmented world perceived through isolated sense organs. (Mukhopadhyay, 2000, p. 74)

Sometimes, eye contact literally is painful for me to achieve. This has become easier for me to achieve however with those in my life with whom I am extremely comfortable. There are certain days, though, where eye contact is not something I am able to achieve, regardless of who the person is. (Rubin, in Biklen, 2005, p. 89)

Olfactory Sensitivities

Individuals with ASD report sensitivities to smell. Some smells may be unbearable, whereas others are pleasing. Intense smells such as perfume or air fresheners may be highly distracting for individu-

als with ASD. It is important to note that many of these smells do not bother individuals without ASD. Therefore, it is critical to examine the environment for potential sensory triggers.

Other Areas of Sensitivities

Additional sensitivities that individuals with ASD report include taste, temperature, pain, vestibular system, and proprioception (Gillingham, 2000). It is critical to become aware of the particular sensitivities an individual with ASD may experience. Variables such as emotion, fatigue, and hunger can greatly affect a person's ability to regulate their sensory system.

Movement Differences

I often can't control my body and make jerky weird movements. I believe the problem is with purposeful movement. Sadly we cannot even move from one place to another when we want to. We compensate by going where a movement takes us and actually use our weird movements to get where we want to go. For example, when I want to move from one area on the keyboard to another I will jerk and have my hand land where I want it to. Movements appear as mental retardation when we can't get our bodies to follow directions. Movement disorders make it appear that we don't understand what is being asked or we are being noncompliant. (Rubin et al., 2001, p. 426)

I cannot seem to tell my right from my left although I know my right from my left. I cannot seem to find my mouth upon command. I have trouble finding where my nose is when I am asked. I find that my breath will not come when I am asked to blow or when I am asked to take a deep breath. I am unable to draw through a straw. I have trouble sticking out my tongue. I cannot seem to spit the water out when brushing my teeth. I cannot purse my lips when I want to drink out of a bottle. I don't seem to get the message to wave or to smile when I should be responding to someone or something. My autism seems to be apparent in my random use of my hands and feet. My habit of biting is a symptom of my being nonverbal and is mostly due to frustration. (Hale & Hale, 1999, p. 60)

They asked him to point at his body parts, but the boy could not do it. Not that he was ignorant of the parts of the human body, but he was unable to point and identify them in his own self. Pointing at objects was difficult too, as he pointed only at the letters on the board and could not generalize it with the other things. Then the doctors asked the other way around. They touched his legs and hands and so on. They asked him to point on the board. This he did with ease. (Mukhopadhyay, 2000, p. 26)

At times, individuals with ASD may move their bodies in ways that seem atypical to individuals without ASD. They might rock, or flap, or jump, or repeatedly touch an object. We might assume that these behaviors are communicative attempts to interact or volitional behaviors that demonstrate a diminished cognitive ability. Movement differences are the least understood characteristic of ASD. However, many researchers (Leary

& Donnellan, 2012; Torres et al., 2013) indicate that our understanding of these movement differences will not only help us better support individuals with ASD but will also play a significant role in objectively measuring and standardizing ASD—its treatment and the tracking of an individual's changes over time.

Donnellan et al. (2006) have defined a movement difference as a difference, interference, or shift in the efficient, effective utilization and integration of movement; a disruption in the organization and regulation of perception, action, posture, language, speech, thought, emotion, and/or memory. Movement differences are manifested in a wide range of behaviors, including the more easily identifiable activities such as unusual gait and posture, constant physical movement, or repetitive rocking. Other movement differences tend to become evident at transition points:

- Starting—difficulty initiating
- Executing—difficulty with the rate, rhythm, target, and so on of movement
- Continuing—difficulty staying on track, not taking alternative paths, and so forth
- Stopping—difficulty terminating a movement; the tendency to perseverate; getting stuck in one sensory mode (e.g., staring into space)
- Combining—difficulty adding a sensory mode or a movement (e.g., listening to someone speak while watching his or her gestures and facial expression, doing two things at once)
- Switching—difficulty letting go of one perception or movement and initiating a new one

Many individuals without ASD also experience movement differences from time to time. However, these movement differences (e.g., intensity, duration, rhythm, rate, frequency, timing) are exacerbated in individuals with ASD, affecting their ability to communicate, relate, and function in their communities. Amos (2018) explored the experiences of individuals with ASD and their families, noting that movement differences were described in numerous ways. Some individuals described them as nonvolitional, tic-like behaviors that were outside of the individuals' control. Others described them as volitional, stress-relieving, and calming movements. Finally, individuals also described them as self-discovered accommodations that allowed them to function more effectively across environments. Individuals also noted the variable performance of movement differences, noting peaks and valleys in performance. For example, parents noted frustration when it appeared their child has mastered a skill only to see it not performed consistently. Individuals with ASD and their parents also noted that movements were often complex and effortful, meaning that automatic movements were difficult for many, leading to delayed habituation. Amos (2018) stressed that the path of true support for those who experience sensory and movement differences must involve mutually explored personal accommodations developed within the context of supportive relationships.

Learning Differences

I think in pictures. Words are like a second language to me. I translate both spoken and written words into full-color movies, complete with sounds, which run like a VCR tape in my head. When somebody speaks to me, his words are instantly translated into pictures. (Grandin, 1995, p. 19)

All the previous described characteristics of ASD can affect an individual's ability to learn. Many individuals with ASD report experiencing learning challenges similar to those with learning disabilities, such as difficulty with input, organization, memory, generalization, and output (Kluth, 2009). Many individuals excel at tasks involving concrete thinking and have more difficulty with abstract thinking, awareness, and judgment. It is critical to remember that lack of cognitive ability might not be the area of challenge. Rather, an individual may not be performing academically due to other challenges of ASD, such as sensory sensitivities, movement differences, or communication skills.

Individuals with ASD also have learning strengths, including precocious and highly developed decoding and word recognition. In addition, many display advanced skill when memorizing chunks of language, including songs; have excellent mathematical skills; or can write beautiful poetry.

Passions, Interests, and Rituals

People with autism like routines, and if those routines are broken it does not mean that we don't understand what is happening it just means that it is harder for us than most to stop our brains from spinning off into their regular patterns. (Rubin, in Biklen, 2005, p. 88)

Intense passions, fascinations, and restricted interests are a key feature of

ASD (Kluth, 2009). Some may have only a few interests over their life, while for others, interests are more variable. The most common topics of fascination across individuals with ASD are trains, cars, transportation systems, machines, weather, natural disasters, geography, animals, drawings, music, pop stars, and television shows (Hippler & Klicpera, 2004; Mercier et al., 2000).

Strict adherence to specific rituals is common in individuals with ASD. These might involve how objects, space, and time are arranged or organized or may involve repetitive types of behavior. Passions, restricted interests, and rituals clearly serve a specific purpose for individuals with ASD. As such, it is critical to understand the role these play in their lives.

FOUNDATIONAL SUPPORTS

Individuals with ASD can be successful in any and every environment. The following section highlights some foundational strategies and supports to support individuals with ASD. Although there are numerous methodologies and packaged programs available to support individuals with ASD, this section focuses on foundational supports that should be involved in every interaction and intervention.

Inclusion and Collaborative Teaming

Inclusion supports and benefits all learners. It stresses interdependence and independence, views all students as capable and complex, values a sense of community, and promotes civil rights and equity (Doyle, 2008; Kluth, 2010; Sapon-Shevin, 2007; Udvari-Solner, 1997). For individu-

als with ASD, access to the least restrictive environments will help them learn and grow. Opportunities to practice and learn from typically developing peers are invaluable for individuals with ASD. Supporting them requires a collaborative team approach. Professionals, parents, peers, and the individuals themselves should all be on the same page when designing supports across the life span.

Relationships and Belonging

Developing, maintaining, and facilitating relationships and belonging are critical for building community for individuals with ASD. Relationships with parents, therapists, teachers, peers, and others should guide all supports for individuals with ASD. When they feel they are in a safe, supportive, and trusting relationship, learning and growth occur. Collaboration and connection with families and other individuals with ASD are key—they are the true experts in ASD.

Social Communication Supports

As many individuals with ASD struggle to communicate and interact socially, communication and social support must be at the forefront of any intervention. It is critical to take the perspective of the individual with ASD and focus on what communication and social skills are important and meaningful to his or her life. Fitting students with ASD into packaged communication or social skills programs does not take into account their individual variability. Our challenge is to determine what supports and strategies work best for each individual with ASD. It is a difficult yet fruitful task.

Sensory and Movement Supports

Understanding each individual's unique sensory system and patterns of movement is critical for truly offering personalized supports and accommodations. This requires that you get to know the individuals you work with by listening and observing. As you become more familiar with and build a relationship with each individual, you can partner as a team to discover the best accommodations, modifications, and adaptations to fit the individual needs of the person you support.

Positive Behavior Supports

It is important to remember that individuals with ASD are trying their best to behave appropriately. Often what looks on the surface like a problem behavior is actually a manifestation of a sensory or movement problem, physical discomfort, inability to communicate effectively, or inability to understand what is being asked and perform the required task (Kluth, 2010). Be sure you spend ample time teaching and reinforcing desired behaviors. When trouble does arise, use strategies that are respectful and promote learning and growth. Behavioral support should not be about control; rather, it should be about collaboratively teaming up to support dreams.

Learning and Environmental Supports

By understanding the many characteristics of ASD, you can help create environments and supports that will enable individuals with ASD to function effectively. Think about the sensory systems of the individuals with ASD whom you support—what types of sensory sensitivities do they have and in what ways can they be accommodated in the environment? Individuals with ASD often report that they learn best when materials are presented clearly and visually. Active learning that provides visuals, examples, manipulatives, and interaction will be most successful. Do not forget to use your most valuable resource: the individuals with ASD. Elicit their perspective on ways they might prefer to receive support. Be creative and flexible in all supports.

CONCLUSION

This chapter presents a general overview of ASD, including definitions, characteristics, and foundational supports. Effective support requires true understanding of each and every individual that you work with. As SLPAs, your growth in understanding will come from working with, listening to, and knowing individuals with ASD in your daily practice.

REFERENCES

American Psychiatric Association. (2013). *Diagnostic and statistical manual of mental disorders* (5th ed.).

Amos, P. (2018). Seeing movement: Implications of the movement sensing perspective for parents. In E. Torres & C. Whyatt (Eds.), *Autism: The movement-sensing perspective* (pp. 295–326). CRC Press.

Baron-Cohen, S. (1989). The autistic child's theory of mind: A case of specific developmental delay. *Journal of Child Psychology and Psychiatry, 30*, 285–297. https://doi.org/10.1111/j.1469-7610.1989.tb00241.x

Barron, J., & Barron, S. (1992). *There's a boy in here.* Simon & Schuster.

Bellini, S. (2006). Social challenges of children and youth with autism spectrum disorders. In E. Boutot & B. Myles (Eds.), *Autism spectrum disorders: Foundations, characteristics, and effective strategies* (pp. 201–222). Pearson.

Bellini, S. (2008). *Building social relationships: A systematic approach to teaching social interaction skills to children and adolescents with autism spectrum disorders and other social difficulties.* Autism Asperger Publishing.

Biklen, D. (2005). *Autism and the myth of the personal one.* New York University Press.

Blackman, L. (1999). *Lucy's story: Autism and other adventures.* Book in Hand.

Blanc, M. (2012). *Natural language acquisition on the autism spectrum: The journey form echolalia to self-generated language.* Communication Development Center.

Bopp, K., Brown, K., & Mirenda, P. (2004). Speech-language pathologists' roles in the delivery of positive behavior support for individuals with developmental disabilities. *American Journal of Speech-Language Pathology, 13,* 5–19. https://doi.org/10.1044/1058-0360(2004/003)

Brady, N. (2000). Improved comprehension of object names following voice output communication aid use: Two case studies. *Augmentative and Alternative Communication, 16,* 197–204. https://doi.org/10.1080/074346100 12331279054

Brien, A., & Prelock, P. (2021). Language and communication in ASD: Implication for intervention. In P. Prelock & R. McCauley (Eds.), *Treatment of autism spectrum disorder: Evidence-based intervention strategies for communication & social interactions* (2nd ed., pp. 51–80). Brookes.

Brown, J., & Whiten, A. (2000). Imitation, theory of mind and related activities in autism: An observational study of spontaneous behavior in everyday contexts. *Autism: The International Journal of Research and Practice, 4,* 185–205. https://doi.org/10.1177/136236130000400 2006

Centers for Disease Control and Prevention. (2021). *Prevalence and characteristics of autism spectrum disorder among children aged 8 years—Autism and developmental disabilities monitoring network, 11 sites, United States, 2018.* https://www.cdc.gov/mmwr/volumes/70/ss/ss7011 a1.htm

Donnellan, A., Leary, M., & Robledo, J. (2006). I can't get started: Stress and the role of movement differences for individuals with the autism label. In G. Baron, J. Groden, G. Groden, & L. Lipsitt (Eds.), *Stress and coping in autism* (pp. 205–245). Oxford University Press.

Doyle, M. (2008). *The paraprofessional's guide to the inclusive classroom: Working as a team* (3rd ed.). Brookes.

Flavell, J., Miller, P., & Miller, S. (1993). *Cognitive development* (3rd ed.). Prentice-Hall.

Gebauer, L., Skewes, J., Horlyck, L., & Vuust, P. (2014). Atypical perception of affective prosody in autism spectrum disorder. *NeuroImage: Clinical, 6,* 370–378. https://doi.org/10.1016/j .nicl.2014.08.025

Gillingham, G. (2000). *Autism: A new understanding!* Tacit.

Grandin, T. (1992). An inside view of autism. In E. Schopler & G. B. Mesibov (Eds.), *High functioning individuals with autism* (pp. 105–126). Plenum.

Grandin, T. (1995). *Thinking in pictures: And other reports from my life with autism.* Doubleday.

Grandin, T., & Scariano, M. (1986). *Emergence: Labeled autistic.* Arena.

Hale, M., & Hale, C. (1999). *I had no means to shout!* 1st Books.

Hall, L. (2009). *Autism spectrum disorders: From theory to practice.* Pearson.

Heflin, L., & Alaimo, D. (2007). *Students with autism spectrum disorder: Effective instructional practices.* Pearson.

Hippler, K., & Klicpera, C. (2004). A retrospective analysis of the clinical case records of "autistic psychopaths" diagnosed by Hans Asperger and his team at the University Children's Hospital, Vienna. In U. Frith & E. Hill (Eds.), *Autism: Mind and brain* (pp. 21–42). Oxford University Press.

Kanner, L. (1943). Autistic disturbances of affective contact. *Nervous Child, 2,* 217–230.

Kluth, P. (2009). *The autism checklist: A practical reference for parents and teachers.* Jossey-Bass.

Kluth, P. (2010). *'You're going to love this kid!' Teaching students with autism in the inclusive classroom* (2nd ed.). Brookes.

Knoblauch, B., & Sorenson, B. (1998). *IDEA's definition of disabilities.* ERIC Digest. ERIC Clearinghouse on Disabilities and Gifted Education.

Koegel, R., & Koegel, L. (1995). *Teaching children with autism: Strategies for initiating positive* interactions and improving learning opportunities. Brookes.

Kolarik, J. (2016). In their own words: Stories from CIP. In M. P. McManmom (Author), *Autism and learning differences: An active learning teaching toolkit* (pp. 455–482). Jessica Kingsley.

Leary, M. R., & Donnellan, A. M. (2012). *Autism: Sensory-movement differences and diversity.* Cambridge Book Review Press.

McDonnell, J. (1993). *News from the border.* Ticknor & Fields.

McKean, T. (1994). *Soon will come the light.* Future Horizons.

Mercier, C., Mottron, L., & Belleville, S. (2000). Psychosocial study on restricted interest in high-functioning persons with pervasive developmental disorders. *Autism, 4*, 406–425. https://doi.org/10.1177/1362361300004004006

Millar, D. (2000). Effects of AAC on the natural speech development of individuals with autism spectrum disorders. In P. Mirenda & T. Iacono (Eds.), *Autism spectrum disorders and AAC* (pp. 171–192). Brookes.

Miller, E., Schuler, A., & Yates, G. (2008). Social challenges and supports from the perspective of individuals with Asperger syndrome and other autism spectrum disabilities. *Autism, 12*(2), 173–190. https://doi.org/10.1177/1362361307086664

Mirenda, P. (2003). Toward functional augmentative and alternative communication: A research review. *Augmentative and Alternative Communication, 16*, 141–151. https://doi.org/10.1044/0161-1461(2003/017)

Mukhopadhyay, T. R. (2000). *Beyond the silence.* National Autistic Society.

Noens, I., & van Berckelaer-Onnes, I. (2005). Captured by details: Sense-making, language and communication in autism. *Journal of Communication Disorders, 38*, 123–141. https://doi.org/10.1016/j.jcomdis.2004.06.002

O'Neil, J. (1999). *Through the eyes of aliens: A book about autistic people.* Jessica Kingsley.

Paul, R., & Sutherland, D. (2005). Enhancing early language in children with autism spectrum disorder. In F. Volkmar, R. Paul, A. Klin, & D. Cohen (Eds.), *Handbook of autism and pervasive developmental disorders* (3rd ed., pp. 925–945). John Wiley.

Prizant, B., & Rydell, P. (1993). Assessment and intervention strategies for unconventional verbal behavior. In J. Reichle & D. Wacker (Eds.), *Communication approaches to challenging behavior: Integrating functional assessment and intervention strategies* (pp. 263–297). Brookes.

Resnick, L., Levine, J., & Teasley, S. (1991). *Perspectives on socially shared cognition.* American Psychological Association.

Robinson, J. (2007). *Look me in the eye: My life with Asperger's.* Crown.

Robledo, J., Strandt-Conroy, K., & Donnellan, A. (2012). An exploration of sensory and movement differences from the perspective of individuals with autism. *Frontiers in Integrative Neuroscience, 6*, 1–13. https://doi.org/10.3389/fnint.2012.00107

Rogers, S. (2000). Interventions that facilitate socialization in children in autism. *Journal of Autism and Developmental Disabilities, 30*, 399–409. https://doi.org/10.1023/A:1005543321840

Rubin, S., Biklen, D., Kasa-Hendrickson, K., Kluth, P., Cardinal, D., & Broderick, A. (2001). Independence, participation, and the meaning of intellectual ability. *Disability and Society, 16*, 425–429. https://doi.org/10.1080/09687590120045969

Sapon-Shevin, M. (2007). *Widening the circle: The power of inclusive classrooms.* Beacon.

Scheuermann, B., & Webber, J. (2002). *Autism: Teaching does make a difference.* Wadsworth/Thomson Learning.

Sinclair, J. (1993). Don't mourn for us. *Our Voice, 1*(3). http://ani.autistics.org/don't_mourn.html

Stiegler, L. (2015). Examining the echolalia literature: Where do speech-language pathologists stand? *American Journal of Speech-Language Pathology, 24*(4), 750–762. https://doi.org/10.1044/2015_AJSLP-14-0166

Therrien, M., Light, J., & Pope, L. (2016). Systematic review of the effects of interventions to promote peer interactions for children who use aided AAC. *Augmentative and Alternative Communication, 32*(2), 81–93. https://doi.org/10.3109/07434618.2016.1146331

Torres, E., Brincker, M., Isenhower, R., Yanovich, P., Stigler, K., Numbereger, J., . . . Jose, J. (2013). Autism: The micro-movement perspective. *Frontiers in Integrative Neuroscience, 7*, 1–26. https://doi.org/10.3389/fnint.2013.00032

Travis, L., Sigman, M., & Ruskin, E. (2001). Links between social understanding and social behavior in verbally able children with autism. *Journal of Autism and Developmental Disorders, 31*, 119–130. https://doi.org/10.1023/A:1010705912731

Udvari-Solner, A. (1997). Inclusive education. In C. Grant & G. Ladson-Billings (Eds.), *Dictionary of multicultural education* (pp. 141–144). Oryx.

Walker, V., & Snell, M. (2013). Effects of augmentative and alternative communication onchallenging behavior: A meta-analysis. *Augmentative and Alternative Communication*, *29*(2), 117–131. https://doi.org/10.3109/07434618.2013.785020

Waterhouse, L., Fein, D., & Modahl, C. (1996). Neurofunctional mechanisms in autism. *Psychological Review*, *103*, 457–489. https://doi.org/10.1037/0033-295X.103.3.457

Wegner, J. (2021). Augmentative and alternative communication strategies: Manual signs, picture communication, and speech-generating devices. In P. Prelock & R. McCauley (Eds.), *Treatment of autism spectrum disorder: Evidence-based intervention strategies for communication & social interactions* (2nd ed., pp. 81–107). Brookes.

White, G. B., & White, M. S. (1987). Autism from the inside. *Medical Hypothesis*, *24*, 223–229. https://doi.org/10.1016/0306-9877(87)90068-5

Williams, D. (1992). *Nobody nowhere*. Avon.

Williams, D. (1994). *Somebody somewhere*. Times Books.

CHAPTER 18

Augmentative and Alternative Communication

Margaret Vento-Wilson

*Just as a dance couldn't possibly be a dance unless people moved
to it, so language doesn't become communication until people
grow to express it back. It has to be a two-way exchange.*

—Staehely (2000, p. 1)

The position statement of the American Speech-Language-Hearing Association (ASHA) asserts, "Communication is the essence of human life and that all people have the right to communicate to the fullest extent possible" (ASHA, 2001, Position Statement, para. 2). For people who are unable to use natural speech to meet their daily communicative needs, this directive presents greater challenges and increased complexity than for those for whom communication occurs through typical development and modalities. Approximately .03% to 1.3% of the U.S. population experiences temporary or permanent challenges in the production and/or comprehension of spoken, written, or signed language (ASHA, n.d.-a; Beukelman & Light, 2020). These percentages translate into a conservative estimate of two million individuals (ASHA, n.d.-a; Sigafoos et al., 2013). Fortunately, through the effective intervention of trained professionals, including speech-language pathology assistants (SLPAs), at least some of the resulting communication barriers may be mitigated through the use of assistive technology (AT) or augmentative and alternative communication (AAC; ASHA, n.d.-a, 2022).

Research conducted by ASHA in 2016 revealed that 45% of speech-language pathologists (SLPs) surveyed provided services to individuals with AAC needs, with the occurrence being slightly higher in hospitals than in school settings. In health care settings, SLPs surveyed reported that 66% of referrals received were for patients who were likely AAC candidates, with the majority of these referrals being from pediatric hospitals (ASHA, 2002). Further, in a recent analysis of caseload distribution in hospitals, SLPs reported spending approximately 3% of their clinical, adult-focused service time with clients using AAC and approximately 6% of their clinical, pediatric-focused service time with children in AAC (ASHA, 2017). In the school setting, between the years 2000 and 2016, the percentage of school-based SLPs with nonverbal students or students using AAC ranged between 48% and 62% (ASHA, 2016). Given the high level of need these figures represent, it is very likely that as an SLPA, you will encounter individuals with AAC needs in your employment and training settings.

As an SLPA, you will be expected to be knowledgeable and competent in AAC concepts and implementation practices. As discussed in Chapter 1, in the area of service delivery, ASHA specifically states that, provided training, supervision, and planning as appropriate, working with individuals who need or use AAC is within an SLPA's scope of practice (ASHA, 2022). The following list provides a general description of the potential roles of an SLPA in AAC intervention (ASHA, 2022; Beukelman et al., 2008):

- Support multimodality intervention
- Prepare low-tech materials
- Integrate low-and high-tech materials into developmental, restorative, or compensatory intervention
- Instruct communication partners in AAC use
- Maintain AAC technology
- Serve as a liaison between AAC commercial companies and related AAC personnel

This chapter provides an overview of AAC concepts and practices. While this topic may initially seem daunting, as you read about and become more familiar with AAC, you may find that this challenging topic offers an opportunity for you to grow as an SLPA and that AAC intervention can, and often does, have a profound effect on the lives of your clients. The journey you are undertaking by reading this chapter parallels the journey your clients undertake, whether they come to you as toddlers with *complex communication needs* (CCNs) or as adults who have had an abrupt or gradual, but nonetheless devastating, loss of speech and language. With the appropriate guidance and support, they too will evolve from novice AAC users into experienced AAC users, with the ability to maintain and develop relationships and remain relevant and involved with their world (Light et al., 2002). Augmentative and alternative communication offers your clients the opportunity to more fully experience that quintessential tool of language, "which is so tightly woven into human experience that it is scarcely possible to imagine life without it" (Pinker, 1994, p. 17).

ASSISTIVE TECHNOLOGY

Assistive technology (AT) can be defined broadly as an item, piece of equipment, or system used as a means to preserve, enhance, or improve the functional capabilities of an individual (Bugaj & Norton-Darr, 2010). However, its primary role is to increase the independence of individuals across their worlds. Examples of AT include the use of eyeglasses, hearing aids, enlarged handles on kitchen utensils, walkers, wheelchairs, and Braille codes on elevator buttons ("What is Assistive Technology," Assistivetechrsl, 2013). Other examples of AT that many people are familiar with today are the use of speech-to-text and the use of reminders on smartphones. Specific to communication, AT can include the use of a broad range of AAC devices or systems (Parette & Sherer, 2004).

AUGMENTATIVE AND ALTERNATIVE COMMUNICATION

The term *AAC* is defined as a system that can be used to temporarily or permanently compensate for the impairments and activity and participation limitations and restrictions of individuals with severe expressive or receptive difficulties with speech, language, or communication (ASHA, n.d.-a; Branson & Demchak, 2009; Davidoff, 2017). Augmentative and alternative communication is also defined as a dynamic, multimodal communication continuum that evolves based on a user's growth and development, the situation, and the communication partner. Its ultimate purpose is to minimize barriers to successful communication and increase communicative competence (Barker et al., 2013; Blackstone et al., 2007; Calculator & Black, 2009). Before delving further into a discussion of AAC, it is essential to understand the distinctions among the terms *speech*, *language*, and *communication*.

Speech is the individual sounds and sound patterns of any given language. It is a vocal production that is comprehended auditorily. Language is symbolic and is used to covey messages through a rule-governed system, which involves syntax, semantics, phonology, morphology, and pragmatics. Language can occur independently of speech, as with American Sign Language (ASL; Figure 18–1), to communicate, either in addition to or instead of spoken language. Communication is the act of conveying a message that establishes a shared understanding between the message sender and the message receiver. Communication can occur without speech or language, such as when two people who speak different languages use gestures or pictures to ask or answer a question. For people with impairments in the production or comprehension of speech, language, or communication, AAC offers the opportunity to create intelligible and comprehensible messages through a combination of symbols and then to use those symbols with their communication partners in multiple settings and circumstances (ASHA, n.d.-a; Barker et al., 2013; Blackstone et al., 2007; Calculator & Black, 2009).

Foundational AAC Concepts

In 2007, Blackstone, Williams, and Wilkins published six principles specific to AAC research and practice. The list reflects extensive collaborative work among AAC users and their families, practitioners, researchers, faculty from universities, policy makers, and AAC developers and manufacturers. The list can be seen in Table 18–1 (Blackstone et al., 2007, p. 192). It is beneficial to keep these principles in mind as you navigate your intervention

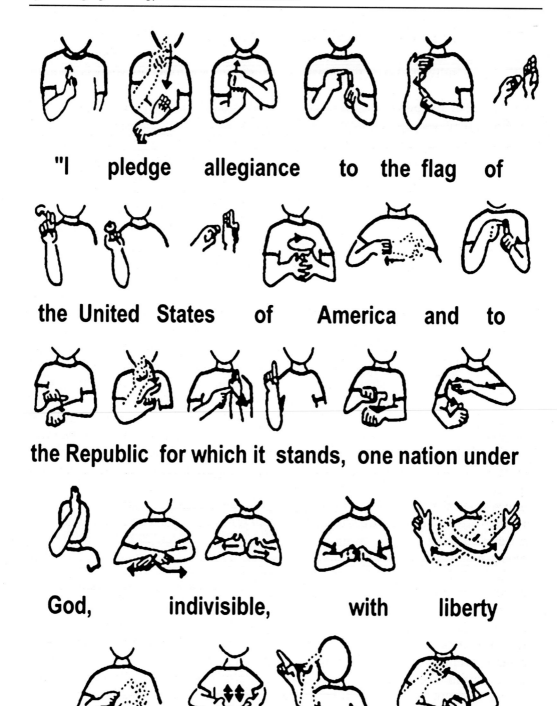

Figure 18–1. The Pledge of Allegiance in American Sign Language. Courtesy of Bing Images, free to share and use commercially.

Table 18–1. Augmentative and Alternative Communication (AAC) Principles

1. People who rely on AAC participate actively in AAC research and practice.

2. Widely accepted theoretical constructs are specifically addressed in the design and development of AAC technologies and instructional strategies.

3. AAC technologies and instructional strategies are designed to support and foster the abilities, preferences, and priorities of individuals with complex communication needs, taking into account motor, sensory, cognitive, psychological, linguistic, and behavioral skills, strengths, and challenges.

4. AAC technologies and instructional strategies are designed so as to recognize the unique roles communication partners play during interaction.

5. AAC technologies and instructional strategies enable individuals with complex communication needs to maintain, expand, and strengthen existing social networks and relationships and to fulfill societal rules.

6. AAC outcomes are realized in practical forms, such as guidelines for clinical practice, design specifications, and commercial products. The social validity of these outcomes is determined by individuals with complex communication needs, their family members, AAC manufacturers, and the broader community.

with AAC users and their families and caregivers.

A second foundational concept integral to AAC intervention is the participation model (Beukelman & Light, 2020) (Figure 18–2), which ASHA has endorsed as a valuable framework for AAC intervention. It is based on a premise of supporting individuals who use AAC in communicating, functioning, and participating in communicative contexts in the same manners as their typically developing peers of the same chronological age. The participation model requires professionals to identify barriers relating to opportunity (i.e., policy, practice, knowledge, skill, attitude) and access (i.e., natural abilities, environmental, AAC systems). Identifying these barriers has the potential to reduce their frequency and level, as well as to increase the participation of AAC users broadly and across contexts (Beukelman & Light, 2020). Further, embedded in the participation model is the idea that AAC and the people who use it are ever evolving, and practitioners must be mindful of both AAC for both today and tomorrow.

The participation model also aligns with ASHA's zero-exclusion policy for AAC services (Brady et al., 2016) and the World Health Organization's (WHO, 2014) International Classification of Functioning (ICF; Figure 18–3), which considers disability as an expected outcome of human diversity. Both of these models reflect the pivotal distinction made between *impairment* and *disability* by the social model of disability (Goering, 2015). In this framework, impairment is conceived of as a bodily state that is nonstandardized, whereas disability is conceived of as disadvantages or participation restrictions caused by disabling characteristics of society—such as the inclusion of ramps versus stairs in a building (Goering, 2015).

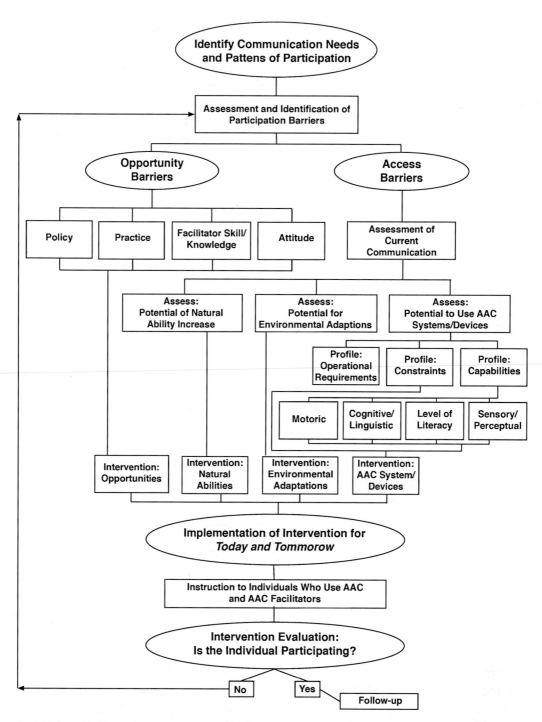

Figure 18–2. The participation model for augmentative and alternative communication (AAC).

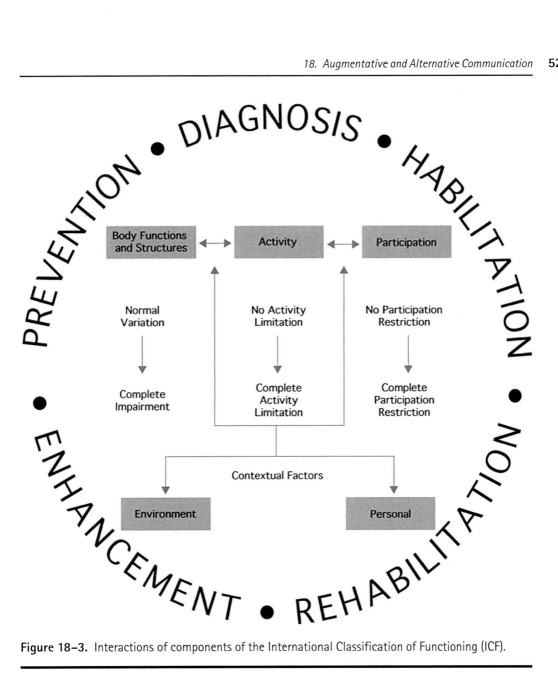

Figure 18–3. Interactions of components of the International Classification of Functioning (ICF).

AAC Users

AAC users are a heterogeneous group of individuals, whose only shared links are the need to replace or enhance their use of natural speech or their ability to comprehend spoken or written language (ASHA, n.d.-a; Blackstone et al., 2009; Davidoff, 2017). An additional factor that contributes to the need for AAC is challenging communicative behavior that (a) is unacceptable in society, (b) involves the use of unusual or reflexive movement, (c) fatigues the user, (d) is so unconventional or idiosyncratic that only familiar communicators can interpret them, (e) is inefficient, or (f) is potentially harmful to the user (ASHA, n.d.-a). Conditions that can cause or contribute to the use of AAC can be congenital or acquired. A nonexhaustive list of these conditions can be found in Table 18–2. When working with individuals who use AAC, it is vital to keep in mind that these impairments do not necessarily signify a concomitant cognitive impairment (Fried-Oken et al., 2012). As Chapter 4 recommends, practitioners should view all individuals as unique in their needs, preferences, and abilities.

Purpose of AAC Intervention

When working with individuals who rely on AAC, it is important to be mindful of the primary purpose of AAC intervention, which extends significantly beyond the directive to find a technical solution to communication problems (Light & McNaughton, 2012). Augmentative and alternative communication intervention involves language organization, strategies, and techniques, as well as the emotional and social issues that surround receptive and expressive language impairments (Cress, 2004). The broadly stated and humanistic purpose of AAC intervention is to enable people to engage efficiently and effectively with others in a variety of situations and contexts of their choice. It allows users to participate in conversations at home and in their communities, learn their native language, and initiate and maintain relationships (Light et al., 2002). According to Light (1988) and Beukelman and Light (2020), the purposes of communicative interaction are:

- Communication of wants and needs
- Information transfer
- Social closeness
- Social etiquette
- Communication with oneself or engagement in inner dialogue

In order to fully accomplish these goals and support communicative inter-

Table 18–2. Common Congenital and Acquired Impairments That May Benefit From Augmentative and Alternative Communication (AAC)

Congenital Impairments	Acquired Impairments
Autism spectrum disorder (ASD)	Acquired apraxia of speech (AOS)
Cerebral palsy (CP)	Amyotrophic lateral sclerosis (ALS)
Childhood apraxia of speech (CAS)	Aphasia
Intellectual disability (ID)	Cancer
Deaf/blind	Cerebral vascular accident (CVA)
	Dysarthria
	Locked-in syndrome
	Multiple sclerosis (MS)
	Primary progressive aphasia (PPA)
	Traumatic brain injury (TBI)

Sources: ASHA, n.d.-a; Beukelman & Light, 2022; Hux et al., 2008.

action, AAC intervention needs to incorporate not just the AAC user but must also consider and integrate family members and other communicative partners —AAC cannot be taught or used in isolation (Cress, 2004).

Myths About AAC Use

One of the basic theoretical underpinnings of AAC is that all individuals have the right to communicate, regardless of the method and regardless of a perceived ability to communicate. Although the effectiveness of AAC has been demonstrated through an extensive body of literature (ASHA, n.d.-a; Beukelman & Light, 2020; Light & McNaughton, 2012), there is a high level of misunderstanding about its assessment and intervention among related professionals, family members, and even users themselves. Table 18–3 identifies some of the more commonly encountered myths and provides research-based data that dispel them and offers support for the use of appropriate AAC assessment and intervention. Although this table highlights many of the myths regarding AAC use, various researchers have suggested that a minimal level of speech comprehension and the ability to use distal gestures, such as pointing, may be suggestive of greater success in AAC use (ASHA, n.d.-a). For individuals with a congenitally based impairment, it is never too early to introduce AAC into comprehensive communication and language intervention (Cress & Marvin, 2003; Romski & Sevcik, 2005). Similarly, for individuals with an acquired impairment, early introduction of compensatory AAC strategies can support remaining verbal comprehension and expression abilities (Hux et al., 2008).

AAC Components

AAC should be thought of as an integrated communication system comprising four primary components or modes rather than a single device: symbols, aids, strategies, and techniques (ASHA, n.d.-a; Beukelman & Light, 2020).

Symbols

Symbols can be graphic (e.g., photographs, text), auditory (e.g., spoken words), gestural (pointing), or tactile (e.g., textures, objects) and can be unaided, such as facial gestures, or aided, such as pictures (ASHA, n.d.-a). The concept of symbols is multifaceted and can be described given their visual relationship to an actual concept (also known as iconicity), their level of stability or transience, and their acquisition hierarchy (ASHA, n.d.-a; Beukelman & Light, 2020).

Iconicity can be thought of as how guessable the symbol is, without assistance (ASHA, n.d.-a). Symbol iconicity ranges from transparent, where the symbol demonstrates a clear relationship to the concept (e.g., a drawing of a house that represents home; Figure 18–4A), to opaque, where the symbol does not demonstrate a clear relationship to the concept without an established meaning (e.g., the ASL sign for home; Figure 18–4B) (Drager & Light, 2010).

Symbol stability refers to how dynamic or static a symbol is. Spoken symbols (i.e., words) and manual signs are very dynamic and transient, whereas graphic symbols are considered static or permanent (Beukelman & Light, 2020). Symbols that are more static and permanent place lower cognitive demands on both the sender and the receiver than do dynamic or transient symbols. Dynamic

Table 18–3. Common Myths and Truths About Augmentative and Alternative Communication (AAC)

Myth	Truth
There are prerequisite skills, cognition levels, and communicative abilities required for AAC assessment and intervention.	Although language and cognition are interrelated, it remains unclear which force drives the other, and without a method of communication, cognition cannot be demonstrated or assessed definitively.
	AAC access has been demonstrated to support the early cognitive and linguistic skills necessary for the development of language.
There is a minimum age for AAC assessment and intervention.	The earliest AAC intervention can apply to a child's behaviors, gestures, cooperative actions, and sounds.
	AAC use benefits infants and toddlers, based on evidence suggesting that a child's early learning experiences in the first 3 years of life are foundational to subsequent brain development.
Language acquisition follows a symbolic representational hierarchy that flows from objects to written words.	During the early phases of language development, symbol type (i.e., iconic or abstract) may not be a significant factor in intervention since, ultimately, all symbols function similarly.
AAC use will interfere with a child's speech or vocal development.	AAC use does not impede vocalizations or oral language. AAC has been shown to encourage vocalizations and oral language by increasing communication opportunities.
	Children typically use the most efficient method of communicating, and with the inherent advantages that speech offers over AAC, children will move to speech when possible.
AAC implementation should be delayed until a consistent verbal communication delay is confirmed over time.	Communication across all modes in the early childhood years should be made available to the child.
	Delaying AAC implementation, when behaviors and physical limitations suggest a risk for impaired speech, can have a negative effect on the long-term development of speech and language.
The introduction of AAC decreases the users' need to work on speech.	Natural speech improvements often correlate with the introduction of AAC.
	AAC users typically use multiple communication modes, including technology, gestures, and natural speech.
Speech, regardless of how limited it is, should be the primary mode of communication.	Children and adults who are left without a reliable means to communicate even their basic wants and needs have the potential to demonstrate behavior problems, social failure, academic challenges, and learned helplessness.
The use of AAC makes individuals look different from their peers.	Rather than inhibiting language production, the implementation of AAC has the potential to inhibit challenging communicative behavior and build more socially acceptable behaviors.
	Ultimately, individuals look more atypical when they are unable to express themselves.
AAC use represents the last resort in speech-language intervention.	Early introduction of AAC fosters communication and language skills, and it diminishes communication failure for both beginning communicators and those with acquired disabilities.
	AAC intervention is holistic in that it addresses improving communication skills across all modes, including verbal skills.

Table 18–3. *continued*

Myth	Truth
AAC, if unsuccessful, can be considered a failure after the implementation of only a limited set of AAC strategies or techniques.	Because AAC is a continuum that may involve a variety of strategies and support levels, multiple attempts may be necessary to find the right combination of strategies, aids, support, and techniques.

Sources: ASHA, n.d.-a; Augmentative and Alternative Communication Connecting Young Kids (YAACK), n.d.; Beukelman & Light, 2020; Beukelman et al., 2007; Branson & Demchak, 2009; Cress & Marvin, 2003; Light & Drager, 2007; National Scientific Council on the Developing Child, 2007; Romski & Sevcik, 2005.

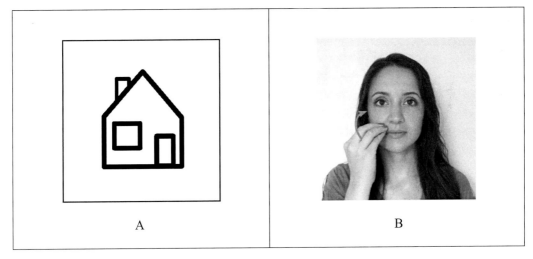

A   B

Figure 18–4. Example of transparent versus opaque symbol iconicity. **A.** Black and white icon of home. Boardmaker. Copyright 2018. Tobii Dynavox, Pittsburgh, PA. All rights reserved. Used with permission. **B.** American Sign Language (ASL) sign for home.

symbols require sustained attention, memory, and sequencing abilities, which can sometimes exceed developing or preserved skills (Fager et al., 2006).

As to acquisition hierarchy, symbols can be arranged in order, given their visual relationship to the actual concept, progressing from real objects (i.e., realia) to a signed representation of a concept (e.g., ASL; ASHA, 2004). Symbols that are more concrete, such as a juice box representing juice, are considered easier to comprehend than more abstract representa-

tions, such as the signed Amerind symbol for more (Figure 18–5; Fried-Oken et al., 2012). Abstract symbols typically require training to use and understand. Box 18–1 contains a generally accepted symbol hierarchy with respect to ease of acquisition, starting with more easily acquired symbols (i.e., objects) and progressing to symbols requiring more effort to acquire (i.e., traditional orthography). Research conducted on symbol use for people with acquired communication impairments suggests that including contextually rich

Box 18–1. Symbol Acquisition Hierarchy

1. Objects
2. Color photographs
3. Black and white photographs
4. Miniature objects
5. Black and white line drawings
6. Blissymbols
7. Traditional orthography

Source: Beukelman & Light, 2020.

---

photographs (Figure 18–6) may lead to more successful expressive and receptive symbol use (Fried-Oken et al., 2012).

On AAC systems, symbols can be arranged in multiple ways, such as alphabet-based methods that use traditional spelling as a means of generating messages. A second way that symbols can be arranged is through single-meaning message generation, where a single graphic icon represents a single word or message, such as when touching an image with a school indicates it is time to go to school. A final method of symbol arrangement is the use of semantic compaction, which is based on iconic encoding with multiple meanings. This concept will be explained more fully in the discussion of vocabulary arrangement (ASHA, n.d.-a).

Aids

Aids, or devices, are used to convey or receive the actual message, such as switch-activated devices or a series of symbols that convey meaning (ASHA, n.d.-a). Augmentative and alternative communication aids can be either aided or unaided, although most AAC users employ multiple communication modalities that incorporate both aided and unaided systems (ASHA, n.d.-a).

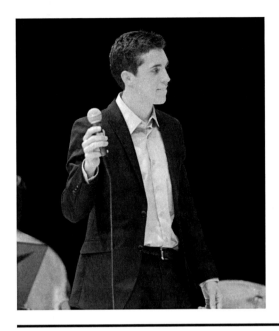

Figure 18–6. Example of a contextually rich photograph.

Unaided Communication. Unaided communication methods involve solely the individual's body (Beukelman & Light, 2020). Unaided communication methods offer an efficient communication method without the need for external devices. Successful unaided communication requires a shared understanding between communication partners of the meaning or situational context represented by a nod, gesture, vocalization, or symbol. This makes communication with unfamiliar partners more difficult, unless the communicative act is transparent or guessable enough to establish a clear meaning. Box 18–2 lists examples of unaided communication. Unaided communication strategies require at least a minimal level of motoric ability. Typical users include people with dysarthria or people who have experienced a stroke or a traumatic brain injury, who are able at least partially to use their preserved cognitive, linguistic, visual, and motoric abilities to convey their messages (ASHA, n.d.-a; Beukelman & Mirenda, 2013).

Aided Communication. Aided communication methods involve the use of tools, equipment, or devices in addition to an individual's body (ASHA, n.d.-a). Aided AAC systems offer increased message length, complexity, speed, and comprehensibility to the communication partner. Aided communication strategies also

> **Box 18–2. Examples of Unaided Communication**
>
> - Speech
> - Eye movements
> - Head nods
> - Gestures
> - Vocalizations
> - Sign language
> - Facial expressions

require at least a minimal level of motoric ability and cognition. It is important to note that there is an inverse relationship between AAC system complexity and the complexity of an individual's communication needs. There is also a direct relationship between reliance on an interlocutor, or communication partner, and the complexity of an individual's communication needs, as seen in Figure 18–7. People with a variety of disorders (e.g., aphasia, apraxia of speech, amyotrophic lateral sclerosis) who are able to use preserved cognitive, linguistic, visual, or motoric abilities to communicate are typical users of aided AAC (Beukelman & Light, 2020).

The class of aided systems can be further broken down into the categories of low-tech and high-tech (Loncke, 2014). Low-tech AAC systems are typically handmade and not computer based. Box 18–3 lists examples of low-tech, aided communication and Appendices 18–A to 18–D describe some of them.

An additional set of aided low-tech communication devices are those that use an electronic component but are limited in their output (Loncke, 2014). Examples of these include:

- Tactile communicators (Appendix 18–E)
- Switch and button communicators (Appendix 18–F)

High-tech AAC systems typically contain microcomputer chips and can be dedicated solely to AAC use or can be a program or app on a nondedicated mobile device or a computer (Beukelman & Light, 2020). They might offer message retrieval and storage, stored or synthetic speech, prediction features, and complex vocabulary (Beukelman & Light, 2020). A significant benefit of AAC systems with speech-generating devices, or voice output, is their ability to enhance communicative interaction between people (Cress

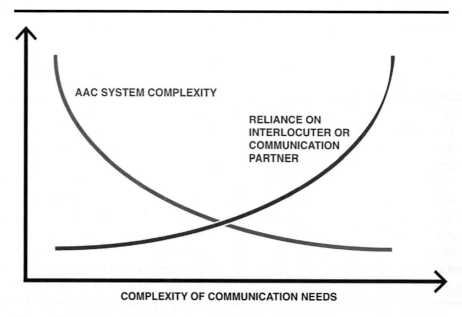

Figure 18–7. Factors influencing augmentative and alternative communication (AAC) intervention and use.

> ## Box 18–3. Examples of Low-Tech Aided Communication
>
> - Paper and pencil (e.g., for use in writing and drawing)
> - Communication books (Appendix 18–A)
> - Eye-gaze boards (Appendix 18–B)
> - Alphabet boards (Appendix 18–C)
> - Choice boards (Appendix 18–D)
> - Real objects
> - Remnant books (e.g., movie tickets, concert programs, menus from recent life events)

& Marvin, 2003). Voice output can be accomplished through stored speech, also called digitized speech, which is similar to a tape recording, and synthesized speech, which is computer generated. The quality of synthesized speech varies based on the system utilized. Stephen Hawking, the British physicist, was probably the most well-known user of a synthetic voice (Figure 18–8). Although Hawking was British, his voice used an American accent, and in 2006 Hawking stated, "I have kept it [the voice] because I have not heard a voice I like better and because I have identified with it" (Sandle, 2018).

AAC users identify the voice quality of AAC systems as being highly important and consider them extensions of the self. Improvements in this technology can have a profound impact on overall quality of life (Mills et al., 2014). Although options for speech output remain limited, recent advances in synthesized speech include voice conversion (Mills et al., 2014), which works by extracting data from a speech corpus and generating a unique synthetic

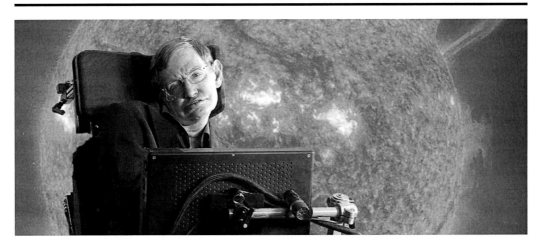

Figure 18–8. Stephen Hawking with his High-Tech Augmentative and Alternative Communication (AAC) system. Courtesy of Bing Images, free to share and use commercially.

voice for each individual. Although still a relatively new technology, as voice conversion techniques continue to develop, there will be more and better choices for AAC users that can produce natural-sounding and intelligible speech. Typically, AAC systems offer a narrow selection of prestored voices, which can be customized by altering loudness, rate, and pitch. Some synthesized voices are very intelligible listeners and others can be robot-like, requiring careful listening. An example of digitized speech is when a classmate or peer prerecords a short phrase (e.g., "Let's go to recess") with an AAC device, which can then be selected and played by the AAC user in a communicative context. Recent advances in technology also allow AAC users, such as those diagnosed with a progressive disease (e.g., amyotrophic lateral sclerosis, multiple sclerosis), to preserve samples of their speech within a computer system to be retrieved at a later date, when they are no longer able to use their natural speech to meet their communicative needs (Mills et al., 2014). VOCALiD is an organization that works to support voice personalization to AAC users through technology (VOCALiD, n.d.). Box 18–4 lists examples of high-tech, aided communication that you can find samples of in Appendices 18–G to 18–J. These are but a few examples of the many high-tech communication devices available to AAC users. As you grow in your skills and experience with AAC, you will no doubt learn about many more options.

Strategies

Because AAC users typically communicate at a fraction of the rate of natural speakers (2 to 15 words per minute versus 200 words per minute), *strategies*, which are used to improve and refine messages and increase the rate of communication, are of high value to AAC users and their communication partners (ASHA, n.d.-a; Beukelman & Light, 2020). Strategies can be used across aided and unaided communication and low- and high-tech devices and may decrease the cognitive and motoric demands on users. Although a complete review of all available strategies is beyond the scope of this chapter, Table 18–4 lists a few examples. Additional methods of refining and improving messages and enhancing the rate of communication are topic identification and partner-focused questions (Beukelman & Light, 2020).

Techniques

Techniques are either direct or indirect selection methods available to users of AAC communication to transmit the mes-

---

Box 18–4. Examples of High–Tech Aided Communication Devices

- Speech-generating devices (SGDs) and voice output communication aids (VOCAs) (Appendix 18–G)
- Text-to-speech devices (Appendix 18–H)
- Computers, iPads, and tablets, with software or apps for communication purposes (Appendices 18–I and 18–J)

Table 18–4. Examples of Augmentative and Alternative Communication Strategies

Strategy	Definition	Example
Encoding	The use of prestored, shortened code to represent a longer message	The use of the letters GG to represent the phrase "Please get my glasses."
Prediction	A dynamic interaction between the AAC user and the AAC device or communication partner that allows for prediction of the balance of a partially formulated message at the letter, word, or phrase level,	Letter: Based on rules of spelling and letter patterns. Word: Based on context and rules of syntax. Phrase: Based on context and topic and sophisticated computer algorithms that incorporate natural language constructs.
Sequencing	When using symbols to communicate and moving beyond the single-symbol level, symbols can be combined to create spontaneous, novel utterances.	An example of a sequenced phrase can be seen in Figure 18–9.

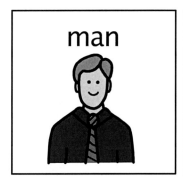 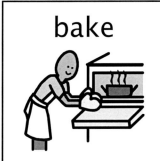 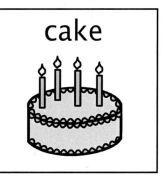

Figure 18–9. Example of symbol sequencing. Boardmaker. Copyright 2018. Tobii Dynavox, Pittsburgh, PA. All rights reserved. Used with permission.

sage itself (ASHA, n.d.-a; Beukelman & Light, 2020).

Direct selection involves an interaction between the motoric abilities of the AAC user and the manual, mechanical, or technological options offered by the communication device. It can be low-tech or high-tech, and allows users to make a direct communication choice via voice, a body part, such as a hand or the head, or some form of technical aid, such as a light pointer, adapted mouse, or a switch. Examples of direct selection techniques are highlighted in Box 18–5 (Beukelman & Light, 2020).

Recent advances in computer technology allow an additional method of direct selection using the eyes, referred to as eye tracking. High-tech devices can track the movements of the eye and register a location on the screen where an AAC user gazes. If the user holds her or his gaze in that position or blinks, the system registers that as a selection (e.g., activation of a symbol on the screen; Fager et al., 2012).

Box 18–5. Examples of Direct Selection Methods

- Eye-gaze
- Physical contact
    - Manual touch or pressure on keyboard or switch
- Pointing (no contact)
- Voice recognition activation

For those individuals without sufficient motoric abilities to make direct selections, *indirect selections* compensate for these limitations. With indirect selection, also called scanning, users make a communication choice through intermediary steps facilitated by their communication partner or the device (Beukelman & Light, 2020). To use indirect selection, the AAC user may make a selection from a series of symbols. For example, symbols can be presented auditorily, as when a communication partner calls out individual letters of the alphabet and waits for confirmation or rejection of a specific letter choice. Symbols can also be presented visually, as when a communication partner points to symbols on a communication board or when a high-tech system highlights a symbol by changing its background color, placing a dark outline around the symbol, and so forth. The AAC user selects a desired symbol using some form of physical confirmation to the listener, such as a head nod or eye-blink, or a tap of the finger, wrist, or head on a switch (Appendix 18–F), which then triggers the AAC device. The speed and timing of the auditory or visual scanning can be individualized to reflect the cognitive, linguistic, visual, auditory, and motoric abilities of the user.

AAC Intervention Guidelines

AAC intervention occurs within the context of a team of stakeholders that includes the AAC users and their families (ASHA, n.d.-a). In addition to you and your supervising SLP, this team of allied professionals can also include general and special education teachers, physical therapists, occupational therapists, and rehabilitation engineers (Beukelman & Light, 2020). As with all other speech-language intervention, AAC intervention revolves around the individualized goals written by an SLP. For your reference, Chapter 7 contains sample AAC objectives. Augmentative and alternative communication intervention looks much like other speech-language intervention except that input and output can be mediated through alternative means, such as vocalizations, signs, objects, or a low- or high-tech device. Best practices suggest focusing on the goal of the intervention rather than modality of production. One of the basic premises of AAC intervention, which mirrors a basic premise of all speech-language intervention, is that it should be functional, take place in naturalistic contexts and situations (Beck et al., 2009), and be led by the AAC user's interests, innate curiosities, actions, and behaviors (Cress & Marvin, 2003; Hourcade et al., 2004; Romski & Sevcik, 2005).

Best practices suggest that the practitioner overlay targeted language or provide a model with natural speech in parallel with symbol manipulation or referencing (Beck et al., 2009; Dada & Alant, 2009). This method of evidence-based intervention, called *augmented input strategies* and *aided language modeling*, has the potential to enhance expressive and receptive language skills. Modeling language allows users to learn, restore, and use language.

An example of this method is when a clinician points to an icon for baby and crib and comments to the child, "Oh look, the baby is sleeping," or when working with adults, asking an individual, "How many grandchildren do you have?" while pointing to icons representing 2 and 3 (Figure 18–10; Beck et al., 2009). When implementing AAC intervention with adults who have cognitive or communication impairments and may have difficulty with symbolic representation (e.g., aphasia), augmented input strategies increase the likelihood of symbol comprehension and communication.

The dynamic aspect of AAC means that users may need to use multiple AAC systems, based on their audience and communication partners. For example, individuals may use vocalizations and signs with familiar communication partners (i.e., at home) and may use a picture-based system with unfamiliar communication partners (i.e., community

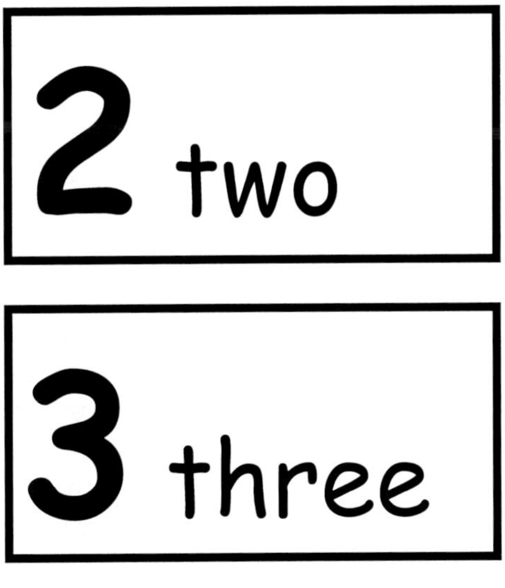

Figure 18–10. Boardmaker choice icons. Boardmaker. Copyright 2018. Tobii Dynavox, Pittsburgh, PA. All rights reserved. Used with permission.

members; ASHA, 2010). Similarly, because AAC is dynamic and multimodal, modifications to the AAC system will likely be needed over the course of intervention. These modifications can involve all components of the AAC system, such as the symbols used and the strategies and techniques employed. For children developing their speech, language, and communication abilities, the AAC components may increase in complexity and the messages increase in length. For adults with acquired conditions, modifications may be required due to speech, language, and communication improvements or due to diminishing capabilities that may accompany degenerative conditions (Beukelman & Ball, 2002).

As discussed in greater detail in Chapter 5, individuals' cultural experiences and background also influence intervention. While much of the research on AAC use has focused on Anglo-European culture, ideals, and values, SLPAs must be aware of the values, ideals, and considerations of other cultures, ethnicities, and languages (ASHA, n.d.-b; Beukelman & Light, 2020) as cultural norms have a significant effect on the implicit and explicit rules of communication and language (Soto, 2012). The concepts of collectivism, cooperation, interdependency, family hierarchies, respect, politeness, and levels of directness within the communication cycle vary across cultures, social communities, customs, and languages and must be considered by SLPAs involved in the implementation of AAC systems. Best practices in AAC implementation allow users to codeswitch, which means to adjust the content and complexity of their communication based on their communication partner/partners, whether they be peers, family members, or health care or educational professionals

(ASHA, n.d.-a). Additional factors to consider include user and family attitudes toward technology and the possible stigmatization of disabilities, rehabilitation services, and education (ASHA, n.d.-a; Beukelman & Light, 2020; Parette & Scherer, 2004). These factors should be carefully considered, especially given the fact that stigmatization is closely associated with abandonment of AT (Parette & Scherer, 2004).

Lastly, vocabulary selection and organization play a key role in AAC intervention. It is generally accepted that both adults and children who rely on AAC benefit when a meaningful, functional, individualized, and motivating vocabulary is available to them. Vocabulary selection is an ongoing process and is typically accomplished with the participation of AAC users and people significant to them, including family, friends, and related professionals such as SLPAs. Assessing vocabulary needs can involve ecological inventories or questionnaires (Fallon et al., 2001), communication diaries, and standardized vocabulary lists (Beukelman & Light, 2020; Van Tatenhove, 2009). Vocabulary selections may depend on where the vocabulary is being used (e.g., home vs. school), age, gender, disease progression, stage of language development, and literacy level (Beukelman & Light, 2020).

Once established, the vocabulary should be broken down into the categories of core and fringe vocabulary for purposes of organization with the AAC device. Core vocabulary refers to words or messages that are highly functional, occur frequently across individuals, and relate to basic functional needs and social exchanges. Fringe vocabulary refers to words or messages that are specific to an individual or context (Beukelman & Light, 2020; Van Tatenhove, 2009). Another perspective on vocabulary types is that core vocabulary comprises a small number of words with broad utility across contexts and fringe vocabulary is composed of a large number of words with specific but limited utility across contexts. As mentioned earlier, it is important to consider individual factors when creating a vocabulary for AAC users. Two significant factors are the individuals' level of language of development and literacy (Davidoff, 2017). Table 18–5 contains examples of core vocabulary for toddlers and adults, although it is not exhaustive. Just as individuals who use AAC to communicate present with unique profiles, their vocabularies too should be individualized.

Once the vocabulary has been defined, it must be organized physically and linguistically to promote efficient and effective communication. Whether creating a communication book or installing software, the vocabulary must be organized based on users' cognitive, com-

Table 18–5. Examples of Core Vocabulary for Toddlers and Adults

Toddler	Adult
All done	Go
Different	Eat
Help	Yes
Mine	No
More	Stop
Not/don't	Home
Stop	Restroom
That	
What	

Sources: Glennen & DeCoste, 1997; Van Tatenhove, 2007.

municative, and motoric abilities; their communication partners' knowledge and experience level; the communicative context; and frequency of use (Beukelman & Light, 2020). Vocabulary can be organized by semantic categories (e.g., people, locations, actions, activities) and syntax (e.g., parts of speech). Box 18–6 (Van Tatenhove, 2007) contains some basic tenants for vocabulary organization.

Helpful Tips

Chapter 5 includes tips for communicating with individuals with disabilities. These recommendations are applicable to AAC users as well. In addition, it is important to keep in mind that AAC users expend a considerable amount of energy and cognitive resources on communication, and they must adapt their communicative choices based on their available resources (Fried-Oken et al., 2012). Best practices suggest the following (Accessible Technology Coalition, 2011):

- Face the person.
- Treat AAC users with the same manners and level of respect you use with others.
- Speak directly to the AAC user; never talk about them with someone else when they are present.
- Communication with the use of AAC takes additional time and energy—allow the AAC user time to compose and communicate their message.
- Do not limit your questions to a simple yes/no format.
- Do not be afraid to ask for clarification.
- Always ask permission to provide assistance or touch their AAC device.
- Be patient when experiencing technological glitches.
- Avoid condescension.
- Remember at all times that a person's silence does not necessarily reflect their desire to communicate.

Box 18–6. Vocabulary Organization

- Place core vocabulary with broad language functions in prominent positions that can be accessed quickly and easily, and place extended vocabulary in secondary positions that may be accessed through multiple steps or on subsequent pages.
- Words or phrases that regulate activities or behaviors (e.g., more, again, help, all gone, all done) should hold prominent positions.
- Words used to comment and relate to others (e.g., fun, good, bad, like) can hold secondary positions.
- The words *yes* and *no* do not need to be in prominent positions if the user has an alternative and reliable method to communicate these ideas.

SUMMARY

We end by reflecting on the words used in the introduction. Having read this chapter, you are now more familiar with the challenges and complexities of AAC. But you are now also more familiar with the ways AAC supports communicative competence, self-expression, and individual agency. While you may still conceive of yourself as a novice in the world of AAC, you have a theoretical foundation from which to approach your work with individuals who rely on AAC. Over time, this theoretical foundation will develop into sound clinical judgment and practice. After that, it is up to you to bridge any remaining gaps that stand between you and the individuals you serve. And I wish you the best of luck in this very important work.

REFERENCES

Accessible Technology Coalition. (2011). *Etiquette in communicating with AAC users.* http://www.access-to-justice.org/pdfs/5_Etiquette_tips.pdf

American Speech-Language-Hearing Association. (n.d.-a). *Augmentative and alternative communication.* http://www.asha.org/Practice-Portal/Professional- Issues/Augmentative-and-Alternative-Communication/

American Speech-Language-Hearing Association. (n.d.-b). *Cultural competence.* https://www.asha.org/Practice-Portal/Professional-Issues/Cultural-Competence//

American Speech-Language-Hearing Association. (n.d.-c.). *International Classification of Functioning, Disability, and Health* (ICF). https://www.asha.org/slp/icf/

American Speech-Language-Hearing Association. (2001). *Scope of practice in speech-language pathology.* Author.

American Speech-Language-Hearing Association. (2002). *2002 Omnibus survey caseload report: SLP.* Author.

American Speech-Language-Hearing Association. (2004). *Roles and responsibilities of speech-language pathologists with respect to augmentative and alternative communication: technical report* [Technical report]. http://www.asha.org/policy

American Speech-Language-Hearing Association. (2010). *Communication services and supports for individuals with severe disabilities: FAQs.* http://www.asha.org/uploadedFiles/Communication-ServicesSevere-Disabilities.pdf

American Speech-Language-Hearing Association. (2016). *Schools survey report: SLP caseload characteristics trends 1995–2016.* https://www.asha.org/uploadedFiles/2016-Schools-SurveySLP-Caseload-Characteristics-Trends.pdf

American Speech-Language-Hearing Association. (2017). *SLP health care survey report: Caseload characteristics and trends 2005–2017.* https://www.asha.org/uploadedFiles/2017-SLP-Health-Care-Survey-Caseload-Characteristics-and-Trends-2005–2017.pdf

American Speech-Language-Hearing Association. (2022). *Speech-language pathology assistant scope of practice* [Scope of practice]. www.asha.org/policy

Assistivetechrsl. (2013). *What is assistive technology (A.T.).* [Video]. Youtube. https://www.youtube.com/watch?v=SIm2MuJUCTE

Augmentative and Alternative Communication (AAC) for Connecting Young Kids (YAACK). (n.d.). *Does AAC impede natural speech?—And other fears.* https://communicationmatrix.org/uploads/5346/YAACK%20posting%20AAC%20does%20not%20im peded%20speech.pdf

Barker, R. M., Akapa, S., Brady, N. C., & Thiemann-Bourque, K. (2013). Support for AAC use in preschool, and growth in language skills, for young children with developmental disabilities. *Augmentative and Alternative Communication, 29*(4), 334–346. https://doi.org/10.3109/07434618.2013.848933

Beck, A. R., Stoner, J. B., & Dennis, M. L. (2009). An investigation of aided language stimulation: Does it increase AAC use with adults with developmental disabilities and complex communication needs? *Augmentative and Alternative Communication, 25*(1), 42–54. https://doi.org/10.1080/07434610802131059

Beukelman, D. R., & Ball, L. J. (2002). Improving AAC use for persons with acquired neurogenic disorders: Understanding human and engineering factors. *Assistive Technology, 14,*

33–44. https://doi.org/10.1080.10400435.2002.10132053

Beukelman, D. R., Ball, L. J., & Fager, S. (2008). An AAC personnel framework: Adults with acquired complex communication needs. *Augmentative and Alternative Communications, 24*(3), 255–267. https://doi.org/10.1080/07434610802388477

Beukelman, D. R., Fager, S., Ball, L., & Dietz, A. (2007). AAC for adults with acquired neurological conditions: A review. *Augmentative and Alternative Communications, 23*(3), 230–242. https://doi.org/10.1080/07434610701553668

Beukelman, D. R., & Light, J. L. (2020). *Augmentative and alternative communication: Supporting children and adults with complex communication needs.* Paul H. Brookes.

Blackstone S., Williams M., & Wilkins D. (2007). Key principles underlying research and practice in AAC. *Augmentative and Alternative Communication, 23*(3), 191–203. https://doi.org/10.1080/07434610701553684

Brady, N., Bruce, S., Goldman, A., Erickson, K., Mineo, B., Ogletree, B., . . . Wilkinson, K. (2016). Communication services and supports for individuals with severe disabilities: Guidance for assessment and intervention. *American Journal on Intellectual and Developmental Disabilities, 121*, 121–138. https://doi.org/10.1352/1944-7558-121.2.121

Branson, D., & Demchak, M. (2009). The use of augmentative and alternative communication methods with infants and toddlers with disabilities: A research review. *Augmentative and Alternative Communications, 25*(4), 274–286. https://doi.org/10.3109/07434610903384529

Bugaj, C. R., & Norton-Darr, S. (2010). *The practical and fun guide to assistive technology in public schools: Building or improving your district's AT team.* International Society for Technology in Education.

Calculator, S. N., & Black, T. (2009). Validation of an inventory of best practices in the provision of augmentative and alternative communication services to students with severe disabilities in general education classrooms. *American Journal of Speech-Language* Pathology, *18*, 329–342. https://doi.org/10.1044/1058-0360(2009/08-0065)

Cress, C. J. (2004). Augmentative and alternative communication and language: Understanding and responding to parent's perspectives. *Topics in Language Disorders, 24*(1), 51–61.

Cress, C. J. & Marvin, C. (2003). Common questions about AAC services in early intervention. *Augmentative and Alternative Communication, 19*(4), 254–272. https://doi.org/10.1080/07434610310001598242

Dada, S., & Alant, E. (2009). The effect of aided language stimulation on vocabulary acquisition in children with little or not functional speech. *American Journal of Speech-Language Pathology, 18*, 50–64. https://doi.org/10.1044/1058-0360(2008/07-0018)

Davidoff, B. E. (2017). AAC with energy—earlier. *The ASHA Leader, 22*, 48–53. https://doi.org/10.1044/leader.FTR2.22012017.48

Drager, K. D., & Light, J. C. (2010). A comparison of the performance of 5-year-old children with typical development using iconic encoding in AAC systems with and without icon prediction on a fixed display. *Augmentative and Alternative Communication, 26*(1), 12–20. https://pubmed.ncbi.nlm.nih.gov/20196700/

Fager, S., Bardach, L., Russell, S., & Higginbotham, J. (2012). Access to augmentative and alternative communication: New technologies and clinical decision-making. *Journal of Pediatric Rehabilitation Medicine, 5*, 53–61. https://doi.org/10.3233/PRM-2012-0196

Fager, S., Hux, K., Beukelman, D. R., & Karantounis, R. (2006). Augmentative and alternative communication use and acceptance by adults with traumatic brain injury. *Augmentative and Alternative Communications, 22*(1), 37–47. https://doi.org/10.1080/07434610500243990

Fallon, K. A., Light, J. C., & Paige, T. K. (2001). Enhancing vocabulary selection for preschoolers who require augmentative and alternative communication (AAC). *American Journal of Speech-Language Pathology, 10*(1), 81–94. https://doi.org/10.1044/1058-0360(2001/010)

Fried-Oken, M., Beukelman, D. R., & Hux, K. (2012). Current and future AAC research considerations for adults with acquired cognitive and communication impairments. *Assistive Technology, 25*, 56–66. https://doi.org/10.1080/10400435.2011.648713

Glennen, S. L., & DeCoste, D. C. (1997). *Handbook of augmentative and alternative communication.* New York, NY: Delmar Cengage Learning.

Goering, S. (2015). Rethinking disability: The social model of disability and chronic disease. *Current Reviews in Musculoskeletal Medicine, 8*, 134–138. https://doi.org/10.1007/s12178-015-9273-z

Hourcade, J., Everhart Pilotte, T., West, E., & Parette, P. (2004). A history of augmentative and alternative communication for individuals with severe and profound disabilities. *Focus on Autism and Other Developmental Disabilities, 19*(4), 235–244. https://doi.org/10.1177/1088 3576040190040501

Hux, K., Weissling, K., & Wallace, S. (2008). Communication-based interventions: Augmentative and alternative communication for people with aphasia. In R. Chapey (Ed.), *Language intervention strategies in aphasia and related neurogenic communication disorders* (pp. 813–836). Lippincott Williams & Wilkins.

Light, J. (1988). Interaction involving individuals using augmentative and alternative communication systems: State of the art and future directions. *Augmentative and Alternative Communication, 4*(2), 66–82. https://doi.org/10.10 80/07434618812331274657

Light, J. C., & Drager, K. (2007). AAC technologies for young children with complex communication needs: State of the science and future research directions. *Augmentative and Alternative Communication, 23*(3), 204–216. https://doi.org/10.1080/07434610701553635

Light, J., & McNaughton, D. (2012). The changing face of augmentative and alternative communication: Past, present, and future challenges. *Augmentative and Alternative Communication, 28*(4), 197–204. https://doi.org/10.3109/0743 4618.2012.737024

Light, J. C., Parsons, A. R., & Drager, K. D. R. (2002). "There's more to life than cookies": Developing interactions for social closeness with beginning communicators who require augmentative and alternative communication. In J. Reichle, D. Beukelman, & J. Light (Eds.), *Exemplary practices for beginning communicators: Implications for AAC* (pp. 187–218). Paul H. Brookes.

Loncke, F. (2014). *Augmentative and alternative communication: Models and applications for educators, speech-language pathologists, psychologists, caregivers, and users.* Plural Publishing.

Mills, T., Bunnell, H. T., & Patel, R. (2014). Toward personalized speech synthesis for augmentative and alternative communication. *Augmentative and Alternative Communication, 30*(3), 226–236. https://doi.org/10.3109/07434618. 2014.924026

National Scientific Council on the Developing Child. (2007). *The timing and quality of early experiences combine to shape brain architecture: Working paper No. 5.* http://developingchild .harvard.edu

Parette, P., & Sherer, M. (2004). Assistive technology use and stigma. *Education and Training in Developmental Disabilities, 39*(3), 271–226.

Pinker, S. (1994). *The language instinct.* William Morris and Company.

Romski, M., & Sevcik, R. A. (2005). Augmentative communication and early intervention: Myths and realities. *Infants & Young Children, 18*(3), 174–185. https://doi.org/10.1097/0000 1163-200507000-0002

Sandle, P. (2018, March 14). Stephen Hawking's voice was his trademark. *Reuters.* https:// www.reuters.com/article/peo ple-hawking-voice/stephen-hawkings-voicewas-his-trade mark-idUSL8N1QW6U2

Sigafoos, J., Schlosser, R. W., & Sutherland, D. (2013). Augmentative and alternative communication. In J. H. Stone & M. Blouin (Eds.), *International encyclopedia of rehabilitation.* https://www.researchgate.net/profile/ David_Beukelman2/publication/230852920_ Augmentative_and_Alternative_Communi cation/links/54871c4d0cf268d28f070dbc/ Augmentative-and-Alternative-Communica tion.pdf

Soto, G. (2012). Training partners in AAC in culturally diverse families. *Perspectives on AAC and Alternative Communication, 21*(4), 144–150. https://doi.org/10.1044/aac21.4.144

Staehely, J. (2000). Prologue: The communication dance. In M. Fried-Oken & H. A. Bersani Jr. (Eds.), *Speaking up and spelling it out: Personal essays on augmentative and alternative communication* (pp. 1–12). Paul H. Brookes.

Van Tatenhove, G. M. (2007). *Normal language development, generative language & AAC.* http:// www.texasat.net/Assets/1--normal-language-- aac.pdf

Van Tatenhove, G. (2009). Building language competence with students using AAC devices: Six challenges. *Perspectives on Augmentative and Alternative Communication, 18*(2), 38–47.

VOCALiD. (n.d.). *VOCALiD.* https://vocalid.ai/

World Health Organization. (2014). *International Classification of Functioning, Disability and Health.* http://www.who.int/classifications/icf/en/

Wu, Y. & Voda, J. A. (1985). User-friendly communication board for nonverbal, severely physically disabled individuals. *Archives of Physical Medicine & Rehabilitation, 66*, 827–828.

APPENDIX 18–A
Example of Communication Book

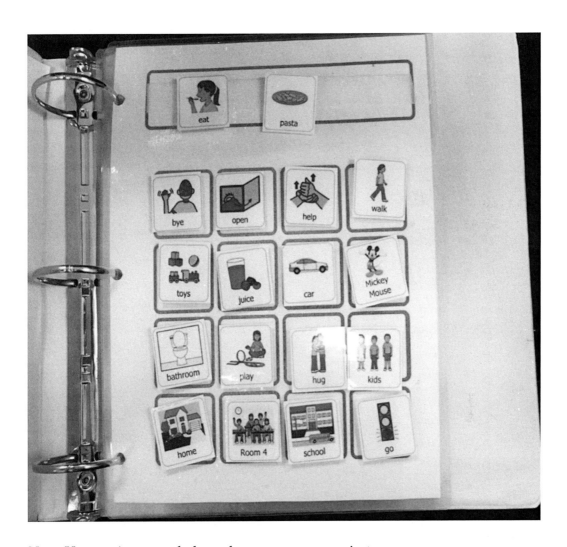

Note. Users point to symbols on the page to communicate.

APPENDIX 18–B
Example of Eye–Gaze Board

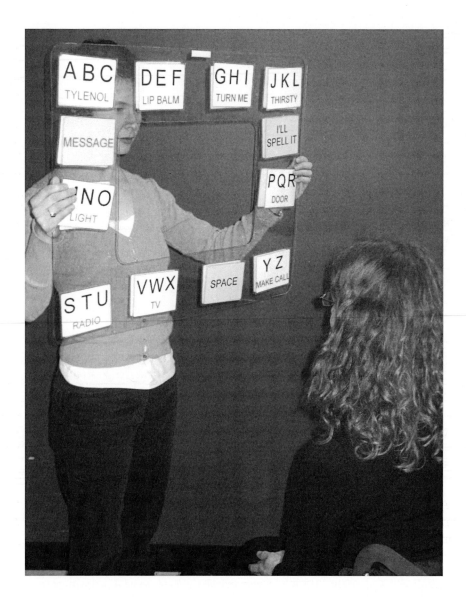

Note. The eye-gaze board is held up between the AAC user and the communication partner. The communication partner places his or her face within the boundaries of the hole in the center of the board and locks gaze with the AAC user before posing a question. The AAC user indicates his or her communication choice by gazing at the desired box and the communication partner confirms the choice verbally.

Source: Courtesy of Bing Images, free to share and use commercially.

APPENDIX 18-C
Example of Alphabet Boards

Traditional Alphabet Board

A	B	C	D	E	F
G	H	I	J	K	L
M	N	O	P	Q	R
S	T	U	V	W	X
Y	Z				
0	1	2	3	4	5
6	7	8	9		

Vowel-Based Alphabet Board (Wu & Voda, 1985)

A	B	C	D		
E	F	G	H		
I	J	K	L	M	N
O	P	Q	R	S	T
U	V	W	X	Y	Z

Note. AAC users communicate messages via alphabet boards by pointing to each letter to form words and phrases or by indicating their choice of auditorily presented letters with an agreed-upon method (e.g., blinking, finger raising, nodding).

APPENDIX 18–D
Example of Choice Board

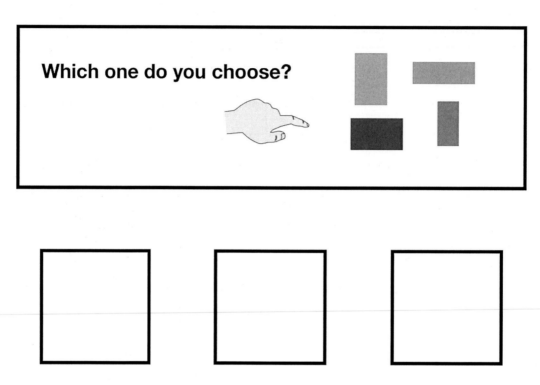

Note. Blank boxes can contain words or visual icons representing items or activities; users indicate a specific choice by pointing to a box(es).

APPENDIX 18–E
Totally Tactile Communicator

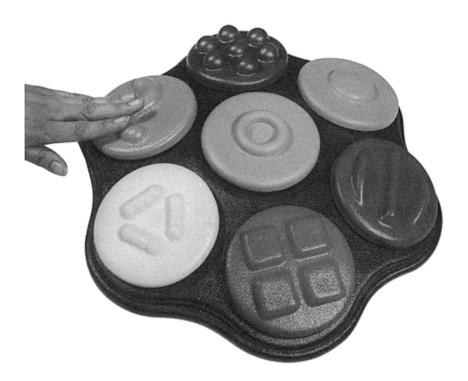

Note. Designed especially for visually impaired users, this communicator features brightly colored plates with raised designs and adjustable activation time (1–12 seconds) that gives users time to feel the plates (i.e., pre-recorded message choices) before activating their message. Features six levels for a total of 36 messages and a total record time of 300 seconds, 7 seconds per message.

Source: Totally Tactile Communicator. Enabling Devices, Hawthrone, NY. Used with express permission: Information available at http://www.enablingdevices.com

APPENDIX 18–F
Example of Switch Communicator
(Big–Talk Triple–Play Sequencer)

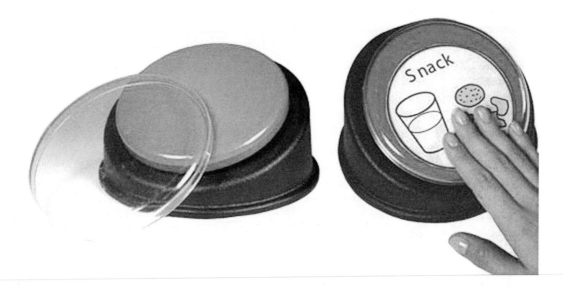

Note. A message is recorded using digitized speech (i.e., recorded human speech). AAC users press a button to play a message in a communicative context. Can also be used as a switch, when attached with a wire to a switch-enabled device. Switch-enabled devices systematically present options to AAC users. When the desired option is highlighted, pressing the switch activates a corresponding symbol on the switch-enabled system. This process is also known as scanning.

Source: Enabling Devices, Hawthorne, NY. Used with express permission. Information available at http://www.enablingdevices.com

APPENDIX 18–G
Speech Generating Device: *GoTalk Express 32*

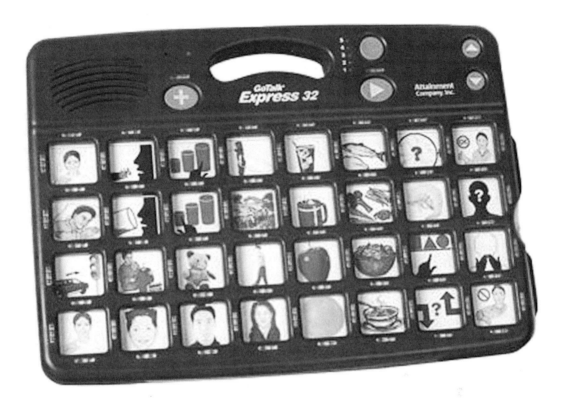

Note. Users select an icon that makes the system play a pre-recorded message (also known as digitized speech).

Source: GoTalk Express 32. Attainment Company, Verona, WI. Used with express permission. Information can be found at http://www.attainmentcompany.com/gotalk-express-32

APPENDIX 18–H
Text–to–Speech Device: *LightwriterSL50TM*

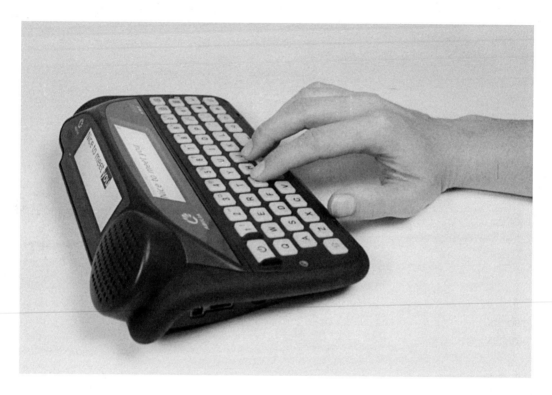

Note. Users type words and the device converts written text into voice output.

Source: LightwriterSL50-Connect. Copyright. Abilia Ltd., Cambridge, England. Used with permission.

APPENDIX 18–1
Visual Scene Display: *Speaking Dynamically Pro* Software

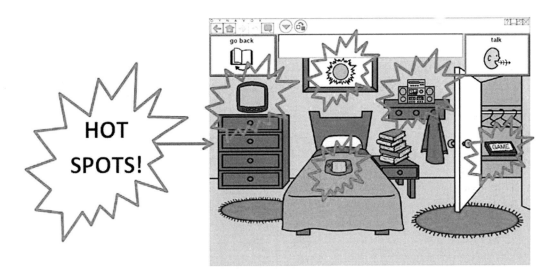

Note. The user selects a "hot spot," and the software is programmed to speak out an associated phrase, such as "T.V." or "I want to play a game," using either digitized or synthesized speech.

Source: Boardmaker. Copyright 2018, Tobii Dynavox, Pittsburgh, PA. All rights reserved. Used with permission.

APPENDIX 18–J
Words For Life Application on an iPad Tablet

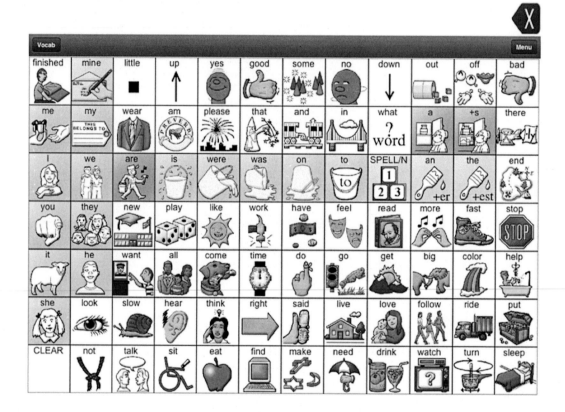

Note. User generates voice output by selecting icon(s).

CHAPTER 19

Adults With Acquired Neurologic Disorders

Jennifer A. Ostergren and Carley B. Crandall

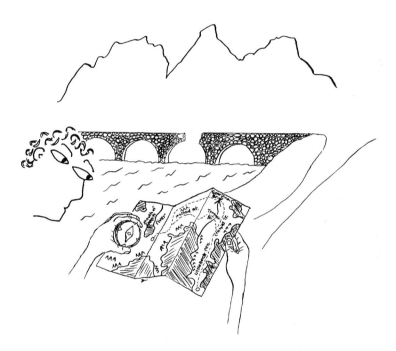

The brain is more than an assemblage of autonomous modules, each crucial for a specific mental function. Every one of these functionally specialized areas must interact with dozens or hundreds of others, their total integration creating something like a vastly complicated orchestra with thousands of instruments, an orchestra that conducts itself, with an ever-changing score and repertoire.

—Oliver Sacks

The topic of this chapter is acquired neurologic disorders and specifically those that occur in adults. This chapter will first cover some foundational knowledge, including important terms and definitions and a general description of the brain and its functions. Key principles helpful to understanding the settings where services are provided for adults with neurologic disorders are discussed. This is followed by a discussion of the nature, scope, and general treatment principles of several common acquired neurologic disorders in adults.

It is important to first highlight that this chapter is by no means exhaustive in providing the critical information you need to effectively serve as a speech-language pathologist assistant (SLPA) for adults with acquired neurologic disorders (and their families). An entire textbook could be written on that topic alone, and there are many such books available. Rather, this chapter serves as a review and reminder of several key principles. Your training as an SLPA has likely been more limited in this topic area, due in part to the very broad scope of the speech-language pathology field. It is impossible to cover every possible disorder, population, and setting where SLPAs are present within the limited scope of training required of SLPAs. In addition, SLPAs are less likely to provide services to adults with neurologic disorders in medical settings than they are to provide services to children in school settings. This is due to differences in the nature and scope of services for adults and also the fee structures and billing options available in each setting.

This chapter is devoted only to adults with acquired neurologic disorders. This is not because children do not acquire neurologic disorders. To the contrary, children also experience acquired neurologic disorders, but the research evidence for children and adults in this area is distinctly different. In children, neurologic disorders impact a developing brain that is acquiring language, cognitive, and motor skill, whereas in adults, acquired neurologic disorders impact language, cognitive, and motor skills that have

already developed. As such, the impacts, outcomes, and intervention approaches are different between adults and children with acquired neurologic disorders. If you are working with a child with an acquired neurologic disorder, you should seek assistance from your supervising speech-language pathologist (SLP) as to the nature of the specific disorder, its impacts, and best practices for intervention. Do not assume that the details discussed in this chapter, specific to adults, are transferable to children, as that is likely not the case given the reasons already stated above.

FOUNDATIONAL KNOWLEDGE

Neurologic disorders are "diseases of the brain, spine and the nerves that connect them. There are more than 600 diseases of the nervous system, such as brain tumors, epilepsy, Parkinson's disease, and stroke as well as less familiar ones such as frontotemporal dementia" (University of California San Francisco [UCSF] Health, n.d., Neurological Disorders, para. 1). Often diseases of this nature are also described using the related terms *neurogenic* (originating in nervous tissue) or *neurological* (of or relating to neurology). Neurologic disorders in adults can be parsed into three categories: developmental (also called congenital), progressive, and acquired (Toronto Acquired Brain Injury Network, 2005). This chapter focuses on the latter, acquired neurologic disorders. Box 19–1 contains a brief description of each type of neurologic disorder.

As might be expected given the essential function of the brain to all human behavior, neurologic disorders can cause a wide range of impairments to physical, cognitive, and psychological functioning

Box 19–1. Categories of Neurologic Disorders

Developmental or Congenital Neurologic Disorders

A neurologic disorder that an individual is born with, such as cerebral palsy, muscular dystrophy, and autism.

Progressive Neurologic Disorders

A neurologic disease with a continuous gradual deterioration of brain function, such as dementia, Alzheimer's disease, and Parkinson's disease.

Acquired Neurologic Disorders

A neurologic disorder resulting from damage to the brain that occurs after birth and is neither developmental nor progressive. Acquired neurologic disorders, also known as acquired brain injury (ABI), encompass both traumatic and nontraumatic brain injuries (Teasdale et al., 2017). Traumatic ABI (sometimes referred to as traumatic brain injury, TBI) occurs as a result of an external force on the brain, such as with a car accident, fall, assault, or sports-related injury. Nontraumatic ABI is damage or alteration in brain function caused by an internal force (Brain Injury Association of America [BIAA], 2012), which means due to a medical problem or disease such as stroke, brain tumor, and/or infection. Table 19–1 lists additional examples of acquired brain injuries.

Table 19–1. Examples of Acquired Brain Injury (Traumatic and Non-Traumatic)

Traumatic Brain Injury Causes	Non-Traumatic Brain Injury Causes
• Falls	• Strokes (Hemorrhage, Blood Clot)
• Assaults	• Infectious Disease (Meningitis, Encephalitis)
• Motor Vehicle Accidents	• Seizures
• Sports/Recreation Injuries	• Electric Shocks
• Abusive Head Trauma (Shaken Baby Syndrome)	• Tumors
• Gunshot Wounds	• Metabolic Disorders
• Workplace Injuries	• Neurotoxic Poisoning (Carbon Monoxide, Lead Exposure)
• Military Actions (Blast Injury)	• Lack of Oxygen (Drowning, Choking, Hypoxic/Anoxic Injury)
	• Drug Overdose

Source: BIAA, 2012, Brain Injury Overview para. 5.

(BIAA, 2012). The quote at the start of this chapter underscores this point, as does the following quote about the brain and its functions (BIAA, 2012):

> The human brain is magnificent and complex. The brain is made up of many parts, each with a specific and important function. It controls our ability to balance, walk, talk, and eat. It coordinates and regulates our breathing, blood circulation, and heart rate. It is responsible for our ability to speak, to process and remember information, make decisions, and feel emotions. Every brain is unique, ever-changing, and extremely sensitive to its environment. (Functions of the Brain, para. 1)

Always remember that a person with a brain injury is a person first. No two people are exactly the same and neither are their neurologic disorders. The effects of an acquired brain injury depend on factors unique to each person and the nature of their injury (BIAA, 2012). Although a detailed discussion of the brain and its function is beyond the scope of this chapter, a brief review of the general makeup of the brain is worthwhile as you consider your role in service as an SLPA for adults with acquired neurologic disorders.

The brain comprises roughly equal-size halves (also known as hemispheres of the brain): a left and a right hemisphere (Figure 19–1). Although they are roughly equal in size, they are not identical, and

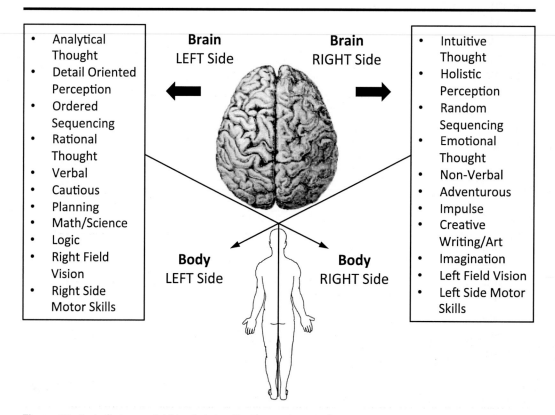

Figure 19–1. Left versus right brain lateralization and control.

they differ in terms of their functions (BIAA, 2012). The right side of the brain controls the left side of the body, while the left side of the brain controls the right side of the body (see Figure 19–1). Common functions associated more with the left hemisphere than the right include analytical, logical, precise, organized, detached, and literal thinking (BIAA, 2012, Functions of the Brain). Common functions ascribed more to the right hemisphere than the left include creative, imaginative, intuitive, conceptual, empathetic, and figurative thinking. These are perhaps false distinctions, however, as the two hemispheres of the brain are highly integrated and collaborate with one another to varying degrees in every important skill and life function. But because certain functions rely more on one hemisphere than the other, different patterns of impairment can result depending on the side of the brain impacted. Table 19–2 summarizes potential impairments as a result of injuries to a specific side of the brain.

Specific structures and regions of the brain affected by acquired neurologic disorders include the brainstem, cerebellum, and the four lobes of the brain (i.e., fron-tal, temporal, parietal, and occipital lobes; Figure 19–2). Certain functions rely more on some of these structures and regions than others. As a result, general patterns of impairment arise when damage occurs in specific areas (BIAA, 2012, Functions of the Brain):

- Frontal lobe damage can impact speaking, motor functions, recall and control of emotions, impulses, and behavior.
- Temporal lobe damage may lead to difficulty with language production and comprehension, memory, social cognition, and complex visual processing.
- Parietal lobe damage can lead to difficulty integrating information from the five primary senses (sight, hearing, taste, smell, and touch), attention, proprioception (sensing where your own body parts are in space), and spatial cognition.
- Occipital lobe damage causes vision problems, like perceiving the size and shape of objects, and color and motion perception.

Table 19–2. Common Characteristics of Injuries to the Right Versus Left Hemispheres of the Brain

Left-Side Brain Injuries	Right-Side Brain Injuries
• Difficulties in understanding language (receptive language)	• Visual-spatial impairments
• Difficulties in speaking or verbal ooutput (expressive language)	• Visual memory deficits
• Catastrophic reactions (depression, anxiety)	• Left neglect (inattention to the left side of the body)
• Difficulty speaking	• Decreased awareness of deficits
• Impaired logic	• Altered creativity and music perception
• Sequencing difficulties	• Loss of "the big picture" type of thinking
• Decreased control over right-sided body movements	• Decreased control over left-sided body movements

Source: BIAA, 2012, Functions of the Brain.

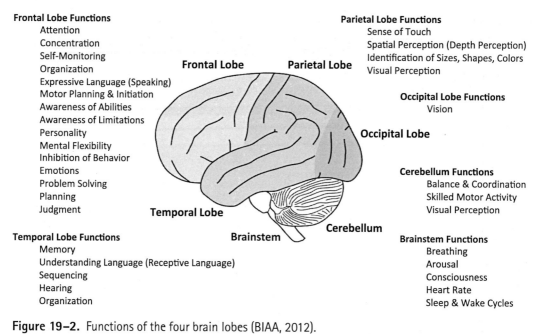

Frontal Lobe Functions
Attention
Concentration
Self-Monitoring
Organization
Expressive Language (Speaking)
Motor Planning & Initiation
Awareness of Abilities
Awareness of Limitations
Personality
Mental Flexibility
Inhibition of Behavior
Emotions
Problem Solving
Planning
Judgment

Temporal Lobe Functions
Memory
Understanding Language (Receptive Language)
Sequencing
Hearing
Organization

Parietal Lobe Functions
Sense of Touch
Spatial Perception (Depth Perception)
Identification of Sizes, Shapes, Colors
Visual Perception

Occipital Lobe Functions
Vision

Cerebellum Functions
Balance & Coordination
Skilled Motor Activity
Visual Perception

Brainstem Functions
Breathing
Arousal
Consciousness
Heart Rate
Sleep & Wake Cycles

Figure 19–2. Functions of the four brain lobes (BIAA, 2012).

- Cerebellar damage may lead to difficulty with coordination of balance and movement.
- Brainstem damage can affect the body's involuntary functions, such as breathing, heart rate, and other functions critical to survival.

SERVICE PROVISION FOR ADULTS WITH NEUROLOGIC DISORDERS

The majority of services provided to adults with acquired neurologic disorders occurs within health care settings, especially in the early stages of recovery, but services are also provided in nonschool private practice settings. Table 19–3 provides a brief description of settings of this nature.

Although the exact numbers are not known, a smaller percentage of SLPAs are employed in health care settings, as compared to school and other non–health-care settings, in part because there are fewer speech-language pathologists (SLPs) in health care settings. A 2021 American Speech-Language-Hearing Association (ASHA) membership and affiliation count found that only 39.4% of certified SLPs were employed in health care settings (ASHA, n.d.-b). In 2002, a survey of ASHA members in health care settings revealed the rarity of SLPA employment in these settings, with 98% of SLP respondents indicating SLPAs were not used in their departments (ASHA, n.d.-a, n.d.-b). This number may be increasing, however, given that a 2021 ASHA membership survey found that 32.9% of SLPs in health care settings reported employing one or more SLP support personnel in their department (ASHA, n.d.-b). Other reasons for a smaller number of SLPAs in health care settings could be the nature

Table 19–3. Health Care and Non-School Private Practice Settings

Health Care Settings	
Acute Hospital	Inpatient care provided in an acute care medical facility
Inpatient Rehab	Free standing rehabilitation hospitals and rehabilitation units in acute care hospitals that are designed to support intensive, interdisciplinary rehabilitation of disabling conditions.
Outpatient	Outpatient services provided in a hospital
Skilled Nursing Facility	Skilled nursing and intermediate or extended care units/facilities. Skilled nursing units are usually either hospital-based or exist in a long-term care facility and require skilled nursing care 24 hours a day. Rehab therapy services may be provided. Intermediate or extended care settings where 24-hour medical supervision is provided, but skilled nursing services are not required.
Non-School Private Practice Settings	
Office Based	Any freestanding speech and hearing clinic or office-based private practice clinic.
Home Health	Speech and language services provided in the home.

Source: ASHA, 2017.

of services provided, the population served, or billing regulations for health care settings. Presently, Medicare policy precludes reimbursement for SLPA services. Private insurance reimbursement for SLPA services is variable based on the insurer (ASHA, n.d.-a).

Some cardinal features of speech-language pathology in health care settings include the use of a World Health Organization (WHO) International Classification framework, patient-centered care, interdisciplinary teams, and use of adult learning principles. Each of these are briefly discussed below.

World Health Organization International Classification Framework

The World Health Organization's (WHO) International Classification of Functioning, Disability and Health (ICF) is integral to understanding the recovery, outcome, and services associated with neurologic disorders. The ICF is biopsychosocial, as it integrates medical, psychological, and social perspectives of disability and function (WHO, 2002, pp. 9, 19). It addresses the concept of disability as something every human being may experience in their life, through a change in health or environment. Figure 19–3 is one representation of the WHO ICF model. As can be seen, disability and functioning are outcomes of the interactions between health conditions (diseases, disorders, and injuries) and contextual factors (personal and environmental; Ostergren, 2017). Personal contextual factors, such as gender, race, education, and coping strategies, are independent of the health condition but may influence how a person functions. Environmental contextual factors are factors outside of the person's control, such as family, work, laws, and

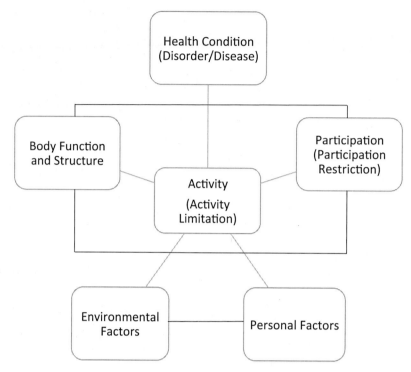

Figure 19–3. World Health Organization (WHO) International Classification of Functioning, Disability and Health (ICF).

cultural norms. There is a synergistic relationship among all three levels of human functioning: functioning of the body or body part(s) (body structure and function), executing tasks or actions (activity), and involvement in life situations (participation). Note that the first of those need not involve the whole person (e.g., a specific body part could be impaired), but the latter two occur at the level of the whole person (e.g., limited activity, restricted participation). As an SLPA, you should be familiar with this framework and its related terminology. It is discussed clinically in health care settings and may be frequently referenced in the resource materials your supervising SLP asks you to read and research on the topic of acquired neurologic disorders.

Patient-Centered Care

Patient-centered care is another key feature of services for adults with acquired neurologic disorders, regardless of the setting where services are provided (Cott, 2004; Ostergren, 2017). Several long-standing principles of patient-centered care include (Picker Institute, n.d.):

■ Respect for patients' values, preferences, and expressed needs
■ Coordination and integration of care
■ Information, communication, and education
■ Physical comfort
■ Emotional support and alleviation of fear and anxiety

■ Involvement of family and
friends
■ Continuity and transition
■ Access to care

In addition, patient-centered principles
also include those listed in Table 19–4.
These are each important factors to consider when providing services to adults
with neurologic disorders. Take a moment
to consider how these factors might influence the services you provide for adults
with acquired neurologic disorders.

Interdisciplinary Teams

The third foundational feature of most
rehabilitation settings for adults with
neurologic disorders is interdisciplinary
teams (Brasure et al., 2013; Ostergren,
2017). The most critical members of any
interdisciplinary team are the individuals with neurologic disorders (and their

Table 19–4. Client-Centered Rehabilitation
Principles from the Client Perspective

Individualization of programs to the needs of each client in order to prepare them for life in the real world
Mutual participation with health professionals in decision-making and goal setting
Outcomes that are meaningful to the client
Sharing of information and education that is appropriate, timely, and according to the clients' wishes
Emotional support
Family and peer involvement throughout the rehabilitation process
Coordination and continuity across multiple service sectors

Source: Cott (2004, pp. 1418-1419); Ostergren (2017).

family members). The composition of
additional team members varies based
on the age of the individual, the nature
of impairments, the stage of recovery,
and specialized training of particular
team members. The team works together
to provide integrated services and identify ways to optimize environmental and
personal factors impacting daily function
(Ostergren, 2017). Examples of potential
team members are listed in Table 19–5.
The table includes you, as a paraprofessional team member.

Adult Learner Principles

It is helpful to consider core tenets of
adult learning pertaining to the services

Table 19–5. Interdisciplinary Team Members

Primary care physician
Rehabilitation nurse
Clinical neuropsychologist
Speech-language pathologist
Audiologist
Rehabilitation psychologist
Behavioral specialist
Dietitian
Educator
Occupational therapist
Physical therapist
Psychiatrist
Social worker
Case manager
Therapeutic recreation specialist
Vocational rehabilitation counselor
Paraprofessionals

Source: Joint Committee on Interprofessional Relations Between
the American Speech-Language-Hearing Association and Division 40 (Clinical Neuropsychology) of the American Psychological
Association (2007, Interdisciplinary Team Membership)..

you provide to this population. An adult learner (Knowles, 1984a, 1984b)

- Has an independent self-concept and can direct his or her own learning
- Has accumulated a reservoir of life experiences that is a rich resource for learning
- Has learning needs closely related to changing social roles
- Is problem-centered and interested in immediate application of knowledge
- Is motivated to learn by internal rather than external factors

Additional aspects of service provision for adults are listed below (Knowles, 1984a, 1984b):

- Adults should be involved in the planning and evaluation of their instruction.
- Adults' experience (including mistakes) provides a basis for learning activities.
- Adults are most interested in learning about subjects that have immediate relevance to their life.
- Adult learning is problem-centered rather than content-oriented.

Take a moment to consider how these principles shape the services you provide as an SLPA working with adults with acquired neurologic disorders (as compared to services for children). Do these principles change specific aspects of your approach? They should, as many of them necessitate that your methods allow for more independence, self-direction, and self-determination. They also require that

you work closely with your supervising SLP to make the function, purpose, and rationale of the services you provide very clear to the adult you are working with. I encourage you to revisit this list frequently as an SLPA who is providing services to adults (not just those with neurologic disorders). Adherence to these principles will mean the difference between successful and unsuccessful treatment services for adult learners.

TREATMENT FOUNDATIONS

Before we discuss treatment approaches specific to given neurologic disorders, it is helpful to first take a 360-degree bird's-eye view of the foundations of treatment of neurologic disorders. Many treatment approaches have common core features and aims. There is a framework that has been adapted from various descriptions of treatment foundations in this area, including the Institute of Medicine's (IOM's) descriptions for cognitive rehabilitation therapy (CRT) for TBI (IOM, 2011). It categorizes treatment approaches as restoration, calibration, or compensation (Figure 19–4). Restoration approaches seek to improve, strengthen, or normalize an impaired function (IOM, 2011). Restoration approaches commonly involve repetition and drills or exercise-like activities, gradually increasing in difficulty and demand, to target an impaired process (IOM, 2011). Treatment in this frame is thought to act as restorative in overcoming damage related to a brain injury. Compensation approaches seek to provide alternative strategies for completing everyday activities, despite residual deficits (IOM, 2011). Compensation approaches are commonly divided into

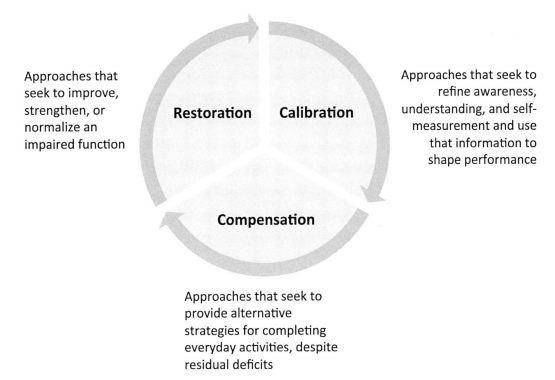

Approaches that seek to improve, strengthen, or normalize an impaired function

Restoration

Calibration

Approaches that seek to refine awareness, understanding, and self-measurement and use that information to shape performance

Compensation

Approaches that seek to provide alternative strategies for completing everyday activities, despite residual deficits

Figure 19–4. Framework of Treatment Approaches for Neurologic Disorders. Ostergren, J. (2017). *Cognitive Rehabilitation Therapy for Traumatic Brain Injury: A Guide for Speech-Language Pathologists.* Copyright 2017. Plural Publishing, Inc. All rights reserved.

internal and external strategy compensation (IOM, 2011). External strategies utilize items external to the individual, such as augmentative and alternative communication (AAC), alarms, notebooks, notes, and calendars. Internal strategies utilize internal processes such as word-finding strategies, mnemonics, visualization, and word association. Lastly, calibration approaches seek to refine awareness, understanding, and self-measurements of performance (e.g., thinking about thinking) and use that information to shape performance. As you learn more about specific approaches in the sections that follow, I encourage you to reflect on these descriptions and identify aspects of spe-

cific techniques that appear to align with one, two, or more of these approaches. Seeing these connections and the underlying themes will increase your understanding of any specific technique.

COMMON NEUROLOGIC DISORDERS

The acquired neurologic disorders discussed in this section are aphasia, right hemisphere brain dysfunction (RHBD), cognitive-communicative disorders associated with TBI, apraxia of speech, and dysarthria. Dysphagia, a disorder of swallowing, is also common, but ASHA's

Scope of Practice for SLPAs has specific limitations on services provided by SLPAs for dysphagia. Specifically, it states that SLPAs may not (ASHA, 2022, Responsibilities Outside the Scope for Speech-Language Pathology Assistants, para. 2):

- Administer or interpret feeding and/or swallowing screenings, checklists, and assessments
- Diagnose communication and feeding/swallowing disorders
- Develop or determine the feeding and/or swallowing strategies or precautions for students, patients, and clients

Some state regulations also limit provisions of services for dysphagia by SLPAs. As such, this chapter does not discuss dysphagia and its treatment. However, as with any personnel providing services to individuals potentially at risk of dysphagia, SLPAs should know the common signs and symptoms of dysphagia and the related topics of aspiration and tube feeding, as discussed in Chapter 6.

Aphasia

Aphasia is defined as an "impairment of language, affecting the production or comprehension of speech and the ability to read and write" (The Stroke Foundation, 2017, Glossary, para. 4). ASHA adds that aphasia is "an acquired neurogenic language disorder resulting from an injury to the brain—most typically, the left hemisphere" (ASHA, n.d.-c, para. 1). While impairments in cognitive skills can co-occur with aphasia, individuals with aphasia generally have intact nonlinguistic cognitive skills, such as memory and executive function. Aphasia involves varying degrees of impairment in four primary areas (ASHA, n.d.-c):

- Spoken language expression
- Spoken language comprehension
- Written expression
- Reading comprehension

Box 19–2 (ASHA, n.d.-c) describes common signs and symptoms of aphasia for each of these impairments. Aphasia is also classified into different types (Table 19–6). Figure 19–5 depicts a decision flow chart about specific presenting features as they relate to these classifications.

The most frequent cause of aphasia is a stroke (National Institute on Deafness and Other Communication Disorders [NIDCD], 2015). Chapter 6 describes in more detail the origins of stroke and its common signs and symptoms. Other causes of aphasia are severe blows to the head, brain tumors, gunshot wounds, brain infections, and progressive neurological disorders, such as Alzheimer's disease (NIDCD, 2015). NIDCD (2015) estimated that there are 180,000 new cases of aphasia per year in the United States and that approximately 1 million people in the United States are living with aphasia. This translates to 1 in 250 people in the United States today (ASHA, n.d.-c).

Research has shown that individuals who receive treatment designed to reduce language impairments associated with aphasia improve to a greater extent than individuals who do not receive treatment (Simmons-Mackie & Kagan, 2007). Treatment is generally provided as early as tolerated (The Stroke Foundation, 2017). Table 19–7 contains a description of common treatment approaches for aphasia. Technology is increasingly advancing the treatment of aphasia, including computer-based software and a variety of low- and high-technology approaches to AAC.

Box 19–2. Common Signs and Symptoms of Aphasia
(ASHA, n.d.-c, Signs and Symptoms)

Impairments in Spoken Language Expression

- Having difficulty finding words (anomia)
- Speaking haltingly or with effort
- Speaking in single words (e.g., names of objects)
- Speaking in short, fragmented phrases
- Omitting small words like *the*, *of*, and *was* (i.e., telegraphic speech)
- Making grammatical errors
- Putting words in the wrong order
- Substituting sounds or words (e.g., *table* for *bed*; *wishdasher* for *dishwasher*)
- Making up words (e.g., jargon)
- Fluently stringing together nonsense words and real words, but leaving out or including an insufficient amount of relevant content

Impairments in Spoken Language Comprehension

- Having difficulty understanding spoken utterances
- Requiring extra time to understand spoken messages
- Providing unreliable answers to "yes/no" questions
- Failing to understand complex grammar (e.g., "The dog was chased by the cat.")
- Finding it very hard to follow fast speech (e.g., radio or television news)
- Misinterpreting subtleties of language (e.g., taking the literal meaning of figurative speech such as "It's raining cats and dogs.")
- Lacking awareness of errors

Impairments in Written Expression (Agraphia)

- Having difficulty writing or copying letters, words, and sentences
- Writing single words only
- Substituting incorrect letters or words
- Spelling or writing nonsense syllables or words
- Writing run-on sentences that do not make sense
- Writing sentences with incorrect grammar

Impairments in Reading (Alexia)

- Having difficulty comprehending written material
- Having difficulty recognizing some words by sight
- Having the inability to sound out words
- Substituting associated words for a word (e.g., *chair* for *couch*)
- Having difficulty reading noncontent words (e.g., function words such as *to, from, the*)

Table 19–6. Types of Aphasia

Aphasia Type	Characteristics
Nonfluent Aphasias	
Broca's	Anomia, short phrase length, agrammatism, impaired prosody and intonation, relatively poor ability to repeat words and phrase, relatively good auditory comprehension, usually associated with right hemiparesis (one-sided weakness) or hemiplegia (one-sided paralysis), and may co-occur with dysarthria and apraxia of speech.
Transcortical Motor	Anomia, impaired initiation of spontaneous speech, short phrase length, preserved ability to repeat words and phrases (unlike in Broca's aphasia), relatively good auditory comprehension, and may co-occur with hemiparesis.
Mixed Nonfluent	Severe anomia, short phrase length, verbal output may be limited to stereotypic utterances, poor ability to repeat words and phrases, relatively poor auditory comprehension, with modality deficits less severe than with global aphasia but more severe than with Broca's aphasia.
Global	Severe deficits in all areas of language comprehension and production; profound anomia with virtually no speech output (may be restricted to stereotypic utterances), very poor auditory comprehension, often associated with right hemiplegia, and may co-occur with severe dysarthria, oral apraxia, apraxia of speech, and dysphagia.
Fluent Aphasias	
Wernicke's	Marked anomia, fluent but often meaningless speech (jargon), well-articulated and prosodic speech consisting of many error types (e.g., phonemic, semantic, and neologistic paraphasias), significant impairment in auditory comprehension, and poor repetition ability.
Transcortical Sensory	Severe anomia, fluent and in many cases meaningless speech (jargon), poor auditory comprehension, persevered ability to repeat words and phrases (unlike in Wernicke's aphasia), with prosodic features relatively preserved.
Conduction	Anomia, fluent output that may be interrupted by word-finding pauses or attempts to self-correct, frequent phonemic paraphasias, significant difficulty with repetition (disproportionate to other impairments), and good auditory comprehension.
Anomic	Significant word-finding difficulties in presence of otherwise fluent and grammatical speech, and relatively or entirely intact auditory comprehension and repetition.

Sources: Brookshire, 2015; Helm-Estabrooks et al., 2014.

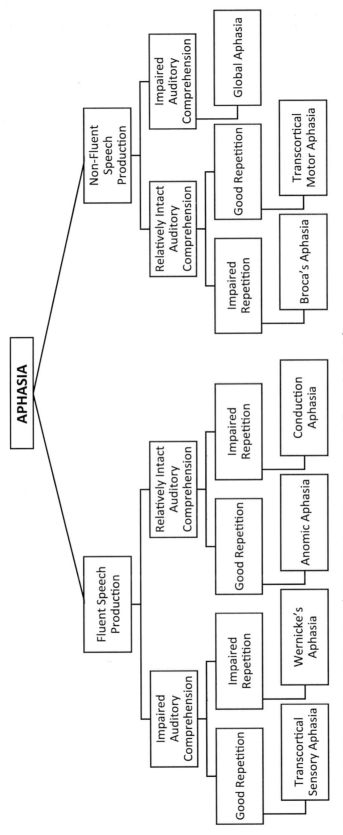

Figure 19–5. Types of Aphasia flow chart (National Aphasia Association, n.d., Types of Aphasia).

Table 19–7. Common Treatment Approaches for Individuals with Aphasia

Treatment Type	General Treatment Goals	Example Approaches
Community Support and Integration	Provide community support and help individuals with aphasia more fully integrate into community life.	*Community Aphasia Groups* Expand opportunities "to socialize, converse, share ideas and feelings, receive support, and learn more about aphasia and aphasia resources" (ASHA, n.d.-c., Community Support and Integration, para. 10) via group treatment with individuals with aphasia (and their family members). *Life Participation Approach to Aphasia (LPAA)* Focuses on long-term management of aphasia and reengaging individuals with aphasia in activities of their choosing by implementing home and community-based treatment.
Constraint-Induced Language Therapy (CILT)	Increase spoken language by discouraging (constraining) use of compensatory communication strategies, such as gestures and writing.	Focus on verbal production without the concurrent use of other communication modalities, via massed practice (multiple trials) and high-intensity training.
Melodic Intonation Therapy (MIT)	Improve expressive language using the prosodic elements of speech (i.e., melody, rhythm, and stress)	Engage undamaged areas of the right hemisphere to facilitate language expression using the intact function of singing (and other visual and tactile cues)
Multimodal Treatment	Use effective and efficient communication strategies as an alternative means of communication.	*Augmentative and Alternative Communication (AAC)* Use aided and unaided communication techniques to supplement or replace spoken language. Examples of aided techniques include picture communication symbols, line drawings, Blissymbols, tangible objects, and speech-generating devices. Examples of unaided techniques include manual signs, gestures, and finger spelling. *Promoting Aphasics' Communication Effectiveness (PACE)* Train individuals and their partners to improve conversation by using any and multiple modes of communication (spoken language, gestures, drawing, writing, partner support) to convey a meaningful and personally relevant message. *Visual Action Therapy (VAT)* Trains individuals with aphasia (commonly global aphasia) to use hand gestures to communicate wants and needs.

Table 19–7. *continued*

Treatment Type	General Treatment Goals	Example Approaches
Partner Approaches	Engage the communication partner in facilitating improved communication.	*Conversational Coaching* Teach verbal and nonverbal communication strategies to individuals with aphasia and their primary communication partners. The SLP serves as a coach, helping the communication partner select and deploy effective communication techniques. *Supported Communication Intervention (SCI)* Teach multimodal communication strategies to communication partners to support the dynamic and social process of communication for the individuals with aphasia.
Script Training	Use intact knowledge of scripts (understanding, remembering, and recalling event sequences of an activity) to facilitate participation in personally relevant activities.	Help the individuals with aphasia create, learn, and automatically use scripted monologues or dialogues during activities of interest.
Syntax Treatments	Improve the grammatical structure for sentence-level deficits.	*Sentence Production Program for Aphasia (SPPA)* Focus on sequential and structured practice of eight specific sentence types. *Treatment of Underlying Forms (TUF)* Treat sentence-level deficits by starting with more complex sentence structures that generalize to less complex sentences that share similar properties.
Word-Finding Treatments	Improve word finding deficit (anomia) in spontaneous utterances.	*Gestural Facilitation of Naming (GES)* Pair verbal expressions with intact gestural abilities to activate word retrieval. *Response Elaboration Training (RET)* Sequentially shape and elaborate on verbal responses using shaping, reinforcement, modeling, and structured cuing. *Semantic Feature Analysis Treatment* Train persons with aphasia in identifying the important semantic features thought to activate the needed semantic network for successful word retrieval. *Verb Network Strengthening Treatment (VNeST)* Improve the production of basic syntactic structures in sentences by targeting retrieval of verbs and their related semantic networks and associations. *Word Retrieval Cuing Strategies* Use structured phonological (beginning sound of a word) and semantic (contextual) cues to prompt word recall.

Source: ASHA, n.d.-b, Treatment Options.

Right Hemisphere Brain Damage

Right hemisphere brain damage (RHBD), also referred to as right hemisphere brain dysfunction or right hemisphere damage, is "an acquired brain injury—usually secondary to stroke or TBI—that causes impairments in language and other cognitive domains that affect communication" (ASHA, n.d.-d). Estimates indicate that 50% to 78% of individuals with RHBD exhibit one or more communication impairments (Lehman Blake et al., 2013) due to cognitive or language deficits.

In the realm of cognition, RHBD can impact attention, memory, and executive control (Lehman Blake et al., 2013). Examples of difficulties stemming from RHBD include the following (ASHA, n.d.-d., Signs and Symptoms, para. 11):

- Reduced sustained attention
- Reduced selective attention (easily distracted)
- Reduced attention to detail
- Unilateral visual neglect—typically, the left side
- Decreased or no awareness of deficits (anosognosia)
- Reduced reasoning and judgment
- Difficulty with sequencing and problem solving
- Impaired executive functioning
- Reduced inhibition
- Reduced recognition of facial expression

In relation to language, RHBD can affect semantic processing of words, discourse processing (including narratives), prosody, and pragmatics. Generally, syntax, grammar, phonological processing, and word retrieval are preserved in RHBD

(ASHA, n.d.-d.). Box 19–3 contains a list of language deficits common to RHBD. Individuals with RHBD may also present with aprosodia, which is reduced (or absence of) normal variations in pitch, loudness, intonation, and rhythm of speech (Blake, 2018). Aprosody combined with reduced emotional expressiveness and diminished facial expressions may also lead to an appearance of flat affect in RHBD.

RHBD results from etiologies (causes) similar to those of aphasia, including stroke, TBI, brain tumors, and other neurological illnesses and injuries (Lehman Blake et al., 2013). Many individuals with RHBD may go untreated, making the exact incidence and prevalence of RHBD unknown. Following stroke, damage to the right hemisphere of the brain occurs in 42% to 49% of patients (ASHA, n.d.-d.).

The most commonly reported treatment areas reported for people with RHBD are difficulties with swallowing and the cognitive functions of memory and problem solving (ASHA, 2017). Disorders of expression, comprehension, and pragmatics are also reported, but to a lesser degree than other cognitive symptoms (ASHA, 2017). Table 19–8 provides a summary of treatment approaches for RHBD.

Cognitive–Communicative Disorders Following Traumatic Brain Injury

Traumatic brain injury, also referred to as neurotrauma, is defined as "a disruption in the normal function of the brain that can be caused by a bump, blow, or jolt to the head or a penetrating head injury" (Centers for Disease Control and Prevention [CDC], 2015, p. 15). An explosive blast can also cause a TBI (CDC, 2015).

Box 19–3. Language Deficits Common to RHBD
(ASHA, n.d.-d., Language)

Discourse Comprehension Deficits

- Difficulty understanding abstract language, figurative language, lexical ambiguities, or information that can be interpreted in multiple ways
- Difficulty making inferences and understanding the global meanings of discourse such as topic, gist, and big picture
- Difficulty understanding jokes, irony, and sarcasm
- Difficulty understanding others' emotions

Discourse Production Deficits

- Verbosity (using more words than needed)
- Egocentric (self-centered) and tangential (peripheral or erratic) comments that digress from the topic
- Focus on irrelevant details
- Disorganized thoughts
- Impulsive and poorly organized responses

Pragmatic Communication Deficits

- Reduced eye contact
- Poor turn taking
- Decreased conversation initiation

Semantic Processing Deficits

- Understanding the metaphorical meaning of words (e.g., "a sea of grief" and "roller coaster of emotions")

TBI can result when the head suddenly and violently hits an object, or when an object pierces the skull and enters brain tissue (National Institute of Neurologic Disorders and Stroke [NINDS], n.d.). TBI can range in severity (from mild to severe). The presence of any of the following clinical signs is considered a disruption in normal brain function after a TBI (Menon et al., 2010):

- Any period of loss of or decreased consciousness
- Any loss of memory for events immediately before (retrograde amnesia) or after the injury (post-traumatic, or anterograde amnesia)
- Muscle weakness, loss of balance and coordination, disruption of vision, change in speech and language, or sensory loss

Table 19–8. Treatment Approaches for RHBD

Treatment Type	General Treatment Goals	Example Approaches
Language Treatment	Improve: • Narrative and conversational discourse • Understanding and managing alternate meanings • Pragmatics	*Narrative and Conversational Discourse Training* Develop skills in making inferences and understanding the topic, gist, and big picture of conversation through either • Guided inference-generating that requires the individual to label, identify, and explain the relationship among items • Macrostructure tasks that require the individual to identify the "big picture" of news stories, picture scenes, or conversations and/or organize information into a logical sequence to support a main idea *Understanding and Managing Alternate Meanings Treatment* Improve the ability to understand lexical ambiguities, generate alternate meanings, and understand nonliteral language through tasks that require the individual to • Group words according to their positive or negative associations • Provide multiple and alternative meanings • Interpret figurative language *Treatment for Pragmatic Deficits* Improve social communication skills through coaching, visual and verbal feedback, video modeling, rehearsal, role-play, and individual and group practice, targeting • Use of appropriate and social and cultural conversational conventions, such as nonverbal cues, turn-taking, organized and on-topic conversation, and social boundaries. • Understanding other peoples' beliefs, attitudes, and emotions and using that understanding to navigate social situations
Prosody	Improve expression and/or interpretation of prosody, such as varying pitch, loudness, and rhythm	*Direct Treatment Approaches for Prosody* Improve conscious control in expression of prosody by using production drills and practice. *Compensatory Treatment Approaches for Prosody* Focus on techniques to compensate for difficulties in expression or interpretation of prosody, such as • Teaching the individual to use cues from the speaker that convey emotions other than prosody, such as word choice, facial expression, and body language • Asking communication partners and the person with RHBD to explicitly state emotions to avoid misunderstanding in expression or interpretation of prosody

Table 19–8. *continued*

Treatment Type	General Treatment Goals	Example Approaches
Attention, Memory, and Executive Function Treatment	Improve attention, memory, and executive functioning deficits	*Attention Treatment* Direct Treatment Approaches for Attention Target sustained, selective, alternating, and/or divided attention deficits, using • Computerized attention training programs • Practice engaging in structured or real-world tasks that require a specific level of attention, gradually increasing the complexity of tasks and type of attention as treatment progresses Metacognitive and Compensatory Strategy Approaches for Attention Help the person understand the nature, scope, and impact of attention deficits through a series of guided exercises with clinician feedback, followed by training in individualized strategies and techniques the person can use to mitigate or minimize the negative impacts of attention deficits on daily tasks. Environmental Modification Approaches for Attention Mitigate and minimize attention deficits by eliminating threats to attention in the environment, such as turning off or moving away from the TV, choosing the best time of day to complete important tasks, or organizing work space and removing distracting items. *Memory Treatment* Provide training and practice in compensating for memory impairments through the use of external and internal strategies, including the following (ASHA, n.d.-h, Attention, Memory, and Executive Function). External Strategies • To-do lists • Notes • Calendars • Alarms and timers • Medication reminders • Journals • Labels Internal Strategies • Mnemonics, such as assigning an abbreviation for information to be recalled (e.g., B.A.D. for bread, aspirin, and detergent to be purchased at the store) • Visualization, repetition, and rehearsal of information to be recalled • Semantic elaboration, such as identifying and describing as many salient features as possible of the information to be remembered or linking the information with preexisting knowledge.

continues

Table 19–8. *continued*

Treatment Type	General Treatment Goals	Example Approaches
Attention, Memory, and Executive Function Treatment *continued*	Improve attention, memory, and executive functioning deficits	*Executive Function* Develop skills for solving problems, thinking flexibly, setting and completing goals, staying on task, and staying organized, including Metacognitive and Compensatory Strategy Approaches for Executive Function Help the person understand the nature, scope, and impact of executive function deficits through a series of guided exercises with clinician feedback, followed by training in individualized strategies and techniques the person can use to mitigate or minimize the negative impacts of deficits in executive function on daily tasks. Environmental Modification Approaches for Executive Function Mitigate and minimize executive function deficits by eliminating threats to them in the environment, such as making sure that items and materials are stored near where they will be used, labeling boxes, drawers, and cabinets to indicate content, color-coding tabs in a file drawer to identify categories (e.g., medical records or bills) to optimize organization and problem solving.

Source: ASHA, n.d.-h. Treatment Options.

- Any alternation in mental state at the time of the injury such as confusion, disorientation, slowed thinking, or difficulty concentrating

It is important to note that concussion, defined as follows (McCrory et al., 2013, pp. 1–2), is also considered TBI:

1. Caused by a direct blow to the head, face, neck, or elsewhere on the body by an "impulsive" force (i.e., the brief force produced when two objects collide).
2. Typically results in the rapid onset of short-lived impairment of neurological function that resolves spontaneously. However, in some cases, symptoms and signs may evolve over a number of minutes to hours.
3. May result in neuropathological changes, but the acute clinical symptoms largely reflect a functional disturbance rather than a structural injury, and as such, no abnormality is seen on standard structural neuroimaging studies.
4. Results in a graded set of clinical symptoms that may or may not involve loss of consciousness.

TBI is classified by the mechanism of primary injury (Ostergren, 2017). Table 19–9 has brief descriptions of primary injuries and their subclassifications related to

Table 19–9. Injury Classifications in Traumatic Brain Injury (TBI)

Primary Brain Injury	
Resulting from initial mechanical forces of the trauma (Greve & Zink, 2009)	
Penetrating/Open–Head Injury:	*High-Velocity Penetrating Brain Injury*
A penetrating brain injury (also known as an open-head injury) occurs when the skull is pierced by an object (NINDS, n.d.)	Resulting from high-velocity objects, such as rifle bullets, artillery shells, and shell fragments, traveling at a high speed penetrating the skull (Kazim et al, 2011; Young et al., 2015).
	Low-Velocity Penetrating Brain Injury
	Results from a penetrating object traveling at a lower rate of speed (as compared to high-velocity projectiles), such as clubs, baseball bats, and knives (Kazim et al., 2011; Young et al., 2015).
Nonpenetrating/Closed–Head Injury:	*Non-Acceleration Head Injuries*
A nonpenetrating brain injury (also known as closed-head injury) occurs as a result of an external force that produces rapid rotation or shaking of the brain within the skull, or an impact to the skull (Koehler & Wilhelm, 2011; NINDS, n.d.).	Resulting from damage to brain tissue primarily from a moving object striking the skull, causing deformation of the skull at the point of impact (McLean & Anderson, 1997). If the force and nature of the object create a fracture to the skull and rupture of the meninges, this is referred to as a penetrating head injury (as above). The skull is slightly elastic, however, and can press inward to some degree, without a penetrating injury.
	Acceleration/Deceleration Head Injuries
	Resulting from damage due to movement of the brain within the skull, from either the moving head striking a stationary or moving object, or when the head is shaken violently.

Source: Ostergren, 2017.

TBI. Not included in the table are blast or explosive injuries to the brain, which are thought to be a unique form of primary injury (Magnuson et al., 2012).

Traumatic brain injury is a major cause of death, especially among young people, and a significant source of lifelong disability (CDC, 2017), so much so that it is often described as a silent epidemic, and unfortunately, the incidence of TBI is on the rise globally (CDC, 2017). Each year in the United States, 2.5 million people sustain a TBI, either as an isolated injury or along with other injuries (CDC, 2017). Every day, 153 people die from injuries related to TBI (CDC, 2017). Falls are the most prevalent cause of TBI in the United States (CDC, 2017); other common sources include motor vehicle accidents and violence.

Individuals with TBI can experience a wide variety of symptoms, including physical, visual, auditory, and vestibular, neurobehavioral, swallowing, and communication impairments (ASHA, n.d.-e). Communication impairments after TBI are common and enduring in nature (Larkins, 2007). They are often attributed to disruptions of attention, memory, executive function, or social cognition (McDonald et al., 2014; Murdoch, 2010). As such, they are described as cognitive-communication disorders, which "encompasses difficulty with any aspect of communication that is affected by disruption of cognition" (ASHA, 2005, para. 1). They are defined as

> a set of communication features that result from underlying deficits in cognition. Communication difficulties can include issues with hearing, listening, understanding, speaking, reading, writing, conversational interaction, and social communication. These disorders may occur as a result of underlying deficits with cognition, that is: attention, orientation, memory, organization, information processing, reasoning, problem solving, executive functions, or self-regulation. (College of Audiologists and Speech-Language

Pathologists of Ontario, CASLPO, 2015, p. 2)

This interconnected relationship between communication and cognition is reflected in Figure 19–6, which shows communication at the center of the processes of attention, memory, executive function, and social cognition (Ostergren, 2017; Strutchen, n.d.). Table 19–10 provides additional examples of communication deficits associated with attention, memory, and executive function following TBI.

One type of treatment for cognitive-communication disorders following TBI is cognitive rehabilitation therapy (CRT). CRT is "a systematic, functionally oriented

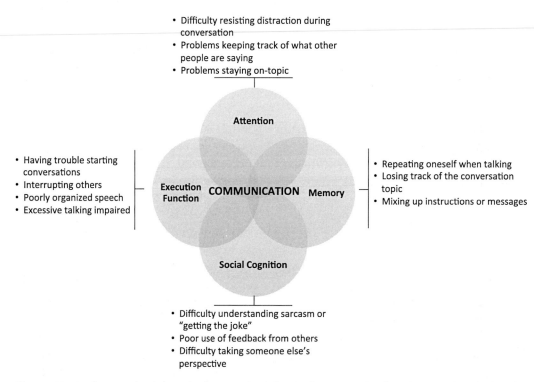

Figure 19–6. Communication at the intersection of attention, executive function, memory, and social communication. Ostergren, J. (2017). *Cognitive Rehabilitation Therapy for Traumatic Brain Injury: A Guide for Speech-Language Pathologists.* Copyright 2017. Plural Publishing, Inc. All rights reserved.

Table 19–10. Communication Deficits Associated With Cognitive Functions Commonly Impaired in TBI

Attention
Difficulty responding appropriately to incoming information
Difficulty learning new information
Difficulty filtering out irrelevant stimuli
Difficulty conversing in situations with distractions, background noise, and multiple participants
Difficulty managing the demands of high-level activity
Difficulty sustaining attention when reading complex and/or lengthy material
Difficulty shifting attention as needed
Difficulty maintaining or changing topics in conversation
Tangential discourse
Social avoidance to compensate for sense of overstimulation

Memory
Difficulty recalling instructions or messages
Difficulty learning new information
Difficulty remembering names of individuals, appointments, directions, and/or location of personal effects
Difficulty recalling details when reading complex and/or lengthy material
Difficulty maintaining topic or remembering purpose of conversation
Repetition of ideas, statements, questions, conversations, or stories
Failure to use compensatory strategies to improve performance on everyday tasks

Executive Function
Lack of coherence in discourse
Lack of organization in planning daily activities
Difficulty implementing plans and actions
Difficulty initiating conversations
Problems recognizing and repairing conversational breakdowns
Inability to determine the needs of communication partners
Difficulty making inferences or drawing conclusions
Difficulty assuming another person's perspective
Difficulty interpreting the behavior of others
Difficulty evaluating validity of information
Verbose; lack of conciseness in verbal expression
Decreased comprehension of abstract language, humor, and/or indirect requests
Difficulty meeting timelines
Difficulty formulating realistic goals
Difficulty recognizing complexity of tasks and need for simplification
Difficulty anticipating consequences of actions
Inappropriate comments

Source: Cornis-Pop et al., 2012, Traumatic Brain Injury.

service of therapeutic cognitive activities, based on an assessment and understanding of the person's brain behavior deficits. Services are directed to achieve functional changes by (1) reinforcing, strengthening, or reestablishing previously learned patterns of behavior, or (2) establishing new patterns of cognitive activity or compensatory mechanisms for impaired neurological systems" (Harley et al., 1992, p. 63). CRT is provided in either individual or group format. It is expected to (ASHA, n.d.-e., Treatment Options):

- Capitalize on strengths and address weaknesses related to underlying structures and functions that affect communication
- Facilitate the individual's activities and participation by assisting the person in acquiring new skills and strategies
- Modify contextual factors that serve as barriers and enhance facilitators of successful communication and participation, including development and use of appropriate accommodations

Table 19–11 summarizes CRT approaches for cognitive-communication disorders. A prominent element of CRT is training in the use of assistive technology for cognition (ATC; Leopold et al., 2015). ATC is designed to "increase, maintain, or improve functional capabilities for individuals whose cognitive changes limit their performance of daily activities" (Scherer, 2012, p. 159). ATC can be divided into low technology, medium technology, and high technology (Sohlberg, 2011). High technology includes the use of increasingly popular mainstream technology such as smartphones and tablet computers. Table 19–12 lists examples of ATC categorized by their level of technology and function (task specific or multifunction).

Table 19–11. Treatment Approaches for Cognitive-Communication Disorders After Traumatic Brain Injury (TBI)

Treatment Type	General Treatment Goals	Example Approaches
Compensatory Strategy Training	Maximize the performance and capitalize on intact skills through either modifying the environment or providing internal and external supports.	Support communication and cognition by identifying, training, and generalizing external and/or internal compensatory strategies. Examples of external strategies are the assistive technology for cognition (ATC) devices and supports listed in Table 19–12. Internal strategies include <ul><li>Mnemonics, such as assigning an abbreviation for information to be recalled (e.g., B.A.D. for bread, aspirin, and detergent to be purchased at the store)</li><li>Visualization, repetition, and rehearsal of information to be recalled</li><li>Semantic elaboration, such as identifying and describing as many salient features as possible of the information to be remembered or associating the information with preexisting knowledge.</li></ul>

Table 19–11. *continued*

Treatment Type	General Treatment Goals	Example Approaches
Computer Assisted Technology (CAT)	Target cognitive processing using commercial software and mobile applications.	Provide consistent feedback to individuals on their performance during cognitive tasks using software or mobile applications that administer repeated trials targeting specific skills or functional tasks, adapted to the individual's performance.
Drill and Practice Training	Establish new networks or stimulate damaged neural networks to restore them using practice and drills for specific skills.	Use repetition of target behaviors to develop new or lost skills and abilities.
Dual Task Training	Improve task complexity by targeting the ability to carry out two competing tasks (typically requiring equal amounts of attention).	Systematic practice and feedback on a combination of two cognitive tasks—a cognitive and motor task, or two motor tasks.
Errorless Learning	Develop new skills or relearn previously developed skills by practicing them without error.	Treatment tasks structure opportunities for repeated practice with a target skill, that • Breaks down the target task into small, discrete steps or units • Provides models before the client is asked to perform the target task • Encourages the client to avoid guessing • Immediately corrects errors and carefully fades prompts once a behavior is established
Metacognitive Skills Training	Improve awareness and self-monitoring of cognitive and communication deficits.	Treatment tasks engage individuals in structured and guided self-reflection and self-regulation in order to facilitate better recognition of problem situations and identification of functional strategies that facilitate success in achieving everyday goals after a TBI.
Social Communication Training	Improve functional conversational skills and success in navigating social situations.	Important components of social communication treatment includes (ASHA, n.d.-a., Treatment Options) • Sharing knowledge with and training everyday communication partners • Selecting highly specific and personal goals and incorporating extensive practice of social behaviors in the situations in which they are required • Situational coaching prior to challenging situations • Situational training to improve social perception and interpretation of others' behaviors to improve self-monitoring of stress • Focusing on social success • Counseling to help an individual identify a sense of self that includes positive social interaction strategies

Source: ASHA, n.d.-a., Treatment Options.

Table 19–12. Sample Assistive Technologies for Cognition Aids Categorized by Function and Level

Task Specific	Multifunctional
Low tech	
Calculator	Sticky notes
Pillbox reminder	Voice mail
Phone dialer	Watch beeps
Alarm clock	Checklists
Electronic speller, thesaurus, dictionary	Answering machines
Oven timer	Appointment calendars
Watch/clock	Car memo pads
Labeler	
Key finder	
Mail sorter baskets	
Map, posted directional signs	
Financial planner	
Posted instructions	
Mid tech	
Camera	Voice recorder/digital recorder
	Cell phone
	Pager
	Data watches
High tech	
Global positioning system (GPS) device	Specialized task guidance systems (Planning and Executive Assistant and Trainer-PEAT, ISSAC, Pocket Coach)
Specialized software programs for facilitated writing, reading, or email	Smartphones
	Personal digital assistants

Source: Sohlberg, 2011, p. 15.

Dysarthria

Dysarthria is broadly defined as "an impaired ability to produce clear speech due to the impaired function of the speech muscles" (The Stroke Foundation, 2017, Glossary, para. 15). More specifically, dysarthria describes a group of neurologic speech disorders with "abnormalities in the strength, speed, range, steadiness, tone, or accuracy of movements required for breathing, phonatory, resonatory, articulatory, or prosodic aspects of speech production" (Duffy, 2013, p. 4). This can be related to sensorimotor problems, such as weakness (paresis), paralysis, incoordination, involuntary movements, or excessive, reduced, or variable muscle tone

(Duffy, 2013). Impairments due to dysarthria range from speech that has mild articulatory imprecision to speech that is totally unintelligible. Box 19–4 lists several common signs of dysarthria (ASHA, n.d.-f). Dysarthria can be one of several types based on the perceptual features of the speaker (Table 19–13).

Anything that causes brain damage can cause dysarthria, including stroke, TBI, and tumors (ASHA, n.d.-f) and a variety of progressive neurologic disorders such as Parkinson's disease, amyotrophic lateral sclerosis (ALS), cerebral palsy, and dementia. The true incidence and prevalence of dysarthria is not known and will vary based on the cause. Research suggests that 8% to 60% of individuals with stroke and 10% to 65% of individuals with TBI present with dysarthria (ASHA, n.d.-g).

Treatment for dysarthria focuses on "facilitating the efficiency, effectiveness, and naturalness of communication" (ASHA, n.d.-g, Treatment). Restoration approaches target the speech production subsystems and compensatory approaches target communication strategies, environmental modifications, and AAC. Medical or surgical interventions are also used to treat dysarthria (ASHA, n.d.-g).

Table 19–14 summarizes of treatment approaches for dysarthria.

Apraxia of Speech

Apraxia is defined as "impaired planning and sequencing of movement that is not due to weakness, incoordination or sensory loss" (The Stroke Foundation, 2017, Glossary, para. 5). There are different forms of apraxia, including limb apraxia, oral apraxia, apraxia of gait, apraxia of swallowing, and apraxia of speech (ASHA, n.d.-h). Often these forms co-occur (ASHA, n.d.-h). Apraxia of speech (AOS) refers to impaired planning and sequencing of speech, including difficulty initiating and executing movements for speech in the absence of weakness in the speech muscles (National Clinical Guideline Centre, 2013). There are two forms of AOS: acquired AOS, caused by damage to the parts of the brain responsible for speaking, and childhood AOS (also known as developmental apraxia of speech, developmental verbal apraxia, or articulatory apraxia), which is present from birth. Consistent with the theme of this chapter, the sections that follow describe acquired AOS.

Box 19–4. Common Signs of Dysarthria

- Slurred or mumbled speech that can be hard to understand
- Slow speech
- Rapid speech
- Quiet speech
- Inability to easily move tongue, lips, and jaw properly
- Robotic or choppy speech
- Changes in voice quality (e.g., hoarseness, breathiness, stuffiness, hypernasality)

Table 19–13. Common Types of Dysarthria and Their Perceptual Characteristics

Dysarthria Type	Perceptual Speech Characteristics
Flaccid	• Continuous breathiness • Diplophonia • Audible inspiration or stridor • Nasal emission • Short phrases • Hypernasality • Rapid deterioration and recovery with rest • Imprecise alternating motion rates (AMRs)
Spastic	• Slow rate • Strained or harsh voice quality • Pitch breaks • Slow and regular AMRs
Ataxic	• Irregular articulatory breakdowns • Excess and equal stress • Distorted vowels • Excessive loudness variation • Irregular AMRs
Hypokinetic	• Monopitch • Monoloudness • Reduced loudness and stress • Tendency for rapid or accelerated rate • Inappropriate silences • Rapidly repeated phonemes • Palilalia • Rapid, "blurred" AMRs
Hyperkinetic	• Prolonged intervals • Sudden forced inspiration or expiration • Transient breathiness • Transient vocal strain or harshness • Voice stoppages/arrests • Voice tremor • Myoclonic vowel prolongation • Intermittent hypernasality • Marked deterioration with increased rate • Inappropriate vocal noises • Intermittent breathy or aphonic segments • Distorted vowels • Excessive loudness variation • Slow and irregular AMRs
Unilateral Upper Motor Neuron	• Slow rate • Imprecise articulation • Irregular articulatory breakdowns • Strained voice quality • Reduced loudness

Source: Duffy, 2013, as cited by ASHA, n.d.-g.

Table 19–14. Treatment Approaches for Dysarthria

Treatment Type	General Treatment Goals	Example Approaches
Speech Production Subsystem Treatment	Treatment approaches that target the speech-production subsystems of • Respiration, • Phonation, • Articulation, and • Resonance	Treatment that focuses on using drills, practice, strength and conditioning training for impacted muscles, postural adjustments, and facilitative techniques to directly target the impacted subsystems of speech.
Communication Strategies	Treatment approaches that target a variety of strategies used by the individual with dysarthria and his/her communication partner to enhance speech intelligibility/comprehensibility.	Treatment focuses on identifying, training, and generalizing strategies in the following areas: Speaker Strategies: • Maintain eye contact • Gaining the listeners attention and introducing the topic before speaking • Using pointing and gesturing to help convey meaning • Looking for signs that the communication partner has not understood the message • Using conversational repair strategies Communication-Partner Strategies: • Being an active listener and making efforts to understand the speaker's message • Asking for clarification information • Providing feedback and encouragement • Optimizing the ability to hear the speaker and to see the speaker's visual communication cues, such as wearing prescribed hearing aids and glasses during conversations
Environmental Modification	Treatment approaches that target identifying and modifying the environment to optimize speech intelligibility/comprehensibility	Treatment aimed at optimizing speech intelligibility/comprehensibility by eliminating threats to it in the environment, such as reducing background noise, ensuring that the environment has good lighting, improving proximity between the speaker and his or her communication partner, and using face-to-face seating for conversations.
Augmentative and Alternative Communication (AAC)	Treatment approaches designed to instruct the speaker in strategies to supplement or replace speech.	Treatment that focuses on training in the use of aided and unaided communication techniques to supplement or replace spoken language. Examples of aided techniques include picture communication symbols, and line drawings. Examples of unaided techniques include manual signs, gestures, and finger spelling. Other AAC approaches for dysarthria include voice amplifiers, artificial phonation devices (e.g., electrolarynx devices and intraoral devices), and oral prosthetics to reduce hypernasality.

Source: ASHA, n.d.-h., Treatment Options.

Acquired forms of AOS often co-occur with dysarthria and aphasia (National Clinical Guideline Centre, 2013). Because of this, and challenges in distinguishing among certain types of errors, there are no reliable data on the incidence and prevalence of acquired AOS in adults (ASHA, n.d.-h; Duffy et al., 2014). When AOS is documented as the primary but not the only communication disorder present, estimates suggest it comprises approximately 7% of all motor speech disorders (Duffy, 2013, as cited in ASHA, n.d.-h).

Treatment approaches for AOS focus on facilitating the efficiency, effectiveness, and naturalness of communication (ASHA, n.d.-h) by either improving speech production or using AAC to enhance communication effectiveness. Treatment for AOS also focuses on minimizing barriers to successful communication, such as (ASHA, n.d.-h, Treatment, para. 5):

- Modifying the environment (e.g., reducing background noise, maintaining eye contact, and decreasing the distance between speaker and listener)
- Informing listeners about the individual's communication needs and his or her preferred method of communication
- Encouraging speakers to use strategies for repairing breakdowns in communication (e.g., repeating, rephrasing, gesturing, writing)

Table 19–15 summarizes common treatment approaches for AOS.

Table 19–15. Common Treatment Approaches for Apraxia of Speech (AOS)

Treatment Type	General Treatment Goals	Example Approaches
Articulatory–Kinematic	Address the symptoms of AOS using the principles of motor programming and planning.	Approaches include elements of the following: • Provide frequent and intensive practice of speech targets • Focus on accurate speech movement • Include external sensory input for speech production (e.g., auditory, visual, tactile, cognitive cues) • Consider practice schedules, such as random versus blocked practice • Provide appropriate types and schedules of feedback regarding performance
Sensory Cueing	Teach movement sequences for speech by incorporating sensory input (e.g., visual, auditory, proprioceptive, and tactile cues).	Provide a variety of sensory feedback (either separately or in combination) on important aspect of motor learning and planning.
Rate and Rhythm Control	Improve speech production by addressing rate and rhythm control (also known as prosodic facilitation).	Increase the length of utterances, decrease dependence on the clinician, and decrease reliance on prosodic patterns by guiding individuals through a gradual progression of steps.
Augmentative and Alternative Communication (AAC)	Supplement or replace speech to facilitate efficiency and effectiveness of communication.	Supplement or replace spoken language with training in the use of aided and unaided communication techniques. Aided techniques include picture communication symbols and line drawings. Unaided techniques include manual signs, gestures, and finger spelling.
Script Training	Facilitate participation in personally relevant activities using intact knowledge of scripts (understanding, remembering, and recalling event sequences of an activity).	Help individuals to create, learn, and automatically use scripted monologue or dialogue during activities of interest.

Source: ASHA, n.d.-h.

REFERENCES

American Speech-Language-Hearing Association. (n.d.-a). *Frequently asked questions: Speech-language pathology assistants.* https://www.asha.org/assistants-certification-program/slpa-faqs/

American Speech-Language-Hearing Association. (n.d.-b). *Executive summary: SLP health care survey 2002.* https://www.asha.org/research/memberdata/

American Speech-Language-Hearing Association. (n.d.-c). *Aphasia.* https://www.asha.org/practice-portal/clinical-topics/aphasia/

American Speech-Language-Hearing Association. (n.d.-d). *Right hemisphere damage.* https://www.asha.org/practice-portal/clinical-topics/right-hemisphere-damage/

American Speech-Language-Hearing Association. (n.d.-e). *Traumatic brain injury in adults.* https://www.asha.org/practice-portal/clinical-topics/traumatic-brain-injury-in-adults/

American Speech-Language-Hearing Association. (n.d.-f). *Dysarthria.* https://www.asha.org/public/speech/disorders/dysarthria/

American Speech-Language-Hearing Association. (n.d.-g). *Dysarthria in adults.* https://www.asha.org/practice-portal/clinical-topics/dysarthria-in-adults/#collapse_1

American Speech-Language-Hearing Association. (n.d.-h). *Acquired apraxia of speech.* https://www.asha.org/practice-portal/clinical-topics/acquired-apraxia-of-speech/#collapse_2

American Speech-Language-Hearing Association. (2005). *Roles of speech-language pathologists in the identification, diagnosis, and treatment of individuals with cognitive-communication disorders: Position statement* [Position statement]. https://www.asha.org/policy/ps2005-00110.htm

American Speech-Language-Hearing Association. (2017). *National Outcomes Measurement System: Adults in healthcare–acute hospital national data report 2017.* National Center for Evidence-Based Practice in Communication Disorders.

American Speech-Language-Hearing Association. (2022). *Speech-language pathology assistant scope of practice.* https://www.asha.org/policy/slpa-scope-of-practice/

Blake, M. L. (2018). *The right hemisphere and disorders of cognition and communication: Theory and clinical practice.* Plural Publishing.

Brain Injury Association of America (BIAA). (2012). *Brain injury basics.* https://www.biausa.org/brain-injury

Brasure, M., Lamberty, G. J., Sayer, N. A., Nelson, N. W., Macdonald, R., Ouellette, J., & Wilt. T. J. (2013). Participation after multidisciplinary rehabilitation for moderate to severe traumatic brain injury in adults: A systematic review. *Archives of Physical Medicine and Rehabilitation, 94*(7), 1398–1420.

Brookshire, R. (2015). *Introduction to neurogenic communication disorders.* Mosby.

Centers for Disease Control and Prevention. (2015). *Report to Congress on traumatic brain injury in the United States: Epidemiology and rehabilitation.* National Center for Injury Prevention and Control; Division of Unintentional Injury Prevention. http://www.cdc.gov/traumatic braininjury/pdf/tbi_report_to_congress_epi_and_rehab-a.pdf

Centers for Disease Control and Prevention. (2017). *TBI: Get the facts.* https://www.cdc.gov/traumaticbrain injury/get_the_facts.html

College of Audiologists and Speech-Language Pathologists of Ontario. (2015). *Practice standards and guidelines for acquired cognitive communication disorders.* http://www.caslpo.com/sites/default/uploads/files/PSG_EN_Acquired_Cognitive_Communication_Disorders.pdf

Cornis-Pop, M., Mashima, P. A., Roth, C. A., MacLennan, D. L., Picon, L. M., Smith Hammond, C., . . . Frank, E. M. (2012). Cognitive-communication rehabilitation for combat related mild traumatic brain injury. *Journal of Rehabilitation Research & Development, 49*(7), xi–xxxi.

Cott, C. A. (2004). Client-centered rehabilitation: Client perspectives. *Disability & Rehabilitation, 26*(24), 1411–1422.

Duffy, J. R. (2013). *Motor speech disorders: Substrates, differential diagnosis, and management.* Elsevier.

Duffy, J. R., Strand, E. A., & Josephs, K. A. (2014). Motor speech disorders associated with primary progressive aphasia. *Aphasiology, 28,* 1004–1017.

Harley, J. P., Allen, C. Braciszewski, T. L., Cicerone, K. D., Dahlberg, C., Evans, S., . . . Smigelski, J. S. (1992). Guidelines for cognitive rehabilitation. *NeuroRehabilitation, 2,* 62–67.

Helm-Estabrooks, N. Albert, M., & Nicholas, N. (2014). *Manual of aphasia and aphasia therapy.* Pro-Ed.

Institute of Medicine. (2011). *Cognitive rehabilitation therapy for traumatic brain injury: Evaluating the evidence.* The National Academies Press. https://doi.org/10.17226/13220

Kazim, S. F., Shamim, M. S., Tahir, M. Z., Enam, S. A., & Waheed, S. (2011). Management of penetrating brain injury. *Journal of Emergencies, Trauma, and Shock, 4*(3), 395–402.

Knowles, M. (1984a). *The adult learner: A neglected species* (3rd ed.). Gulf.

Knowles, M. (1984b) *Andragogy in action.* Jossey-Bass.

Larkins, B. (2007). The application of the ICF in cognitive-communication disorders following traumatic brain injury. *Seminars in Speech and Language, 28*(4), 334–342.

Lehman Blake, M., Frymark, T., & Venedictov, R. (2013). An evidence-based systematic review on communication treatments for individuals with right hemisphere brain damage. *American Journal of Speech-Language Pathology, 22*, 146–160.

Leopold, A., Lourie, A., Petras, H., & Elias, E. (2015). The use of assistive technology for cognition to support the performance of daily activities for individuals with cognitive disabilities due to traumatic brain injury: The current state of the research. *NeuroRehabilitation, 37*(3), 359–378.

Magnuson, J., Leonessa, F., & Ling, G. (2012). Neuropathology of explosive blast traumatic brain injury. *Current Neurology and Neuroscience Reports, 12*(5), 570–579.

McCrory P., Meeuwisse, W. H., Aubry, M., Cantu, B., Dvorák, J., Echemendia, R. J., . . . Turner, M. (2013). Consensus statement on concussion in sport: The 4th international conference on concussion in sport held in Zurich, November 2012. *British Journal of Sports Medicine, 47*, 250–258.

McDonald, S., Togher, L., & Code, C. (2014). *Social and communication disorders following traumatic brain injury*. Psychology Press.

Menon, D. K., Schwab, K., Wright, D. W., Maas, A. I., & Demographics and Clinical Assessment Working Group of the International and Interagency Initiative toward Common Data Elements for Research on Traumatic Brain Injury and Psychological Health. (2010). Position statement: Definition of traumatic brain injury. *Archives of Physical Medicine and Rehabilitation, 91*(11), 1637–1640.

Murdoch, B. E. (2010). Speech-language disorders associated with traumatic brain injury. In B. E. Murdoch (Ed.), *Acquired speech and language disorders: A neuroanatomical and functional neurological approach* (2nd ed., pp. 118–152). Wiley-Blackwell.

National Aphasia Association. (n.d.). *Aphasia definitions*. https://www.apha sia.org/aphasia-definitions/

National Clinical Guideline Centre. (2013). *Stroke rehabilitation: Long-term rehabilitation after stroke* (Clinical Guideline 162). National Institute for Health and Care Excellence.

National Institute of Neurologic Disorders and Stroke. (2015). *Traumatic brain injury: Hope through research* (NIH Publication No. 152478). https://www.ninds.nih.gov/Disorders/Patient-Caregiver-Education/Hope-Through-Research/Traumatic-Brain-Injury-Hope-Through

National Institute on Deafness and Other Communication Disorders. (2015). *NIDCD fact sheet: Aphasia* (NIH Pub. No. 97–4257). https://www.nidcd.nih.gov/sites/default/files/Documents/health/voice/Aphasia 6-1-16.pdf

Ostergren, J. (2017). *Cognitive rehabilitation therapy for traumatic brain injury: A guide for speech-language pathologists*. Plural Publishing.

Picker Institute. (n.d.). *Principles of patient-centered care*. http://cgp.pick erinstitute.org/?page_id=1319

Scherer, M. J. (2012). *Assistive technologies and other supports for people with brain impairment*. Springer.

Simmons-Mackie, N., & Kagan, A. (2007). Application of the ICF in aphasia. *Seminars of Speech and Language, 28*(4), 244–253.

Sohlberg, M. (2011). Assistive technology for cognition. *ASHA Leader, 16*(2), 14.

Strutchen, M. A. (n.d.). *Social communication and traumatic brain injury (TBI): A guide for professionals*. Traumatic Brain Injury Model System at TIRR Memorial Hermann Brain Injury Research Center. http://www.tbicommunity.org/resources/publications/professional_education_social_comm.pdf

The Stroke Foundation. (2017). *Clinical guidelines for stroke management 2017*. https://informme.org.au/Guidelines/Clinical-Guidelines-for-Stroke-Management-2017

Teasdale, R., Cullen, N., Marshall, S., Janzen, S., & Bayley, M. (2017). *Evidence-based review of moderate to severe acquired brain injury: Introduction and methodology*. https://www.abiebr.com/sites/default/files/modules/Module%201_V12_Intro.pdf

Toronto Acquired Brain Injury Network. (2005). *Definition of acquired brain injury*. http://www.abinetwork.ca/definition

University of California San Francisco Health. (n.d.). *Neurological disorders*. https://www.ucsfhealth.org/conditions/neurological_disorders/

World Health Organization. (2002). *Towards a common language for functioning, disability and health: ICF*. http://www.who.int/classifications/icf/training/icfbeginnersguide.pdf

Young, L., Rule, G. T., Bocchieri, R. T., Walilko, T. J., Burns, J. M., & Ling, G. (2015). When physics meets biology: Low and high-velocity penetration, blunt impact, and blast injuries to the brain. *Frontiers in Neurology, 6*(89), 1–19.

Index